Applied
Pharmacology
for the Dental Hygienist

8th EDITION

Applied
Pharmacology
for the Dental Hygienist

Elena Bablenis Haveles, BS Pharmacy, PharmD, RPh
Adjunct Associate Professor of Pharmacology
Gene W. Hirschfeld School of Dental Hygiene
College of Health Sciences
Old Dominion University
Norfolk, Virginia

ELSEVIER

2-9-22
ww
#83.99

ELSEVIER

3251 Riverport Lane
St. Louis, Missouri 63043

APPLIED PHARMACOLOGY FOR THE DENTAL
HYGIENIST, EIGHTH EDITION   ISBN: 978-0-323-59539-1

Notices

Practitioners and researchers must always rely on their own experience and knowledge in
evaluating and using any information, methods, compounds or experiments described herein.
Because of rapid advances in the medical sciences, in particular, independent verification of
diagnoses and drug dosages should be made. To the fullest extent of the law, no responsibility is
assumed by Elsevier, authors, editors or contributors for any injury and/or damage to persons or
property as a matter of products liability, negligence or otherwise, or from any use or operation
of any methods, products, instructions, or ideas contained in the material herein.

Library of Congress Control Number: 2018962845

Content Strategist: Joslyn Dumas
Content Development Manager: Ellen Wurm-Cutter
Content Development Specialist: Elizabeth McCormac and Laura Klein
Publishing Services Manager: Shereen Jameel
Senior Project Manager: Karthikeyan Murthy
Design Direction: Margaret Reid

Printed in Canada

Last digit is the print number: 9   8   7   6   5   4   3

  Working together
to grow libraries in
developing countries

www.elsevier.com • www.bookaid.org

Celeste M. Abraham, BS, DDS, MS
Associate Clinical Professor
Periodontics
Texas A&M University College of Dentistry
Dallas, Texas

Jocelyne King, HD, Diploma in Dental Hygiene, Registrant of CDHO
Collège Boréal, Écoles des sciences de la santé (ESS)
Collège Boréal, Sudbury, ON
Sudbury, ON, Canada

Elizabeth Morch, RDH AGDDE Med.
Registrant: College of Dental Hygienists of BC
Faculty
Dental Programs
Camosun College
Victoria, BC, Canada

Amilia Peskir, HD, BSc, CPEC
Diploma in Dental Hygiene from John Abbott College
License with L'Ordre des hygieniestes dentaire du Québec
    (license in good standing with the Order of Dental
    Hygienists of Québec)
BSc General Agriculture, major Microbiology from McGill
    University
Diploma in Education from the University of Sherbrooke
Teacher
Dental Hygiene
John Abbott College
Sainte-Anne-de-Bellevue, Québec, Canada (H9X 3L9)

Paula D. Silver, BS Biology, PharmD.
Medical Instructor
MA/LPN/RN
ECPI University
Newport News, Virginia

Rebecca G. Tabor, RDH, MEd
Associate Professor
Allied Health
Western Kentucky University
Bowling Green, Kentucky

To my husband, Paul, and sons, Andrew and Harry

PREFACE

Knowledge of pharmacology is imperative to the success of a dental hygiene student. *Applied Pharmacology for the Dental Hygienist*, Eighth Edition, is written with the specific needs of the dental hygienist in mind to help ensure your success in this subject matter.

Society is information-conscious, and it is expected that the dental hygienist be knowledgeable about medications. Dental hygienists are called on to complete medication and health histories, administer certain medications, provide counseling about oral hygiene, and, in some states, prescribe medication and provide counseling about medications.

The primary goal of this book remains to produce safe and effective dental hygienists and to offer them the tools that they need to continue to learn throughout their lifetimes. This textbook provides the dental hygienist with the necessary knowledge of pharmacology to assess for medical illness, adverse reactions, and drug interactions that may affect oral health care and treatment. It is not intended that the dental hygienist take the place of the dentist in providing the patient with information about the various medications but that the hygienist will work with the dentist in providing appropriate patient care.

INTENDED AUDIENCE

The primary intended audience of this specific textbook is the dental hygiene student. However, practicing dental hygienists and dentists may find this book useful for a quick review of pharmacology. The information may also benefit dental students as a classroom text or resource.

IMPORTANCE TO THE PROFESSION

Continual learning after the completion of a formal education is especially critical in the dynamic area of pharmacology. New drugs are constantly being discovered and synthesized. New effects of old drugs are identified. New diseases and drugs for the treatment of those diseases are being studied. Today's dental hygiene student will need to be able to access new information about new drugs and intelligently communicate with others (professionals and patients) using the unique medical and pharmacologic vocabularies. It is hoped that this textbook will also help dental hygiene students to accomplish the following goals:

1. Students should achieve an understanding of the need and importance of obtaining and using appropriate reference material when needed. When confronted with a patient taking a new or unfamiliar drug, the dental hygiene student will use the appropriate references to learn about the effects of the drug. Pharmacology is a field in which new information is constantly becoming available.
2. Students should develop the ability to find the necessary information about drugs with which they are not familiar. The textbook encourages the use of the current reference sources that will be available where dental hygienists practice.
3. Students should develop the ability to apply that information to their clinical dental patients within a reasonable time.

ORGANIZATION

The material has been organized to create a readable and clinically applicable resource in pharmacology that specifically addresses the needs of the dental hygiene student. The textbook is divided into four sections:

PART ONE: General Principles includes general information about pharmacology, pharmacokinetics, drug action and handling, adverse reactions, prescription writing, autonomic pharmacology, the role of the dental hygienist, and pharmacology in oral health care.

PART TWO: Drugs Used in Dentistry includes the pharmacology of nonopioid analgesics, opioid analgesics, antibiotics, antifungals, antiviral drugs, antianxiety drugs, local anesthetics, and general anesthetics with a special emphasis on nitrous oxide. It also has chapters on the treatment of oral conditions and dental hygiene-related disorders. Each chapter focuses on dental-related adverse effects, how the drug may affect oral health care, and the specific dental hygiene considerations.

PART THREE: Drugs That May Alter Dental Treatment includes the more common disease states or medical conditions that patients may present with, as well as how those medications or the disease states themselves can affect oral health care. Each chapter also focuses on dental-related adverse effects, how the drug may affect oral health care, and specific dental hygiene considerations.

PART FOUR: Special Situations includes significant information on treating emergency situations, women who are pregnant or lactating, patients with substance abuse issues, and those patients self-treating with herbal remedies or supplements. Each chapter also focuses on dental-related adverse effects, how the drug may affect oral health care, and specific dental hygiene considerations.

KEY FEATURES

This book includes many features and learning aids to assist the student studying pharmacology:

- Dental Hygiene Focus: Although pharmacologic basics are covered overall and for specific types of drugs, interactions of clinical interest in oral health care are incorporated throughout the book. These sections offer explanations on why certain drugs are used or contraindicated in a dental treatment plan, providing students with targeted information they will need for practice.
- Consistent Presentation: Information about each drug varies, but all drugs are presented using a similar format so that sections can be easily identified. Each drug group is discussed and includes the group's indications (for what purpose the drugs are used), pharmacokinetics (how the body handles the drugs), pharmacologic effects (what the drugs do), adverse reactions (bad things the drugs do), drug interactions (how the drugs react with other drugs in the body), and the dosage of the drugs (how much is indicated).
- Academic Skills Assessment: Review questions are included at the end of each chapter, and answers are available to instructors. These questions help students to assess their knowledge and gauge comprehension of chapter material.
- Clinical Case Study: A clinical case with questions is included at the end of each chapter and answers are available to instructors. These cases and questions help students to assess their knowledge and gauge comprehension of chapter material by means of clinical application of the material.
- Key Terminology: Key terms are bolded throughout and appear in color within chapter discussions; each term is defined in a back-of-book glossary. The language of pharmacology is new to many

dental hygiene students, and the in-text highlights draw students' attention to terms they may need to review. The glossary provides a centralized, quick, and handy reference.

- Summary Tables and Boxes: Throughout, concepts are summarized in boxes and tables to accompany narrative discussions, providing easy-to-read versions of text discussions that support visual learners and serve as useful tools for review and study.
- Note Boxes: Boxes are interspersed throughout text discussions to briefly convey important concepts, indications, contraindications, memory tools, warnings, and more. They are easy to see and provide quick statements or phrases that are easy to remember.
- Dental Hygiene Considerations Boxes: Each chapter concludes with a compilation of the most relevant dental-specific information, which is summarized in terms of how that chapter's content specifically relates to the day-to-day practice of dental hygiene. These sections help to explain to students the need for an understanding of pharmacology and its importance in helping them achieve maximal oral health for their patients.
- Writing Level: Certain content areas and tables throughout the book have been simplified to better explain difficult concepts, such as receptors and metabolism. Pharmacology is a complex subject matter, and this book attempts to present information in a way that helps to ensure that students can fully comprehend the content and apply it to the practice of dental hygiene.
- Art Program: Approximately one-third of the images are new to this edition, and many of those that appeared in the previous edition have been updated and improved. The new images are more targeted and visually appealing and help support text discussions so that students can see key concepts at work.
- Reference Citations: Chapters contain bibliographical information as necessary, directing students to targeted sources of information where additional dental-related information can be located.
- Appendixes: Resources such as the *What If* scenarios that quickly outline situations in which relatively quick assessments and decisions are required and the calculation of children's dosages highlight additional information that proves useful in the clinical environment.
- Drug Index: A separate index covers the mention of all the drugs discussed within the book, allowing readers to quickly access targeted information about specific drugs or drug classes.

ANCILLARIES

A companion Evolve website has been created specifically for Applied Pharmacology for the Dental Hygienist and can be accessed directly from http://evolve.elsevier.com/Haveles/pharmacology. The following resources are provided:

For the Instructor

- TEACH Instructor's Resource (TIR)—A complete and detailed course-planning resource includes the following features, all designed around standard 50-minute classes:
  - Lesson Plans with detailed content mapping to chapter objectives, case scenarios, and activities for inside and outside the classroom
  - Lecture Outlines consisting of PowerPoint slides with talking points
  - Answer Keys and rationales to the Clinical Skills Assessments in the textbook
- Test Bank—Approximately 900 objective-style questions—multiple-choice, true/false, matching, and short-answer—are provided, with accompanying rationales for correct answers and page-number references for remediation.
- Image Collection—All of the book's images, organized by chapter with correlating figure numbers to the textbook, are available for download into PowerPoint or other presentations and materials.
- Color Pill Atlas—Labeled color image for the pills most commonly prescribed is included.

For the Student

- Practice Quizzes—Approximately 600 questions are provided in an instant-feedback format to allow students to assess their understanding of content and prepare for examinations. Rationales and page-number references are provided for remediation.
- Drug Guides—The major groups and specific drugs covered within each chapter are organized and summarized in terms of classification and mechanism of action for a quick study tool.
- Case Studies—Case presentations are followed by thought questions that deal with drug indications, contraindications, interactions, and more. Answers are provided.

Elena Bablenis Haveles

ACKNOWLEDGMENTS

Thank you to my peers and administrators at the Gene W. Hirschfeld School of Dental Hygiene, Old Dominion University, for their support.

To my father, Harry C. Bablenis, thank you for always believing in me and encouraging me to be my very best.

To my children, Andrew and Harry, many thanks for picking up the slack at home so that I could edit this book and keep up with our hectic schedules.

To my husband, Paul, thank you for your guidance and support as I try to juggle this and everything else in our lives. I love you.

EBH

HOW TO BE SUCCESSFUL IN PHARMACOLOGY

Before the lecture, read the syllabus outline for the subject to be covered during the class period. Become familiar with the vocabulary. Guess what might be said about the various topics. Think of what has been said in pharmacology about the topic; look at your pharmacology notes to see what you already know about the topic. Skim the textbook chapter(s) assigned to identify areas to be covered.

Attend class, take notes in your syllabus, and ask yourself questions about what was said. Compare what was said with what you previously thought about the topic.

Reread your lecture notes before the next class. Add and complete things you remember from class. Ask fellow classmates for clarification if you have questions. Read notes from previous classes.

Read the textbook assignment. Note especially those areas discussed in class. Let the textbook assignment answer questions you might have had in class. Answer general course objectives in the front of your syllabus for the drug group covered.

Look up in a medical dictionary any words for which you do not know the meaning. Construct a vocabulary list for each subject. Pay attention to the derivatives of the unknown medical word—its stem, prefixes, and suffixes.

Use active learning when studying. Be able to determine what portion of your study time is spent in active learning. Use the examples below to classify your study methods.

- Active: Writing things down, making up flash cards, speaking out loud, discussing the concepts with classmates, asking each other questions, giving a lecture (to your parrot) without notes, making a video or audio recording of your performances (for your own practice), or writing everything you know about a drug on an empty blackboard.
- Not active: Looking over notes, reading the book, listening in lecture, and reviewing your notes.

Did you answer the Academic Skills Assessment questions and the Clinical Case Study questions? These questions and cases are included at the end of each chapter so the learner can check to see if he or she knows the answers to these questions. It is a review for your benefit. Answers are only available through your instructor.

Did you think about what the information may mean to the dental hygienist? Trying to understand why things happen will make learning more efficient and more fun, too. What problems might be encountered when treating a patient taking this medication? How can the chance that something untoward will happen be minimized?

Did you think of examples in "real life"? By thinking of real-life examples, readers can transform a topic into a picture in their brain. For example, the "fight or flight" response associated with the sympathetic nervous system can be visualized as a caveman, his eyes big and his heart pounding, being chased by a hungry tiger.

USE OF OBJECTIVES TO FOCUS STUDYING

Find out what the objectives are for your pharmacology class. These are some objectives that may give you an idea about the organization of the material.

Goals for **commonly prescribed dental drugs** include the following:
- State the therapeutic use(s) for each drug group.
- Discuss the mechanism of action of the drug, when applicable.
- Explain the important pharmacokinetics for the drug group.
- List and describe the major pharmacologic effects associated with the drug group. State and discuss the important adverse reactions or side effects and their management or minimization.
- Describe any contraindications/cautions to the use of the drug group.
- Recognize clinically significant drug–drug, drug–disease, and drug–food interactions.
- Describe "patient instructions" for each drug group that could be prescribed.

Goals for drugs patients may be taking that can alter dental treatment:
- Determine the "dental implications" of each drug group for the management of dental patients using that drug group.
- Determine whether any dental drugs are likely to have drug interactions with these groups.
- State change(s) in the treatment plans that would be required for patients taking medications.

CONTENTS

PART I General Principles

1 Information, Sources, Regulatory Agencies, Drug Legislation, and Prescription Writing, 2
   History, 2
   Role of the Dental Hygienist, 2
      Medication/Health History, 2
      Medication Administration, 3
      Emergency Situations, 3
      Appointment Scheduling, 3
      Nonprescription Medication, 3
      Nutritional or Herbal Supplements, 3
   Sources of Information, 3
      Printed Resources, 3
      Computer and Online Resources, 4
   Drug Names, 4
      Drug Substitution, 5
   Federal Regulations and Regulatory Agencies, 5
      Harrison Narcotic Act, 5
      Food and Drug Administration, 5
      Federal Trade Commission, 5
      Drug Enforcement Administration, 5
      Omnibus Budget Reconciliation Act, 5
   Clinical Evaluation of a New Drug, 5
   Drug Legislation, 6
      History, 6
      Scheduled Drugs, 6
      Package Inserts, 6
      Black Box Warning, 6
      Labeled and Off-Label Uses, 7
      Orphan Drugs, 7
      Drug Recall, 7
   Prescription Writing, 7
      Measurement, 7
      Prescriptions, 7
      Role of the Dental Hygienist and Patient Adherence to Medication Therapy, 9
   Dental Hygiene Considerations, 10
   Academic Skills Assessment, 10
   Clinical Applications, 10

2 Drug Action and Handling, 11
   Characterization of Drug Action, 11
      Log Dose-Effect Curve, 11
      Potency, 11
      Efficacy, 11
      Therapeutic Index, 12
   Mechanism of Action of Drugs, 12
      Receptors, 13
   Pharmacokinetics, 14
      Passage Across Body Membranes, 14
      Absorption, 14
      Distribution, 15
      Redistribution, 16
      Metabolism (Biotransformation), 16
   Clinical Pharmacokinetics, 18
      Half-Life, 18
      Kinetics, 18
   Factors that Alter Drug Effects, 18
   Routes of Administration and Dose Forms, 19
      Routes of Administration, 19
      Dosage Forms, 23
   Dental Hygiene Considerations, 23
   Academic Skills Assessment, 23
   Clinical Case Study, 23

3 Adverse Reactions, 24
   Definitions and Classifications, 24
   Clinical Manifestations of Adverse Reactions, 25
      Exaggerated Effect on Target Tissues, 25
      Effect on Nontarget Tissues, 25
      Effect on Fetal Development (Teratogenic Effect), 25
      Local Effect, 25
      Drug Interactions, 25
      Hypersensitivity (Allergic Reaction), 26
      Idiosyncrasy, 27
      Interference With Natural Defense Mechanisms, 27
   Toxicologic Evaluation of Drugs, 27
   Recognizing Adverse Drug Effects, 28
   Dental Hygiene Considerations, 28
   Academic Skills Assessment, 28
   Clinical Case Study, 29

PART II Drugs Used in Dentistry

4 Autonomic Drugs, 31
   Autonomic Nervous System, 31
      Anatomy, 31
      Parasympathetic Autonomic Nervous System, 31
      Sympathetic Autonomic Nervous System, 31
      Functional Organization, 32
      Neurotransmitters, 32
   Parasympathetic Autonomic Nervous System, 35
      Cholinergic (Parasympathomimetic) Agents, 35
      Anticholinergic (Parasympatholytic) Agents, 37
      Nicotinic Agonists and Antagonists, 39
   Sympathetic Autonomic Nervous System, 39
      Sympathetic Autonomic Nervous System Receptors, 39
      Adrenergic (Sympathomimetic) Agents, 40
      Adrenergic Blocking Agents, 42
      Neuromuscular Blocking Drugs, 43
   Dental Hygiene Considerations, 43
      Cholinergic Drugs, 43
      Anticholinergic Drugs, 43
      Adrenergic Agonists, 43
   Academic Skills Assessment, 44
   Clinical Case Study, 44

5 Nonopioid (Nonnarcotic) Analgesics, 45
   Pain, 45
   Classification, 45
   Salicylates, 45
      Acetylsalicylic Acid, 45
      Nonacetylated Salicylates, 50

Nonsteroidal Antiinflammatory Drugs, 50
  Chemical Classification, 50
  Mechanism of Action, 50
  Pharmacokinetics, 50
  Pharmacologic Effects, 51
  Adverse Reactions, 51
  Drug Interactions, 52
  Contraindications and Cautions, 52
  Precautions, 52
  Therapeutic Uses, 52
  Specific Nonsteroidal Antiinflammatory Drugs, 53
Acetaminophen, 54
  Pharmacokinetics, 54
  Pharmacologic Effects, 54
  Adverse Reactions, 54
  Drug Interactions, 55
  Uses, 55
  Doses and Preparations, 55
Drugs Used to Treat Gout, 56
  Colchicine, 56
  Febuxostat, 56
  Allopurinol, 56
  Probenecid, 56
  Other Drugs, 56
Drugs Used to Treat Arthritis, 56
  Disease-Modifying Antirheumatic Drugs, 56
  Biologic Response Modifiers, 57
Dental Hygiene Considerations, 57
Academic Skills Assessment, 57
Clinical Case Study, 57

6 Opioid (Narcotic) Analgesics and Antagonists, 58
History, 58
Classification, 58
Mechanism of Action, 58
Pharmacokinetics, 58
Pharmacologic Effects, 59
  Analgesia, 59
  Sedation and Euphoria, 59
  Cough Suppression, 60
  Gastrointestinal Effects, 60
Adverse Reactions, 60
  Respiratory Depression, 60
  Nausea and Emesis, 61
  Constipation, 61
  Miosis, 61
  Urinary Retention, 61
  Central Nervous System Effects, 61
  Cardiovascular Effects, 61
  Biliary Tract Constriction, 61
  Histamine Release, 61
  Pregnancy and Nursing Considerations, 61
  Addiction, 61
  Allergic Reactions, 62
  Drug Interactions, 63
Specific Opioids, 63
  Opioid Agonists, 63
  Mixed Opioids, 65
  Opioid Antagonists, 65
  Full Agonist/Reuptake Inhibitors, 66
Dental Use of Opioids, 66
Chronic Dental Pain and Opioid Use, 67
  Patient Concerns Regarding Opioid Use, 67

Dental Hygiene Considerations, 67
Academic Skills Assessment, 67
Clinical Case Studies, 67

7 Antiinfective Agents, 68
Dental Infection "Evolution", 68
Definitions, 69
Infection, 69
Resistance, 69
Indications for Antimicrobial Agents, 70
  Therapeutic Indications, 70
  Prophylactic Indications, 70
General Adverse Reactions and Disadvantages
  Associated with Antiinfective Agents, 70
  Superinfection (Suprainfection), 70
  Allergic Reactions, 70
  Drug Interactions, 70
  Gastrointestinal Complaints, 72
  Pregnancy Considerations, 72
  Dose Forms, 72
  Cost, 72
Penicillins, 72
  Pharmacokinetics, 72
  Mechanism of Action, 73
  Spectrum, 73
  Resistance, 73
  Adverse Reactions, 73
  Uses, 74
  Specific Penicillins, 74
Cephalosporins, 75
  Pharmacokinetics, 75
  Spectrum, 75
  Mechanism of Action, 75
  Adverse Reactions, 75
  Uses, 76
Macrolides, 76
  Erythromycin, 76
  Azithromycin and Clarithromycin, 77
Tetracyclines, 77
  Pharmacokinetics, 77
  Spectrum, 77
  Adverse Reactions, 77
  Drug Interactions, 78
  Uses, 79
Clindamycin, 79
  Pharmacokinetics, 79
  Spectrum, 79
  Adverse Reactions, 79
  Uses, 80
Metronidazole, 80
  Pharmacokinetics, 80
  Spectrum, 80
  Adverse Reactions, 80
  Drug Interactions, 80
  Uses, 81
Rational Use of Antiinfective Agents in
  Dentistry, 81
  Stages of Infection, 81
  Failure of Antiinfective Therapy, 81
Antimicrobial Agents for Nondental Use, 81
  Vancomycin, 81
  Aminoglycosides, 82
  Sulfonamides, 82

Sulfamethoxazole-Trimethoprim, 83
Nitrofurantoin, 83
Quinolones (Fluoroquinolones), 83
Antituberculosis Agents, 84
Isoniazid, 84
Rifampin, 85
Pyrazinamide, 85
Ethambutol, 85
Topical Antibiotics, 85
Neomycin, Polymyxin, and Bacitracin, 85
Mupirocin, 85
Antibiotic Prophylaxis Used in Dentistry, 86
Prevention of Infective Endocarditis, 86
Prosthetic Joint Prophylaxis, 87
Noncardiac Medical Conditions, 88
Dental Hygiene Considerations, 88
Academic Skills Assessment, 88
Clinical Case Study, 88
Bibliography, 89

8 Antifungal and Antiviral Agents, 90
Antifungal Agents, 90
Nystatin, 90
Imidazoles, 90
Antiviral Agents, 92
Herpes Simplex, 92
Acquired Immunodeficiency Syndrome, 94
Chronic Hepatitis, 96
Dental Hygiene Considerations, 97
Academic Skills Assessment, 97
Clinical Case Study, 97

9 Local Anesthetics, 98
History, 98
Ideal Local Anesthetic, 98
Chemistry, 98
Mechanism of Action, 98
Action on Nerve Fibers, 98
Ionization Factors, 99
Pharmacokinetics, 99
Absorption, 99
Distribution, 101
Metabolism, 101
Excretion, 101
Pharmacologic Effects, 101
Peripheral Nerve Conduction (Blocker), 101
Antiarrhythmic, 101
Adverse Reactions, 101
Toxicity, 102
Local Effects, 102
Malignant Hyperthermia, 102
Pregnancy and Nursing Considerations, 102
Allergy, 102
Composition of Local Anesthetic Solutions, 103
Local Anesthetic Agents, 103
Amides, 103
Esters, 105
Other Local Anesthetics, 105
Vasoconstrictors, 105
Overview, 105
Drug Interactions, 107
Choice of Local Anesthetic, 107

Topical Anesthetics, 108
Amides, 109
Esters, 110
Precautions in Topical Anesthesia, 110
Doses of Local Anesthetic and Vasoconstrictor, 110
Dental Hygiene Considerations, 111
Academic Skills Assessment, 111
Clinical Case Study, 111

10 General Anesthetics, 112
History, 112
Mechanism of Action, 112
Overview, 112
Stages and Planes of Anesthesia, 112
Adverse Reactions, 113
General Anesthetics, 113
Classification of Anesthetic Agents, 113
Induction Anesthesia, 113
Induction and Maintenance Anesthesia, 115
Nitrous Oxide, 115
Halogenated Hydrocarbons, 117
Balanced General Anesthesia, 117
Dental Hygiene Considerations, 117
Academic Skills Assessment, 117
Clinical Case Study, 118

11 Antianxiety Agents, 119
Definitions, 119
Benzodiazepines, 120
Chemistry, 120
Pharmacokinetics, 120
Mechanism of Action, 121
Pharmacologic Effects, 121
Adverse Reactions, 121
Abuse and Tolerance, 122
Drug Interactions, 123
Medical Uses, 123
Management of the Dental Patient Taking Benzodiazepines, 124
Barbiturates, 124
Chemistry, 125
Pharmacokinetics, 125
Mechanism of Action, 125
Pharmacologic Effects, 125
Adverse Reactions, 125
Long-Term Use, 125
Contraindications, 125
Drug Interactions, 125
Uses, 125
Nonbenzodiazepine-Nonbarbiturate Sedative-Hypnotics, 126
Buspirone, 126
Nonbenzodiazepine Receptor Hypnotics, 126
Zolpidem, 126
Zaleplon, 126
Eszopiclone, 126
Melatonin Receptor Agonist, 126
Melatonin, 127
Orexin Receptor Antagonist, 127
Centrally Acting Muscle Relaxants, 127
Pharmacologic Effects, 127
Individual Centrally Acting Muscle Relaxants, 127
Miscellaneous Agents, 127

Baclofen, 127
Tizanidine, 128
Dantrolene, 128
General Comments About Antianxiety Agents, 128
Analgesic-Sedative Combinations, 128
Special Considerations, 128
Precautions, 128
Dental Hygiene Considerations, 129
Academic Skills Assessment, 129
Clinical Case Study, 129

Part III   Drugs That May Alter Dental Treatment

12   Drugs for the Treatment of Cardiovascular Diseases, 131
Dental Implications of Cardiovascular Disease, 131
Contraindications to Treatment, 131
Vasoconstrictor Limit, 132
Periodontal Disease and Cardiovascular Disease, 132
Heart Failure, 132
Treatment of Heart Failure, 132
Angiotensin II Receptor Neprilysin Inhibitor, 134
I$_f$ Channel Inhibitor, 134
Cardiac Glycosides, 134
Digitalis Glycosides, 134
Antiarrhythmic Agents, 135
Automaticity, 135
Arrhythmias, 135
Antiarrhythmic Agents, 135
Antianginal Drugs, 136
Angina Pectoris, 136
Nitroglycerin-Like Compounds, 136
β-Adrenergic Blocking Agents, 138
Calcium Channel Blocking Agents, 138
Ranolazine, 138
Angiotensin-Converting Enzyme Inhibitors, 139
Angiotensin Receptor Blockers, 139
Dental Implications, 139
Antihypertensive Agents, 139
Patient Evaluation, 141
Treatment of Hypertension, 141
Diuretic Agents, 142
Angiotensin Receptor Blockers, 146
Direct Renin Inhibitors, 146
Calcium Channel Blocking Agents, 147
β-Adrenergic Blocking Agents, 147
α$_1$-Adrenergic Blocking Agents, 148
Central α-Adrenergic Agonists, 149
Peripheral Adrenergic Neuron Antagonist, 149
Management of the Dental Patient Taking Antihypertensive Agents, 149
Antihyperlipidemic Agents, 149
3-Hydroxy-3-Methylglutaryl Coenzyme A Reductase Inhibitors, 150
Inhibitors of Intestinal Absorption of Cholesterol, 151
Niacin, 152
Cholestyramine, 152
Fibric Acid Derivatives, 152
Proprotein Convertase Subtilisin/Kexin Type 9 Inhibitors, 152
Fish Oils, 152

Dental Implications of Elevated Cholesterol Levels, 152
Drugs That Affect Blood Coagulation, 152
Anticoagulants, 152
Parenteral Anticoagulants, 153
Low-Molecular-Weight Heparin, 153
Oral Anticoagulants, 153
Factor Xa Inhibitors, 154
Direct Thrombin Inhibitor, 155
Thienopyridines, 155
Clopidogrel, 155
Ticlopidine, 155
Prasugrel, 155
Ticagrelor, 155
Streptokinase and Alteplase, 155
Dipyridamole, 155
Pentoxifylline, 156
Drugs That Increase Blood Clotting, 156
Hemostatic Agents (Fibrinolytic Inhibitors), 156
Dental Hygiene Considerations, 156
Academic Skills Assessment, 156
Clinical Case Study, 156
References, 157

13   Drugs for the Treatment of Gastrointestinal Disorders, 158
Gastrointestinal Drugs, 158
Gastrointestinal Diseases, 158
Dental Implications, 159
Drugs Used to Treat Gastrointestinal Diseases, 159
Histamine$_2$-Blocking Agents, 159
Proton Pump Inhibitors, 160
Mixed Anti-Infective Therapy for Ulcer Treatment, 160
Antacids, 161
Miscellaneous Gastrointestinal Drugs, 161
Laxatives and Antidiarrheals, 161
Agents Used to Manage Chronic Inflammatory Bowel Disease, 163
Celiac Disease, 163
Dental Hygiene Considerations, 164
Academic Skills Assessment, 164
Clinical Case Study, 164
14   Drugs for the Treatment of Seizure Disorders, 165
Epilepsy, 165
Generalized Seizures, 165
Partial (Focal) Seizures, 166
Drug Therapy of Patients with Epilepsy, 166
General Adverse Reactions of Antiepileptic Agents, 167
Gastrointestinal Distress, 167
Valproate, 167
Lamotrigine, 168
Levetiracetam, 168
Oxcarbazepine, 168
Carbamazepine, 168
Phenytoin, 170
Ethosuximide, 171
Benzodiazepines, 171
Other Antiepileptic Agents, 172
Dental Treatment of the Patient with Epilepsy, 172
Nonseizure Uses of Antiepileptics, 172

Neurologic Pain, 172
Psychiatric Use, 172
Dental Hygiene Considerations, 172
Academic Skills Assessment, 172
Clinical Case Study, 173

15   Drugs for the Treatment of Central Nervous System Disorders, 174
Psychiatric Disorders, 174
Antipsychotic Agents, 175
Mechanism of Action, 175
Pharmacologic Effects, 175
Drug Interactions, 177
Uses, 178
Dental Implications, 178
Antidepressant Agents, 179
Selective Serotonin Reuptake Inhibitors, 179
Serotonin-Norepinephrine Reuptake Inhibitors, 180
Tricyclic Antidepressants, 180
Monoamine Oxidase Inhibitors, 181
Other Antidepressants, 181
Suicide and Antidepressants, 182
Dental Implications, 182
Drugs for Treatment of Bipolar Disorder, 182
Lithium, 182
Antiepileptic Drugs, 182
Second-Generation Antipsychotics, 183
Dental Hygiene Considerations, 183
Academic Skills Assessment, 183
Clinical Case Study, 183

16   Adrenocorticosteroids, 184
Mechanism of Release, 184
Classification, 184
Definitions, 184
Routes of Administration, 185
Mechanism of Action, 185
Pharmacologic Effects, 185
Adverse Reactions, 185
Metabolic Changes, 186
Infections, 186
Central Nervous System Effects, 186
Peptic Ulcer, 186
Impaired Wound Healing and Osteoporosis, 186
Ophthalmic Effects, 186
Electrolyte and Fluid Balance, 187
Adrenal Crisis, 187
Dental Effects, 187
Uses, 187
Medical Uses, 187
Dental Uses, 188
Corticosteroid Products, 188
Dental Implications, 189
Adverse Reactions, 189
Steroid Supplementation, 190
Topical Use, 190
Dental Hygiene Considerations, 191
Academic Skills Assessment, 191
Clinical Case Study, 191
Reference, 191

17   Drugs for the Treatment of Respiratory Disorders and Allergic Rhinitis, 192
Respiratory Diseases, 192
Asthma, 192
Chronic Obstructive Pulmonary Disease, 192
Drugs Used to Treat Respiratory Diseases, 195
Metered-Dose Inhalers, 195
Sympathomimetic Agents, 196
Corticosteroids, 196
Leukotriene Modifiers, 197
Cromolyn, 198
Methylxanthines, 198
Antimuscarinic, 198
Anti-Immunoglobulin E Antibodies, 198
Interleukin-5 Antibody Antagonists, 198
Agents Used to Manage Upper Respiratory Infections, 198
Dental Implications of the Respiratory Drugs, 199
Allergic Rhinitis, 199
Pharmacologic Effects, 200
H_1-Receptor Blocking Effects, 201
Other Effects (Unrelated to H_1-Blocking Effects), 201
Adverse Reactions, 201
Central Nervous System Depression, 201
Anticholinergic Effects, 201
Dental Hygiene Considerations, 202
Academic Skills Assessment, 202
Clinical Case Study, 203

18   Drugs for the Treatment of Diabetes Mellitus, 204
Pancreatic Hormones, 204
Diabetes Mellitus, 204
Types of Diabetes, 204
Dental Implications of Diabetes, 205
Systemic Complications of Diabetes, 207
Evaluation of the Dental Patient With Diabetes, 207
Goals of Therapy, 208
Drugs Used to Manage Diabetes, 208
Insulins, 208
Oral Antidiabetic Agents, 209
Treatment of Hypoglycemia, 214
Glucagon, 214
Dental Hygiene Considerations, 214
Academic Skills Assesment, 214
Clinical Case Study, 214
Bibliography, 214

19   Drugs for the Treatment of Other Endocrine Disorders, 215
Pituitary Hormones, 215
Anterior Pituitary, 215
Posterior Pituitary, 217
Thyroid Hormones, 217
Iodine, 217
Hypothyroidism, 217
Hyperthyroidism, 217
Female Sex Hormones, 218
Estrogens, 219
Progestins, 220
Hormonal Contraceptives, 220

Male Sex Hormones, 221
  Androgens, 221
Other Agents That Affect Sex Hormone
  Systems, 222
  Clomiphene, 222
  Leuprolide, 222
  Tamoxifen, 222
  Danazol, 223
  Aromatase Inhibitors, 223
Dental Hygiene Considerations, 223
Academic Skills Assessment, 223
Clinical Case Study, 223

20 Antineoplastic Drugs, 225
Use of Antineoplastic Agents, 225
Mechanisms of Action, 225
Classification, 227
Adverse Drug Effects, 227
  Bone Marrow Suppression, 227
  Osteonecrosis, 227
  Gastrointestinal Effects, 230
  Dermatologic Effects, 230
  Hepatotoxicity, 230
  Nephrotoxicity, 230
  Immunosuppression, 230
  Germ Cells, 230
  Oral Effects, 230
Combinations, 231
Dental Implications, 231
Dental Hygiene Considerations, 232
Academic Skills Assessment, 232
Clinical Case Study, 232

PART IV Special Situations

21 Emergency Drugs, 234
General Measures, 234
  Steps Indicated, 234
  Preparation for Treatment, 234
Categories of Emergencies, 235
  Lost or Altered Consciousness, 235
  Respiratory Emergencies, 236
  Cardiovascular System Emergencies, 236
  Other Emergency Situations, 239
  Drug-Related Emergencies, 239
Emergency Kit for the Dental Office, 239
  Drugs, 239
  Equipment, 242
Dental Hygiene Considerations, 243
Academic Skills Assessment, 243
Clinical Case Study, 243

22 Pregnancy and Breastfeeding, 244
General Principles, 244
  Two Main Concerns, 244
  History, 244
Pregnancy, 244
  Pregnancy Trimesters, 244
  Teratogenicity, 245
  US Food and Drug Administration Pregnancy
    Categories, 245
Breastfeeding, 246

Dental Drugs, 246
  Local Anesthetic Agents, 246
  Epinephrine, 246
  Analgesics, 246
  Antiinfective Agents, 249
  Antianxiety Agents, 250
Dental Hygiene Considerations, 251
Academic Skills Assessment, 251
Clincial Case Study, 251

23 Substance Use Disorders, 252
General Considerations, 252
  Definitions, 252
  Psychological Dependence, 253
  Physical Dependence, 253
  Tolerance, 253
Central Nervous System Depressants, 254
  Ethyl Alcohol, 254
  Nitrous Oxide, 257
  Opioid Analgesics, 258
  Opioid Street Drug, 259
Sedative-Hypnotics, 259
  Pattern of Abuse, 259
  Management of Acute Overdose and
    Withdrawal, 260
Central Nervous System Stimulants, 260
  Cocaine, 260
  Amphetamines, 260
  Caffeine, 261
  Tobacco, 261
Psychedelics (Hallucinogens), 262
  Lysergic Acid Diethylamide, 263
  Phencyclidine, 263
  Marijuana, 263
Identifying the Substance User, 263
The Impaired Dental Hygienist, 264
Dental Hygiene Considerations, 264
Academic Skills Assessment, 264
Clinical Case Study, 264

24 Natural/Herbal Products and Dietary Supplements, 265
Limited Regulation, 265
  Dietary Supplement Health and Education Act, 265
  Package Labeling, 266
Safety of Herbal and Nutritional Products, 266
  Oral Adverse Effects, 266
Drug Interactions, 266
Standardization of Herbal Products, 267
Good Manufacturing Practice, 268
Herbal Supplements Used in Oral Health Care, 269
  Acemannan, 269
  Essential Oil Mouth Rinse, 269
  Oil of Cloves (Eugenol), 269
  Triclosan, 269
  Xylitol, 269
Dental Hygiene Considerations, 270
Academic Skills Assessment, 270
Clinical Case Study, 270

25 Oral Conditions and Their Treatment, 271
Infectious Lesions, 271
  Acute Necrotizing Ulcerative Gingivitis, 271
  Herpes Infections, 271
  Candidiasis (Moniliasis), 273

Angular Cheilitis/Cheilosis, 274
Alveolar Osteitis, 275
Immune Reactions, 275
Recurrent Aphthous Stomatitis, 275
Lichen Planus, 276
Miscellaneous Oral Conditions, 276
Geographic Tongue, 276
Burning Mouth or Tongue Syndrome, 276
Inflammation, 277
Pericoronitis, 277
Postirradiation Caries, 277
Root Sensitivity, 277
Actinic Lip Changes, 277
Stomatitis, 277
Drug-Induced Oral Side Effects, 277
Xerostomia, 277
Sialorrhea, 277
Hypersensitivity-Type Reactions, 278
Oral Lesions That Resemble Autoimmune-Type Reactions, 279
Stains, 279
Gingival Enlargement, 279
Osteonecrosis of the Jaw, 279
Agents Commonly Used to Treat Oral Lesions, 279
Corticosteroids, 279
Palliative Treatment, 280

Dental Hygiene Considerations, 281
Academic Skills Assessment, 281
Clinical Case Study, 281
26 Hygiene-Related Oral Disorders, 282
Dental Caries, 282
Prevention, 282
Gingivitis, 288
Prevention, 288
Tooth Hypersensitivity, 288
Pathophysiology, 289
Treatment, 289
Dental Hygiene Considerations, 290
Academic Skills Assessment, 291
Clinical Case Study, 291
Reference, 291
Bibliography, 291

Appendix A: Medical Acronyms, 292
Appendix B: Medical Terminology, 295
Appendix C: What If…, 297
Appendix D: Oral Manifestations: Xerostomia and Taste Changes, 302
Appendix E: Children's Dose Calculations, 305
Glossary, 306
Drug Index, 315
Index, 327

PART I

General Principles

Chapter 1

*Information, Sources, Regulatory Agencies,
Drug Legislation, and Prescription Writing, 2*

Chapter 2

Drug Action and Handling, 11

Chapter 3

Adverse Reactions, 24

Information, Sources, Regulatory Agencies, Drug Legislation, and Prescription Writing

http://evolve.elsevier.com/Haveles/pharmacology

LEARNING OBJECTIVES

1. Discuss the history of pharmacology and its relationship to the dental hygienist.
2. List where detailed and updated information on medications can be found.
3. Define the ways in which drugs are named and the significance of each.
4. Define generic equivalence and how it is related to drug substitution.
5. Describe the acts and agencies within the federal government designed to regulate drugs.
6. Identify the four phases of clinical evaluation involved in drug approval and the five schedules of drugs.
7. Discuss the history of drug legislation, including:
   - List the five schedules of controlled substances.
   - Explain package inserts and black box warnings.
   - Differentiate between labeled and off-label uses.
   - Explain orphan drugs and drug recalls.
8. Prescription writing. Become familiar with the basics of prescription writing as well as describing the parts of the prescription and prescription label regulations.

Pharmacology is derived from the Greek prefix *pharmaco-*, meaning "drug" or "medicine," and the Greek suffix *-logy*, meaning "study." Therefore pharmacology is the study of drugs and their interactions with living cells and systems. Drugs are chemical substances that are used in the diagnosis, treatment, or prevention of disease or other abnormal conditions. They can be used in both humans and animals. Drugs include synthetically derived compounds, vitamins, and minerals as well as herbal supplements—although these last substances are marketed not as drugs but as food supplements. In addition to pharmacology, the dental hygienist should know about its related disciplines, as listed and defined in Table 1.1.

HISTORY

In the beginning, plants were discovered to produce beneficial effects.

Pharmacology had its beginning when our human ancestors noticed that ingesting certain plants altered body functions or awareness. The first **pharmacologist** was a person who became more astute in observing and remembering which plant products produced predictable results. From this humble beginning, a huge industrial and academic community concerned with the study and development of drugs has evolved. Plants from the rain forest and chemicals from tar have been searched for the presence of drugs. The agents discovered and found to be useful are then prescribed and dispensed through the practice of medicine, dentistry, pharmacy, and nursing. Health care providers who can write prescriptions include physicians (for humans), veterinarians (for animals), dentists (for dental problems), and optometrists (for eye problems). Physicians' assistants, nurse practitioners, pharmacists, and dental hygienists can prescribe drugs under certain guidelines and in certain states.

ROLE OF THE DENTAL HYGIENIST

Knowledge of a patient's medication/health history is necessary to provide optimal oral health care.

In today's ever-changing health care environment, it is important that the dental hygienist know more than the name and color of a medication. Patients rely on the dental hygienist to provide them with the correct information regarding their medication and oral health care. Although dental hygienists do not normally prescribe drugs, it is important that they have knowledge of pharmacology and its related disciplines to provide more effective care for the patient.

Medication/Health History

As a result of the many breakthroughs in medicine and pharmacy research, more and more diseases can be treated; therefore, more and more people are taking medication. More often than not, the dental hygienist is the first health professional in the dental practice to assess the patient's medication history. Obtaining a medication/health history is the first step in safely treating a patient. Patients may be taking any number of medications that interact with medications used in oral health care or that may adversely affect oral health. An understanding of the actions, indications, adverse reactions, and therapeutic uses of these drugs can help determine potential effects on dental treatment. Comparing the medical conditions of the patient with the medications he or she is taking often raises questions in the interview. Examples include the risk of xerostomia in patients taking calcium channel blockers for hypertension and the increased risk of gingival bleeding in patients taking an aspirin each day to prevent a heart attack or stroke which will be further addressed in Chapter 12. A detailed health/medication history allows the dental hygienist to provide the best possible health care to the patient (Box 1.1).

TABLE 1.1 Disciplines Related to Pharmacology

Area of Pharmacology	Definition
Pharmacotherapy	The use of medications to treat different disease states
Pharmacodynamics	The study of the action of drugs on living organisms
Pharmacokinetics	The study of what the body does to a drug; the measurement of the absorption, distribution, metabolism, and excretion of drug from the body
Pharmacy	The practice of compounding, preparing, dispensing, and counseling of patients about their medications
Toxicology	The study of the harmful effects of drugs on living tissues

BOX 1.1 Obtaining a Medication History

1. Do you take any medications for_____?
   - Heart/high blood pressure/angina
   - Lungs/asthma/Chronic Obstructive Pulmonary Disease (COPD)
   - Diabetes/sugar
   - Ulcer/reflux/heartburn
   - Mental health issues
   - Arthritis
   - Seizures
2. What are the names of your medicines and how many times a day do you take them?
3. How many times a day did your health practitioner tell you to take them?
4. Have you taken your medicine today?
5. Do you take any medicine that you can buy without a prescription? For example,
   - Acetaminophen, aspirin, ibuprofen, naproxen
   - Antihistamines/decongestants
   - Omeprazole (Prilosec OTC), lansoprazole (Prevacid 24HR), omeprazole/sodium bicarbonate (Zegerid OTC), nizatidine (Axid AR), famotidine (Pepcid AC), cimetidine (Tagamet HB), ranitidine (Zantac 75)
6. Do you take any herbal supplements? If so, please tell me their names and why you are taking them.
7. Have you noticed any problems (side effects) when you take your medicine?
8. Do you have any allergies to medicine? If yes, what medicine?
9. What happened to you when you took the medicine?

Medication Administration

Because the dental hygienist administers certain drugs in the office, knowledge of these agents is crucial. For example, the oral health care provider commonly applies topical fluoride (Chapter 26), and in some states, both the dentist and the dental hygienist administer local anesthetics and nitrous oxide (Chapter 10). In-depth knowledge of these agents is especially important because of their frequent use.

Emergency Situations

The ability to recognize and assist in dental emergencies requires knowledge of certain drugs, all of which will be discussed in greater detail in Chapter 21. The indications for these drugs and their adverse reactions must be considered. For example, in a patient having an anaphylactic reaction, epinephrine must be administered quickly.

Appointment Scheduling

Patients taking medication for systemic diseases may require special handling in the dental office. For example, asthmatic patients who experience dental anxiety should schedule their appointments early in the morning, when they are not rushed or under pressure, in order to avoid an asthma attack (Chapter 17). Diabetic patients should schedule their appointments 90 minutes after meals and medication administration. Certain patients may need to take medication before their appointments (Chapter 18). Patients with a history of infective endocarditis need to be premedicated with antibiotics before some of their dental or dental hygiene appointments (Chapter 7).

Nonprescription Medication

More and more patients are self-treating with nonprescription drugs. Also, nonprescription or over-the-counter (OTC) products may be recommended for certain patients. The study of pharmacology will assist the oral health care provider in making an intelligent selection of an appropriate OTC product. Although patients tend to forget that OTC products are drugs, knowledge of pharmacology will allow the dental hygienist to evaluate the patient for therapeutic OTC drug effects and adverse effects.

Nutritional or Herbal Supplements

Many patients self-treat or are prescribed nutritional or herbal supplements for any number of disease states, as will be further discussed in Chapter 24. Although the vast majority of these supplements do not carry US Food and Drug Administration (FDA) approval for treating disease states, patients still use them. These supplements are drugs and can cause adverse effects and interact with other drugs.

SOURCES OF INFORMATION

> Always keep reference guides or electronic devices close by so you can quickly look up information regarding medication therapy.

Many different medications are available, and it is important for the dental hygienist to know where to look for information about prescription medications, nonprescription medications, and herbal supplements. There are many sources, including reference texts, association journals, and the Internet, where pertinent drug information can be found. Box 1.2 reviews the different sources of information.

Printed Resources

Each publication type can be selected according to its lack of bias, its publication date (when the current edition was released), its readability (vocabulary, simplicity of explanations, and presence of visual aids), its degree of detail (all you want to know and much more, just the right amount of information, or not enough to understand what is being said), and its price. Some publications are specific for disease states, geriatric or pediatric patients, drug interactions, or prescription drugs or nonprescription drugs. Reference books can be updated monthly, quarterly, and annually. Every dental office should have at least one reference book that lists the names of both prescription and OTC drugs. Further, a standard pharmacology textbook would be helpful in understanding the reference books. Because of the continual release of new drugs, a recent edition (not more than 1 or 2 years old) of a reference book is needed.

BOX 1.2 Pharmacologic References and Resources Recommended for the Dental Office

Drug Information Reference Books
American Hospital Formulary Service (AHFS) Drug Information
United States Pharmacopeia-Drug Information (USP-DI)
Drug Facts and Comparison
Physicians' Desk Reference (PDR)
Handbook of Nonprescription Drugs: An Interactive Approach to Health Care
PDR for Nonprescription Drugs, Supplements, and Herbs
PDR for Herbal Medicines
Natural Products: A Case-Based Approach for Health Care Professionals
Merck Manual for Medical Information
Drug Interaction Facts
Goodman and Gilman's The Pharmacologic Basis of Therapeutics

Dental Drug Reference Books
Mosby's Dental Drug Reference
Lexi-Comp's Drug Information Handbook for Dentistry

Selected Journals
Journal of Dental Hygiene
Dimensions in Dental Hygiene
Registered Dental Hygienist (RDH) Magazine
Pharmacy Today
Drug Topics
New England Journal of Medicine
Journal of the American Dental Association

Websites
www.epocrates.com
www.davis'sdrugguide.com
www.lexicomp.com
www.pdr.net
www.rxlist.com
www.drugs.com
www.fda.gov/medwatch
www.medscape.com
www.mayoclinic.com
www.nlm.nih.gov/medlineplus/

Newsletters
Pharmacist Letter
The Medical Letter

Computer and Online Resources

Although books serve as the usual source of information on drugs, many health care providers are using electronic resources, such as computer software and Internet-based services. Computer tablets and smart phones are also being used more and more for recording and storing patient information, calculating drug doses, and consulting medication information databases. Many online resources are available; they include *Davis's Drug Guide* (http://www.drugguide.com/ddo/), Epocrates (www.epocrates.com), and Lexi-Comp (www.lexicomp.com). These sites have applications (apps) that can be downloaded to smart phones as well as computer-based online sites. Lexi-comp also has apps specific for dentistry. In addition, many pharmacology textbooks include CD-ROMs that supplement the written material.

Journals are another source of information that provide the dental hygienist with the most current information regarding medication and oral health care therapy. More than 3000 journals are available online and can be accessed through Medline (www.medline.com) and PubMed (www.pubmed.com), as well as at specific journal websites.

In addition, the practicing pharmacist can be a source of information. It is particularly important for the dental professional to establish a professional relationship with a local pharmacist, who may assist him or her in understanding the possible effects of a new drug on a patient.

DRUG NAMES

It is important for the dental hygienist to understand the ways in which a drug can be named, because he or she must be able to discuss drugs with both the patient and the provider of the patient's care. The ability to refer to a drug's name(s) is complicated by the fact that all drugs have at least two names, and many have more.

When a particular drug is being investigated by a company, it is identified by its chemical name, which is determined by its chemical structure. If the structure is unknown at the time of investigation, a code name, usually a combination of letters and numbers, is assigned to the product (e.g., RU-486). Often the code name is used even when the chemical structure is identified and named. It is much easier to speak and write the code name than the full name of the chemical structure.

> Each drug has only one generic name but may have several trade names.

If a compound is found to be useful and it is determined that the compound will be marketed commercially, the pharmaceutical company discovering the drug gives the drug a trade name (e.g., Motrin). This name, which is capitalized, is usually chosen so that it can be easily remembered and promoted commercially. This trade name, registered as a trademark under the Federal Trademark Law, is the property of the registering company. The trade name is protected by the Federal Patent Law for 20 years from the earliest claimed filing date, plus patent term extensions. Although the brand name is technically the name of the company marketing the product, it is often used interchangeably with the trade name.

Before any drug is marketed, it is given a generic name that becomes the "official" name of the drug. For each drug, there is only one generic name (e.g., ibuprofen), selected by the United States Adopted Name Council, and the name is not capitalized. This Council selects a generic name that hopefully does not conflict with other drug names. However, the names of several marketed drugs have been changed because they were confused with the names of other drugs that had already been marketed. After the original manufacturer's patents have expired, other companies can market the **generic drug** under a trade name of their choosing (e.g., Advil). Fig. 1.1 compares the chemical, generic, and trade names of ibuprofen.

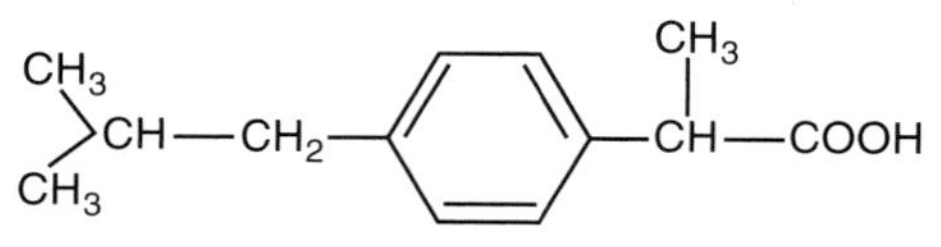

Chemical Name: (±)-2-(p-isobutylphenyl) propionic acid
Generic Name: Ibuprofen
Trade: Motrin, Advil

Fig. 1.1 A comparison of the chemical, generic, and trade names of ibuprofen.

Drug Substitution

> For dental drugs, generic substitution provides equivalent therapeutic results at a reduced cost.

In the discussion of generic and trade names, the question of generic equivalence and substitution arises. Are the various different generic products equivalent? Once the patent of the original drug expires, other companies can market the same compound under a generic name. In 1984, Congress passed the Drug Price Competition and Patent Term Restoration Act, which allowed generic drugs to receive expedited approval. The FDA still requires that the active ingredient of the generic product enter the bloodstream at the same rate as the trade name product. The variation allowed for the generic name product is the same as for the reformulations of the brand name product. For the few drugs that are difficult to formulate and have narrow therapeutic indexes, no differences exist between the trade name product and the generic product; therefore, generic substitution drugs give equivalent therapeutic results and provide a cost savings to the patient.

Drugs can be judged "similar" in several ways. When two formulations of a drug meet the chemical and physical standards established by the regulatory agencies, they are termed *chemically equivalent*. If the two formulations produce similar concentrations of the drug in the blood and tissues, they are termed *biologically equivalent*. If they prove to have equal therapeutic effects in a clinical trial, they are termed *therapeutically equivalent*. A preparation can be chemically equivalent yet not biologically or therapeutically equivalent. These products are said to differ in their bioavailability. Before generic drugs are marketed, they must be shown to be biologically equivalent, which would make them therapeutically equivalent.

FEDERAL REGULATIONS AND REGULATORY AGENCIES

Many agencies are involved in regulating the production, marketing, advertising, labeling, and prescribing of drugs.

Harrison Narcotic Act

In 1914 the Harrison Narcotic Act established regulations governing the use of opium, opiates, and cocaine. Marijuana laws were added in 1937. Before this law, mixtures sold OTC could contain opium and cocaine. These mixtures were promoted to be effective for many "problems."

Food and Drug Administration

The FDA, which is part of the Department of Health and Human Services (DHHS), grants approval so that drugs can be marketed in the United States. Before a drug can be approved by the FDA, it must be determined to be both safe and effective. The FDA requires physical and chemical standards for specific products and quality control in drug manufacturing plants. It determines which drugs may be sold by prescription or OTC and regulates the labeling and advertising of prescription drugs. Because the FDA is often more stringent than regulatory bodies in other countries, drugs are often marketed in Europe and South America before they are available in the United States.

Federal Trade Commission

The Federal Trade Commission (FTC) regulates the trade practices of drug companies and prohibits the false advertising of foods, nonprescription (OTC) drugs, and cosmetics.

Drug Enforcement Administration

The Drug Enforcement Administration (DEA) of the Department of Justice administers the Controlled Substances Act of 1970. This federal agency regulates the manufacture and distribution of substances that have a potential for abuse, including opioids (narcotics), stimulants, and sedatives.

Omnibus Budget Reconciliation Act

The newest federal regulation concerning drugs is the Omnibus Budget Reconciliation Act (OBRA) of 1990. It mandates that, beginning January 1, 1993, pharmacists must provide patient counseling and a prospective drug utilization review (DUR) for Medicaid patients. Although this federal law covers only Medicaid patients, state boards of pharmacy are interpreting this law to apply to all patients. Dental patients who have their prescriptions filled at a pharmacy should receive counseling from the pharmacist about their prescriptions.

CLINICAL EVALUATION OF A NEW DRUG

It takes almost 12 years from the time a drug is synthesized in the laboratory to its availability on pharmacy shelves, at a cost of more than 350 million dollars. Before a discovered or synthesized compound is approved for marketing, it must pass through many steps (Fig. 1.2). Animal studies begin by measuring both the acute and chronic toxicity. The median lethal dose is determined for several species of animals. Long-term animal studies continue, including a search for teratogenic effects. Toxicity and pharmacokinetic properties are also noted. This process, referred to as *preclinical testing*, usually lasts about 3 years. After the preclinical trials have been completed, an investigational new drug application (INDA) must be filled out and submitted before any clinical trials can be performed.

Clinical studies of drugs involve the following four phases:

Phase 1: Small and then increasing doses are administered to a limited number of healthy human volunteers, primarily to determine safety. This phase determines the biologic effects, metabolism, safe dose range in humans, and toxic effects of the drug.

Phase 2: Larger groups of humans are given the drug and any adverse reactions are reported to the FDA. The main purpose of phase 2 is to test effectiveness.

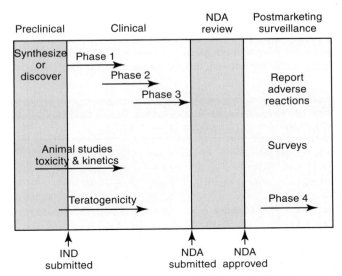

Fig. 1.2 Development of a new drug. *IND*, Investigational new drug; *NDA*, new drug application.

Phase 3: More clinical evaluation takes place involving a large number of patients who have the condition for which the drug is indicated. During this phase, both safety and efficacy must be demonstrated. Dosage is also determined during this phase.

Phase 4: This phase involves postmarketing surveillance. The toxicity of the drug that occurs in patients taking the drug after it is released is recorded. Several drugs in recent years have been removed from the market only after phase 4 has shown serious toxicity.

DRUG LEGISLATION

History

The Food and Drug Act of 1906 was the first federal law to regulate interstate commerce in drugs. The Harrison Narcotic Act of 1914 and its amendments provided federal control over narcotic drugs and required registration of all practitioners prescribing narcotics.

The Food and Drug Act was rewritten and became the Food, Drug, and Cosmetic Act of 1938. This law and its subsequent amendments prohibited interstate commerce of drugs that have not been shown to be safe and effective. The Durham-Humphrey Law of 1952 is a particularly important amendment to the Food, Drug, and Cosmetic Act because it required that certain types of drugs be sold by prescription only. This law required that these drugs be labeled as follows: "Caution: Federal law prohibits dispensing without prescription." The law also prohibits the refilling of a prescription unless directions to the contrary are indicated on the prescription. The Drug Amendments of 1962 (Kefauver-Harris Bill) made major changes in the Food, Drug, and Cosmetic Act. Under these amendments, manufacturers were required to demonstrate the effectiveness of drugs, to follow strict rules in testing, and to submit to the FDA any reports of adverse effects from drugs already on the market. Manufacturers were also required to list drug ingredients by generic name in labeling and advertising and to state adverse effects, contraindications, and efficacy of a drug.

The Drug Abuse Control Amendments of 1965 required accounting for drugs with a potential for abuse such as barbiturates and amphetamines.

The Controlled Substance Act of 1970 replaced the Harrison Narcotic Act and the Drug Abuse Control Amendments to the Food, Drug, and Cosmetic Act. The Controlled Substances Act is extremely important because it sets current requirements for writing prescriptions for drugs often prescribed in dental practice.

Scheduled Drugs

Federal law divides controlled substances into five schedules according to their abuse potential (Table 1.2). The rules for prescribing these agents, whether prescriptions can be telephoned to the pharmacist and whether refills are allowed, differ depending on the drug's schedule.

New drug entities are evaluated and added to the appropriate schedule. Drugs on the market may be moved from one schedule to another if changes in abuse patterns are discovered.

The current requirements for prescribing controlled drugs (Controlled Substance Act of 1970) are as follows:

- Any prescription for a controlled substance requires a DEA number.
- All Schedule II through IV drugs require a prescription.
- Any prescription for Schedule II drugs must be written in pen or indelible ink or typed. A designee of the dentist, such as the dental hygienist, may write the prescription, but the prescriber must personally sign the prescription in ink and is responsible for what any designee has written.
- Schedule II prescriptions cannot be telephoned to the pharmacist (except at the discretion of the pharmacist for an emergency supply to be followed by a written prescription within 72 hours).
- Because Schedule II prescriptions cannot be refilled, the patient must obtain a new written prescription to obtain more medication.
- Certain states require the use of "triplicate" or "duplicate" prescription blanks for Schedule II drugs. These blanks, provided by the state, are requested by the dentist. After a prescription is written, the dentist keeps one copy and gives two copies to the patient. The patient presents these two copies to the pharmacist, who must file one copy and send the other to the State Board of Pharmacy. These consecutively numbered blank prescription pads provide additional control for Schedule II drugs.
- Prescriptions for Schedule III and IV drugs may be telephoned to the pharmacist and may be refilled no more than five times in 6 months, if so noted on the prescription.

Package Inserts

Package inserts (PIs) contain literature about the drug and is negotiated between the manufacturer and the FDA. The PI provides information regarding the chemical makeup of the drug, FDA-approved indications for use, contraindications, warnings, adverse reactions, drug interactions, dose and administration, and how it is supplied. PIs now contain a "Highlights of Prescribing Information" section that summarizes key information. This section is followed by the "Table of Contents" and the "Full Prescribing Information" main section. The labeling changes were made because the existing labeling was too complicated and too long, and so finding important information took an unacceptably long time. The PI for any new drug or being rewritten for a new indication for an existing drug must include the new formatting.

Black Box Warning

A black box warning is about a drug that the FDA has required a manufacturer to prominently display in a box in the PI. The intent of the black box is to draw attention to the specific warning and make sure

TABLE 1.2	Schedules of Controlled Substances		
Schedule	**Abuse Potential**	**Examples**	**Handling**
I	Highest	Heroin, LSD, marijuana, hallucinogens	No accepted medical use; experimental use, only in research
II	High	Oxycodone, morphine, amphetamine, secobarbital, hydrocodone (alone or in combination with ibuprofen or acetaminophen)	Written prescription with provider's signature only; no refills
III	Moderate	Codeine mixtures (Tylenol #3)	Prescriptions may be telephoned; no more than five prescriptions in 6 months
IV	Less	Diazepam (Valium), tramadol (ultram)	Prescriptions may be telephoned; no more than five prescriptions in 6 months
V	Least	Some codeine-containing cough syrups	Can be bought over-the-counter in some states

LSD, Lysergic acid diethylamide.

that both the prescriber and patient understand the serious safety concerns associated with that drug. Generally the FDA uses black box warnings to bring attention to potentially fatal, life-threatening, or disabling adverse effects of different medications.

Some examples of black box warnings include:

January 13, 2011: Manufacturers of prescription drug products that contain acetaminophen are asked to limit the strength of acetaminophen to no more than 325 mg per tablet, capsule, or other dosing unit. In addition, the FDA has required that a black box warning label be included on all packaging for acetaminophen products highlighting the potential for severe liver damage and a warning highlighting the potential for allergic reactions (e.g., swelling of the face, mouth, and throat, difficulty breathing, itching, and rash).

November 14, 2007: Manufacturer of the prescription drug product rosiglitazone agreed to add new information to an existing black box warning regarding the potential increase in the risk of heart attacks for patients taking rosiglitazone.

March 2, 2006: Long-acting β_2-agonists containing salmeterol xinafoate (Serevent Diskus) and fluticasone propionate/salmeterol xinafoate (Advair Diskus) now carry the warning that their use may increase the risk of asthma-related deaths.

Labeled and Off-Label Uses

The FDA approves the use of drugs for specific indications, which are listed or labeled on the PI of the drug. Any information or use outside the labeled indications is considered *off-label*. Prescribers are allowed to use a drug for an off-label use if good medical practice justifies such use, the use is well-documented in the medical literature, and the drug meets the current standard of medical care. However, drug manufacturers are not allowed to bring up off-label uses when speaking with the prescribing practitioner or patient, nor can they distribute written material regarding off-label uses.

Orphan Drugs

Orphan drugs are developed to specifically treat rare medical conditions. Rare medical conditions with *orphan* status are diseases that occur in less than 200,000 people in the United States. The assignment of orphan status to a disease and to any drug developed to treat that disease has resulted in medical breakthroughs that may never have occurred because of the cost associated with the research and development of new drugs.

Drug Recall

Medications can be recalled from use by the manufacturer itself, at the request of the FDA, or by FDA order under statutory authority. Medications are recalled if there is reasonable probability that their use will have serious adverse health consequences or death. Patients taking a drug that is recalled should call their health care providers about the best course of action.

PRESCRIPTION WRITING

Dental hygienists need to become familiar with the basics of prescription writing for the following reasons:

- Correctly written prescriptions save time for the office personnel, the dentist, and the pharmacist who must call to clarify an incorrectly written prescription.
- Prescriptions written carefully are less likely to result in mistakes.
- A record of the prescription should be included in the patient's record.
- Prescriptions should be written out and Latin abbreviations should be avoided to minimize the risk for errors.

Some drug abusers ("shoppers") search for dental offices that might provide them with prescriptions for controlled substances or prescription blanks that they can use to forge their own prescriptions. Every dental office should keep prescription blanks in a secure place. The prescriber's DEA number should not be printed on the prescription blanks but should be written in only when needed. The dental hygienist should watch to see that prescription blanks are not scattered around the office. If the dentist practices in a state that requires "triplicate" or "duplicate" prescription blanks for Schedule II prescriptions, pads for those prescriptions must be stored under lock and key to prevent them from being stolen.

Measurement
Metric System

> The metric system is the primary measuring system for compounding and dispensing medication.

In pharmacy, the primary measuring system is the metric system. Solid drugs are dispensed by weight (milligrams [mg]) and liquid drugs by volume (milliliters [mL]). It is rarely necessary to use units other than the milligram or the milliliter in prescription writing; occasionally grams (gm) or micrograms (μg) are used. In addition to the milliliter, the liter (L) is also used to measure volume.

Household Measures

Although clinicians will direct the pharmacist to dispense a liquid preparation in milliliters, the pharmacist generally converts metric measurements into a convenient household unit of measurement to be included in the directions to the patient. Liquids are converted into teaspoonfuls (tsp or t; 1 tsp equals 5 mL) and tablespoonfuls (tbsp or T; 1 tbsp equals 15 mL). The pharmacist supplies a calibrated oral syringe or dropper for infants and younger children. Most liquid dose forms come with calibrated dosing cups for both adults and children. Household utensils should not be used. The dosing cups are available in 2.5-, 5-, and 10-mL volumes with milliliters marked along their lengths.

Prescriptions
Format

The parts of the prescription are divided into three sections. They are the heading, body, and closing (Fig. 1.3).

Heading. The heading of the prescription contains the following information:

- Name, address, and telephone number of the prescriber (printed on the prescription blank)
- Name, address, age, and telephone number of the patient (written)
- Date of prescription (not a legal prescription unless filled in with date); often missing

The name, address, and telephone number of the prescriber are important when the pharmacist must contact the prescribing clinician for verification or questions. The date is particularly important because it allows the pharmacist to intercept prescriptions that may not have been filled at the time of writing. For example, a prescription for an antibiotic written 3 months before being presented to the pharmacist might be used for a different reason from that the dentist originally intended. Likewise, a prescription for a pain medication that is even a few days old requires the pharmacist to question the patient as to why the prescription is being filled so long after it was written. The age of the patient enables the pharmacist to check for the proper dose.

Body. The body of the prescription contains the following information:

- The Rx symbol
- Name and dose size or concentration (liquids) of the drug

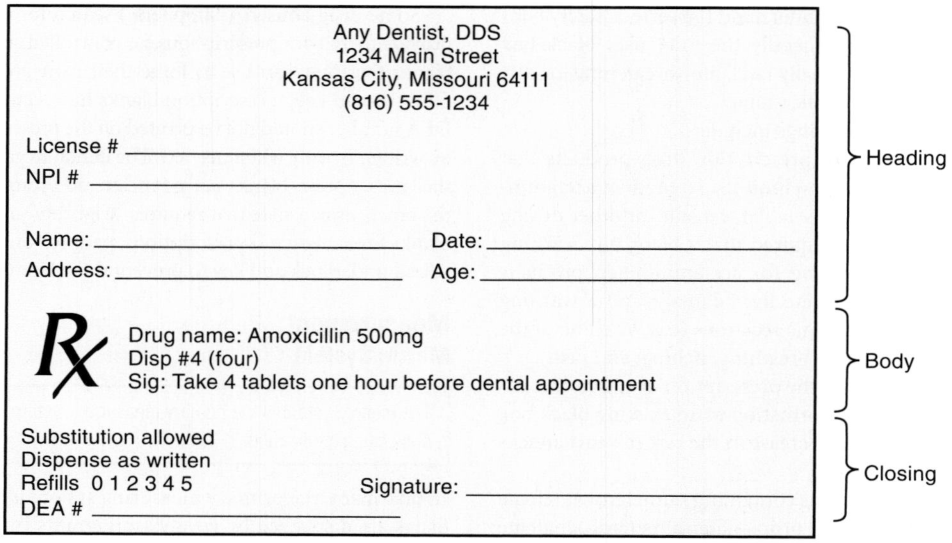

Any Dentist, DDS
1234 Main Street
Kansas City, Missouri 64111
(816) 555-1234

License # _____

NPI # _____

Name: _____ Date: _____

Address: _____ Age: _____

$R\!\!\!/\,_{\!X}$ Drug name: Amoxicillin 500mg
Disp #4 (four)
Sig: Take 4 tablets one hour before dental appointment

Substitution allowed
Dispense as written
Refills 0 1 2 3 4 5   Signature: _____
DEA # _____

} Heading

} Body

} Closing

Fig. 1.3 A typical prescription form.

- Amount to be dispensed
- Directions to the patient

The first entry after the Rx symbol is the name of the drug being prescribed. This is followed by the size (milligrams) of the tablet or capsule desired. In the case of liquids, the name of the drug is followed by its concentration (milligrams per milliliter [mg/mL]). The second entry is the quantity to be dispensed—that is, the number of capsules or tablets or milliliters of liquid. In the case of tablets and capsules, the word "Dispense" is often replaced with #, the symbol for a number. When writing prescriptions for opioids or other controlled substances, the prescriber should add in parentheses the number of tablets or capsules written out in longhand. This practice reduces the possibility that an intended 8 could become an 18 or 80 at the discretion of an enterprising patient. Directions to the patient are preceded by the abbreviation "Sig:" (Latin for *signa*, "write"). The directions to the patient must be completely clear and explicit and should include the amount of medication and the time, frequency, and route of administration. The pharmacist will transcribe any Latin abbreviations (Table 1.3) into English on the label when the prescription is filled.

Closing. The closing of the prescription contains the following:
- Prescriber's signature
- DEA number, if required
- Refill instructions

After the body of the prescription, space is provided for the prescriber's signature. Certain states have more than one place to sign. Certain institutions also provide a space on which to print the prescriber's name. This is not necessary for dentists with their own prescription blanks. If there are several dentists in one office, the names of all the dentists in the practice should be included on the prescription blanks. Then the individual dentist should check a box or circle his or her name so the pharmacist will know who signed the prescription.

Prescription Label Regulations

In addition, the law requires that all prescriptions be labeled with the name of the medication and its strength. Fig. 1.4 is a sample prescription label. This labeling allows easy identification by other practitioners or quick identification in emergency situations. One should note that the name, address, and telephone number of the pharmacy; the patient's and dentist's names; the directions for use; the name and strength of the medication; and the original date and the date filled

TABLE 1.3 Abbreviations Commonly Used in Prescriptions

Abbreviation	Definition
a or $\bar{a}$	before
ac	before meals
bid	twice a day
$\bar{c}$	with
cap	capsule
d	day
disp	dispense
gm	gram
gr	grain
gtt	drop
h	hour
hs	at bedtime
$\bar{p}$	after
pc	after meals
PO	by mouth
prn	as required, if needed
q	every
qid	four times a day
$\bar{s}$	without
sig	write (label)
$\overline{ss}$	one half
stat	immediately (now)
tab	tablet
tid	three times a day
ud	as directed

(refilled) are required. The quantity of medication dispensed (number of tablets) and the number of refills remaining are noted as well. If a generic drug is prescribed, then the generic name of the drug and the manufacturer's are also required to be shown on the label. If the trade drug is used, only the trade name must be shown.

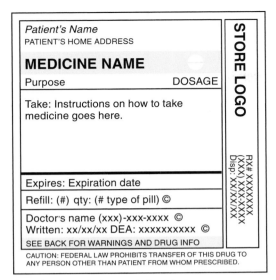

Fig. 1.4 Sample of a typical prescription label.

In most states, before a dentist can legally write a prescription for a patient, the following two criteria must be met:

Patient of record: The person for whom the prescription is being written is a patient of record (no next-door neighbors or relatives, unless they are also patients of record).

Dental condition: The condition for which the prescription is being prescribed is a dental or related condition (no birth control pills or thyroid replacement drugs).

Abbreviations. A few Latin abbreviations are used in prescription writing to save time. The abbreviations also make alteration of a prescription by the patient more difficult. In some cases they are necessary to get all the required information into the space on the prescription form. Some abbreviations that may be useful are shown in Table 1.3. If abbreviations are used on a prescription, they should be clearly written.

For example, the three abbreviations qd (every day), qod (every other day), and qid (four times a day) can look quite similar, and choosing the wrong one could be disastrous.

Electronic and Fax Prescribing

Electronic prescribing (e-prescribing) is the electronic transmission of a prescription to a pharmacy, which reduces the incidence of errors in reading handwritten prescriptions and the patient's ability to tamper with a prescription. Electronic prescriptions are uploaded to a transaction hub, which provides the common link between the prescriber and the pharmacy, thereby reducing the risks associated with traditional prescription writing. Once in the hub, the information is sent to the pharmacy benefits manager, who assesses patient eligibility. Once this step has been completed, the prescription is sent to the pharmacy, which in turn notifies the prescriber of receipt of the prescription (Fig. 1.5). A written record of the prescription is kept in the patient's record. Prescriptions can also be faxed to a pharmacy. The inclusion of e-prescribing in the Medicare Modernization Act of 2003 (MMA) gave momentum to its use in provider practices across the country. The MMA expanded Medicare to include a drug benefit program (Medicare Part D), which began in 2006.

Role of the Dental Hygienist and Patient Adherence to Medication Therapy

Patient adherence to medication therapy is vital to the success of therapy. Adherence to therapy implies that the patient takes the medication as prescribed. Many different factors can contribute to nonadherence to therapy; they include poor understanding of the disease and a need for medication, fear of medication side effects, distrust of health care professionals, economic factors, and forgetfulness. Also, the longer the duration of therapy and the higher the number of times a day the patient must take a prescription, the higher the risk for nonadherence to medication therapy.

The dental hygienist should be able to answer the patient's questions about the prescription and should make sure that the patient knows how to take the medication prescribed (how long and when), what

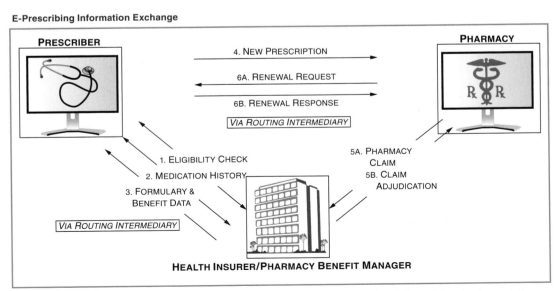

Fig. 1.5 Electronic Prescription Processing. (Source: *RAND, A Toolset for E-Prescribing Implementation, Santa Monica, Calif. (forthcoming).)*

precautions to observe (drug interactions, possible side effects, driving limitations), and the reason for taking the medication. Information about the consequences of nonadherence should be included. A patient who is informed about the prescribed medication is more likely to adhere to therapy. A patient should never get home and not know which drug is the antibiotic (for infection) and which is the analgesic (for pain). Side effects, such as drowsiness and stomach upset, should be noted on the label.

DENTAL HYGIENE CONSIDERATIONS

1. The dental hygienist should understand the importance of obtaining a patient health/medication history.
2. The dental hygienist should have an in-depth understanding of pharmacology because many dental hygienists are now licensed to administer local anesthetics and nitrous oxide.
3. The dental hygienist should be able to explain to the patient how to take a prescription or nonprescription medicine.
4. The dental hygienist should discuss the name of the drug prescribed, what it is used to treat or prevent, the dose, the amount prescribed, and how often it should be taken.
5. The dental hygienist should also tell the patient what to do if the patient feels that he or she is experiencing a side effect or allergic reaction.
6. The dental hygienist should have the patient repeat back what he or she has been told. This step should help determine whether there are any knowledge gaps.
7. The dental hygienist should answer any questions that the patient may have.

ACADEMIC SKILLS ASSESSMENT

1. Define the term *pharmacology*.
2. Explain why the oral health care provider should have a knowledge of pharmacology.
3. Explain the importance of conducting health/medication histories.
4. Why should a dental practice keep more than one type of reference book?
5. Discuss the most important features of a good reference book.
6. Define and give an example of the following terms:
   a. Chemical name
   b. Trade name
   c. Brand name
   d. Generic name
7. Explain why a list of the most current drugs should be available in every dental office.
8. Name three federal regulatory agencies and state the major responsibility of each.
9. Explain the various stages of testing through which a drug must pass before it is marketed for the general public.
10. List the information required in a prescription.
11. Explain two precautions that should be taken in the dental office to discourage drug abusers.
12. List the components of the Controlled Substance Act.

CLINICAL APPLICATIONS

Toula Pappas is new to your practice. She is 40 years old and has three children. Because this is her first appointment, you must conduct the medication/health history.

1. What types of questions would you ask during a medication/health history?
2. What is the importance of the medication/health history?
   During the history you learn that Mrs. Pappas is a healthy individual whose only prescribed medication is esomeprazole 40 mg once daily. Upon further questioning, you learn that Mrs. Pappas self-treats with an occasional acetaminophen or ibuprofen.
3. Where can you look up information regarding esomeprazole.
4. What is a good reference source for over-the-counter (OTC) medications?
5. Why might Mrs. Pappas take the OTC drugs?
   Mrs. Pappas returns for another visit and is prescribed an antibiotic for an abscess. The prescription reads as follows: Amoxicillin 250 mg Sig: 1 tid for 10 days.
6. Please explain this prescription to Mrs. Pappas.

Drug Action and Handling

LEARNING OBJECTIVES

1. Differentiate dose, potency, and efficacy in the context of the actions of drugs.
2. Explain the pharmacologic effect of a drug.
3. Discuss the major steps of pharmacokinetics: absorption, distribution, metabolism, and excretion.
4. Explain how altering absorption, distribution, metabolism, and excretion can affect clinical pharmacokinetics.

5. Explain how half-life relates to clinical pharmacokinetics.
6. Provide an example of factors that may alter the effect of a drug.
7. Summarize the various routes of drug administration and the common dosage forms used.

A *drug* is a biologically active substance that can modify cellular function. A general understanding of drug action is important and will allow the dental hygienist to make informed decisions regarding possible drug interactions or adverse reactions for the patient. This chapter discusses the action of drugs in the body and methods of drug administration. Chapter 3 considers the problems or adverse reactions these drugs can cause. By understanding how drugs work, what effects they can have, and what problems they can cause, the dental hygienist can better communicate with the patient and other health care providers about medications the patient may be taking or may need to have prescribed for dental treatment.

CHARACTERIZATION OF DRUG ACTION

Dose-response curve, potency, and *efficacy* are terms used to measure drug response or action.

Log Dose-Effect Curve

When a drug exerts an effect on biologic systems, it is possible to measure the response to the dose of the drug given. If the dose of the drug is plotted against the intensity of the effect, a curve will result (Fig. 2.1). If this curve is replotted using the log of the dose (log dose) versus the response, another curve is produced from which the potency and efficacy of a drug's action may be determined (Fig. 2.2).

Potency

> *Potency*—related to the amount of drug needed to produce an effect.

The potency of a drug is a function of the amount of drug required to produce an effect. The potency of a drug is shown by the location of that drug's curve along the log-dose axis (*x*-axis). The curves in Fig. 2.3 illustrate two drugs with different potencies. The potency of drug A is greater because the dose required to produce its effect is smaller. The potency of B is less than that of A because B requires a larger dose to produce its effect.

For example, both meperidine and morphine have the ability to treat severe pain, but approximately 100 mg of meperidine would be required to produce the same action as 10 mg of morphine. In Fig. 2.4, the curve for drug B (meperidine) is to the right of the curve for drug A (morphine) because the dose of meperidine needed to produce pain relief is larger (10 times larger) than that of morphine. The potency of the drug should not be an issue as long as appropriate doses of medication are used. Less potent drugs require higher doses to produce therapeutic effects, whereas more potent drugs can reach toxic levels at lower doses. Review the proper dose of each drug before it is prescribed to the patient.

Efficacy

> *Efficacy*—related to the maximal effect of a drug regardless of dose.

Efficacy is the maximum intensity of effect or response that can be produced by a drug. Administering more drug will not increase the efficacy of the drug but can often raise the probability of an adverse reaction. The efficacy of a drug increases as the height of the curve increases (Fig. 2.5). The efficacy of the drugs whose curves are illustrated in Fig. 2.5 is shown by the height of the curve when it plateaus (levels out horizontally). It is shaded from least (*light*) to most (*dark*) potent. The efficacy of any drug is a major descriptive characteristic indicating its action. For example, the efficacy of drug B (meperidine) and that of drug A (morphine) are about the same because both drugs relieve severe pain.

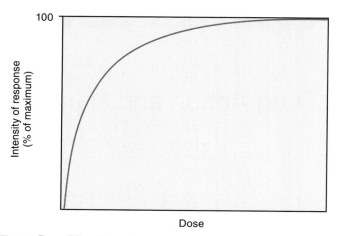

Fig. 2.1 Dose-Effect Curve. The x-axis (horizontal) represents an increasing dose of the drug, and the y-axis (vertical) represents an increasing effect of the drug.

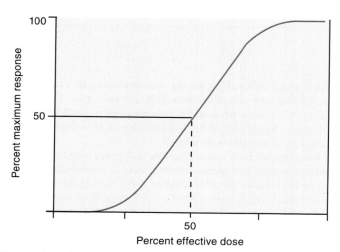

Fig. 2.2 Log Dose-Effect Curve. As the dose is increased (going to the *right* on the x-axis), the effect (the y-axis) is zero at first, then there is a small effect, and finally the effect quickly increases. Around the dose where the line is increasing sharply is the therapeutic range of the compound. Finally, the curve plateaus (flattens out). This is the maximum response a drug can exhibit.

Therapeutic Index

The therapeutic index (TI) is a ratio of the median lethal dose (LD_{50}) to the median effective dose (ED_{50}) and is expressed as follows:

$$TI = LD_{50} / ED_{50}$$

Because death is the end point when one is measuring the lethal dose, LD_{50} is the dose that causes death in 50% of test animals. The ED_{50} is the dose required to produce the desired clinical effect in 50% of test animals. The greater the TI, the safer the drug. Drugs with a lower TI (closer to zero) require careful monitoring to avoid toxic reactions. An example of a drug with a low TI is digoxin, a drug used to treat heart failure.

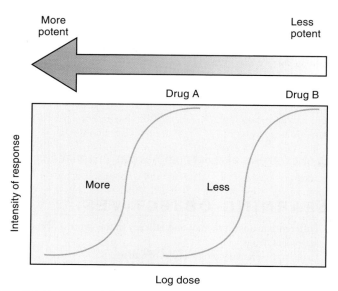

Fig. 2.3 Potency of Agent. The *arrow* is shaded in proportion to increasing potency. *Dark shading,* very potent; *light shading,* of low potency.

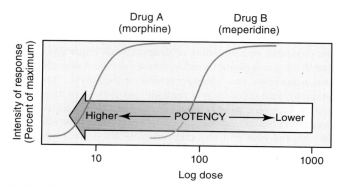

Fig. 2.4 Comparison of Log Dose-Effect Curves for Morphine and Meperidine.

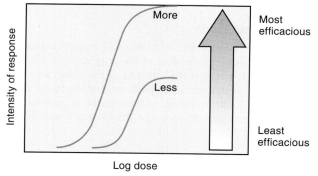

Fig. 2.5 Efficacy of Agent.

MECHANISM OF ACTION OF DRUGS

After drugs have been distributed to their sites of action, they elicit a pharmacologic effect. The pharmacologic effect occurs because of a modulation in the function of an organism. Drugs do not impart a new function to the organism; they merely produce either the same action as an endogenous agent or block the action of an endogenous agent. This signaling mechanism has two functions: amplification of the signal and flexible regulation. The presence of very fine controls to modulate the body's function allows the regulation of certain reactions, slowing or speeding them.

Receptors

Once a drug passes through the biologic membrane, it is carried to many different areas of the body, or sites of action, to exert its **therapeutic effects** or adverse effects. For the drug to exert its effects, it must bind with the receptor site on the cell membrane. Drug receptors appear to consist of many large molecules that exist either on the cell membrane or within the cell itself (Fig. 2.6). More than one receptor type or identical receptors can be found at the site of action. Usually a specific drug binds with a specific receptor in a lock-and-key fashion. Many drug-receptor interactions consist of weak chemical bonds, and the energy formed during this interaction is very low. As a result, the bonds can be formed and broken easily. Once a bond is broken, another drug molecule immediately binds to the receptor.

Different drugs often compete for the same receptor sites. The drug with the stronger affinity for the receptor will bind to more receptors than the drug with the weaker affinity (Fig. 2.7). More of the drug with the weaker affinity will be required to produce a pharmacologic response. Drugs with stronger affinities for receptor sites are more potent than drugs with weaker affinities for the same sites.

Agonists and Antagonists

When a drug combines with a receptor, it alters the function of the organism. It may produce enhancement or inhibition of the function. Drugs that combine with the receptor may be classified as either agonists or antagonists (Fig. 2.8).

Agonist. An *agonist* is a drug that (1) has affinity for a receptor, (2) combines with the receptor, and (3) produces an effect. Naturally occurring neurotransmitters are agonists.

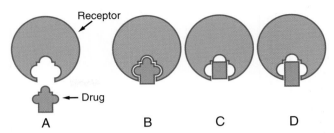

Fig. 2.7 (A) Drugs act by forming a chemical bond with specific receptor sites, similar to a lock and key. (B) The better the "fit," the better the response. Drugs with complete attachment and response are called *agonists*. (C) Drugs that attach but do not elicit a response are called *antagonists*. (D) Drugs that attach and elicit a small response but that also block other responses are called partial agonists. (From Clayton BD, Willihnganz M. *Basic Pharmacology for Nurses*. 16th ed. St. Louis: Mosby; 2013.)

Antagonist. An *antagonist* counteracts the action of the agonist. The following are three different types of antagonists:

A *competitive antagonist* is a drug that (1) has affinity for a receptor, (2) combines with the receptor, and (3) produces no effect. Its presence causes a shift to the right in the dose-response curve (see Fig. 2.8). The antagonist competes with the agonist for the receptor, and the outcome depends on the relative affinities and concentrations of each agent. If the concentration of the agonist is increased, the competitive antagonism can be overcome, and vice versa.

Noncompetitive antagonists bind to a receptor site that is different from the binding site for the agonist. Its presence reduces the maximal response of the agonist (see Fig. 2.8).

A *physiologic antagonist* has affinity for a different receptor site than the agonist. Its presence decreases the maximal response of the agonist by producing an opposite effect via different receptors.

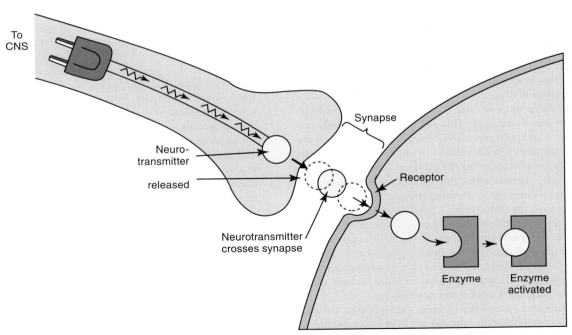

Fig. 2.6 The neurotransmitter is transmitting the message (like electricity) across the synapse (space where nerve is absent). The neurotransmitter then interacts with the receptor (shaped to fit together), which then may signal an enzyme to be synthesized or activated. *CNS*, Central nervous system.

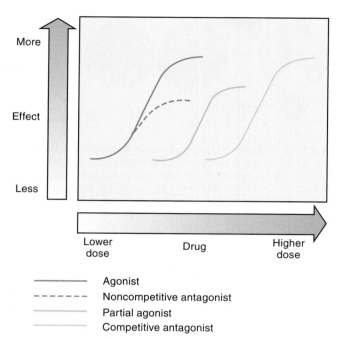

Agonist
Noncompetitive antagonist
Partial agonist
Competitive antagonist

Fig. 2.8 Agonists and Antagonists and Their Interactions.

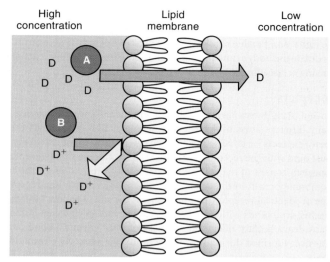

Fig. 2.9 Passage of Drug (*D*) and Metabolite (*D*+) Through Membranes. (A) Lipid-soluble, un-ionized: drug easily passes through the cell membrane from area of high to low drug concentration. (B) Water-soluble ionized drug cannot pass through the cell membrane.

PHARMACOKINETICS

Pharmacokinetics is the study of how a drug enters the body, circulates within the body, is changed by the body, and leaves the body. Factors that influence the movement of a drug are divided into four major steps: absorption, distribution, metabolism, and excretion (ADME).

Passage Across Body Membranes

The amount of drug passing through a cell membrane and the rate at which a drug moves are important in describing the time course of action and the variation in individual response to a drug. Before a drug is absorbed, transported, distributed to body tissues, metabolized, and subsequently eliminated from the body, it must pass through various membranes, such as cellular membranes, blood capillary membranes, and intracellular membranes. Although these membranes have variable functions, they share certain physicochemical characteristics that influence the passage of drugs across them.

These membranes are composed of lipids (fats), proteins, and carbohydrates. The membrane lipids make the membrane relatively impermeable to ions and polar molecules. Membrane proteins make up the structural components of the membrane and help move the molecules across the membrane during the transport process. Membrane carbohydrates are combined with either proteins or lipids. The lipid molecules orient themselves so that they form a fluid bimolecular leaflet structure with the hydrophobic (lipophilic) ends of the molecules shielded from the surrounding aqueous environment and the hydrophilic ends in contact with the water. The various proteins are embedded in and layered onto this fluid lipid bilayer, forming a mosaic. Studies of the ability of substances to penetrate this membrane have indicated the presence of a system of pores or holes through which lower-molecular-weight and smaller chemicals can pass.

The physicochemical properties of drugs that influence the passage of drugs across biologic membranes are lipid solubility, degree of ionization, and molecular size and shape. The mechanisms of drug transfer across biologic membranes are passive transfer and specialized transport.

Passive Transfer

Lipid-soluble substances move across the lipoprotein membrane by a passive transfer process called **simple diffusion**. This type of transfer is directly proportional to the concentration **gradient** (difference) of the drug across the membrane and the degree of lipid solubility. For example, a highly lipid-soluble compound attains a higher concentration at the membrane site and readily diffuses across the membrane into an area of lower concentration (Fig. 2.9). A water-soluble agent has difficulty passing through a lipoprotein membrane.

Specialized Transport

Certain substances are transported across cell membranes by processes that are more complex than simple diffusion and filtration. These processes are as follows:

Active transport is a process by which a substance is transported against a concentration gradient or electrochemical gradient. This action is blocked by metabolic inhibitors. Active transport is believed to be mediated by transport "carriers" that furnish energy for the transportation of the drug.

Facilitated diffusion does not move against a concentration gradient. This phenomenon involves the transport of some substances, such as glucose, into cells. It has been suggested that the process of pinocytosis may explain the passage of macromolecular substances into the cells.

Absorption

Absorption is the process by which drug molecules are transferred from the site of administration to the circulating blood. This process requires the drug to pass through biologic membranes.

The following factors influence the rate of absorption of a drug:
- The physicochemical factors discussed previously.
- The site of absorption, which is determined by the route of administration. For example, one advantage of the oral route is the large absorbing area presented by the intestinal mucosa.
- The drug's solubility. Drugs in solution are more rapidly absorbed than insoluble drugs.

Effect of Ionization

Drugs that are weak electrolytes dissociate (separate) in solution and equilibrate into an un-ionized form and an ionized form. The un-ionized, or uncharged, portion acts like a nonpolar, lipid-soluble compound that readily crosses body membranes (see Fig. 2.9). The ionized portion will pass across these membranes with greater difficulty because it is less lipid soluble.

The pH of the tissues at the site of administration and the dissociation characteristics (pKa) of the drug will determine the amount of drug present in the ionized and un-ionized states. The proportion in each state will determine the ease with which the drug will penetrate the tissues.

Weak acids. When the pH at the site of absorption increases, the hydrogen ion concentration simply falls. This results in an increase in the ionized form (A^-), which cannot easily penetrate tissues.

Conversely, if the pH of the site falls, the hydrogen ion concentration will rise. This results in an increase in the un-ionized form (HA), which can more easily penetrate tissues.

Weak bases. If the pH of the site rises, the hydrogen ion concentration falls. The drop results in an increase in the un-ionized form (B), which can more easily penetrate tissues. Conversely, if the pH of the site falls, the hydrogen ion concentration rises, resulting in an increase in the ionized form (BH^+), which cannot easily penetrate tissues. In summary, weak acids are better absorbed when the pH is less than the pKa, whereas weak bases are better absorbed when the pH is greater than the pKa.

This dissociation also explains the fact that in the presence of infection, the acidity of the tissue increases (and the pH decreases) and the effect of local anesthetics decreases. In the presence of infection, the $[H^+]$ increases because of accumulating waste products in the infected area. The increase in $[H^+]$ (decrease in pH) leads to an increase in ionization and a decrease in penetration of the membrane. This decreased penetration reduces the clinical effect of the local anesthetic.

Oral Absorption

The dose form of a drug is an important factor influencing absorption of drugs administered via the oral route. Unless the drug is administered as a solution, the absorption of the drug in the gastrointestinal tract involves a release from a dose form such as a tablet or capsule. This release requires the following steps before absorption can take place:

1. *Disruption:* The initial disruption of a tablet coating or capsule shell is necessary.
2. *Disintegration:* The tablet or capsule contents must disintegrate (break apart).
3. *Dispersion:* The concentrated drug particles must be dispersed (spread) throughout the stomach or intestines.
4. *Dissolution:* The drug must be dissolved (in solution) in the gastrointestinal fluid.
   A drug in solution skips these four steps, so it usually has a quicker onset of action.

Absorption From Injection Site

Absorption of a drug from the site of injection depends on the solubility of the drug and the blood flow at that site. For example, drugs with low water solubility, such as some penicillin salts, are absorbed very slowly after intramuscular injection. Absorption at injection sites is also affected by the dosage form. Drugs in suspension are absorbed much more slowly than those in solution. Certain insulin preparations are formulated in suspension form to decrease their absorption rate and prolong their action. Drugs that are least soluble will have the longest duration of action.

Distribution
Basic Principles

All drugs occur in two forms in the blood: bound to plasma proteins and the free drug. The free drug is the form that exerts the pharmacologic effect. The bound drug is a reservoir (place to store) for the drug. The proportion of drug in each form depends on the properties of that specific drug (percentage protein bound). Within each compartment (e.g., blood, brain), the drug is split between the bound drug and the free drug. Only the free drug can pass across cell membranes.

For a drug to exert its activity, it must be made available at its site of action in the body. The mechanism by which this is accomplished is distribution, which is the passage of drugs into various body fluid compartments such as plasma, interstitial fluids, and intracellular fluids. The manner in which a drug is distributed in the body will determine how rapidly it produces the desired response; the duration of that response; and, in some cases, whether a response will be elicited at all.

Drug distribution occurs when a drug moves to various sites in the body, including its site of action in specific tissues. However, drugs are also distributed to areas where no action is desired (nonspecific tissues). Some drugs, because of their characteristics, are poorly distributed to certain regions of the body. Other drugs are distributed to their sites of action and then redistributed to other tissue sites. The distribution of a drug is determined by several factors, such as the size of the organ, the blood flow to the organ, the solubility of the drug, the plasma protein-binding capacity, and the presence of certain barriers (blood-brain barrier, placenta).

Distribution by Plasma

After a drug is absorbed from its site of administration, it is distributed to its site of action by the blood plasma. Therefore the biologic activity of a drug is related to the concentration of the free, or unbound, drug in the plasma. Drugs are bound reversibly to plasma proteins such as albumin and globulin. The drug that is bound to the protein does not contribute to the intensity of the drug action because only the unbound form is biologically active. The bound drug is considered a storage site. If one drug is highly bound, another administered drug that is highly bound may displace the first drug from its plasma protein-binding sites, increasing the effect of the first drug. This is one mechanism of drug interaction.

Blood-Brain Barrier

The tissue sites of distribution should be considered before administration. For example, for drugs to penetrate the central nervous system (CNS), they must cross the blood-brain barrier. The passage of a drug across this barrier is related to the drug's lipid solubility and degree of ionization. The endothelium of this barrier contains a cell layer and a basement membrane. The welding of the endothelial cells together prevents the formation of clefts, gaps, or pores that might allow the penetration of certain drugs. To diffuse transcellularly, the drug must penetrate the epithelial and basement membrane cells. Thiopental, a highly lipid-soluble, nonionized drug, easily penetrates the blood-brain barrier to gain access to the cerebrospinal fluid and induce sleep within seconds after intravenous administration.

Placenta

The passage of drugs across the placenta involves simple diffusion in accordance with their degree of lipid solubility. Although the placenta may act as a selective barrier against a few drugs, most drugs pass easily across the placental barrier. Lipid-soluble drugs penetrate this membrane most easily. Therefore when agents are administered to the mother, they are concomitantly administered to the fetus. The term *barrier* is a misnomer when used to describe the placenta.

Enterohepatic Circulation

Drugs are typically absorbed via the intestines, are distributed through the serum, pass to specific and nonspecific sites of action, come to the liver, and are metabolized before being excreted via the kidneys. When a drug undergoes enterohepatic circulation, the process varies. The steps are the same until the drug is metabolized. At that point, the metabolite is secreted via the bile into the intestine. The metabolite is broken down by enzymes and releases the drug. The drug is then absorbed again, and the process continues. After being taken up by the liver the second time, these drugs are again secreted into the bile. This circular pattern continues, with some drug escaping with each passing. This process prolongs the effect of a drug. If the enterohepatic circulation is blocked, the level of the drug in the serum falls.

Redistribution

Redistribution of a drug is the movement of a drug from the site of action to nonspecific sites of action. A drug's duration of action can be affected by its redistribution from one organ to another. If redistribution occurs between specific and nonspecific sites, a drug's action will be terminated. For example, thiopental produces sleep within seconds, but the effect is terminated within a few minutes. This is because the drug is first distributed to the CNS (sleep), is subsequently redistributed through the plasma to the muscle (action terminated), and finally reaches the fat depots of the body (no action still).

Metabolism (Biotransformation)

> Drug metabolism produces compounds that are more polar (ionized) and more easily excreted.

Metabolism, which is also known as *biotransformation*, is the body's way of changing a drug so that it can be more easily excreted by the kidneys. Many drugs undergo metabolic transformation, or change, most commonly in the liver. The metabolite (metabolic product) formed is usually more polar (ionized) and less lipid soluble than its parent compound. This means that renal tubular reabsorption of the metabolite will be reduced because reabsorption favors lipid-soluble compounds. Metabolites are also less likely to bind to plasma or tissue proteins and less likely to be stored in fat tissue. Decreases in renal tubular reabsorption, binding to the plasma or tissue proteins, and fat storage cause the metabolite to be excreted more easily. Drug metabolism is an enzyme-dependent process that has developed through evolution.

Drugs can be metabolized in any of the three following ways (Fig. 2.10):

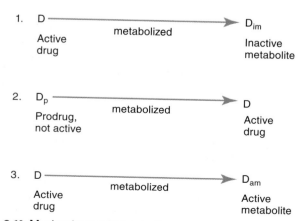

Fig. 2.10 Mechanisms of Metabolism.

Active to inactive: By metabolism, an inactive compound may be formed from an active parent drug. This is the most common type of reaction in drug biotransformation. Agents that interfere with the metabolism of certain drugs will increase the blood level of the drugs whose metabolism is inhibited. An example is doxycycline. Doxycycline, the active compound, is metabolized by the liver into an inactive metabolite.

Inactive to active: An inactive parent drug may be transformed into an active compound. The inactive compound is then termed a *prodrug*. Interference with the metabolism of this drug delays its onset of action because it will be harder for the active compound to be formed. For example, acyclovir is an antiviral agent. To be effective, it must be taken into the cell and converted to its active metabolite.

Active to active: An active parent drug may be converted to a second active compound, which is then converted to an inactive product. The total effect of such a drug would be the addition of the effect of the parent drug plus the effect of the active drug metabolite. When an active metabolite is formed, the action of the drug is prolonged. For example, diazepam (Valium), an active antianxiety agent, is metabolized into its active metabolite, desmethyldiazepam. Diazepam's action is prolonged because of its own effect combined with that of its active metabolite.

First-Pass Effect

When drugs are given orally, they are absorbed through the intestinal wall and then pass through the hepatic (liver) portal circulation, which can inactivate some drugs. This is termed the *first-pass effect* because the drug passes through the liver first before it circulates in the systemic circulation. During the drug's first pass through the liver, it is metabolized (the amount metabolized varies) and the amount of drug available to produce a systemic effect is reduced. Drugs with a high first-pass effect have a larger oral-to-parenteral dose ratio. This means that the dose required when given orally for an equivalent effect is much greater than the dose needed when used parenterally. Because morphine has a high first-pass effect, the oral dose needed to produce an equivalent effect is much larger than its parenteral dose.

Phase I reactions. In phase I reactions, lipid molecules are metabolized by three processes, oxidation, reduction, and hydrolysis, which require very little energy. Oxidative reactions are the most common type of phase I reactions. Phase I reactions are carried out by the microsomal or cytochrome P-450 enzymes, which are also known as the *mixed-function oxidases,* in the liver. The concentration of these enzymes can be affected by drugs and environmental substances. Phase I metabolism may be affected by other drugs that alter microsomal enzyme inhibition or induction.

Phase II reactions. Phase II reactions involve conjugation with any of the following agents: glucuronic acid, sulfuric acid, acetic acid, or an amino acid. The most common conjugation occurs with glucuronic acid. This conjugation is termed glucuronidation. Glucuronic acid, which is a substance normally occurring in the body, may be transferred to a drug molecule that has an appropriate functional group to accept it. Functional groups that may be involved include ethers, alcohols, aromatic amines, and carboxylic acid. This mechanism, either alone or in combination with a phase I reaction, allows the body to convert a lipid-soluble drug to a more polar compound. The enzymes that mediate the conjugation are termed transferases.

Cytochrome P-450 Induction and Inhibition

The cytochrome P-450 microsomal enzyme system can be induced to speed up drug metabolism or inhibited to reduce or slow down drug metabolism. Because drugs that cause enzyme induction cause other drugs to be more quickly metabolized, the metabolized drugs have

TABLE 2.1 Selected Cytochrome P-450 (CYP) Isoenzymes: Substrates, Inhibitors, and Inducers

Number	Substrate	Inhibitors	Inducers
CYP 2D6	Imipramine Amitriptyline Fluoxetine Haloperidol Codeine Oxycodone Hydrocodone	Cimetidine Fluoxetine Paroxetine Haloperidol	Dexamethasone Rifampicin
CYP 3A4	Carbamazepine Lidocaine Clarithromycin Erythromycin Venlafaxine Atorvastatin Simvastatin Alprazolam Diazepam	Corticosteroids Grapefruit juice Omeprazole Clarithromycin Ketoconazole Itraconazole Fluoxetine	Carbamazepine Phenytoin Barbiturates
CYP2C9	Ibuprofen Fluoxetine Fluvastatin	Fluconazole Miconazole	Rifampicin Secobarbital

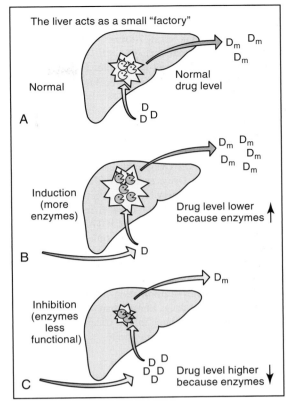

Fig. 2.11 Alteration of Drug Metabolism Induction and Inhibition. Enzyme induction and inhibition alter the blood levels of drugs (D) metabolized by the hepatic enzymes. (A) Normal. The liver is metabolizing drugs at the normal rate producing the normal effects. (B) Induction. With enzyme induction (stimulation), increase in the enzymes causes the drug to be more quickly metabolized, and blood level of the drug and its effect are decreased (assuming that the metabolite is inactive). Induction = effect. (C) Inhibition. With enzyme inhibition, the metabolism of drugs is slower (due to weaker enzymes) and the blood level of the drug that is metabolized is increased. Inhibition = effect. D_m, Drug metabolite.

reduced pharmacologic effects. Research has shown that the hepatic enzymes can be divided into many categories, or types of *isoenzymes*. Examples of isoenzymes are cytochrome P-450 2D6 and cytochrome P-450 3A4. Table 2.1 lists examples of drugs that are substrates of these enzymes and drugs that either induce or inhibit the isoenzymes. For example, phenobarbital stimulates the production of microsomal enzymes that normally metabolize the anticoagulant warfarin. Thus administering phenobarbital to a patient taking warfarin can decrease warfarin's anticoagulant response because the metabolism of the anticoagulant is stimulated by phenobarbital (Fig. 2.11).

Inhibition of the metabolism of certain drugs may occur through several mechanisms. With inhibition, the blood levels and action of the drugs metabolized by these enzymes are increased. Examples of drugs that inhibit the metabolism of other drugs are erythromycin and cimetidine. Inhibiting the microsomal enzymes would result in an increase in the effect of the drugs metabolized by the liver enzymes (see Table 2.1).

Excretion

Although drugs may be excreted by any of several routes that have direct access to the external environment, renal (kidney) excretion is the most important. Extrarenal routes include the lungs, bile, gastrointestinal tract, sweat, saliva, and breast milk. Drugs may be excreted unchanged or as metabolites.

Renal route. Elimination of substances via the kidney can occur by the following three routes:

Glomerular filtration: Either the unchanged drug or its metabolites are filtered through the glomeruli and concentrated in the renal tubular fluid. This filtration process depends on the amount of plasma protein binding and the glomerular filtration rate. Bound drugs cannot be filtered and remain in the systemic circulation. Most drugs are managed by this mechanism.

Active tubular secretion: Active secretion transports the drug from the bloodstream across the renal tubular epithelial cells and into the renal tubular fluid. Glomerular filtration and active tubular secretion

are relatively nonselective, and several compounds, both exogenous and endogenous (naturally occurring), can compete for transport.

Passive tubular diffusion: With most drugs, passive tubular diffusion (also termed *passive reabsorption*) plays a part in regulating the amount of drug in the tubular fluid. This process favors the reabsorption of un-ionized, lipid-soluble compounds. The more ionized, less lipid-soluble metabolites have more difficulty penetrating the cell membranes of the renal tubules and are likely to be retained in the tubular fluid and eliminated in the urine. This process is also influenced by the urinary pH, which affects the amount of ionized and un-ionized drug in the tubular fluid. Alteration in the pH of the urine can favor drug excretion in cases of poisoning or can inhibit it when a prolongation of the drug's effect is desired. Weakly ionized acids or bases are excreted in the following fashion:

Alkaline urine: When the tubular urinary pH is more alkaline than the plasma, weak acids are excreted more rapidly and weak bases are excreted more slowly.

Acid urine: When tubular urine is more acid, weak acids are excreted more slowly and weak bases are excreted more rapidly.

Extrarenal routes. Certain drugs may be partially or completely eliminated via routes other than the kidney, or by the lungs. Gases used in general anesthesia are excreted across the lung tissue by a process of simple diffusion. Alcohol is also partially excreted from the lungs. (One can smell alcohol on someone's breath if the person has been drinking alcohol.) This fact is used in testing a driver's breath for the presence of alcohol (i.e., with the Breathalyzer).

Biliary excretion. Some drug metabolites formed in the liver are excreted via the bile into the intestinal tract and eliminated in the feces. Thus enterohepatic circulation, discussed earlier, prolongs a drug's action.

Saliva. Drugs can also be excreted into the saliva. After drugs are excreted in the saliva, they are usually swallowed, and their fate is the same as that of drugs ingested orally.

Gingival crevicular fluid. Drugs may also be excreted in the gingival crevicular fluid (GCF). Drugs excreted in the GCF produce a higher level of drug in the gingival crevices, which can increase their usefulness in the treatment of periodontal disease. Some drugs, such as the tetracyclines, are concentrated in the GCF. This means that the drug level of tetracycline in the GCF is several times (four or more times) higher than the blood level. This property makes the systemic use of a drug more effective within the gingival sulcus than one that is not thus concentrated.

Other. Two minor routes of elimination are through breast milk and sweat. The distribution of drugs in milk may be a potential source of undesirable effects for the nursing infant. Chapter 22 discusses dental drugs that can be given to nursing mothers.

CLINICAL PHARMACOKINETICS

Half-Life

The half-life ($t_{1/2}$) of a drug is the amount of time that passes for its concentration to fall to half (50%) of its original blood level. A drug with a short half-life is quickly removed from the body and its duration of action is short. A drug with a long half-life is slowly removed from the body and its duration of action is long.

It takes approximately four to five half-lives for a drug to be considered eliminated from the body. Because only 3% to 6% remains after four or five half-lives, respectively, we can say that the drug is essentially gone. Conversely, it takes about four or five half-lives of repeated dosing for a drug's level to build up to a steady state (level amount) in the body. If the half-life of a drug is 1 hour, then in 4 or 5 hours the drug would be mostly gone from the body. In 4 hours, 94% of the drug would be gone. However, if the half-life of a drug is 60 hours, then it would take 240 (10 days) to 300 hours (12 days) for that drug to be eliminated from the body. Even after a drug with a long half-life is discontinued, its effect can take several days to dissipate, depending on its half-life.

Kinetics

Kinetics is the mathematical representation of the way in which drugs are removed from the body. The most common mechanism is first-order kinetics (Fig. 2.12). Drugs that demonstrate first-order kinetics are eliminated from the body at a constant percentage per unit of time. Once a drug is given orally and steady state is achieved, plasma blood levels equal the levels eliminated. Plasma blood levels and elimination are proportional to the dose administered.

A few drugs, such as aspirin and alcohol, exhibit zero-order kinetics. With zero-order kinetics, the rate of metabolism remains constant over time, and the same amount of drug is metabolized per unit of time regardless of dose. Zero-order kinetics occurs because the enzymes that metabolize these drugs can become saturated at usual therapeutic doses. If the dose of the drug is increased, the metabolism cannot increase above its maximum rate. With small doses, drugs with zero-order kinetics can be metabolized without buildup. With high

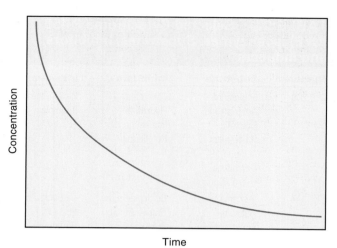

Drug elimination is equal to drug plasma concentration

Fig. 2.12 First-Order Kinetics. Half-life constant throughout the usual doses. Half of the dose of the drug in the body is removed with each half-life. *1, 2 ... 5,* Number of half-lives that have passed.

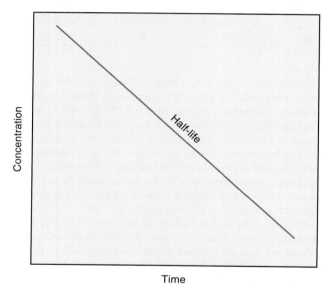

With zero-order kinetics, drug elimination mechanisms become saturated. The drug is more quickly metabolized with a small dose and metabolism does not increase with a larger dose.

Fig. 2.13 Zero-Order Kinetics. Large dose (A). Small dose (B). Disappearance of a drug whose metabolism is saturable. With a small dose (B), the drug is metabolized more quickly than when a large dose (A) is given. With a large dose, the metabolism cannot increase, so it takes a long time for the body to clear the drug. The half-life varies with the dose of the drug.

doses, the metabolism of the drug cannot increase and the duration of action of the drug can be greatly prolonged (Fig. 2.13). Small changes in the dosages of these drugs may produce a large change in their serum concentrations, leading to unexpected toxicity.

FACTORS THAT ALTER DRUG EFFECTS

When a drug is administered, the following factors may influence or modify the drug's effect:

Patient adherence: Through either lack of understanding or lack of motivation, patients often take medications incorrectly or not at all. Sometimes this may result from faulty communication, inadequate patient education, or the patient's health belief system. Thus poor patient adherence can be an important factor in a therapeutic failure.

Psychologic factors: The attitude of the prescriber and the dental staff can affect the efficacy of the drug prescribed. A placebo is a dose form that looks like the active agent but contains no active ingredients (the "sugar pill"). The magnitude of the placebo effect depends on the patient's perception, and there is large individual variation. Health care providers can maximize a drug's effect to achieve an improved therapeutic result by explaining the effectiveness of the drug.

Tolerance: A patient may exhibit tolerance to many drugs, including the sedatives-hypnotics and the opioids. *Drug tolerance* is defined as the need for an increasingly larger dose of the drug to obtain the same effects as the original dose or the decreased effect produced after repeated administration of a given dose of the drug. When a patient becomes tolerant to one drug, tolerance to other drugs with similar pharmacologic actions occurs. This is termed *cross-tolerance.* If tolerance develops, a normal sensitivity to the drug's effect may be restored by cessation of use of the drug.

Pathologic state: Patients with disease may respond to the administration of medication differently from other patients. For example, patients with hyperthyroidism are extremely sensitive to the toxic effects of epinephrine. Hepatic or renal disease influences the metabolism and excretion of drugs, potentially leading to an increased duration of drug action. With repeated doses in patients with such diseases, the serum level of a drug may become toxic.

Time of administration: The time a drug is administered, especially in relation to meals, alters the response to that drug. Certain drugs with a sedative action are best administered at bedtime to minimize the sedation experienced by the patient.

Route of administration: The effect of the route of administration on the onset and duration of action of a drug was discussed previously.

Sex: The sex of the patient can alter a drug's effect. Women may be more sensitive than men to certain drugs, perhaps because of their smaller size or their hormones. Pregnancy alters the effect of certain drugs. Women of childbearing age should avoid teratogenic drugs, and the oral health care provider should determine whether a patient is pregnant before administering any agent.

Genetic variation: Many differences in patient response to drugs have been associated with variations in the ability to metabolize certain drugs. This difference may account for the fact that certain populations have a higher incidence of adverse effects to some drugs—they have a genetic predisposition.

Drug interactions: A drug's effect may be modified by previous or concomitant administration of another drug. There are many mechanisms by which drug interactions may modify a patient's therapeutic response to treatment.

Age and weight: The dose of a drug administered to children should be smaller than the adult dose. Age or weight has been suggested as a method of calculating a child's dose. Because of the great variability of weight in relation to age, the child's weight should be used to determine the child's dose. Because a child is not just a small adult, it is best to follow the manufacturer's recommendations for children's dosing. Older adults may respond differently from younger patients to drugs. Whether this is solely because of changes in renal or liver function or whether being elderly predisposes to this sensitivity is controversial.

Environment: The environment contains many substances that may affect the action of drugs. Smoking induces enzymes, so higher doses of benzodiazepines are needed to produce the same effect in a smoker than in a nonsmoker. Some chemical contaminants, such as pesticides and solvents, can have an effect on a drug's action.

Other: The action of drugs can be altered by the patient-provider interaction. If the patient "believes" in the substance or process (drug/herb/incantation) being used, the patient's opinion will enhance the drug's effect. The attitude of both the patient and the provider can alter the physiology of the body. These actions may account for the positive effect of many mental exercises (e.g., meditation).

ROUTES OF ADMINISTRATION AND DOSE FORMS

Routes of Administration

> *Route*—various ways a drug can be administered.

The route of administration of a drug affects both the onset and the duration of response. As previously explained, *onset* refers to the time it takes for the drug to begin to have its effect. Duration is the length of a drug's effect. The routes of administration can be classified as enteral or parenteral (Table 2.2). Drugs given by the enteral route are placed directly into the gastrointestinal tract by oral or rectal administration. Parenteral administration bypasses the gastrointestinal tract and includes various injection routes, inhalation, and topical administration. In practice, the term *parenteral* usually refers to an injection.

Although oral administration is considered the safest, least expensive, and most convenient route, the parenteral route has certain advantages. The injection results in fast absorption, which produces a rapid onset and a more predictable response than oral administration. The parenteral route is useful for emergencies, the treatment of unconscious patients, those who are uncooperative, or patients with nausea. Some drugs must be administered by injection to remain active. The disadvantages of the parenteral route include the facts that asepsis must be maintained to prevent infection, an intravascular injection can occur by accident, administration by injection is more painful, it is difficult to remove the drug, adverse effects may be more pronounced, and self-medication is difficult. Parenteral therapy is also more dangerous and more expensive than oral medication. Fig. 2.14 illustrates several common forms of drug administration.

Oral Route

> *Oral*—the most common and most popular route of administration in the United States.

The oral route of administration is the simplest way to introduce a drug into the body. It allows the use of many different dose forms to obtain the desired results; tablets, capsules, and liquids are conveniently given. An advantage of this route is the large absorbing area present in the small intestine. Oral administration produces a slower onset of action than parenterally administered agents. One disadvantage of this route is that stomach and intestinal irritation may result in nausea and vomiting. Another disadvantage is that certain drugs, such as insulin, are inactivated by gastrointestinal tract acidity or enzymes.

Drug blood levels obtained after oral administration are less predictable than those after parenteral administration. The presence of food in the stomach, the pathologic condition of the gastrointestinal tract, the effects of gastric acidity, and passage through the hepatic

TABLE 2.2   Routes of Administration

Route	Dosage Form	Reason for Use	Examples
Enteral			
PO	Tablets, capsules, troches, syrup, suspensions	Easy to take Undergoes first-pass metabolism	Antibiotics, NSAIDs, acetaminophen, cough syrups
Rectal	Suppository	Patient inability to take oral medications	Glycerin suppositories, antinauseants
Topical			
Epicutaneous	Cream, ointment, gel	Direct application to the skin provides a local effect	Hydrocortisone cream Antifungal cream Estrogen
Transdermal patch	Patch	Dosing over an extended period eliminates the need for repeated oral dosing	Nitroglycerin, scopolamine, fentanyl, nicotine
Inhalation	Oral, nasal	Rapid drug response Can have local effects (the lungs) or general effects (anesthesia)	Albuterol inhaler, oral steroid inhalers, nitrous oxide, steroid nasal sprays, decongestant sprays
Sublingual	Tablets	Rapid drug response (mucous membrane allows for rapid absorption)	Nitroglycerin tablets
Buccal	Tablets	Rapid drug response (mucous membrane allows for rapid absorption)	Fentanyl buccal tablets
Subgingival	Drug-impregnated gels or strips	Act locally with minimal systemic effects	Antibiotics Chlorhexidine
Parenteral			
IV		Post the most rapid drug response Bypasses first-pass metabolism 100% is absorbed into the bloodstream	Antibiotics Medical emergency drugs
IM			Antibiotics Antipsychotics
SQ		Gaining systemic access through SQ tissue avoids liver enzymes that would inactivate the drug	Insulin
Intradermal		Avoids liver enzymes that would inactivate the drug	Tuberculin test Influenza vaccination
Intrathecal		Avoids the blood-brain barrier Localized to the cerebrospinal fluid	Spinal anesthesia Analgesia
Intraperitoneal		Localized effect in the peritoneum	Local anesthesia Chemotherapy

IM, Intramuscular; *IV,* intravenous; *NSAIDs,* nonsteroidal antiinflammatory drugs; *PO,* oral; *SQ,* subcutaneous.

portal circulation can alter blood levels. Drug interactions can occur when two drugs are present in the stomach. The oral route necessitates greater patient cooperation.

Rectal Route

Drugs may be given rectally as suppositories, creams, or enemas. Rectal administration can be used if a patient is vomiting or unconscious. This route may be used for either a local (e.g., for hemorrhoids) or a systemic (e.g., antiemetic) effect. Because most drugs are poorly and irregularly absorbed when administered rectally, this route is not often used to achieve a systemic drug effect. In addition, patient acceptance of this route is poor.

Intravenous Route

Intravenous administration produces the most rapid drug response, with an almost immediate onset of action. Because the injection is made directly into the blood, the absorption phase is bypassed. Another advantage of the intravenous route is that it produces a more predictable response than oral administration because factors that affect drug absorption have been eliminated. It is also the route of choice for an emergency situation. The disadvantages of administration include

phlebitis due to local irritation, drug irretrievability (drug is immediately absorbed and cannot be easily treated with an antidote), allergy, and side effects related to high plasma concentrations of the drug.

Intramuscular Route

Absorption of drugs injected into the muscle occurs because of the high blood flow through skeletal muscles. Somewhat irritating drugs may be tolerated if given by the intramuscular route. This route may also be used for injection of suspensions to provide a sustained effect. Injections are usually made in the deltoid region or gluteal mass.

Subcutaneous Route

The subcutaneous route involves the injection of solutions or suspensions of drugs into the subcutaneous areolar tissue to gain access to the systemic circulation. If irritating solutions are injected subcutaneously, sterile abscesses may result. Insulin is commonly administered by this route.

Intradermal Route

Small amounts of drugs, such as local anesthetics, can be injected into the epidermis of the skin to provide local anesthesia. With this type of

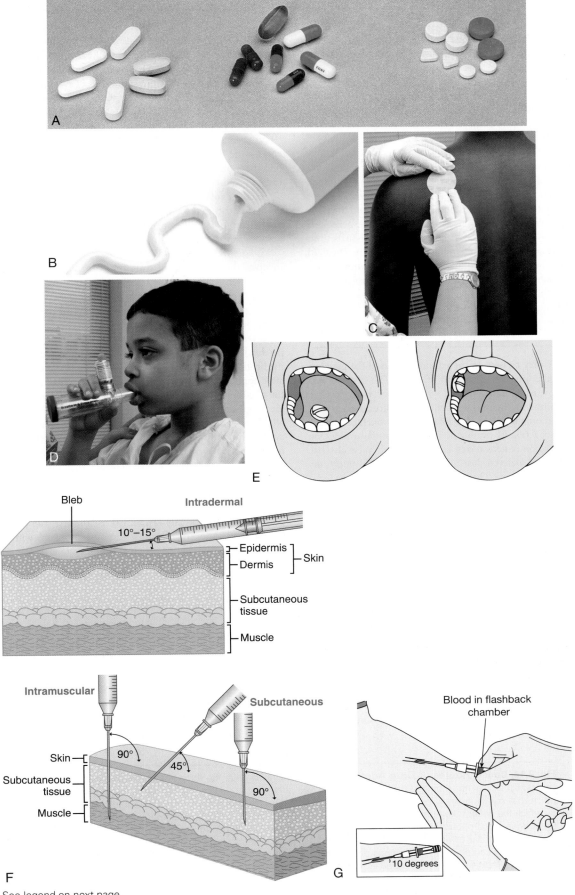

Fig. 2.14 See legend on next page.

injection, a small bump (bleb) rises as the liquid is injected just under the skin. The tuberculosis skin test is performed using the intradermal route.

Intrathecal Route

Intrathecal administration involves the injection of solutions into the spinal subarachnoid space. It may be used for spinal anesthesia or for the treatment of certain forms of meningitis.

Intraperitoneal Route

The intraperitoneal route involves placing fluid into the peritoneal cavity, where exchange of substances can occur. A drug may be absorbed through the mesenteric veins. This route of administration is also used for peritoneal dialysis. In this case, the substances are passing from the body to the fluid. Large volumes of fluids are slowly run into the peritoneal cavity. A waiting period of several hours allows the waste products from the body to be exchanged with the fluid in the peritoneal cavity. The fluid is removed, and the body's waste products are carried out with it. This process is used as a substitute for the kidney in patients with renal failure.

Inhalation Route

> *Inhalation route*—used for local or systemic effects.

The inhalation route may be used in the administration of the gaseous, microcrystalline, liquid, or powdered form of drugs. This route of administration may be used for either local or systemic effects. An example involves inhalers utilized for their local effects, such as those used to treat asthma. After inhalation, the drug is deposited on the bronchiolar endothelium and exerts its action by producing bronchodilation or reducing inflammation. Inhalation of aerosolized liquid in fine droplets also has a local effect. Today's oral metered-dose inhalers contain hydrofluorocarbons that do not harm the ozone. These inhalers contain finely powdered drugs that are also inhaled into the lungs. One advantage of the use of the powdered form is that inhalation must continue until the visible powder is gone. General anesthetics in the form of volatile liquids such as isoflurane or gases such as nitrous oxide (N_2O) and oxygen are examples of the use of the inhalation route for systemic effects. This route of administration is popular for the abuse of many drugs (smoked or even inhaled) because of the quick onset of action and the fact that no needles are required.

Topical Route

Topical routes consist of application to body surfaces. Topical applications are administered to the skin, to the oral mucosa, and even sublingually (under the tongue). The inhalation route could even be called topical. Drugs used topically may be intended to have either local or systemic effects.

Because most drugs do not penetrate intact skin, application to the skin is generally used for local effects. Corticosteroids are applied to inflamed or irritated skin. Intravaginal creams or suppositories and solutions or suspensions instilled into the eye or ear are other ways to administer topical agents for local effects.

Rarely, systemic (unintended) side effects can occur from the topical administration of drugs for their local effect. One example is the administration of topical corticosteroids over a large proportion of the body, which may result in symptoms of systemic toxicity (Cushing Syndrome). If an occlusive dressing (commercial plastic wrap or a plastic suit) is used or if the surface is abraded, inflamed, or sloughing, the chance of side effects increases dramatically. In the oral cavity, interruptions in the mucous membranes or mucosal inflammation increases the likelihood of a systemic effect. Local anesthetics sprayed into the mouth may be adsorbed and produce a blood level equivalent to that produced by intravenous administration.

Examples of drugs applied topically for a systemic effect include transdermal patches and sublingual (SL) spray or tablet administration. Drugs that often produce allergic reactions should not be administered topically because sensitization occurs more readily than when used orally.

Subgingival strips and gels. A dental-specific topical application involves the placement of drug-impregnated strips or gels subgingivally. Systemic effects are minimized because small doses can be used when drugs are administered via this route. Doxycycline gel (Atridox) and a chlorhexidine-containing chip (PerioChip) are examples of agents administered into the gingival crevice.

Transdermal patch. Transdermal drug delivery systems (drug patches) are designed to provide continuous controlled release of medication through a semipermeable membrane over a given period after application of drug to the intact skin. This approach eliminates the need for repeated oral dosing. Examples of patches on the market are scopolamine (Transderm-Scop), nitroglycerin (Transderm-Nitro, Nitrodisc, Nitro-Dur), clonidine (Catapres-TTS), estrogens (Estraderm, Climara), fentanyl (Duragesic), testosterone (Androderm), and nicotine (NicoDerm, Nicobid) transdermal patches.

Most patches consist of several layers. Beginning with the skin, the layers are as follows: adhesive (to stick to the skin), membrane (to control the rate of drug release), drug reservoir (where the drug is stored), and a backing that is impenetrable to the drug (to keep the drug from evaporating into the air) (Fig. 2.15). Before use, the protective backing must be removed. The most common problems with transdermal patches are local irritation, erythema, and edema. These problems can

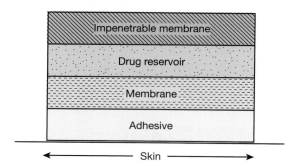

Fig. 2.15 Layers of a Transdermal Patch.

Fig. 2.14, Cont'd Routes of Drug Administration. (A) Oral route in the form of pills, tablets, capsules, or liquids. (B) Topical route by application on the surface of the mucosa or skin. (C) Transdermal route, through a patch that continuously releases a controlled quantity of a medication through the skin. (D) Inhalation route, by which the patient breathes in a gaseous substance. (E) Sublingual route, by placement of medication under the tongue (absorption takes place through the oral mucosa). (F) Injection route. The type of drug determines how the injection is given: subcutaneous, directly under the skin; intramuscular, into a muscle; intradermal, into the skin. (G) Example of an intravenous push medication administration. (A, C, D from Proctor DB, Adams AP. *Kinn's the Medical Assistant: An Applied Learning Approach.* 12th ed. St. Louis: Saunders; 2014; E from Clayton BD, Willihnganz M. *Basic Pharmacology for Nurses.* 16th ed. St. Louis: Mosby; 2013; F from Fuller JK. *Surgical Technology: Principles and Practice.* 5th ed. St. Louis: Saunders; 2010; G from Clayton BD, Stock YN, Harroun RD. *Basic Pharmacology for Nurses.* 14th ed. St Louis: Mosby; 2007.)

be minimized by rotating the location of the patch. Patches are designed to be changed daily, every few days, or weekly, depending on the drug.

Topical anesthesia. Topical anesthetics are applied directly to the mucous membranes and rapidly absorbed into the systemic circulation, providing the patient with injection-free local anesthesia. An example of this type of anesthesia is the combination of lidocaine and prilocaine (Oraqix).

Sublingual and buccal routes

SL—"under the tongue" for systemic effects.

Two ways in which drugs can be applied topically are the SL and buccal routes. The mucous membranes of the oral cavity provide a convenient absorbing surface for the systemic administration of drugs, which can be placed under the tongue (SL) or on other areas of the oral mucosa (buccal pouch). Absorption of many drugs into the systemic circulation occurs rapidly. An example of this effect is the fast onset of action of nitroglycerin SL tablets to treat acute anginal pain. Drugs that are susceptible to degradation by the gastrointestinal tract and even by the liver, such as testosterone, are safely administered as SL tablets because they avoid both the first-pass effect and gastrointestinal acid and enzymes.

Dosage Forms

Table 2.2 lists the usual dosage forms. The most commonly used dosage forms in dentistry are the tablet and capsule given orally. Liquid solutions or suspensions are often prescribed for children. Sometimes drugs are given in solution or suspension when a liquid form is desired, especially for children. For injection, the drug may be in solution, such as a local anesthetic, or in a suspension, such as procaine penicillin G, when a longer duration of action is desired. Mouthwashes containing alcohol are also recommended by dental health care workers. Elixirs (contain alcohol) and syrups (contain sugar) are children's dosage forms.

DENTAL HYGIENE CONSIDERATIONS

1. Various factors can affect drug absorption, and the dental hygienist should be aware of them.
2. The most common factors affecting drug absorption include patient compliance, or adherence to medication therapy. Lack of health insurance, misunderstanding of the reason for the medication, or a lack of faith in the health care system can lead to noncompliance.
3. Patient age and pathologic state can affect drug metabolism. As a result, lower doses and slower dose increases may be necessary. All this information can be obtained by determining the patient's age and conducting a health history.
4. Lower protein stores can lead to the storage of less medication in protein, which puts the patient at risk for toxicity. This problem is most common in elderly patients, who by virtue of their age have lower protein stores.
5. The dental hygienist should also understand drug potency so that the appropriate medication and dose are prescribed.

ACADEMIC SKILLS ASSESSMENT

1. Define and differentiate between the potency and efficacy of a drug.
2. Describe the dose-response curve using the terms ED_{50} (effective dose) and LD_{50} (lethal dose).
3. Define the term *pharmacokinetics*. Name the four categories involved.
4. Define the major routes of drug administration, including the following:
   a. Oral
   b. Intravenous
   c. Inhalation
   d. Topical
5. State the dose forms most often used in dentistry.
6. Explain the influence of pH on the dissociation characteristics of weak acids and weak bases.
7. Explain each of the steps involved in oral absorption as follows:
   a. Disruption
   b. Disintegration
   c. Dispersion
   d. Dissolution
8. Define the $t_{1/2}$, or half-life, of a drug and state its significance.
9. Although an elderly patient appears healthy and weighs 110 pounds, what are your concerns regarding drug distribution in this patient?
10. Define the following terms:
    a. Agonist
    b. Competitive antagonist
    c. Physiologic antagonist
11. What are the different ways in which drugs can be metabolized?
12. State the major route of drug excretion.
13. Explain how metabolism can be altered by an effect on liver microsomal enzymes.

CLINICAL CASE STUDY

Mrs. Fannie Smith, 72 years old, has been coming to your practice for several years. A detailed medication/health history reveals a healthy 130-pound woman whose only medication is hydrochlorothiazide 25 mg every morning for high blood pressure. She also takes an occasional ibuprofen for arthritis pain. She presents today for her regular oral health maintenance checkup.

1. What are your concerns regarding drug distribution in a 72-year-old woman?
2. As a dental hygienist, how can you assess liver and renal function without requesting liver and renal function tests?
3. Mrs. Smith has a cavity, which needs to be addressed. What would be the route of administration for delivering a local anesthetic?
4. What are the advantages and disadvantages of parenteral drug administration?
5. Mrs. Smith takes hydrochlorothiazide and ibuprofen. What are the advantages and disadvantages of orally administered drugs?
6. What factors should be taken into account when medications are prescribed to elderly patients?
7. What would be the more appropriate time of day for Mrs. Smith to take her hydrochlorothiazide and why? How does this timing affect drug absorption?
8. How can the dental hygienist help minimize any adverse reactions or drug interactions in Mrs. Smith?

Adverse Reactions

http://evolve.elsevier.com/Haveles/pharmacology

LEARNING OBJECTIVES

1. Define an adverse drug reaction and name five categories of reaction.
2. Discuss the risk-to-benefit ratio of the use of a drug for therapeutic effect and its potential adverse reactions.
3. Explain how the toxic effects of drugs are evaluated.
4. Discuss the importance of recognizing adverse drug effects.

Although drugs may act on biologic systems to accomplish desired effects, they lack absolute specificity in that they can act on many different organs or tissues. This lack of specificity is the reason for undesirable or adverse drug reactions. No drug is free from producing some adverse effects in a certain number of patients. It is estimated that between 5% and 10% of the patients hospitalized annually in the United States are admitted because of adverse reactions to drugs. Also, during their hospitalizations, 10% to 20% of patients experience adverse reactions to drugs.

The dental hygienist is in a good position to observe any adverse reactions to or undesirable effects of drugs administered in the dental office. Adverse reactions to drugs prescribed by the patient's physician can be identified in the health history. The dental hygienist should question the patient about any potential oral manifestations of drugs. For example, if the patient is taking phenytoin (Dilantin), questions about enlargement of the patient's gums should be explored. Because many drugs can produce xerostomia, complaints of dry mouth should direct the dental hygienist to examine the patient's medications. Knowledge of the typical adverse drug reactions can help dental hygienists identify, minimize, or prevent these types of reactions. Because of the rapport between a patient and the dental hygienist, the patient often reveals important facts about the health history or asks questions concerning medications prescribed. The dental hygienist must know the terms used to describe adverse reactions to discuss a drug's undesirable effect accurately with other health professionals. For example, allergy refers to a specific type of reaction to a drug but does not include a complaint of excessive gas, or *flatulence.*

DEFINITIONS AND CLASSIFICATIONS

Unfortunately every drug has more than one action. The clinically desirable actions are termed *therapeutic effects,* and the undesirable reactions are termed adverse effects. Dividing a drug's effects into two categories is artificial because whether an effect is adverse or therapeutic depends on the indication for which the drug is being used. For example, when an antihistamine used to relieve hay fever causes drowsiness, the drowsiness can be considered an adverse effect.

However, if the antihistamine were being used to induce sleep (over-the-counter [OTC] sleep aid), drowsiness would be considered the therapeutic effect.

An adverse drug reaction is a response to a drug that is not desired, is potentially harmful, and occurs at usual therapeutic doses. It may be an exaggeration of the desired response, an expected but undesired response, an allergic reaction, a cytotoxic reaction, or an effect on the fetus. Often, adverse drug reactions are divided into the following categories:

Toxic reaction: A toxic reaction is an extension of the pharmacologic effect resulting from a drug's effect on the target organs. In this instance, the amount of the desired effect is excessive.

Side effect: A side effect is a dose-related reaction that is not part of the desired therapeutic outcome. It occurs when a drug acts on nontarget organs to produce undesirable effects. The terms *side effect* and *adverse reaction* are often used interchangeably. The upset stomach produced by ibuprofen is an adverse reaction when ibuprofen is given to manage pain.

Idiosyncratic reaction: An idiosyncratic reaction is a genetically related abnormal drug response. Certain populations, because of their genetic constitution, are more susceptible to certain adverse reactions to specific drugs. Eskimos metabolize certain drugs faster than other populations; therefore a larger dose of those drugs (e.g., isoniazid) would be needed in an Eskimo patient.

Drug allergy: A drug allergy is an immunologic response to a drug resulting in a reaction such as a rash or anaphylaxis. This response accounts for less than 5% of all adverse reactions. Unlike other adverse reactions, allergic reactions are neither predictable nor dose related.

Interference with natural defense mechanisms: Certain drugs, such as adrenocorticosteroids, can reduce the body's ability to fight infection. Drugs that interfere with the body's defenses cause a patient to get infections more easily and have more trouble fighting them.

The importance of distinguishing among different types of adverse effects can be shown using aspirin as an example. Aspirin can cause adverse reactions such as gastric upset or pain. At higher doses, aspirin can predictably produce toxicity, such as tinnitus

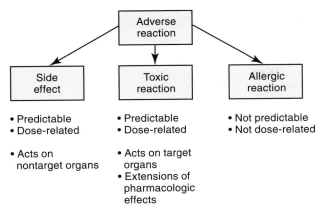

Fig. 3.1 Classification of Common Adverse Reactions.

and hyperthermia (elevated temperature). Another type of reaction to aspirin is allergic, often involving a rash or difficulty in breathing (asthma-like reaction). These differences are significant and become pertinent when one is discussing an adverse reaction with another health professional. Patients who experience allergic reactions to a medication should not receive that medication or similar medications. Side effects such as gastrointestinal upset, although bothersome, are not reasons to avoid prescribing a medication. It can be given. However, if the gastrointestinal upset is too much for the patient to tolerate, another drug should be considered. It is important to describe in the patient's chart the patient's "problem" in enough detail so that side effects can be separated from allergic reactions. Fig. 3.1 describes the types of adverse reactions and notes whether they are predictable or dose-dependent.

CLINICAL MANIFESTATIONS OF ADVERSE REACTIONS

Before a drug is used, there must be an assessment of its risks versus its benefits (risk-to-benefit ratio). This means that the beneficial effect of the drug must be weighed against its potential for adverse reactions. For example, one would compare the drug's therapeutic effect (e.g., controlling seizures) with its potential to cause an adverse reaction (e.g., birth defects). In a real-life example, one should compare the therapeutic effect of certain drugs to produce weight loss with their potential for the serious adverse reactions such as primary pulmonary hypertension (which is fatal in 50% of patients) and cardiac valvular damage.

Exaggerated Effect on Target Tissues

An exaggerated effect on its target tissue or organ is considered an extension of the therapeutic effect caused by the overreaction of a sensitive patient or by the use of a dose that is too large. For example, a patient may experience exaggerated hypoglycemia when given a therapeutic dose of an oral hypoglycemic agent for the treatment of diabetes. The patient's plasma glucose level may fall too low because of an unusual sensitivity to the drug, the dose administered was too high for that patient, or the patient took the drug but did not eat. Occasionally this type of adverse reaction may result from liver or kidney disease. Because the disease interferes with the drug's metabolism or excretion, the drug's action may be enhanced or prolonged.

Effect on Nontarget Tissues

The effect on nontarget organs or tissues is caused by the nontherapeutic action of the drug. These reactions can occur at usual doses, but they appear more often at higher doses. For example, aspirin may produce gastric upset in usual therapeutic doses; however, with higher doses, salicylism—characterized by tinnitus, disturbances of the acid-base balance, and confusion—can result. Toxic reactions can affect many parts of the body. A reduction in the dose of a drug usually reduces these adverse reactions.

Effect on Fetal Development (Teratogenic Effect)

The word *teratogenic* comes from the Greek prefix *terato*, meaning "monster," and the suffix *genic*, meaning "producing" or "producing a malformed fetus." The relationship between drugs and congenital abnormalities has been recognized since the middle of the 20th century. In 1961, thalidomide, an OTC drug marketed in Europe, was found to cause phocomelia (short arms and legs) in the exposed fetus. In some cases, only one dose of this drug had the effect. This incident reinforced the fact that more studies were needed to determine the effects of drugs on pregnant women. For new drugs, many more studies on animals and their reproductive capacity are conducted before the drugs are put on the market. Although more information is now available about the safety of drugs in pregnant women, sufficient information is still lacking.

The US Food and Drug Administration (FDA) has recently eliminated the FDA pregnancy categories of A, B, C, D and X and replaced them with narrative sections and subsections to better educate the patient about any risks associated with drug use and pregnancy and lactation (Figure 22.1).

Although no drug can be considered "completely safe" for administration to a pregnant woman, many of the drugs used in dentistry are considered to be among the safest. These include the antibiotics penicillin and erythromycin, the pain medication acetaminophen (Tylenol), and the local anesthetic lidocaine. Even these drugs should be administered only if there is a clear need. Elective dental procedures should be conservatively addressed. Drugs used in dentistry that are contraindicated during pregnancy include tetracycline, the benzodiazepines, and metronidazole. The use of nonsteroidal antiinflammatory drugs (NSAIDs) should be avoided. The teratogenic potential for dental drugs is discussed in Chapter 22.

Also, dental patients do not always announce that they are pregnant, so it is important to ask any woman of childbearing age (between approximately 11 and 63 years of age [a 63-year-old French woman gave birth in 1997]) whether she is pregnant. Problem drugs should be avoided as early as possible during the pregnancy. The greatest risk from exposure to drugs occurs before the pregnancy status is known.

Local Effect

Local reactions are characterized by local tissue irritation. Occasionally, injectable drugs can produce irritation, pain, and tissue necrosis at the site of injection. Topically applied agents can cause irritation at the site of application. Drugs taken orally can produce gastrointestinal symptoms such as nausea or dyspepsia because of their local actions on the gastrointestinal tract.

Drug Interactions

Although drug interactions are not adverse effects, they can lead to adverse effects. A drug interaction can occur when the effect of one drug is altered by another drug. Such an interaction may result in undesirable effects such as toxicity and lack of efficacy. Drug interactions can

TABLE 3.1   Selected Drug Interactions

Type of Interaction	Increased Blood Levels	Lower Blood Levels	Enhanced Drug Effect	Blocking of Drug Effect	Worsening of Illness
Drug-drug	Anticonvulsants can decrease the metabolism of many drugs and each other, leading to increased plasma levels of these drugs Macrolides raise the plasma levels of many drugs	Anticonvulsants can increase the metabolism of many drugs and each other, leading to decreased plasma levels of these drugs Histamine H_2–receptor blockers lower the plasma levels of many drugs	Benzodiazepines and first-generation antihistamines (increased sedation)	Epinephrine blocks the action of histamine during an allergic reaction	
Drug-food	Grapefruit can increase the plasma blood levels of antibiotics, benzodiazepines, calcium channel blockers, and warfarin	Dairy products can decrease the absorption of tetracycline			
Drug-disease	Hepatic dysfunction, renal dysfunction, and heart failure can all slow down drug metabolism and elimination from the body				Beta blockers can cause an asthma attack in a susceptible person Celecoxib can cause gastrointestinal bleeding in persons with peptic ulcer disease Uncontrolled hyperthyroidism can cause increased sensitivity to epinephrine Hypothyroidism can cause increased sensitivity to opioid analgesics

also have beneficial effects. Whenever a drug is prescribed or suggested to a dental patient, the chance of drug interactions must be considered. The likelihood that a drug interaction would occur increases with the number of drugs a patient is taking. Drug interactions are not limited to interactions between legally prescribed drugs but also with alcohol and other drugs of abuse. These interactions are discussed in further detail in Chapter 23. Drug-food and drug-disease interactions may also occur. Table 3.1 gives examples of the different drug interactions.

Hypersensitivity (Allergic Reaction)

A hypersensitivity reaction occurs when the immune system of an individual responds to the drug administered or applied. One example of an allergic (hypersensitivity) reaction is hives in a patient who has taken a drug. For a drug to produce an allergic reaction, it must act as an antigen and react with an antibody in a previously sensitized patient. This reaction is neither dose-dependent nor predictable. For an allergic reaction to occur, an ingested drug must be metabolized to a reactive metabolite known as a hapten. Such a hapten can act as an antigen after combining with proteins in the body. The antigen formed then stimulates the production of an antibody. With subsequent exposure to the drug, the antibodies formed react with the antigen (drug or metabolite) administered and elicit an antigen-antibody reaction. This reaction triggers a series of biochemical and physiologic events that can be life threatening.

Drug allergy can be divided into the following four types of reactions, depending on the type of antibody produced or the cell mediating the reaction (Table 3.2):

Type I reactions are mediated by immunoglobulin E (IgE) antibodies. When a drug antigen binds to IgE antibody, histamine, leukotrienes, and prostaglandins are released, producing vasodilation, edema, and the inflammatory response. The targets of this reaction are the bronchioles, resulting in anaphylactic shock; the respiratory system, resulting in rhinitis and asthma; and the skin, resulting in urticaria and dermatitis. Because these reactions can occur relatively quickly after drug exposure, they are known as *immediate* hypersensitivity reactions. Anaphylaxis is an acute life-threatening allergic reaction characterized by hypotension, bronchospasm, laryngeal edema, and cardiac arrhythmias, which can occur within a few minutes up to less than 1 hour after drug administration. Drugs used in dentistry that have produced fatal anaphylaxis include the penicillins, ester local anesthetics, and aspirin. Unexpected anaphylaxis may occur, such as after a patient has been given a dose of penicillin by injection. Oral penicillin can also produce anaphylaxis, but that is much less common.

Type II, or cytotoxic/cytolytic, reactions are complement-dependent reactions involving either IgG or IgM antibodies. The antigen-antibody complex is fixed to a circulating blood cell, resulting in lysis. Examples of this reaction are penicillin-induced hemolytic anemia and methyldopa-induced autoimmune hemolytic anemia.

Type III, or immune-complex disease, reactions involve aggregations of antigens and antibodies. Usually there are more antibodies than antigens. When there is a large amount of antigens or the body's immune system is not clearing antigens, the antigen/antibody ratio increases. When the number of antibodies is comparable to the amount of antigens, an immune-complex can form. In this case a single antibody can bind to multiple antigens, which are in turn bound to multiple antibodies. This "clump" of antibodies and antigens deposits in tissue, causing inflammation by activating complement and attracting neutrophils. The reaction is manifested as serum sickness and includes urticarial skin eruptions, arthralgia,

TABLE 3.2 Hypersensitivity Reactions

Type	Mediator	Reaction	Typical Time of Onset	Example
I (immediate, anaphylactic)	Antibody	Immunoglobuin (Ig) E antibody is induced by allergen and binds to mast cells and basophils. After encountering the antigen again, the fixed IgE becomes cross-linked, inducing degranulation and release of mediators (e.g., histamine)	Minutes	Penicillin allergy Anaphylaxis Allergic urticaria Food allergies (nuts, shellfish) Hay fever Allergic Rhinitis Bee stings Allergic Conjunctivitis
II (cytotoxic)	Antibody	Antigens on a cell surface combine with antibody; this leads to complement-mediated lysis (e.g., transfusion of Rh reactions or autoimmune hemolytic anemia).	Hours to days	Aspirin- or antibiotic- induced hemolytic anemia Neutropenia Transfusion reactions
III (immune complex)	Antibody	Antigen-antibody immune complexes are deposited in tissues, complement is activated, and polymorphonuclear cells are attracted to the site, causing tissue damage	2–3 weeks	Drug induced-serum sickness (penicillins, sulfonamide) Post-streptococcal glomerulonephritis Rheumatoid arthritis Systemic lupus erythematosus
IV (delayed)	Cell	Helper T lymphocytes sensitized by an antigen release lymphokines on second contact with the same antigen. The lymphokines induce inflammation and activate macrophages that in turn release various mediators	2–3 days	Contact dermatitis Poison oak/ivy, tuberculosis tests Topical benzocaine, lidocaine Stevens-Johnson Syndrome, Toxic epidermal necrolysis

IgE, Immunoglobulin E.
Modified from Levinson WE. *Review of Medical Microbiology and Immunology.* 14th ed. New York: McGraw-Hill Medical; 2014.

arthritis, lymphadenopathy, and fever. This type of reaction can be caused by the penicillins and sulfonamides. Type III reactions usually develop 4 to 10 days after exposure and can become chronic if there is continued exposure to the antigen.

Type IV, or delayed hypersensitivity, reactions are mediated by sensitized T lymphocytes and macrophages. When the cells contact the antigen, an inflammatory reaction is produced by lymphokines, neutrophils, and macrophages. An example of a type IV reaction is allergic contact dermatitis caused by topical application of a drug. Topical benzocaine, penicillin, poison oak, and poison ivy can produce this type of reaction. Reaction to jewelry containing nickel is another example.

Idiosyncrasy

An idiosyncratic reaction is one that is neither a drug's side effect nor an allergic reaction. Some idiosyncrasies have been found to be genetically determined abnormal reactions, whereas others may be the result of an immunologic mechanism. About 10% of black males can experience severe hemolytic anemia when given the antimalarial drug primaquine. The reason is a deficiency in the enzyme glucose-6-phosphate dehydrogenase (G6PD), which is required to metabolize the drug.

Interference With Natural Defense Mechanisms

A drug's effect on the body's defense mechanisms can result in an adverse reaction. Long-term systemic administration of corticosteroids can lead to decreased resistance to infection. Because periodontal disease involves both infection and an immune response, drugs that are immunosuppressive can exacerbate a patient's poor oral health.

TOXICOLOGIC EVALUATION OF DRUGS

LD$_{50}$ kills one-half of the subjects.
ED$_{50}$ produces a response in one-half of the subjects.

Optimally, evaluations of the toxic effects of drugs are based on experiments performed with animals and clinical trials conducted in humans. Animal experiments can often elicit adverse reactions that could occur in humans, but unfortunately drug reactions in animals do not always predict reactions in humans. The *lethal dose* (LD$_{50}$), one measure of the toxicity of a drug, is the dose of a drug that kills 50% of the experimental animals. The *median effective dose* (ED$_{50}$) is the dose required to produce a specified intensity of effect in 50% of the animals. Fig. 3.2 shows a plot of the dose of a

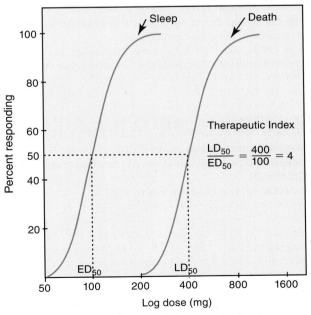

Fig. 3.2 Dose-Response Curve and Therapeutic Index.

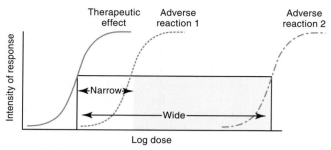

Fig. 3.3 Difference Between Narrow and Wide Therapeutic Indexes.

drug against the percentage of maximum response (sleep or death) in animals. A dose-response curve is then obtained. The value on the dose axis that corresponds to the 50% intensity level on the response axis can be read directly from the curve. This figure illustrates the ED_{50} and LD_{50}.

Because all drugs are toxic at some dose, the LD_{50} is meaningless unless the ED_{50} is also known. The ratio LD_{50}/ED_{50} is the therapeutic index (TI) of a drug:

$$nTI = \frac{LD_{50}}{ED_{50}}$$

If the value of the TI is small (narrow TI), then toxicity is more likely. If the TI is large (wide TI), then the drug will be safer (Fig. 3.3). A drug with a wide TI will have a large LD_{50} and a small ED_{50} (the distance between these curves is large). A TI of greater than 10 is usually needed to produce a therapeutically useful drug. The TI derived from animal studies determines both the LD_{50} and the ED_{50} from a variety of animals.

RECOGNIZING ADVERSE DRUG EFFECTS

It is important for the dental hygienist to educate the patient regarding potential adverse drug effects. A careful explanation of the potential adverse effect and its presenting symptoms helps the patient better manage his or her health care. A patient who knows what to expect has a much clearer picture of what is going on if an adverse effect occurs. Some adverse effects are common, such as headache and upset stomach, and normally do not require medical attention. Nausea can usually be alleviated by taking the drug with food or milk. Sedation can be minimized by taking the drug at bedtime. Other effects may require medical attention. Once the patient has a better understanding of the different side effects, he or she will be better able to communicate what is happening to the health care professional.

If a patient is reporting a suspected adverse drug effect, the dental hygienist should first determine what drugs the patient is taking. Once a list of drugs is identified, it is important to determine which drug or drugs may be causing the adverse effect. If the patient is taking multiple drugs, the dental hygienist should determine when the patient is taking each drug. Also, it is important to determine whether the patient's symptoms occurred after beginning drug therapy and how long after the patient took the drug the symptoms were first noted.

Depending on the symptoms reported, therapy with that particular drug may have to be stopped and the patient evaluated for further symptoms. If appropriate, drug therapy can be started again and the patient observed for any other adverse effects.

DENTAL HYGIENE CONSIDERATIONS

1. Know the difference between a side effect, toxic effect, and allergic reaction.
2. If the patient has stated that he or she has had an allergic reaction to a medication, always ask the patient to explain what happened.
3. Remember that an allergic reaction to a medication usually means that the patient should not receive that medication or any other medication in the same chemical class.
4. Side effects, although bothersome, usually do not prevent the patient from taking the medication. The medication may have to be taken with food or milk or at bedtime. If the patient cannot tolerate the side effect, another drug can be used.
5. Make sure that the patient understands how to take the medication in order to avoid toxic reactions.
6. Always explain what adverse effects the patient could experience and what the patient should do if he or she experiences them.
7. Always ask female patients from puberty to menopause if there is a possibility that they may be pregnant. This precaution is to avoid exposing the developing fetus to medications.

ACADEMIC SKILLS ASSESSMENT

1. Name four classifications of adverse drug reactions.
2. Describe the problem with identifying teratogenic agents (see also Chapter 22).
3. Describe the types of adverse reactions.
4. Explain the four mechanisms by which an allergic reaction can occur.
5. Describe why the risk-to-benefit ratio is important and helpful in deciding whether to administer a drug to a patient.

CLINICAL CASE STUDY

Joanna Hernandez, 45 years old, presents to your office with complaints of swollen, aching gums. A thorough examination reveals an infection around one of her molars, which will require antibiotic treatment. Ms. Hernandez also requests something for pain. You then refer to Ms. Hernandez's dental record and see that she is allergic to penicillin and ibuprofen.

1. What information would you like to know regarding the allergies to penicillin and ibuprofen?
2. How would allergies affect what is prescribed to Ms. Hernandez?

Upon further questioning, you find out that Ms. Hernandez experienced breathing problems, rash, and edema the last time she took penicillin. Her primary care provider told her that she was allergic to penicillin and that she should not take it again. The allergy to ibuprofen sounded more like a side effect. It made Ms. Hernandez feel nauseous and gave her heartburn.

3. What is the difference between the therapeutic and adverse effect of a drug?
4. Compare and contrast side effects, allergic reactions, toxic reactions, and idiosyncratic reactions.

PART II

Drugs Used in Dentistry

Chapter 4
Autonomic Drugs, 31

Chapter 5
Nonopioid (Nonnarcotic) Analgesics, 45

Chapter 6
Opioid (Narcotic) Analgesics and Antagonists, 58

Chapter 7
Antiinfective Agents, 68

Chapter 8
Antifungal and Antiviral Agents, 90

Chapter 9
Local Anesthetics, 98

Chapter 10
General Anesthetics, 112

Chapter 11
Antianxiety Agents, 119

Autonomic Drugs

http://evolve.elsevier.com/Haveles/pharmacology

LEARNING OBJECTIVES

1. Identify the major components and functional organization of the autonomic nervous system.
2. Discuss the major neurotransmitters in the sympathetic autonomic nervous system and the importance of receptors.
3. Discuss the pharmacologic effects, adverse reactions, contraindications, and dental considerations of cholinergic agents, which act on the parasympathetic nervous system.

4. Discuss the pharmacologic effects, adverse reactions, contraindications, and dental considerations of anticholinergic agents, which act on the parasympathetic nervous system.
5. Discuss the pharmacologic effects, adverse reactions, contraindications, and dental considerations of adrenergic agents and list several specific adrenergic agents.
6. Explain the workings of adrenergic blocking agents and neuromuscular blocking agents.

The dental hygienist should become familiar with the autonomic nervous system (ANS) drugs for three reasons. First, certain ANS drugs are used in dentistry. For example, both the vasoconstrictors added to some local anesthetic solutions and the drugs used to increase salivary flow are ANS drugs. Second, some ANS drugs produce oral adverse reactions. For example, the anticholinergic drugs cause xerostomia.

> Autonomic nervous system (ANS) drug effects are important because many other drugs have the same effects.

Third, members of other drug groups have effects similar to those of the ANS drugs. Antidepressants and antipsychotics are drug groups with autonomic side effects, specifically anticholinergic effects. An understanding of the effects of the autonomic drugs on the body will facilitate an understanding of the action of other drug groups that have autonomic effects. Before the ANS drugs can be understood, the normal functioning of the ANS must be reviewed. The physiology of the ANS is therefore reviewed first.

AUTONOMIC NERVOUS SYSTEM

The ANS functions largely as an automatic modulating system for many bodily functions, including the regulation of blood pressure and heart rate, gastrointestinal tract motility, salivary gland secretions, and bronchial smooth muscle. This system relies on specific neurotransmitters (chemicals that are released to send messages) and a variety of receptors to initiate functional responses in the target tissues. Before ANS pharmacology is discussed, the anatomy and physiology of this system are reviewed.

Anatomy

The ANS has two divisions, the sympathetic autonomic nervous system (SANS) and the parasympathetic autonomic nervous system (PANS). Each consists of afferent (sensory) fibers (What's happening?), central integrating areas (Let's coordinate all this info! Hey, what did you find out?), efferent (peripheral) motor preganglionic fibers (This is what's happening, i.e., the heart is beating too slow), and postganglionic motor fibers (Heart, begin beating!).

The preganglionic neuron (Fig. 4.1) originates in the central nervous system (CNS) and passes out to form the ganglia at the synapse with the postganglionic neuron. The space between the preganglionic and postganglionic fibers is termed the *synapse* or synaptic cleft. The postganglionic neuron originates in the ganglia and innervates the effector organ or tissue.

Parasympathetic Autonomic Nervous System

Cell bodies in the CNS give rise to the preganglionic fibers of the parasympathetic division. They originate in the nuclei of the third, seventh, ninth, and tenth cranial nerves (CN III, VII, IX, and X) and the second through fourth sacral segments (S2 to S4) of the spinal cord. The preganglionic fibers of the PANS are relatively long and extend near to or into the innervated organ. The distribution is relatively simple for the third, seventh, and ninth cranial nerves, whereas the tenth or vagus nerve has a complex distribution. There usually is a low ratio of synaptic connections between preganglionic and postganglionic neurons, leading to a discrete response when the PANS is stimulated. The postganglionic fibers, originating in the ganglia, are usually short and terminate on the innervated tissue.

Sympathetic Autonomic Nervous System

The cell bodies that give origin to the preganglionic fibers of the SANS span from the thoracic (T1) to the lumbar (L2) portion of the spinal

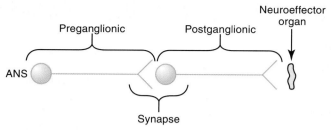

Fig. 4.1 Typical efferent nerve. The preganglionic fiber originates in the brain. It ends at the synapse where the neurotransmitter carries the message to the postganglionic fiber. A group of synapses make up a ganglion. The postganglionic fiber releases a neurotransmitter to send the message to an effector organ. *ANS,* Autonomic nervous system.

cord (sometimes referred to as the "in-between" distribution, that is, between the two locations of the innervation of the PANS). This arrangement produces a more diffuse effect in the SANS. The preganglionic fibers exit the cord to enter the sympathetic chain located along each side of the vertebral column. Once a part of the sympathetic chain (groups of nerves a few inches from the vertebral column), preganglionic fibers form multiple synaptic connections with postganglionic cell bodies located up and down the sympathetic chain. Thus a single SANS preganglionic fiber often synapses with numerous postganglionic neurons, producing a more diffuse effect in the SANS. The postganglionic fibers then terminate at the effector organ or tissues.

The adrenal medulla is also innervated by the sympathetic preganglionic fibers. It functions much as a large sympathetic ganglion, with the glands in the medulla representing the postganglionic component. When the SANS is stimulated, the adrenal medulla releases primarily epinephrine and a small amount of norepinephrine (NE) into the systemic circulation. A diffuse response is produced when the SANS is stimulated because of the high ratio of synaptic connections between the preganglionic and postganglionic fibers and because the adrenal medulla, when stimulated, releases epinephrine into the bloodstream.

Functional Organization

> Divisions of the parasympathetic autonomic nervous system (PANS) and sympathetic autonomic nervous system (SANS) often produce opposite effects, such as yin and yang.

In general, the divisions of the ANS, the parasympathetic and the sympathetic, tend to act in opposite directions (Fig. 4.2). The parasympathetic division of the ANS is concerned with conservation of the body processes. Both digestion and intestinal tract motility are greatly

influenced by the PANS. The sympathetic division is designed to cope with sudden emergencies such as the "fright-or-flight" or "fight-or-flight" situation. In most but not all instances, the actions produced by each system are opposite: one increases the heart rate and the other decreases it; one dilates the pupils of the eye and the other constricts them. The receptors being innervated for each function may be different. For example, both the PANS and the SANS stimulate muscles in the eye that change the size of the pupil. The SANS stimulates the radial smooth muscles (out from the pupil, such as sun rays), producing an increase in pupil size. When the pupils are dilated, the effect is termed *mydriasis*). The PANS stimulates the circular smooth muscles (such as a bull's-eye), producing a decrease in pupillary size. When pupils are constricted, the effect is termed *miosis*.

Almost all body tissues are innervated by the ANS, with many but not all organs receiving both parasympathetic and sympathetic innervation. The response of a specific tissue to stimuli at any one time will be equal to the sum of the excitatory and inhibitory influences of the two divisions of the ANS (if a tissue receives both innervations). Table 4.1 summarizes the effects of the ANS on major tissues and organ systems.

In addition to the dual innervation of tissues, there is another way in which the two divisions of the ANS can interact. Sensory fibers in one division can influence the motor fibers in the other. Thus, although in an isolated tissue preparation the stimulation of one of the divisions would produce a specific response, in the intact body a more complex and integrated response can be expected. The net effect would be a combination of the direct and indirect effects.

Neurotransmitters

> Neurotransmitters are similar to carrier pigeons: they carry messages.

Communication between nerves or between nerves and effector tissue takes place through the release of chemical neurotransmitters across the synaptic cleft. Neurotransmitters are released in response to the nerve action potential (or pharmacologic agents in certain cases) to interact with a specific membrane component: the receptor. Receptors are usually found on the postsynaptic fiber and the effector organ but may be located on the presynaptic membrane as well (Table 4.2). The interaction between neurotransmitter and receptor is specific and is rapidly terminated by disposition of the neurotransmitter. There are several specific mechanisms by which the neurotransmitter produces an effect on the receptor.

Disposition of the neurotransmitter occurs most often by either its reuptake into the presynaptic nerve terminal or its enzymatic breakdown. Nerves in the ANS contain the necessary enzyme systems and other metabolic processes to synthesize, store, and release neurotransmitters. Thus

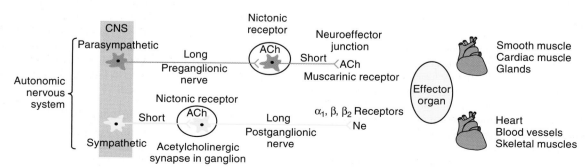

Fig. 4.2 The main components of the autonomic nervous system. *ACh,* Acetylcholine; *CNS,* central nervous system.

TABLE 4.1 Effects of the Autonomic Nervous System (ANS) on Effector Organs

Organ	Aspect	Parasympathetic ANS	Receptor(s)	Sympathetic ANS
Eye	Lens (ciliary muscle)	Contraction (near vision)	β_2	Relaxation (distant vision)
	Iris	Contraction miosis	α_1	Contraction
				Radial muscle mydriasis
Cardiovascular system	Heart force (inotropic)		β_1, β_2	Increase in force
	Heart, sinoatrial node rate (chronotropic)	Decreases heart rate	β_1, β_2	Increase in heart rate
Blood vessels, smooth muscles	Coronary		$\alpha_1, \beta_1, \beta_2$	Constriction (α), dilation (β)
	Skin/mucosa		α_1, α_2	Constriction
	Skeletal muscle	Dilation	α_1	Constriction
			β_2	Dilation
	Abdominal viscera		α_1	Constriction
			β_2	Dilation
	Salivary glands	Dilation	α_1, β_2	Constriction
Lungs	Bronchial smooth muscle	Contraction	β_2	Relaxation
	Secretions: bronchial, nasopharyngeal		α_1, β_1	Secretion increase/decrease
Gastrointestinal tract/ genitourinary tract	Motility/tone	Contracts, increases	$\alpha_1, \alpha_2,$ β_1, β_2	Relaxation
Stomach, intestine, bladder	Sphincters	Relaxation	α_1	Contraction
	Secretions from gastrointestinal tract	Stimulation	α_2	Inhibition
	Secretion from salivary glands	Increase profuse and watery	α	Viscous, thickened
	Uterus		α_1, β_2	Relaxation
Endocrine	Pancreas, acini	Secretion	α_1	Decreases secretions
	Pancreas, islet cells		α_2	Decreases secretions
	Adrenal medulla	Secretion epinephrine/norepinephrine		
Skin	Sweat	Secretion, generalized		Secretion, local
	Pilomotor muscles		α_1	Contraction
Liver	Glycogen synthesis		α_1	Glycogenolysis
			β_2	Gluconeogenesis
Other	Adipose tissue		$\alpha_2, \beta_1, \beta_2$	Lipolysis
	Male sex organs	Erection	α_1	Ejaculation
	Skeletal muscle		β_2	Contraction

TABLE 4.2 Types of Cholinergic Receptors

Receptor Site	Location	Neurotransmitter	Stimulating Agent	Blocking Agent
Muscarinic	Muscarinic cholinergic	Acetylcholine	Muscarine	Atropine
Nicotinic	Nicotinic cholinergic	Acetylcholine	Nicotine	Hexamethonium
Somatic-skeletal muscle	Cholinergic somatic	Acetylcholine	Nicotine	d-Tubocurarine (curare)

drugs can modify ANS activity by altering any of the events associated with neurotransmitters: (1) synthesis, (2) storage, (3) release, (4) receptor interaction, and (5) disposition. The specificity of the neurotransmitters and receptors dictates the tissue response, which occurs as follows:

Between the preganglionic and postganglionic nerves: Acetylcholine (ACh) is the neurotransmitter in the synapse (ganglion) formed between the preganglionic and postganglionic nerves. Nerves that release ACh are termed *cholinergic.* Because this synapse is also stimulated by nicotine, it is also termed *nicotinic* in response.

Between postganglionic nerves and the effector tissues:

PANS: The neurotransmitter released from the postganglionic nerve terminal is ACh; it is also termed *cholinergic.* Because the postsynaptic tissue responds to muscarine, it is identified as muscarinic. Thus the cholinergic synapses are distinguished from one another.

SANS: NE is the transmitter substance released by the postganglionic nerves; it is designated as adrenergic.

Neuromuscular junction: Although not within the ANS, the neuromuscular junction (Fig. 4.3) of skeletal muscle releases the neurotransmitter ACh and is termed *cholinergic.* Figs. 4.4–4.6 illustrate the PANS, SANS, and neuromuscular junction.

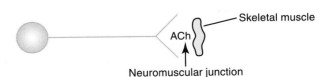

Fig. 4.3 The neuromuscular junction of skeletal muscle releases acetylcholine. *ACh,* Acetylcholine.

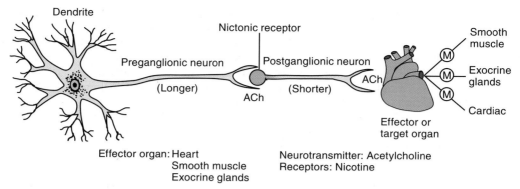

Fig. 4.4 The Parasympathetic nervous system. *ACh,* Acetylcholine.

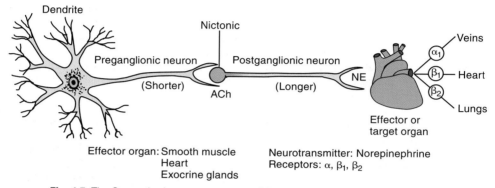

Fig. 4.5 The Sympathetic nervous system. *ACh,* Acetylcholine; *NE,* norepinephrine.

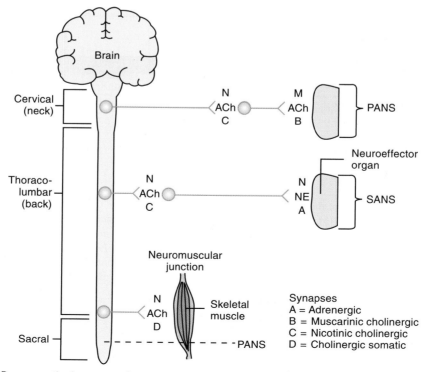

Fig. 4.6 Parasympathetic autonomic nervous system *(PANS),* sympathetic autonomic nervous system *(SANS),* and neuromuscular junction. *ACh,* Acetylcholine; *NE,* norepinephrine.

PARASYMPATHETIC AUTONOMIC NERVOUS SYSTEM

ACh has been identified as the principal mediator in the PANS. When an action potential travels along the nerve, it causes the release of the stored ACh from the synaptic storage vesicles, and if sufficient ACh is released, it initiates a response in the postsynaptic tissue. If the postsynaptic tissue is a postganglionic nerve, depolarization with generation of an action potential occurs in that neuron. In the postganglionic parasympathetic fibers, the postsynaptic tissue is an effector organ and the response is the same as that of the neurotransmitter. The action of the released ACh is terminated by hydrolysis by acetylcholinesterase to yield the inactive metabolites choline and acetic acid (or acetate) (Fig. 4.7).

> There are three acetylcholine (ACh) receptor sites:
> - The parasympathetic autonomic nervous system (PANS)
> - Ganglions
> - The neuromuscular junction

Once ACh is released from the presynaptic neuron into the synaptic cleft, it can bind to either muscarinic or nicotinic receptor sites. Small doses of ACh bind to muscarinic receptors and duplicate the effects of the chemical substance muscarine. Large doses bind to nicotinic receptors and duplicate the effects of nicotine, a chemical substance found in cigarettes. Nicotinic receptors are found in the neuromuscular junction, parasympathetic nervous system, sympathetic nervous system, adrenal medulla, and CNS, whereas muscarinic receptors are found only in the parasympathetic nervous system, sympathetic nervous system, and CNS. The amount of neurotransmitter released, the size of the synaptic cleft, and the postganglionic site determine which receptor site is activated.

Cholinergic (Parasympathomimetic) Agents

Depending on their mechanism of action (Table 4.3), the cholinergic (parasympathomimetic) agents are classified as direct-acting (acts on

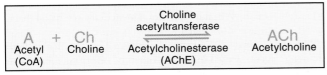

Fig. 4.7 Formula for Acetylcholine.

receptor) or indirect-acting (causes release of neurotransmitter). The direct-acting agents (Fig. 4.8) include the choline derivatives and pilocarpine. The choline derivatives include both ACh and other, more stable choline derivatives. These derivatives of ACh possess activity similar to PANS stimulation but have a longer duration of action and are more selective.

The indirect-acting (see Fig. 4.8) parasympathomimetic agents or cholinesterase inhibitors act by inhibiting the enzyme cholinesterase.

When the enzyme that normally destroys ACh is inhibited, the concentration of ACh builds up (it is not being destroyed), resulting in PANS stimulation.

Pharmacologic Effects

Cardiovascular effects. The cardiovascular effects associated with the cholinergic agents are the result of both direct and indirect actions. The direct effect on the heart produces a negative chronotropic and negative inotropic action. A decrease in cardiac output is associated with these agents.

The cholinergic agents' effects on the smooth muscles around the blood vessels result in relaxation and vasodilation, producing a decrease in total peripheral resistance. The indirect effect of these agents is an increase in heart rate and cardiac output. Because the direct and indirect effects of these agents on the heart rate and cardiac output are opposite, the resulting effect depends on the concentration of the drug present. Generally there is bradycardia and a decrease in blood pressure and cardiac output.

Gastrointestinal effects. The cholinergic agents excite the smooth muscle of the gastrointestinal tract, producing an increase in activity, motility, and secretion.

Effects on the eye. The cholinergic agents produce miosis and cause cycloplegia—a paralysis of the ciliary muscles of the eye that results in the loss of visual accommodation. Because intraocular pressure is also decreased, these agents are useful in the treatment of glaucoma.

Effects on the brain. Acetylcholinesterase inhibitors increase ACh concentrations in the brain, which boosts cholinergic neurotransmission in the forebrain and compensates for the loss of functioning brain cells.

Adverse Reactions

> Salivation
> Lacrimation
> Urination
> Defecation

TABLE 4.3	Cholinergic (Parasympathomimetic) Agents		
Type	**Classification**	**Drug Name**	**Therapeutic Use**
Direct-acting	Choline esters	Bethanechol (Urecholine)	Urinary retention not due to urinary tract obstruction
	Other	Pilocarpine (Isopto Carpine)	Glaucoma
	Other	Pilocarpine (Salagen)	Xerostomia
Indirect-acting	Reversible agents	Physostigmine (Antilirium)	Some drug overdoses
		Neostigmine (Prostigmin)	Myasthenia gravis, reversible nondepolarizing muscle relaxants
		Pyridostigmine (Mestinon)	
		Edrophonium (Tensilon)	
		Donepezil (Aricept)	Mild, moderate, severe AD dementia
		Galantamine (Razadyne)	Mild to moderate AD dementia
		Rivastigmine	
	Irreversible organophosphates	Malathion, parathion	Agricultural insecticides
		Sarin (GB)	No known therapeutic uses
		Tabun	

AD, Alzheimer disease.

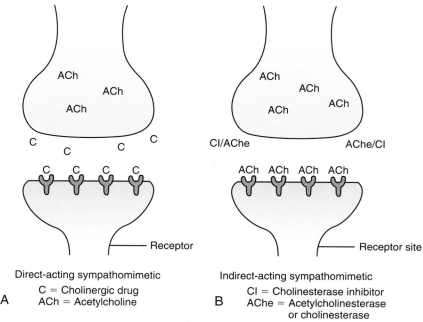

Fig. 4.8 (A) Direct-acting parasympathomimetics (cholinergic drugs). Cholinergic drugs resemble acetylcholine and act directly on the receptor. (B) Indirect-acting parasympathomimetics (cholinesterase inhibitors). Cholinesterase inhibitors inactivate the enzyme acetylcholinesterase (cholinesterase), thus permitting acetylcholine to react to the receptor. (Adapted from Kee JL, Hayes ER, McCuiston LE. *Pharmacology: A Nursing Process Approach.* 6th ed. St. Louis: Saunders; 2009.)

The adverse reactions associated with the administration of the cholinergic agents are essentially extensions of their pharmacologic effects. When large doses of these agents are ingested, the resultant toxic effects are described by the acronym SLUD: *s*alivation, *l*acrimation, *u*rination, and *d*efecation. With even larger doses, neuromuscular paralysis can occur as a result of the effect on the neuromuscular junction. CNS effects, such as confusion, can be seen if toxic doses are administered.

The treatment of an overdose of cholinesterase inhibitors, such as the insecticides or organophosphates (parathion), includes a combination of pralidoxime (pra-li-DOX-eem) (2-PAM, Protopam) and atropine. Pralidoxime regenerates the irreversibly bound ACh receptor sites that are bound by the inhibitors (knocks them off like a prizefighter), and atropine blocks (competitively) the muscarinic effects of the excess ACh present.

Contraindications

The relative contraindications to or cautions with the use of the cholinergic agents stem from these agents' pharmacologic effects and adverse reactions. They include the following:

Bronchial asthma: Cholinergic agents may cause bronchospasms or precipitate an asthmatic attack.

Hyperthyroidism: Hyperthyroidism may increase the risk of atrial fibrillation.

Gastrointestinal tract or urinary tract obstruction: If either the gastrointestinal tract or the urinary tract is obstructed and a cholinergic agent is given, an increase in secretions and motility could cause pressure and the system could "back up."

Severe cardiac disease: The reflex tachycardia that can result from administration of cholinergic agents may exacerbate a severe cardiac condition.

Myasthenia gravis treated with neostigmine: Patients with myasthenia gravis should not be given irreversible cholinesterase inhibitors because neostigmine occupies the enzyme, and the irreversible agent would not function.

Peptic ulcer: Cholinergic agents stimulate gastric acid secretion and increase gastric motility. This action could exacerbate an ulcer.

Uses

The direct-acting agents are used primarily in the treatment of glaucoma, a condition in which the intraocular pressure is elevated. Occasionally, they are used to treat myasthenia gravis, a disease resulting in muscle weakness from an autoimmune reaction that reduces the effect of ACh on the voluntary muscles. The urinary retention that occurs after surgery is also treated with the choline esters (see Table 4.3).

Pilocarpine (pye-loe-KAR-peen) (Salagen), a naturally occurring cholinergic agent, is used in the treatment of xerostomia, but its success may be limited because of the myriad of potential side effects. Common side effects from pilocarpine include perspiration (sweating), nausea, rhinitis, chills, and flushing. Pilocarpine is available in 5-mg tablets. The usual dose of pilocarpine is 5 mg three times a day (tid). This can be obtained by giving one 5-mg tablet tid. Pilocarpine is also available as ophthalmic solution in strengths of 1%, 2% and 4%. It is used topically in the eye to treat glaucoma. Several strengths (e.g., 2%) are available as generic preparations.

The indirect-acting cholinergic agents, the cholinesterase inhibitors, are divided into groups on the basis of the speed of reversibility of their binding to the enzyme. Edrophonium is rapidly reversible, whereas physostigmine and neostigmine are slowly reversible. These agents are used to treat glaucoma and myasthenia gravis.

Physostigmine (fi-zoe-STIG-meen) (Antilirium) has been used to treat reactions caused by several different kinds of drugs. Acute toxicity from the anticholinergic agents (e.g., atropine) and other agents that have anticholinergic action (e.g., the phenothiazines, tricyclic antidepressants, and antihistamines) has been treated with physostigmine.

Indirect-acting reversible acetylcholinesterase inhibitors are also being used to treat Alzheimer disease (AD) dementia. They have been shown to produce modest improvements in dementia symptoms but do not slow down, stop, or reverse disease progression.

Donepezil (Aricept) is has been approved by the US Food and Drug Administration (FDA) for the treatment of mild, moderate, and severe AD dementia, whereas galantamine (Razadyne, Razadyne ER) and Rivastigmine (generics and Exelon Patch) are FDA-approved to treat mild to moderate AD dementia. The more common side effects of all of these drugs are gastrointestinal and include nausea, vomiting, and diarrhea. These drugs can also cause bradycardia, so caution should be exercised when patients taking these drugs rise from the dental treatment chair.

The cholinesterase inhibitors developed for use as insecticides and chemical warfare agents are essentially irreversible and are called the *irreversible cholinesterase inhibitors*. Members of this group include parathion, malathion, and sarin (which has been used in a terrorist attack on a subway in Japan, where it poisoned passengers).

Anticholinergic (Parasympatholytic) Agents

The anticholinergic agents prevent the action of ACh at the postganglionic parasympathetic nerve endings. The release of ACh is not prevented but the receptor site is competitively blocked by the anticholinergics (Fig. 4.9). Thus the anticholinergic drugs block the action of ACh on smooth muscles (e.g., intestines), glandular tissue (e.g., salivary glands), and the heart. These agents are called *antimuscarinic agents* because they block the muscarinic receptors and not the nicotinic receptors.

Pharmacologic Effects

Central nervous system effects. Depending on the dose administered, the anticholinergics can produce CNS stimulation or depression. For example, usual therapeutic doses of scopolamine more often cause sedation, whereas atropine in high doses can cause stimulation. Atropine and scopolamine are tertiary agents, and propantheline (proe-PAN-the-leen) (Pro-Banthine) and glycopyrrolate (Robinul) are quaternary agents (Fig. 4.10). Because of their water solubility, quaternary agents do not penetrate the CNS well. The tertiary agents are lipid soluble and can easily penetrate the brain. The quaternary agents cause fewer CNS adverse reactions because they are less likely to enter the brain.

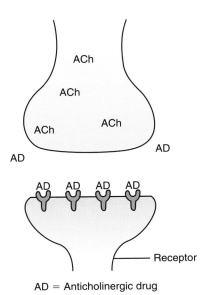

AD = Anticholinergic drug

Fig. 4.9 Anticholinergic response. The anticholinergic drug occupies the receptor sites, blocking acetylcholine. *ACh,* Acetylcholine. (Adapted from Kee JL, Hayes ER, McCuiston LE. *Pharmacology: A Nursing Process Approach.* 6th ed. St. Louis: Saunders; 2009.)

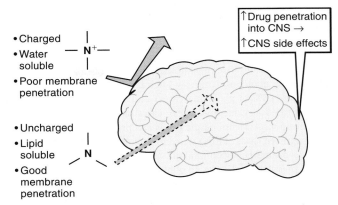

Fig. 4.10 Anticholinergics, brain penetration. Quaternary amines are charged and hydrophilic (water-soluble), so they cannot easily penetrate the brain. Tertiary amines are uncharged and lipophilic (lipid-soluble), so they easily penetrate the brain. *CNS,* Central nervous system.

Effects on exocrine glands. The anticholinergics affect the exocrine glands by reducing the flow and the volume of their secretions. These glands are located in the respiratory, gastrointestinal, and genitourinary tracts. This effect is used therapeutically in dentistry to decrease salivation and create a dry field for certain dental procedures, such as obtaining a difficult impression.

Effects on smooth muscle. Anticholinergics relax the smooth muscle in the respiratory and gastrointestinal tracts. Ipratropium is an anticholinergic inhaler used to treat asthma. The effect of anticholinergics on gastrointestinal motility has given rise to the name "spasmolytic agents." If these drugs are used repeatedly, constipation can result. By delaying gastric emptying and decreasing esophageal and gastric motility, the anticholinergics may exacerbate the condition. The smooth muscle in the respiratory tract is relaxed by the anticholinergic agents, causing bronchial dilation. This effect is used to treat asthma.

Effects on the eye. The parasympatholytics have two effects on the eye, mydriasis and cycloplegia. **Cycloplegia** refers to paralysis of the ciliary muscles of the eye, which results in the loss of visual accommodation. The effects of cycloplegia and mydriasis are useful in preparing the eye for ophthalmologic examinations. For eye examinations, **mydriasis** dilates the pupil so that the retina can be examined, and cycloplegia allows for proper measurements to make glasses. These effects occur when the drug is given topically or systemically.

Cardiovascular effects. With large therapeutic doses, the anticholinergic agents can produce vagal blockade, resulting in tachycardia. This effect has been used therapeutically to prevent cardiac slowing during general anesthesia. With small doses, bradycardia predominates. This variable response in the heart rate occurs because heart rate is a function of both direct (increased heart rate) and indirect (decreased heart rate) effects.

Adverse Reactions

The adverse reactions associated with the anticholinergics are essentially extensions of their pharmacologic effects. They include **xerostomia** (see Appendix D for a discussion of drugs that cause xerostomia and a discussion of artificial salivas), blurred vision, **photophobia**, tachycardia, fever, and urinary and gastrointestinal stasis. **Hyperpyrexia** (elevated temperature) and hot, dry, flushed skin caused by a lack of sweating are also seen. Hyperpyrexia is treated symptomatically.

Anticholinergic toxicity can cause signs of CNS excitation, including delirium, **hallucinations**, convulsions, and respiratory depression.

Contraindications

Specific contraindications to or cautions about the use of the anticholinergic agents are as follows.

Glaucoma. Anticholinergics are the only ANS drug group that can cause an acute rise in intraocular pressure in patients with angle-closure glaucoma (narrow angle). Glaucoma is divided into angle-closure (5% of glaucoma cases) and open-angle (wide-angle) glaucoma (95% of glaucoma cases); cases of angle-closure glaucoma are uncommon. Anticholinergic drugs can precipitate an acute attack in unrecognized cases of this rare condition. If angle-closure glaucoma is diagnosed, emergency ophthalmic surgery must be performed to relieve the pressure on the eye. In contrast, the patient with open-angle glaucoma who is currently receiving treatment with eye drops (many types) can be given a few doses of anticholinergic agents with impunity.

Prostatic hypertrophy. Because the anticholinergic agents can exacerbate urinary retention, older men with prostatic hypertrophy (many men older than 50 years) who already have difficulty urinating should not be given these drugs. Acute urinary retention that may require catheterization could occur.

Intestinal or urinary obstruction or retention. Constipation or acute urinary retention can be precipitated by the use of anticholinergic agents in susceptible patients. Constipation can be exacerbated, especially in patients with chronic constipation. (Such patients should not be given an opioid [narcotic] for pain control.)

Cardiovascular disease. Because anticholinergic agents have the ability to block the vagus nerve, resulting in tachycardia, patients with cardiovascular disease should be given these agents with caution.

Uses

Table 4.4 lists examples of anticholinergic (parasympatholytic) agents as well as their usual oral doses and routes of administration.

Preoperative medication. The anticholinergic agents are used preoperatively for two reasons. First, they inhibit the secretions of saliva and bronchial mucus that can be stimulated by general anesthesia. Second, they have the ability to block the vagal slowing of the heart resulting from general anesthesia.

Treatment of gastrointestinal disorders. Many types of gastrointestinal disorders associated with increased motility or acid secretion have been treated with anticholinergic agents. For example, patients with gastric ulcers are sometimes treated with the anticholinergic agents, although there is little proof of their effectiveness. Both nonspecific diarrhea and hypermotility of the colon have also been treated with these agents. In the doses used, it is difficult to prove that the anticholinergic agents are effective for these purposes.

Treatment of overactive bladder. Anticholinergic drugs are currently first-line therapy for treating overactive bladder (OAB). These drugs are thought to work by inhibiting acetylcholine/muscarinic receptors in the detrusor muscle of the bladder, which prevents contraction, thereby allowing the bladder to fill completely. Once this happens, patients experience a reduction in the urgency and frequency to urinate with a return to normal bladder function.

Ophthalmologic examination. Because of the ability of anticholinergic agents to cause mydriasis and cycloplegia, they are commonly used topically before examinations of the eye. Producing mydriasis allows full visualization of the retina. Cycloplegia is useful to relax the lens so that the proper prescription for eyeglasses may be determined.

Reduction of Parkinson-like movements. Before the advent of levodopa, anticholinergic agents were commonly used to reduce the tremors and rigidity associated with Parkinson disease. Patients treated with these agents predictably experienced the side effects dry mouth and blurred vision. At present anticholinergic agents are used only occasionally in combination with levodopa for the treatment of Parkinson disease.

TABLE 4.4   Examples of Anticholinergic (Parasympatholytic) Agents

Category	Agent	Strengths*	Route of Administration
Tertiary			
Natural alkaloids	Atropine	0.4 mg	PO
		0.4 mg/ml	IV
		1% sol	ophth
	Scopolamine	0.4 mg	PO
	Transderm-Scop	1 mg	transdermal patch
		0.25%	ophth
Synthetic esters	Dicyclomine (Bentyl)	20; 10 mg/5 mL (syrup)	PO
Quaternary			
Esters	Ipratropium (Atrovent)	—	Inhalation
	Propantheline (Pro-Banthine)	15	PO
Vasoselective			
	Tolterodine (Detrol,	1, 2	PO
	Detrol LA)	2, 4 (LA)	PO
	Oxybutynin (Ditropan	5	PO
	Ditropan XL	5, 10, 15	Patch
	Oxytrol	3.9	Gel
	Gelnique)	10%	PO
	Trospium chloride		
	Sanctura	20	PO
	Sanctura SR	60	PO
	Solifenacin (VESIcare)	5, 10	PO
	Darifenacin (Enablex)	7.5, 15	PO
	Fesoterodine (Toviaz)	4, 8	PO

*Usual oral dose (mg).
Ophth, Ophthalmic; Intravenous (IV) *PO,* oral.

The phenothiazines, used to treat psychoses, can produce extrapyramidal (Parkinson-like) side effects (see Chapter 15). These include abnormal mouth and tongue movements, rigidity, tremor, and restlessness. Anticholinergic agents, such as trihexyphenidyl (trye-hex-ee-FEN-I-dill; Artane) and benztropine (BENZ-troe-peen; Cogentin), are often administered concurrently with the phenothiazines to reduce rigidity and tremor.

Motion sickness. Scopolamine, because of its CNS-depressant action, is used to treat motion sickness. Transdermal scopolamine is applied behind the ear to prevent motion sickness before boating trips.

Drug Interactions

The most important drug interaction associated with the anticholinergic agents is an additive anticholinergic effect. The anticholinergic effects of other agents—such as the phenothiazines, antihistamines, and tricyclic antidepressants—can be additive with those of the parasympatholytics. Mixing more than one drug group possessing anticholinergic effects can lead to symptoms of anticholinergic toxicity, including urinary retention, blurred vision, acute glaucoma, and even paralytic ileus. Dental office personnel must pay careful attention to the medications the patient is taking to rule out excessive anticholinergic effects.

Nicotinic Agonists and Antagonists

Nicotine, which is present in cigarettes, is so toxic that one drop on the skin is rapidly fatal. In low doses, it produces stimulation through depolarization. At high doses, it produces paralysis of the ganglia, resulting in respiratory paralysis. Peripherally, it increases blood pressure, heart rate, and gastrointestinal motility and secretions. Nicotine constricts the blood vessels and reduces blood flow to the extremities. Nicotine is addicting, and withdrawal symptoms can occur. It is also used as an insecticide.

SYMPATHETIC AUTONOMIC NERVOUS SYSTEM

The major neurotransmitters in the SANS are NE and epinephrine. They are synthesized in the neural tissues and stored in synaptic vesicles. NE is the major neurotransmitter released at the terminal nerve endings of the SANS. With stimulation, epinephrine is released from the adrenal medulla and distributed throughout the body via the blood.

The term *catecholamine* is made up of two terms that relate to the structure of such drugs. *Catechol* refers to 1,2-dihydroxybenzene; *amine* refers to the chemical structure, NH_2. NE, epinephrine, and dopamine are endogenous sympathetic neurotransmitters that are catecholamines. Isoproterenol (Isuprel) is an *exogenous catecholamine*; this term is used to refer to the epinephrine contained in a lidocaine-with-epinephrine solution.

The adrenergic drugs can be classified by their mechanisms of action (Fig. 4.11) as follows:

Direct-acting: Epinephrine, NE, and isoproterenol produce their effects directly on the receptor site by stimulating the receptor.

Indirect-acting: The indirect-acting agents, such as amphetamine, release endogenous NE, which then produces a response. Depletion of the endogenous NE with reserpine diminishes the response to these agents.

Mixed-acting: Mixed-acting agents, such as ephedrine, can either stimulate the receptor directly or release endogenous NE to cause a response.

NE's action is terminated primarily by reuptake into the presynaptic nerve terminal by an amine-specific pump. The NE taken up in this manner is stored for reuse. In addition, two enzyme systems, mono-amine oxidase (MAO) and catechol-*O*-methyltransferase (COMT), are involved in the metabolism of a portion of both epinephrine and NE.

Sympathetic Autonomic Nervous System Receptors

As early as 1948, the existence of at least two types of adrenergic receptors, termed *alpha* (α) and *beta* (β), was recognized. The activation of α-adrenergic receptors (α-receptors) causes a different response from that to the activation of β-adrenergic receptors (β-receptors). More subreceptor types are now known.

α-Receptors

The stimulation of the α-receptors results in smooth-muscle excitation or contraction, which then causes vasoconstriction. Because α-receptors are located in the skin and skeletal muscle, vasoconstriction of the skin and skeletal muscle follows stimulation. Drugs that block the action of neurotransmitters on the α-receptors are referred to as α-adrenergic blocking agents.

β-Receptors

There are at least two types of β-receptors, β_1 and β_2. Excitation of β_1-receptors causes stimulation of the heart muscle, resulting in a positive chronotropic effect (increased rate) and a positive inotropic effect (increased strength). The β_1-receptor controls the heart (one can remember the receptor that controls the heart by remembering that humans have only one heart) (Fig. 4.12). Other actions thought to be associated primarily with β_1-receptor stimulation include metabolic effects on glycogen formation.

The stimulation of the β_2-receptors results in smooth-muscle relaxation. Because the blood vessels of the skeletal muscle are innervated by β_2-receptors, stimulation causes vasodilation. Relaxation of the smooth muscles of the bronchioles, also containing β_2-receptors, results in bronchodilation. Stimulation of β_2-receptors produces bronchodilation in the lungs (one can remember the receptor that controls the lungs by remembering that humans have two lungs) (see Fig. 4.12). Drugs with this effect have been used in the treatment of asthma. The type of receptor found in a given tissue determines the effect that adrenergic agents have on that tissue (see Table 4.1).

Agents that block β-receptor effects are called β-adrenergic blocking agents, or β-blockers. Some (e.g., propranolol) are nonspecific, blocking both β_1-receptors and β_2-receptors, whereas others are more selective, blocking primarily β_2-receptors.

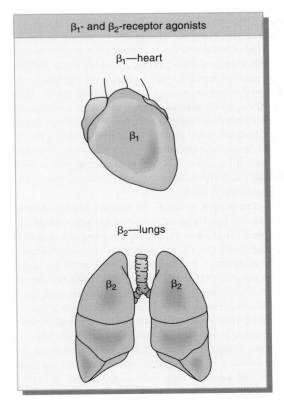

Fig. 4.12 β-Receptors: β1 and β2.

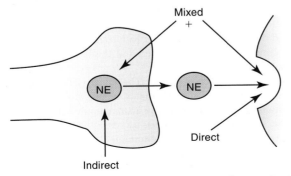

Fig. 4.11 Sympathetic autonomic nervous system: direct-, mixed-, and indirect-acting adrenergic agents. *NE*, Norepinephrine.

TABLE 4.5	Examples of Adrenergic Receptor Agonists (Sympathomimetic Adrenergic Agonists)		
Type	**Drug**	**Receptors**	**Indications**
Endogenous catecholamines	Epinephrine (Adrenalin) (Primatene) (EpiPen)	α/β	Anaphylaxis, asthma
	Norepinephrine (Levophed)	α/β	Hypotension
α_1-Selective	Phenylephrine (Neo-Synephrine)	α_1	Hypotension, nasal congestion
	Tetrahydrozoline (Tyzine, Visine)	α	Conjunctivitis, rhinitis
	Oxymetazoline (Afrin, Neo-Synephrine 12 h, OcuClear)	α	Conjunctivitis, nasal congestion
α_2-Selective	Clonidine (Catapres)	α_2	Hypertension
	Methyldopa (Aldomet)	α	Hypertension
β-Nonselective	Isoproterenol (Isuprel)	β	Heart block, bronchospasm
β_1-Selective	Dobutamine (Dobutrex)	$\beta_1 > \beta_2$	Cardiac decompensation
β_2-Selective	Albuterol (Proventil, Ventolin)	$\beta_2 > \beta_1$	Asthma
	Metaproterenol (Alupent)	$\beta_2 > \beta_1$	Asthma
β_3-Selective	Mirabegron (Myrbetriq)	β_3	Overactive bladder
Miscellaneous indirect-acting	Amphetamine	CNS/α/β	ADHD, narcolepsy
	Dextroamphetamine (Dexedrine)	CNS/α/β	ADHD, narcolepsy
	Amphetamine aspartate, sulfate, saccharate, and sulfate (Adderall)	CNS/α/β	ADHD, narcolepsy
	Methamphetamine (Desoxyn)	CNS/α/β	ADHD, obesity
	Methylphenidate (Ritalin)	CNS/α/β	ADHD
	Ephedrine	α/β	Methamphetamine precursor
	Pseudoephedrine (Sudafed)	α/β	Nasal congestion

ADHD, Attention-deficit hyperactivity disorder; *CNS,* central nervous system.

Adrenergic (Sympathomimetic) Agents

Adrenergic agents play an important part in the treatment of anaphylaxis and asthma and are added to local anesthetic solutions (vasoconstrictors) to prolong their action. Table 4.5 lists some adrenergic agents.

Pharmacologic Effects

When one is discussing the pharmacologic effects of the adrenergic drugs, it is important to note the proportions of α-receptor and β-receptor activity each possesses. For example, epinephrine has both α-receptor and β-receptor activity, NE and phenylephrine stimulate primarily α-receptors, and isoproterenol acts mainly on β-receptors. Although the effects of these agents depend on their ability to stimulate various receptors, the general actions of the adrenergic agents are discussed with specific reference to α-receptor or β-receptor effects as applicable.

Central nervous system effects. The sympathomimetic agents, such as amphetamine, produce CNS excitation, or alertness. With higher doses, anxiety, apprehension, restlessness, and even tremors can occur.

Cardiovascular effects

Heart. The general effect of the sympathomimetics, such as epinephrine, on the heart is to increase its force and strength of contraction. The final effect on blood pressure is a combination of the direct and the indirect effects. NE, primarily an α-agonist, produces vasoconstriction that increases peripheral resistance, resulting in an increase in blood pressure. With an increase in blood pressure, the vagal reflex decreases the heart rate. Epinephrine, an α- and β-agonist, constricts the α-receptors and dilates the β-receptors. This produces a widening of the pulse pressure (systolic blood pressure minus diastolic blood pressure) with an increase in systolic and a decrease in diastolic blood pressures. Isoproterenol, primarily a β-agonist, produces vasodilation (lowers peripheral resistance), which triggers an increase in heart rate (vagal reflex).

Vessels. The vascular responses observed with the sympathomimetics depend on the location of the vessels and whether they are innervated by α-receptors, β-receptors, or both. Agents with α-receptor effects produce vasoconstriction primarily in the skin and mucosa (which are innervated with α-receptor fibers), whereas agents with β-receptor effects will produce vasodilation of the skeletal muscle (which is innervated with β-receptor fibers). The resultant effect on the total peripheral resistance is an increase for an agent with α-receptor effects and a reduction for an agent with β-receptor effects.

Blood pressure. The sympathomimetic effect on the blood pressure is generally an increase. With epinephrine, which has both α-receptor–stimulating and β-receptor–stimulating properties, there is a rise in systolic pressure and a decrease in diastolic pressure. With NE, there is a rise in both systolic and diastolic pressures. With isoproterenol, there is little change in systolic pressure but a decrease in diastolic pressure.

Effects on the eye. The sympathomimetic agents have at least two effects on the eye: a decrease in intraocular pressure, which makes them useful in the treatment of glaucoma, and mydriasis.

Effects on the respiratory system. Sympathomimetic agents cause a relaxation of the bronchial smooth muscle because of their β-receptor effect. This has made them useful in the treatment of asthma and anaphylaxis.

Metabolic effects. The hyperglycemia resulting from β-receptor stimulation can be explained on the basis of increased glycogenolysis and decreased insulin release. Fatty acid mobilization, lipolysis, and gluconeogenesis are stimulated and the basal metabolic rate is increased.

Effects on the salivary glands. The mucus-secreting cells of the submandibular glands and sublingual glands are stimulated by the sympathomimetic agents to release a small amount of thick, viscous saliva. Because the parotid gland has no sympathetic innervation (only parasympathetic) and the sympathomimetics produce vasoconstriction, the flow of saliva is often reduced, resulting in xerostomia.

Effects on the bladder. β_3-receptor stimulation of the detrusor muscle of the bladder relaxes the bladder, which allows it to fill completely with urine before sending the message to the brain that urination is necessary.

Adverse Reactions

The adverse reactions associated with the adrenergic drugs are extensions of their pharmacologic effects. Anxiety and tremors may occur, and the patient may have palpitations. Serious arrhythmias can result. Agents with an α-adrenergic action can also cause a dramatic rise in blood pressure. The sympathomimetic agents should be used with caution in patients with angina, hypertension, or hyperthyroidism.

Contraindications

Sympathomimetic drugs should not be used in persons with uncontrolled hypertension, angina, or hyperthyroidism. These drugs stimulate α- and β-receptors in the heart and would further raise blood pressure and heart rate in persons with already increased blood pressure and heart rates. This effect could lead to arrhythmias or a myocardial infarction.

Uses

Vasoconstriction

Prolonged action. The sympathomimetic agents are used in dentistry primarily because of their vasoconstrictive action on the blood vessels. Agents with an α-adrenergic effect (vasoconstriction) are often added to local anesthetic solutions. These vasoconstrictors prolong the action of the local anesthetics and reduce their potential for systemic toxicity.

Hemostasis. The adrenergic agents have been used in dentistry to produce hemostasis. Epinephrine can be applied topically or infiltrated locally around the bleeding area. Epinephrine-containing retraction cords, used to stop bleeding and to retract the gingiva before an impression is taken, can produce problems such as systemic toxicity. Epinephrine is quickly absorbed after topical application if the tissue is injured. The total amount of epinephrine given by all routes must be noted to prevent an overdose.

Decongestion. Sympathomimetic agents are often incorporated into nose drops or sprays (see Table 4.5) to treat nasal congestion. These agents provide symptomatic relief by constricting the vessels and reducing the swelling of the mucous membranes of the nose. Within a short time, the congestion can return; this is a condition called rebound congestion. With repeated local use of such agents, systemic absorption can cause problems even greater than rebound congestion. Systemic decongestants or topical intranasal steroids are now preferred.

Cardiac effects

Treatment of shock. The value of the adrenergic agents in the treatment of shock is controversial. These drugs will elevate a lowered blood pressure, but correcting the cause of shock is more important. Some agents with both α- and β-adrenergic receptor effects (e.g., epinephrine) are used.

Treatment of cardiac arrest. The sympathomimetic agents, especially epinephrine, are used to treat cardiac arrest.

Bronchodilation. The use of the sympathomimetic agents in the treatment of respiratory disease stems from their action as bronchodilators. Patients with asthma or emphysema are often treated with adrenergic agents to provide bronchodilation. In the treatment of anaphylaxis, when bronchoconstriction is predominant, epinephrine is the drug of choice.

Overactive bladder. Mirabegron, a β₃ agonist is used to treat the symptoms of urge urinary incontinence, urgency, and urinary frequency associated with OAB.

Central nervous system stimulation. Amphetamine-like agents have been used and abused as "diet pills." They are indicated for the treatment of attention-deficit disorder (ADD) and narcolepsy.

Adrenergic agonists with some specificity for CNS stimulation are used for both legitimate and illegitimate purposes.

Methylphenidate (meth-ill-FEN-I-date) (Ritalin) and dextroamphetamine (dex-troe-am-FET-a-meen) (Dexedrine) are adrenergic agents used to treat ADD in both children and adults. These agents, given to hyperactive children and adults, reduce impulsivity and increase attention span. Some children with ADD exhibit excessive motor activity—turn around in the chair, stand up from the chair, grab dental instruments, squirt water, and ask about everything. Side effects exhibited with the use of these agents include insomnia and anorexia. ADD has also been known as *attention-deficit hyperactivity disorder* (ADHD) and *minimal brain dysfunction* (MBD), and children with the disorder have been referred to as *hyperkinetic* children.

Diethylpropion (dye-eth-il-PROE-pee-on; Tenuate) is an adrenergic drug that is used as a "diet pill." Uses for weight loss, to produce euphoria, and for "staying awake" are not legitimate medical uses for adrenergic agents. Truck drivers have used these agents to keep themselves awake for long hours. Hallucinations and psychosis resulting from the use of the drugs make these truck drivers dangerous.

Narcolepsy, a disease in which spontaneous deep sleep can occur at any time, is treated with the sympathomimetic amines. Tolerance to the effect does not seem to occur.

Specific Adrenergic Agents

Epinephrine. The drug of choice for acute asthmatic attacks and anaphylaxis, epinephrine (Epi) (ep-i-NEF-rin; Adrenalin), may be administered by both the intravenous and subcutaneous routes. It is also used in patients with cardiac arrest. It is added to local anesthetic solutions to delay absorption and reduce systemic toxicity (see Chapter 9). Epinephrine should be stored in amber-colored containers and placed out of the reach of sunlight because light causes deterioration. As it deteriorates, epinephrine first turns pink, then brown, and finally precipitates. Solutions of epinephrine with any discoloration or precipitate should be discarded immediately. (One should check the expiration date too.)

Phenylephrine. Phenylephrine (fen-ill-EF-rin; Neo-Synephrine) causes primarily α-receptor stimulation, which produces vasoconstriction in the cutaneous vessels. This leads to increases in total peripheral resistance and in systolic and diastolic pressures. A reflex vagal bradycardia also results. Phenylephrine is used as a mydriatic and in nose sprays (Neo-Synephrine) or drops to relieve congestion.

Levonordefrin. Levonordefrin (lee-voe-nor-DEF-rin; Neo-Cobefrin), a derivative of NE, is a vasoconstrictor often added to local anesthetic solutions. Although claims made for this drug include less CNS excitation and cardiac stimulation, a higher dose is required to produce vasoconstriction equal to that achieved with epinephrine. Therefore it is difficult to distinguish levonordefrin's effects from those of other vasoconstrictors. Its effects resemble those of α-receptor stimulation.

Ephedrine and pseudoephedrine. In contrast to the catecholamines, ephedrine and pseudoephedrine (soo-doe-e-FED-rin; Sudafed) are effective when taken orally and have a longer duration of action. They have both α- and β-receptor activity. Their mechanism of action is mixed; that is, they have both direct action and indirect action. Ephedrine is often used in combination with other agents for patients with asthma as nonprescription remedies. Pseudoephedrine is also present in over-the-counter (OTC) products designed for the treatment of the common cold or allergies such as pseudoephedrine (Sudafed). The newest use of these agents is to "cook" them to produce methamphetamine, which is used illicitly. For this reason, their availability has been restricted by federal law. Ephedrine, in any form (herbal or chemical), is no longer available in dietary supplements; its use as such is illegal in the United States. Pseudoephedrine is now kept "behind the counter" with a pharmacist. Those wishing to purchase pseudoephedrine must be above 18 years of age and must go to the pharmacy to purchase it. In most states, the patient must produce legal identification and sign a log. There is also a limit as to how much a person can purchase each month.

Dopamine. Dopamine (DOE-pa-meen; Intropin) is a neurotransmitter in parts of the CNS. It is both an α-agonist and a β-agonist and is used primarily in the treatment of shock. It is a precursor of NE and epinephrine synthesis, as shown in Fig. 4.13. Dopamine first acts on the β-receptors of the heart, producing a positive chronotropic and inotropic effect. In higher doses, it stimulates the α-receptors, producing vasoconstriction. However, it exerts an unusual vasodilating effect in certain vessels and produces an increase in blood flow to the renal, splanchnic, cerebral, and coronary vessels. Ventricular arrhythmias and hypotension can occur.

Dipivefrin. Dipivefrin (dye-PIV-e-frin) (Propine) and epinephrine are sympathomimetic ophthalmics that are used to treat glaucoma. They decrease the production of aqueous humor (β-receptor effect), increase its outflow (β-receptor effect), and produce mydriasis (primarily α-receptor effect). Dipivefrin, a prodrug, is metabolized in vivo to epinephrine. It may produce fewer side effects than epinephrine because it penetrates into the eye better and is used to treat chronic open-angle glaucoma.

Adrenergic Blocking Agents

Adrenergic blocking agents can block all the adrenergic receptors (α- and β-blockers), just the α-receptors (α-blockers), just the β-receptors (β-blockers), or just α_1-receptors (α_1-blockers), α_2-receptors (α_2-blockers), β_1-receptors (β_1-blockers), or β_2-receptors (β_2-blockers) (Table 4.6).

α-Adrenergic Blocking Agents

The α-adrenergic blocking agents competitively inhibit the vasoconstricting effects (α-receptor effects) of the adrenergic agents. This reduces the sympathetic tone in the blood vessels, producing a decrease in the total peripheral resistance. The resulting decrease in blood pressure stimulates the vagus, thereby producing a reflex tachycardia. Patients who are pretreated with α-blocking agents and given epinephrine exhibit a predominance of β-effects (vasodilation), which lowers blood pressure. This effect is termed epinephrine reversal because the blood pressure goes down instead of going up. The α-adrenergic blockers also block the mydriasis that adrenergic agents normally cause.

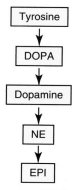

Fig. 4.13 Synthesis of epinephrine *(EPI)* from tyrosine, including the intermediate steps involving dopamine. *DOPA,* 3,4 dihydrophenylalanine; *NE,* norepinephrine.

| Tyrosine |
| DOPA |
| Dopamine |
| NE |
| EPI |

TABLE 4.6 Examples of Adrenergic Receptor Antagonists (Sympatholytics, Adrenergic Blockers)

Receptor	Examples
α-Adrenergic Receptor Antagonists	
$\alpha_1 > \alpha_2$	Phentolamine (Regitine)
$\alpha_1 >>> \alpha_2$	Phenoxybenzamine (Dibenzyline)
α_2	Prazosin (Minipress)
α Partial agonist and antagonist	Yohimbine
	Ergot
β-Adrenergic Receptor Antagonists (L = low, I = intermediate, H = high ISA)	
Nonspecific (nonselective) β	Propranolol (Inderal)
Specific (selective) $\beta_1 > \beta_2$	Acebutolol (Sectral)
	Atenolol (Tenormin)
α- and β-Adrenergic Antagonists	
α, β	Labetalol (Normodyne, Trandate)

ISA, Intrinsic sympathetic activity.

The agents phenoxybenzamine (fen-ox-ee-BEN-za-meen; Dibenzyline) and phentolamine (fen-TOLE-a-meen; Regitine) are α-blockers. They are used in the treatment of peripheral vascular disease in which vascular spasm is a common feature (e.g., Raynaud syndrome) and in the diagnosis and treatment of pheochromocytoma, a catecholamine-secreting tumor of the adrenal medulla.

Other examples of α_1-adrenergic blocking agents are tolazoline (toe-LAZ-a-zeen; Priscoline), prazosin (PRA-zoe-sin; Minipress), terazosin (ter-AY-zoe-sin; Hytrin), and doxazosin (dox-AY-zoe-sin; Cardura), which are competitive blockers of the α-receptor. They are effective in the treatment of hypertension and are discussed in Chapter 12. These agents are also indicated in the management of vasospasm in Raynaud disease and in the treatment of benign prostatic hypertrophy (to increase ease of urination).

β-Adrenergic Blocking Agents

The β-blocking drugs competitively block the β-receptors in the adrenergic nervous system. Their generic names end in *olol,* so they can be easily recognized. Because β-receptor stimulation produces vasodilation, bronchodilation, and tachycardia, β-blockers would block these effects, producing bradycardia and, in asthmatics, possible bronchoconstriction. Their exact effect is determined by the tone in the sympathetic nervous system. The β-blockers may be either nonspecific (nonselective), such as propranolol (proe-PRAN-oh-lole; Inderal), or specific (selective) such as atenolol (a-TEN-oh-lole; Tenormin). The specific β-blockers have more activity on the heart and blood vessels (β-receptors) than on the lungs (β-receptors). This specificity, or selectivity, produces fewer side effects. The selective β-blockers also have a lower chance of causing drug interactions.

Propranolol (Inderal) is a β-blocker that depresses the heart (negative chronotropic and inotropic effect), produces bronchoconstriction, and can cause hypoglycemia. It is used in the treatment of arrhythmias (for its quinidine-like effect), angina, hypertension, and migraine headache prophylaxis. Diseases in which tachycardia occurs, such as hyperthyroidism and pheochromocytoma, can be symptomatically treated with propranolol. The β-blockers are discussed in Chapter 12.

α- and β-Blocking Agents

Labetalol (la-BET-a-lole; Normodyne, Trandate) has both α- and β-blocking action. Because the β-blockers are designated using the suffix *-olol,* this α- and β-blocker uses the suffix *-alol.* It is a selective α-blocker and a nonselective β-blocker. It is indicated for the treatment of hypertension and produces a fall in blood pressure without reflex tachycardia.

Neuromuscular Blocking Drugs

The neuromuscular blocking drugs are agents that affect transmission between the motor nerve endings and the nicotinic receptors on the skeletal muscle. These blocking agents act either as antagonists (nondepolarizing) or as agonists (depolarizing).

Nondepolarizing (Competitive) Blockers

Indigenous people living along the Amazon have used poison arrows when hunting animals. The poison is the neuromuscular blocking drug curare, or *d*-tubocurarine. This nondepolarizing blocker combines with the nicotinic receptor and blocks the action of ACh. The depolarization of the membrane is inhibited, and muscle contraction is blocked. These competitive blockers can be overcome by the administration of cholinesterase inhibitors such as neostigmine. Current examples are vecuronium and pancuronium.

Neuromuscular blocking drugs cause paralysis of the small facial muscles, followed by paralysis of the fingers, limbs, extremities, and trunk. The function of the muscles involved in respiration is lost, beginning with the intercostal muscles. The last function lost is the most primitive diaphragmatic breathing. Nature has planned that loss of function is in the order of least important to most important (the diaphragm). The duration of action of these drugs ranges between 20 minutes and 2 hours, depending on the dose.

Depolarizing Agents

Depolarizing agents, such as succinylcholine (suk-sin-ill-KOE-leen), attach to the nicotinic receptor and, similar to ACh, cause depolarization. The constant stimulation of the receptor causes the sodium channel to open, producing depolarization (phase I). Transient fasciculations of the muscles result. With time, the receptor cannot transmit any further impulses, and repolarization occurs as the sodium channel closes (phase II). A flaccid paralysis is produced by resistance to depolarization.

Succinylcholine produces muscle fasciculations followed by paralysis. The paralysis lasts only a few minutes because succinylcholine is broken down by plasma cholinesterase.

Succinylcholine can cause cardiac arrhythmias, hyperkalemia, and increased intraocular pressure. When it is used in general anesthesia in conjunction with halothane, succinylcholine precipitates malignant hyperthermia in susceptible patients (heredity). The drug of choice for malignant hyperthermia is dantrolene (Dantrium). Sometimes a small dose of curare is administered before the administration of succinylcholine to block the fasciculations of the succinylcholine, thus reducing postoperative muscle pain.

DENTAL HYGIENE CONSIDERATIONS

Cholinergic Drugs

- Dental hygienists need to encourage patients to use good oral hygiene to help with the effects of increased salivation from cholinergic drugs.
- The dental hygienist should raise a patient into the sitting position slowly and have the patient rise slowly from the dental chair to help minimize the hypotensive effects of cholinergic drugs.

Anticholinergic Drugs

Xerostomia
- Xerostomia can be minimized with meticulous oral hygiene, including brushing and flossing.
- Patients should also drink plenty of water and keep a glass of water by the bedside at night.
- Patients should avoid prescription and nonprescription mouth rinses that contain alcohol because alcohol can exacerbate dry mouth.
- Caffeinated beverages can also exacerbate dry mouth.
- Fruit juices and sodas contain sugar, which can increase the patient's risk for caries.
- Have the patient chew tart sugarless gum or suck on tart sugarless candy to help minimize dry mouth.

Tachycardia
- Always check the patient's pulse and blood pressure, especially before a procedure that may require epinephrine.

Sedation
- Caution should be used if another sedating drug, such as an opioid analgesic, is necessary.
- The patient should have someone drive him or her to and from the appointment.

- The patient should avoid any activity that requires careful thought or concentration.

Adrenergic Agonists

Tachycardia
- The patient's blood pressure and pulse rate should be checked at each visit, especially if epinephrine or levonordefrin is required.
- Patients with uncontrolled hypertension or uncontrolled hyperthyroidism should not receive these drugs.

Central Nervous System Excitation and Tremors
- The CNS effects of adrenergic agents can be exacerbated in a patient with existing CNS health issues or with hyperthyroidism.
- Both can be avoided or minimized with detailed medication/health histories and lower doses of a vasoconstrictor.

Drug Interactions
- Many OTC cough and cold products contain adrenergic agonists, which can interact with vasoconstrictors, leading to increased blood pressure.
- Check the patient's blood pressure and pulse rate.
- Such interactions can be avoided by carefully questioning the patient about his or her use of OTC drugs.

Oral β-Adrenergic Agonists
- Oral β-adrenergic agonists have the ability to raise blood pressure and heart rate, especially when used in combination with a vasoconstrictor.
- This effect can be avoided or minimized by measuring the patient's blood pressure and pulse rate before administering a vasoconstrictor.
- Ask specific questions about the patient's medications and health.

ACADEMIC SKILLS ASSESSMENT

1. Compare and contrast the parasympathetic and sympathetic nervous systems. Include neurotransmitters, receptor sites, and effects on innervated organs.
2. Explain the difference in mechanism of action between the direct-acting and indirect-acting cholinergic agents.
3. Describe the pharmacologic effects of the cholinergic agents on the heart, gastrointestinal tract, and eye.
4. State two major uses of the cholinergic agents.
5. Describe a unique dental use for pilocarpine.
6. Describe the pharmacologic effects of the anticholinergic agents on the exocrine glands, smooth muscle, and eye.
7. List the adverse reactions associated with the anticholinergic agents.
8. State the contraindications to and cautions for the use of anticholinergic agents and explain their relationship to the pharmacologic effects of these agents.
9. State the major therapeutic uses of the anticholinergic agents.
10. State the pharmacologic effect of the adrenergic agents on the eye, bronchioles, and salivary glands.
11. State the therapeutic uses of the adrenergic agents, especially in dentistry.
12. Explain the limits to the accepted medical uses of the amphetamine-like agents. Explain why ephedrine tablets are bought by the case by some individuals.
13. Name the pharmacologic class to which atenolol (Tenormin) belongs. Describe the effects that make β-blockers useful in the treatment of arrhythmias, angina, and hypertension.
14. Differentiate between "selective" and "nonselective" β-blockers. Name a difference important to the dental health team (drug interaction).

CLINICAL CASE STUDY

Harry Karteris, 83 years old, has been coming to your dental practice for almost 40 years. He was diagnosed with Parkinson disease about 5 years ago. Mr. Karteris is currently taking benztropine mesylate for the disease and acetaminophen for general aches and pains. Unfortunately, since he started taking benztropine mesylate, he has begun to have problems with his teeth.

1. What is benztropine mesylate, and what are some of its clinical uses?
2. What are some of the contraindications to medications such as benztropine mesylate?
3. What are some of the adverse reactions associated with benztropine mesylate?
4. What should Mr. Karteris be told about the dental adverse reactions associated with his medication?
5. What drugs prescribed in a dental office would interact with benztropine mesylate?
6. What should Mr. Karteris be told if one of these interacting medications (i.e., sedating drugs) must be prescribed for him?

Nonopioid (Nonnarcotic) Analgesics

LEARNING OBJECTIVES

1. Describe pain and its purpose and main components.
2. Discuss the classification of analgesic agents and the chemistry, pharmacokinetics, pharmacologic effects, adverse reactions, toxicity, drug interactions, and uses of aspirin.
3. Define the term *nonsteroidal antiinflammatory drug* and discuss the chemistry, pharmacokinetics, pharmacologic effects, adverse reactions, toxicity, drug interactions, and uses of these drugs, giving several examples of these.
4. Discuss the properties, pharmacologic effects, adverse reactions, drug interactions, uses, and dosing of acetaminophen.
5. Explain the disease known as *gout* and summarize the drugs used to treat it.
6. Explain the disease known as rheumatoid arthritis and summarize the mechanism of action of the classes of drugs used to treat it.

Pain control is of great importance in dental practice. Pain often brings the patient to the dental office. Conversely, pain can be the factor that keeps the patient from seeking dental care at the appropriate time. Thus dental treatment is often rendered on inflamed, hypersensitive tissues of a patient who suffers from mental fatigue after enduring pain for a length of time.

The dental hygienist must be able to recognize and evaluate a patient's need for medication to control pain. Because pain is such a complex phenomenon, the entire patient must be considered before the type of medication that may be needed is determined.

PAIN

The sensation of pain is the means by which the body is made urgently aware of the presence of tissue damage. Pain represents a protective reflex for self-preservation. Just as the hand is quickly removed from a hot object, a painful dental abscess brings the patient to the dental office seeking professional assistance for its resolution. Pain is a diagnostic symptom of an underlying pathologic condition. Although the relief of pain is an immediate objective, only by treatment of the underlying cause is the ultimate resolution achieved.

The two components of pain are perception and reaction. Perception, the physical component of pain, involves the message of pain that is carried through the nerves eventually to the cortex. Reaction, the psychologic component of pain, involves the patient's emotional response to the pain. Although individuals are surprisingly uniform in their perception of pain, they vary greatly in their reaction to it. A decrease in the pain threshold (a greater reaction to pain) has been said to be associated with emotional instability, anxiety, fatigue, youth, certain nationalities, female gender, and fear and apprehension. The pain threshold is raised by sleep, sympathy, activities, and analgesics (Fig. 5.1). As a result, analgesic therapy must be selected for the individual. A level of discomfort that may not require drug treatment in one person may demand extreme therapy in another. Although some patients undergoing routine exodontia require no postoperative medication, even the strongest analgesics do not completely control postoperative extraction pain in others.

CLASSIFICATION

The analgesic agents can be divided into two groups, the nonopioids, also called *nonnarcotic analgesics,* and the opioids, also called *narcotic analgesics.*

An important difference between the nonopioid and the opioid analgesics (narcotic analgesics) is their sites of action. Nonopioid analgesics act primarily at the peripheral nerve endings, although their antipyretic effect is mediated centrally. Opioids act primarily within the central nervous system (CNS).

Another difference between the opioids and the nonopioid analgesic agents is their mechanism of action. The action of the nonopioid analgesic agents is related to their ability to inhibit prostaglandin synthesis. The opioids affect the response to pain by depressing the CNS (the reaction). The side effect profiles of the two groups also differ.

The nonopioids can be divided into the salicylates (aspirin-like group), acetaminophen, and the nonsteroidal antiinflammatory drugs (NSAIDs) (Box 5.1). Aspirin, a member of the salicylates, is discussed first.

SALICYLATES

Since antiquity, extracts of willow bark containing salicin have been used to reduce fever. Over the years, many other salicylates (sa-LI-si-lates) have been synthesized, but aspirin is the most useful salicylate for analgesia. Box 5.2 lists some analgesic and some topical salicylates. Because aspirin is the prototype salicylate, it is discussed first.

Acetylsalicylic Acid

Chemistry

Acetylsalicylic acid (aspirin, ASA) is broken down into acetic acid (HA) and salicylic acid (SA) (Fig. 5.2). Acetic acid imparts the characteristic vinegar odor to a bottle of aspirin. Therefore the degree of breakdown

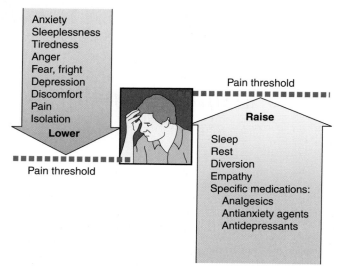

Fig. 5.1 Factors that alter the pain threshold. Sleep raises the threshold and fear lowers it. (From McKenry L, Tessier Ed, Hogan MA. *Mosby's Pharmacology in Nursing.* 22nd ed. St. Louis: Mosby; 2006.)

BOX 5.1	**Selected Nonopioid Analgesics**

Salicylates
Aspirin
Choline salicylate
Diflunisal
Magnesium salicylate
Salsalate

Nonsteroidal Antiinflammatory Drugs (NSAIDs)
Etodolac
Ibuprofen
Ketoprofen
Naproxen

Nonsalicylate/Nonnarcotic
Acetaminophen

BOX 5.2	**Salicylates**

Oral
Aspirin
Choline salicylate (Arthropan)
Diflunisal (Dolobid)
Magnesium salicylate (Doan's Pills)
Salsalate (Disalcid)
Sodium salicylate combination (Trilisate)

Topical
Methyl salicylate, oil of wintergreen (toxic by mouth) (Icy Hot, BENGAY)
Salicylic acid (Compound W, DuoFilm)
Trolamine salicylate (Myoflex)

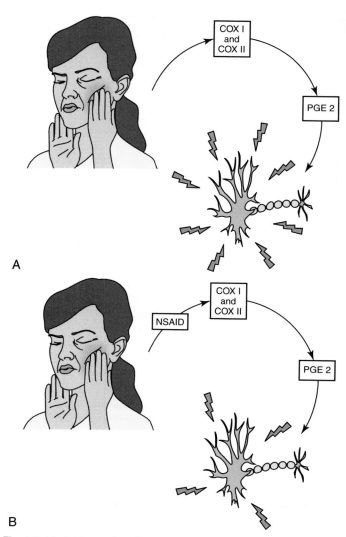

A

B

Fig. 5.2 Model for nociceptive pain. (A) Tissue injury triggers cyclooxygenase II *(COX II)* in peripheral tissue to convert arachidonic acid to prostaglandin E_2 *(PGE$_2$)*, resulting in stimulation of the nociceptor in peripheral nerves to send a signal for pain to the central nervous system. (B) Nonsteroidal antiinflammatory drug *(NSAID)* interfering with COX II–mediated prostaglandin synthesis.

Mechanism of Action

The mechanism of aspirin's analgesic, antipyretic, antiinflammatory, and antiplatelet effects is related to its ability to inhibit prostaglandin synthesis. Aspirin inhibits the enzyme cyclooxygenase (COX I and COX II, prostaglandin synthase) by acetylating serine, which results in inhibition of the production of prostaglandins. Fig. 5.3 shows the synthesis of the prostaglandins and leukotrienes from arachidonic acid. Prostaglandins, which are lipids that are synthesized locally by inflammatory stimuli, can sensitize the pain receptors to substances such as bradykinin. Prostaglandins can also lower the pain threshold to painful stimuli, cause inflammation and fever, and affect vascular tone and permeability, resulting in edema.

Therefore a reduction in prostaglandins results in a reduction in pain. Because aspirin blocks the synthesis of prostaglandins by nonselectively blocking cyclooxygenase, it is more effective if given before the painful stimuli are experienced. Because of this mechanism, aspirin is more effective against "throbbing" pain (caused by inflammation and common in dentistry) than against "stabbing" pain (direct effect on nerve endings).

of aspirin can be roughly determined by smelling a bottle of aspirin tablets. (If one thinks "phew" when opening an aspirin bottle, it is time to purchase a new bottle.) In addition, SA is a strong keratolytic agent (used to remove plantar warts from the bottom of feet) and may cause additional adverse gastrointestinal (GI) effects if degraded aspirin is administered orally.

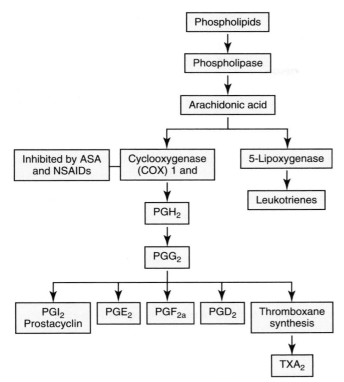

Fig. 5.3 Synthesis of prostaglandins (PGs) and leukotrienes (LTs) and the sites of action of aspirin (ASA) and nonsteroidal antiinflammatory drugs (NSAIDs) that interfere with prostaglandin synthesis. TXA2, thromboxane A2.

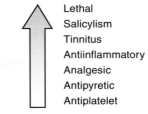

Lethal
Salicylism
Tinnitus
Antiinflammatory
Analgesic
Antipyretic
Antiplatelet

Fig. 5.4 Pharmacologic effects and adverse reactions of aspirin from low to high doses.

Because of its easy accessibility and long history of use, aspirin's worth as an analgesic is often unrecognized by the lay public.

Antipyretic effect. The ability of aspirin to reduce fever (antipyretic effect) results from its inhibition of prostaglandin synthesis in the hypothalamus. Hypothalamic prostaglandin synthesis is caused by elevated blood values of leukocyte pyrogens induced by inflammation. Increased hypothalamic prostaglandin levels produce higher body temperature. Therefore the inhibition of hypothalamic prostaglandin synthesis results in a return to more normal body temperature. Aspirin reduces fever by inducing peripheral vasodilation and sweating. Although it reduces an elevated temperature, it has no effect on normal body temperature. In fact, in toxic doses aspirin causes hyperthermia (see the section on Adverse Reactions).

Antiinflammatory effect. Aspirin's antiinflammatory effect is derived from its ability to inhibit prostaglandin synthesis (COX I and COX II). The prostaglandins are potent vasodilating agents that also increase capillary permeability. Therefore aspirin causes decreased erythema and swelling of the inflamed area. This antiinflammatory action is useful in dental patients because inflammation is a significant part of most dental pain. Patients with arthritis may be given large doses of aspirin to provide symptomatic relief of pain and inflammation in the joints.

Uricosuric effect. Although large doses (>3 g/day) of aspirin can produce a uricosuric effect, small doses (<1 g/day) produce uric acid retention. Aspirin can also counteract the uricosuric effect of probenecid (proe-BEN-e-sid) (Benemid), which is used to treat gout. Aspirin is no longer used as a uricosuric agent because more effective agents are available to treat gout.

Antiplatelet effect. Aspirin irreversibly binds to platelets. Its antiplatelet effect has been shown to be clinically effective for secondary myocardial infarction prevention in adults, the primary prevention of coronary artery disease, and the treatment of an ischemic event or the prevention of a further ischemic event. The effect of aspirin on platelets depends on the dose taken. Depending on the dose, aspirin can inhibit either prostacyclin (inhibits platelet aggregation) or thromboxane A2 (stimulates platelet aggregation). Fig. 5.5 demonstrates that inhibition of thromboxane A2 would prevent clotting because thromboxane A2 promotes clotting. Further studies are needed to determine aspirin's usefulness and dose in preventing clotting events in different patient populations.

Adverse Reactions

In sufficiently high doses, aspirin can have a variety of undesirable effects. Some of aspirin's side effects can be minimized but not eliminated. Precautions for and contraindications to the administration of aspirin are listed in Table 5.1.

Gastrointestinal effects

Gastric effects are common.

Aspirin's most common side effect is related to the GI tract, which may take the form of simple dyspepsia, nausea, vomiting, or gastric

Pharmacokinetics

Aspirin is rapidly and almost completely absorbed from the stomach and small intestine, producing its peak effect on an empty stomach in 30 minutes (90 minutes for salicylate). The buffered tablet reaches its peak in about 20 minutes (salicylate). Before a tablet of aspirin can be absorbed, it must be dispersed and dissolved. Addition of a buffer to the tablet facilitates this process. This facilitation is borne out by the somewhat quicker peak of action and higher blood levels attained with buffered aspirin preparations. Buffered aspirin has a higher proportion of the aspirin in the ionized form, which should make absorption slower, but this is offset by the increase in the rate of dissolution, which is facilitated. This difference in absorption has not been shown to translate into a clinically significant quicker effect.

Aspirin is widely distributed into most body tissues and fluids. It is poorly bound to plasma proteins. It is hydrolyzed to salicylate in the mucosa of the GI tract and on first pass through the liver. The half-life of unhydrolyzed aspirin is about 15 minutes. The half-life of hydrolyzed aspirin is dose-dependent. With small doses, the half-life is 2 to 3 hours; with higher doses, a half-life of 15 to 30 hours can be attained. The half-life varies with the dose because a constant amount rather than a constant percentage of the drug is metabolized per hour. This type of metabolism is called *zero-order kinetics* (see Chapter 2).

Pharmacologic Effects

Analgesic effect. Aspirin's analgesic effect has been repeatedly demonstrated in many clinical trials. In fact, new drugs are often compared in analgesic strength to aspirin. Aspirin typically relieves mild-to-moderate pain such as that due to arthritis, headache, or toothache. Aspirin's effects by dose are illustrated in Fig. 5.4.

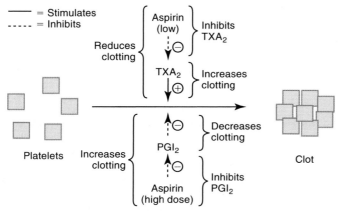

Fig. 5.5 The effects and mechanisms of action of aspirin, thromboxane *(TXA₂)*, and prostacyclin *(PGI₂)* Synthesis.

bleeding. These adverse effects result from direct gastric irritation and inhibition of prostaglandins. Because prostaglandins are responsible for inhibition of gastric acid secretion and stimulation of the cytoprotective mucus in the stomach, aspirin counteracts these effects. In high doses, aspirin's stimulation of the chemoreceptor trigger zone in the CNS can also produce nausea and vomiting. Salicylates may exacerbate preexisting ulcers, gastritis, or hiatal hernia.

Bleeding. At usual therapeutic doses, aspirin irreversibly interferes with the clotting mechanism by reducing platelet adhesiveness caused by interfering with adenosine diphosphate (ADP) release. The bleeding time is prolonged, and each platelet is affected until new platelets are formed (4–7 days). Replacement of all of the affected platelets is not required to produce normal clotting. After about 20% of the platelets have been replaced with newly formed platelets, clotting will have returned to normal after about 36 hours. Therefore, with lower doses of aspirin, 1.5 days should be enough to obtain normal clotting. With large doses of aspirin, the half-life is prolonged. Aspirin inhibits the production of prothrombin, resulting in hypoprothrombinemia. Three other mechanisms—the local irritant effects on the stomach, the decrease in platelet stickiness, and the loss of protective mucosa—magnify adverse effects on the stomach. Salicylate-induced gastric bleeding is painless. With a small loss of blood, aspirin does not produce significant bleeding. Salicylates

may exacerbate preexisting conditions such as ulcers, gastritis, hiatal hernia, and gastrointestinal esophageal reflux disease (GERD).

Reye's syndrome. In children and adolescents with either chickenpox or influenza, the use of aspirin has been epidemiologically associated with Reye's (pronounced "reyz") syndrome. In place of aspirin, acetaminophen is used in pediatrics for both its analgesic and its antipyretic actions. Reye's syndrome is associated with hepatotoxicity and encephalopathy, commonly fatal.

Hepatic and renal effects. Rarely, aspirin can produce hepatotoxicity. Renal papillary necrosis and interstitial nephritis leading to dialysis is associated with use of certain analgesics. It may be caused by the concomitant administration of aspirin and acetaminophen.

Pregnancy and nursing considerations. Although animal studies have shown that aspirin can cause birth defects, human studies have demonstrated only a slight positive correlation between long-term aspirin ingestion and congenital abnormalities. With aspirin abuse, there is an increased risk of stillbirth, neonatal death, and decreased birth weight. With near-term, high-dose administration of aspirin, gestation can be prolonged, parturition delayed, and risk of hemorrhage in the newborn and mother increased. Even premature closure of the patent ductus arteriosus (hole in the fetal heart) has been reported. Although salicylates are excreted in the breast milk, usual occasional therapeutic doses of aspirin do not present a problem for the healthy nursing infant.

Hypersensitivity (allergy)

> True aspirin allergy is uncommon.

The incidence of true aspirin allergy is less than 1% (0.2%–0.4%). Many patients with "allergy to aspirin" in their charts, on questioning, actually have stomach problems rather than true allergy. In the patient's chart, it is important to differentiate aspirin's adverse reactions from its hypersensitivity reactions. Adequate questioning of patients who "claim" to be allergic to aspirin is needed; patients with true aspirin hypersensitivity cannot be given any of the other NSAIDs because of some cross-hypersensitivity. Allergic reactions can vary from rash, wheezing, urticaria, and angioneurotic edema to anaphylactic shock. When a true aspirin allergy exists, any aspirin-containing products should be avoided.

Some people with asthma cannot take aspirin or NSAIDs because of the aspirin hypersensitivity triad known as Samter's triad. This triad consists of *aspirin hypersensitivity, asthma,* and *nasal polyps.* It occurs in about 30% to 40% of people who have asthma and nasal polyps.

TABLE 5.1 Precautions for and Contraindications to the Administration of Aspirin

Disease or Condition	Drug Used	Possible Effects of Aspirin
Myocardial infarction, atrial fibrillation, valve replacement	Warfarin (Coumadin)	Increases anticoagulant effect of warfarin
Peptic ulcer (heartburn), gastroesophageal reflux disease (GERD)	Histamine H₂ blockers (e.g., cimetidine)	Gastric irritant effect
Gout	Probenecid (Benemid)	Antagonizes uricosuric effect of probenecid
Arthritis, cancer, psoriasis	Methotrexate (MTX)	Increases toxicity of methotrexate
Rheumatic fever, arthritis	Large doses of aspirin	Do not add more aspirin if patient is taking large doses already
Hemophilia	Factor VIII	Gastric bleeding
Hypoprothrombinemia		Bleeding
Vitamin K deficiency, alcoholism		Bleeding
G6PD deficiency		Hemolysis
Diabetes	Oral hypoglycemics	Hypoglycemia

This reaction is thought to be the result of the shunting of the products of arachidonic acid from the production of prostaglandins to the leukotrienes and is thought to be a potential mechanism for this hypersensitivity. These patients exhibit cross-hypersensitivity involving aspirin and other agents, including the NSAIDs, and they should not be given any NSAIDs.

Toxicity

An overdose of aspirin can have harmful effects and even cause death.

Symptoms. When the blood level of salicylates reaches a certain point, a toxic reaction, referred to as salicylism, occurs. It is characterized by tinnitus (ringing in the ears), headache, nausea, vomiting, dizziness, and dimness of vision. Hyperthermia and electrolyte imbalance can also occur. With higher blood levels, stimulation of respiration leads to hyperventilation, which produces respiratory alkalosis. Compensatory alkalosis results in renal loss of bicarbonate, sodium, and potassium. Both respiratory acidosis and metabolic acidosis ensue. The cause of death from aspirin poisoning is usually acidosis and electrolyte imbalance.

Prevention

> Toxicity prevention requires the use of childproof containers.

Children are the primary victims of accidental poisoning. The lethal dose of aspirin is greater than 500 mg/kg of body weight. The education of parents regarding the potential for poisoning and proper storage and childproof containers for over-the-counter (OTC) aspirin have significantly reduced accidental poisonings in children.

Treatment. Treatment of aspirin poisoning includes removing excess drug in the stomach by inducing emesis or administering activated charcoal to absorb the aspirin. Other symptoms are treated symptomatically. For example, hyperthermia is treated with cooling baths or "blankets," acidosis with sodium bicarbonate, hypokalemia with potassium, and hypoglycemia with intravenous (IV) glucose. Box 5.3 lists the patient instructions for aspirin.

Drug Interactions

The drug interactions of aspirin are listed in Table 5.1. Some of the more notable are briefly discussed in the following paragraphs.

Warfarin: The drug interaction between aspirin and warfarin can result in bleeding. Warfarin (WAR-far-in), an oral anticoagulant, is highly protein-bound. If aspirin is administered to a patient taking warfarin, it can displace the warfarin from its binding sites, thus increasing its anticoagulant effect. In addition, aspirin affects both platelets and the GI tract. Bleeding and hemorrhage may result from these interactions.

Probenecid: Aspirin interferes with the uricosuric effect of probenecid (proe-BEN-e-sid). Aspirin has been reported to precipitate an acute attack of gout. One should avoid giving aspirin to patients taking probenecid.

Methotrexate: Methotrexate (meth-oh-TREX-ate; MTX) is an antineoplastic drug used to treat certain kinds of cancer and autoimmune diseases (arthritis, psoriasis). Aspirin can displace MTX from its protein-binding sites and can also interfere with its clearance. The displacement and interference result in increased serum concentration and MTX toxicity such as bone marrow depression.

Sulfonylureas: Higher doses of salicylates (more than 2 g) may produce a hypoglycemic effect. One proposed mechanism involves the displacement of the sulfonylureas from their plasma protein–binding sites by aspirin. This hypoglycemic effect can also be observed with insulin.

Antihypertensives: Aspirin reduces the antihypertensive effect of many antihypertensives, including angiotensin-converting enzyme (ACE) inhibitors, β-blockers, and thiazide and loop diuretics. Several doses of aspirin over a few days are needed for this reduction to occur. Aspirin's effect on renal function, resulting in water and sodium retention, may contribute to this effect.

Uses

General uses. One use of aspirin is to provide analgesia for mild-to-moderate pain. It is the analgesic against which new analgesics are measured for efficacy. Its antipyretic effect is useful in the control of fever, but it should be avoided in children (Reye syndrome). Its antiinflammatory action is useful in the treatment of inflammatory conditions such as rheumatic fever and arthritis.

Low-dose aspirin therapy. Because of its effect on platelet aggregation (inhibition), aspirin is used to prevent unwanted clotting. Clinical trials have shown that daily use of aspirin as a secondary preventive measure can reduce all-cause mortality by 18% and myocardial infarctions by 30% in persons with known cardiovascular (CV) disease. Aspirin can be of benefit to persons who have already had a stroke, heart attack, angina, or peripheral vascular disease as well as those who have had angioplasty or bypass surgery. Low-dose aspirin therapy (75–325 mg) is recommended for these patients unless there are contraindications to therapy.

Patients experiencing a myocardial infarction are usually advised by emergency responders to chew one low-dose aspirin at the onset of symptoms. Patients should call 911 first and wait for their instructions before taking the aspirin tablet. The aspirin tablet can be administered once the emergency responder is present, in the ambulance, or in the emergency room. Again, this measure is indicated only in patients who do not have aspirin allergies, hypersensitivity, or other contraindications.

Aspirin can also be used as preventive therapy in persons who have not experienced a heart attack or stroke but are at increased risk for these events. The US Preventative Service Task Force recommends that men with no history of heart disease or stroke aged 45 to 79 years of age take a low-dose aspirin tablet each day to prevent myocardial infarction and that women with no history of heart attack or stroke aged 55 to 79 do the same to prevent stroke. However, the benefit of aspirin therapy must outweigh the risk of the many adverse effects associated with aspirin therapy, especially GI bleeding.

Doses and Preparations

The usual adult dose of aspirin for the treatment of pain or fever is 325 to 650 mg every 4 to 6 hours. The dose for arthritis is 3000 to 4000 mg/day in divided doses. For prevention of myocardial infarction, the dose is 75 to 325 mg/day. The dose for children greater than 12 years of age is 300 to 650 mg every 4 to 6 hours (not to exceed 4 g/day). However, aspirin should not be given to children under the age of 18 unless under the direct supervision of a doctor.

BOX 5.3 Patient Instructions for Use of Aspirin

- Take with a full glass of water.
- Take with food, milk, or an antacid to minimize gastrointestinal irritation.
- Do not use more than one nonsteroidal antiinflammatory drug (NSAID) concurrently.
- Do not take over-the-counter (OTC) analgesics with aspirin.
- Do not give to children younger than 18 years of age because of the risk of Reye syndrome.
- Aspirin use can prolong bleeding time.
- If the pain does not subside within 24 hours, call the dentist.

TABLE 5.2   Selected Over-the-Counter (OTC) Aspirin-Containing Products

	Aspirin		Ingredients	
Type of Aspirin	Selected Brand Name(s)	Amount of Aspirin (mg)	Other	Approximate Amount (mg)
Regular	Bayer	500, 325	None	
	St. Joseph	81	None	
	Bayer, low dose	81	None	
Enteric coated	Ecotrin	500, 325	None	
	Ecotrin, low dose	81	None	
Buffered tablets	Bayer Aspirin Plus	500	Buffered with calcium carbonate	Each tablet contains 140 mg of calcium
Combinations	Excedrin tablets	250	Caffeine	65
			Acetaminophen	250
	Anacin	400	Caffeine	32

Many types of preparations containing aspirin are available by prescription and OTC (Table 5.2). Some of these types are as follows:

Regular aspirin. Single-entity forms of aspirin include the commonly used 325-mg (5-grain) tablet and the 81-mg flavored children's tablet. Many brand name and generic products are available in all strengths.

Enteric-coated aspirin. Aspirin can be formulated with a coating that dissolves in the intestine rather than in the stomach. The advantage of such enteric-coated aspirin is that gastric symptoms are reduced. The disadvantage is that these products can be erratically absorbed, resulting in unreliable blood levels. The onset of action is too long to make them useful for acute dental pain. They have limited use in treatment of chronic arthritis when gastric irritation is a problem. They can be used when daily aspirin is used for clot prevention.

Combinations

With buffer. Although claimed to have fewer GI side effects, buffered tableted preparations have never been shown to do so. They are absorbed at a slightly quicker rate. The liquid buffered preparations do produce less GI irritation, but they contain sodium, which is relatively contraindicated in patients with high blood pressure.

With another analgesic. Aspirin can be combined with an opioid analgesic or acetaminophen. Caffeine is part of this combination. Mixing aspirin with an opioid can allow a decrease in the amount of the opioid in the product and therefore will reduce its side effects.

With sedatives. Adding a sedative to aspirin can make it more effective if anxiety is a substantial component of the pain. Prescribing a separate antianxiety agent would give the prescriber more control, however, and is preferred.

With caffeine. Caffeine potentiates the analgesic effect of aspirin and other analgesics. The addition of 130 mg of caffeine is equivalent to increasing the dose of the analgesic by one-third or more. Most proprietary preparations contain about half this much caffeine. (However, one can always take two tablets of most analgesics.)

Nonacetylated Salicylates
Common Agents

Sodium, choline, *magnesium* salicylate and salicylamide, and salsalate are other salicylates. These drugs do not interfere with platelet aggregation, are rarely associated with GI bleeding, and are well tolerated by persons with asthma. Also, there is no cross-sensitivity with aspirin. However, there are no well-controlled studies demonstrating the comparative efficacy of nonacetylated salicylates for treating chronic pain. Their efficacy as analgesic agents and the appropriate doses for analgesia must be determined. Magnesium is contraindicated in patients with renal disease, and sodium in those with CV disease. Salicylamide is a weak analgesic. Salsalate is made up of the combination of two SAs.

Diflunisal

Diflunisal (dye-FLOO-ni-sal; Dolobid) is a nonacetylated salicylate classified as an NSAID. Its peak action occurs 2 to 3 hours after ingestion, and its half-life is 8 to 12 hours in the normal patient. It is as effective as the other NSAIDs in the treatment of pain. Like other NSAIDs, diflunisal can be administered before a dental procedure to delay the onset of postsurgical pain. Because of its long half-life, it is dosed only two or three times daily. The general comments relating to the NSAIDs also apply to diflunisal. Its antipyretic effect is not clinically useful.

NONSTEROIDAL ANTIINFLAMMATORY DRUGS

NSAIDs have important applications in dentistry. Their mechanism of action and many of their pharmacologic effects and adverse reactions resemble those of aspirin. Many prescribers agree that the NSAIDs are the most useful drug group for the treatment of dental pain. The availability of OTC NSAIDs gives the dental health hygienist several products that can be recommended for purchase. Whether a prescription should be written for an NSAID or an OTC NSAID depends on appraisal of the patient's attitudes. The difference between a prescription and OTC NSAID is the strength. OTC products are usually lower doses than the prescription product.

Chemical Classification

NSAIDs are divided into several chemical derivatives: propionic acids, acetic acids, fenamates, pyrazolones, oxicams, and others. Table 5.3 lists selected NSAIDs by chemical classification, pharmacokinetic parameters, analgesic dose, and dosing interval.

Mechanism of Action

Like aspirin, NSAIDs inhibit the enzyme cyclooxygenase (COX, or prostaglandin synthase), resulting in a reduction in the formation of prostaglandin precursors and thromboxanes from arachidonic acid (see Fig. 5.3). Many of the actions and the adverse reactions of the NSAIDs result from their inhibition of prostaglandin synthesis.

All of the currently available NSAIDs inhibit both COX I and COX II. COX I is a widely distributed constitutive (present at all times) enzyme responsible for the adverse reactions of the NSAIDs, such as stomach problems, reduced renal function, fluid retention, and reduced platelet adhesiveness. COX II is an inducible enzyme that is synthesized only when inflammation occurs. COX II is also expressed in the kidneys, where it helps maintain perfusion.

Pharmacokinetics

Most NSAIDs peak in about 1 to 2 hours. The effect of food on absorption of the NSAIDs approved to treat pain—ibuprofen, the naproxens, and diflunisal—is to reduce the rate but not the extent of their absorption.

TABLE 5.3 Nonselective Nonsteroidal Antiinflammatory Drugs: Peak, Half-Life, and Analgesic and Maximum Doses

Drug Name(s)	Peak (h)	Half-Life (h)	Analgesic Dose (mg) and Interval	Maximum Daily Dose (mg)
Propionic Acid Derivatives				
Ibuprofen (generic, Motrin)	1–2	1.8–2.5	400 q4–6h	2400
Ibuprofen OTC (generic, Motrin, Advil)			200–400 q4–6h	1200
Flurbiprofen (generic, Ansaid)	1.5	5.7	100 q12	300
Fenoprofen (Nalfon)	1–2	2–3	200 q4–6h	3200
Naproxen (Naprosyn)	2–4	12–15	250 q6–8h or 500 q12h	1000
Naproxen sodium (Anaprox)	1–2	12–13	275 q6–8h or 550 q12h	1100
Naproxen sodium OTC (generic, Aleve)			220 q8–12h	660
Ketoprofen (Orudis)	0.5–2	2–4	50 q6 or 75 q8	300
Acetic Acid Derivatives				
Diclofenac (Cataflam)	1	1–3	50 q8–12	200
Etodolac (generic)	1–2	7.3	200–400 q6–8h	1000
Ketorolac (generic, Toradol)*	0.5–1	2.4–8.6	10 q4–6h (PO)	40
Nonacidic Agent				
Nabumetone (generic, Relafen)	3–6	(22.5–30)*	500 or 750 q8–12	2000
Fenamic Acid Derivatives				
Meclofenamate (generic, Meclomen)	0.5–1	2–3	50–100 q4	400
Mefenamic acid (generic, Ponstel)	2–4	2–4	500 stat, 250 q6h	1250
Salicylates				
Diflunisal (generic, Dolobid)†	2–3	8–12	500 q8–12h	1500
Oxicams				
Meloxicam (generic, Mobic)	5–10	15–20	7.5–15 qd	15

*For short-term (<5 days) treatment following the use of the parenteral form.
†Salicylate.
OTC, Over-the-counter; *stat,* immediately.

Oral antacids have no effect on absorption of the NSAIDs except for diflunisal (antacids reduce absorption). These agents are metabolized in the liver and excreted by the kidney. The half-lives of the individual agents are listed in Table 5.3.

Pharmacologic Effects

The analgesic, antipyretic, and antiinflammatory actions of the NSAIDs result from the same mechanism as aspirin's inhibition of prostaglandin synthesis, the inhibition of COX. NSAIDs are useful for treating dysmenorrhea (painful menstruation) because an excess of prostaglandins in the uterine wall produces painful contractions. In the treatment of gout, the action of the NSAIDs is related to their analgesic and antiinflammatory actions but is independent of their effect on serum uric acid.

Adverse Reactions

Gastrointestinal Effects

GI irritation, pain, and bleeding problems leading to tarry stools can occur with all NSAIDs. The prostaglandins stimulate the production of cytoprotective mucus that protects the stomach against gastric acid secretion. Prostaglandin inhibitors such as NSAIDs can interfere with the normal protective mechanisms in the stomach and increase acid secretion, causing symptoms or even an ulceration or perforation. A prostaglandin, misoprostol (mye-soe-PROST-ole) or prostaglandin E_2 (Cytotec, PGE_2), is available to prevent NSAID-induced ulcers.

Central Nervous System Effects

The dose-dependent CNS side effects of NSAIDs include sedation, dizziness, confusion, mental depression, headache, vertigo, and convulsions. Because of the CNS effects of the NSAIDs, patients taking them should be cautioned about driving an automobile. These agents are not addicting, tolerance does not develop, and no withdrawal syndrome can be induced.

Blood Clotting

The NSAIDs reversibly inhibit platelet aggregation because they inhibit thromboxane A_2 production. In contrast to that of aspirin, an NSAID's effect remains only as long as the drug is present in the blood: 1 day for ibuprofen, 4 days for naproxen, and 2 weeks for oxaprozin.

Cardiovascular Effects

There have been reports of an increased risk of serious CV events such as myocardial infarction and stroke in patients taking some NSAIDs. The risks appear to be highest with diclofenac and lowest with naproxen. The risk appears to increase with higher doses of celecoxib but otherwise appears to be similar to that with nonselective NSAIDs.

Renal Effects

All NSAIDs, including celecoxib, inhibit renal prostaglandins, decrease renal blood flow, cause fluid retention, and may cause hypertension and renal failure in some patients, especially the elderly. Renal effects of the NSAIDs include renal failure, cystitis, and an increased incidence of urinary tract infections. The NSAIDs have little effect on the patient with normal kidney function; however, in those with renal disease, decreases in both renal blood flow and glomerular filtration rate can occur. NSAIDs have precipitated renal insufficiency. In patients with decreased renal function, peripheral edema with fluid retention has been noted.

Oral Effects

Oral manifestations of NSAIDs reported include ulcerative stomatitis, gingival ulcerations, and dry mouth.

Other Effects

Other adverse effects associated with the NSAIDs are muscle weakness, ringing in the ears, hepatitis, hematologic problems, and blurred vision. Celecoxib has been associated with cholestatic jaundice, which may be related to sulfonamide allergy. Celecoxib is contraindicated in persons with sulfonamide allergies.

Hypersensitivity Reactions

Like aspirin, the NSAIDs can induce a wide range of hypersensitivity reactions, including hives or itching, angioneurotic edema, chills and fever, Stevens-Johnson syndrome, exfoliative dermatitis, and epidermal necrolysis. Anaphylactoid reactions including bronchospasm (wheezing) have been reported.

Pregnancy and Nursing Considerations

> NSAIDs contraindicated in pregnancy.

Like aspirin, the NSAIDs given late in pregnancy can prolong gestation, delay parturition, and produce dystocia or premature closure of the ductus arteriosus. The uterine prostaglandins are responsible for parturition and closure of the ductus arteriosus. Fenoprofen, ibuprofen, and naproxen have not been shown to be teratogenic in animal studies, Their use during pregnancy or lactation should only be considered after serious discussion between the patient and her practitioner regarding the potential for any adverse effects to the baby. Diflunisal, tolmetin, and mefenamic acid have been shown to be teratogenic in animals.

Ibuprofen has not been detected in breast milk, whereas fenoprofen and mefenamic acid are present in small quantities. Again, the risk versus benefit for these drugs during pregnancy or lactation should be discussed by the health care practitioner and their patient. Small amounts of both naproxen (1% of serum) and diflunisal (5% of serum) are excreted in breast milk.

Drug Interactions

The drug interactions of the NSAIDs are summarized in Table 5.4. Interactions for each NSAID continue to be under investigation for

TABLE 5.4 Selected Drug Interactions of the Nonsteroidal Antiinflammatory Drugs

Drug	Potential Outcome
Lithium	Increased effect of lithium
Methotrexate (MTX)	Increased effect of MTX leads to bone marrow toxicity
Diuretics	Reduced antihypertensive effect
Angiotensin-converting enzyme (ACE) inhibitors	Reduced antihypertensive effect
β-Blockers	Reduced antihypertensive effect
Digoxin	Increased digoxin effect

their clinical significance and presence. Lithium toxicity has been reported in patients taking lithium for bipolar affective disorders who also take NSAIDs. These agents may increase the effect of digoxin, a drug used for congestive heart failure. Digoxin's narrow therapeutic index is one reason for caution. NSAIDs have been shown to reduce the effect of agents used as antihypertensives, such as diuretics, ACE inhibitors, and β-blockers. Probenecid can raise serum levels of NSAIDs. These agents can increase the toxicity of cyclosporine and MTX. Before patients are given NSAIDs, drug interactions should be checked.

Contraindications and Cautions

The contraindications to and cautions for using an NSAID (Table 5.5) are related to their adverse reactions. Patients with asthma, CV or renal diseases with fluid retention, coagulopathies, peptic ulcer, and ulcerative colitis should be given NSAIDs cautiously if at all.

All NSAIDs have been associated with the development of acute kidney injury. This risk is higher in those patients who are hypovolemic, who have a viral illness, or who may be taking ACE inhibitors or angiotensin receptor blockers alone or in combination with diuretics. For this reason, renal function should be monitored in patients at risk for renal disease and NSAID use should be avoided in these patients.

All NSAIDs contain block box warnings for the following events:

Cardiovascular disease: All NSAIDs may increase the risk of serious CV thrombotic events, myocardial infarction, and stroke, all of which may be fatal. The risk may increase with a longer duration of use, and in patients with CV disease or risk factors for CV disease.

GI effects: All NSAIDs increase the risk for serious GI events, including bleeding, ulceration, and perforation of the stomach or intestine, which may be fatal. Severe GI events can occur at any time and without warning, and elderly patients are at a higher risk.

Patients also at higher risk for adverse reactions to NSAIDs include those with renal function impairment or a history of previous hypersensitivity to aspirin or other NSAIDs and geriatric patients, who are more prone to adverse hepatic or renal reactions. Box 5.4 lists the patient instructions for NSAIDs.

Precautions

Preexisting asthma. Patients with asthma may have aspirin hypersensitivity which can cause severe bronchospasm that can be fatal. Since cross-sensitivity between aspirin and NSAIDs have been reported, NSAIDs should not be used in patients with known aspirin hypersensitivity reaction. NSAIDs should be used with caution in persons with preexisting asthma.

Therapeutic Uses
Medical

Depending on the specific NSAID and the clinical trials that have been conducted, medical use of NSAIDs involves many conditions. Osteoarthritis, rheumatoid arthritis (RA), gouty arthritis, fever, dysmenorrhea, and pain are indications for the NSAIDs. Accepted unlabeled indications for which NSAIDs are often prescribed include bursitis and tendonitis.

Dental

NSAIDs are useful in the management of dental pain. Many studies that have compared the analgesic efficacy of the NSAIDs with that of the opioid analgesics find that they are equivalent in many clinical situations. For example, usual analgesic doses of NSAIDs have been shown to be as effective as 650 mg of aspirin or acetaminophen plus 60 mg of codeine and even as effective as the intermediate-strength opioid combinations (oxycodone plus aspirin or acetaminophen). In usual prescription doses, NSAIDs can be shown to be statistically significantly better than codeine alone, aspirin, acetaminophen, or placebo.

TABLE 5.5 Contraindications to and Cautions for the Use of Aspirin and Nonsteroidal Antiinflammatory Drugs (NSAIDs)

Drugs	Disease	Comments
Aspirin: small doses	Prevent clotting, heart disease	May use NSAIDs, continue aspirin
Aspirin: high doses	Rheumatic fever	Aspirin lowers blood level of NSAIDs
Lithium	Bipolar (manic) disorder	NSAIDs reduce lithium clearance, causing potential lithium toxicity
H₂ blockers Proton pump inhibitors	Peptic ulcer, gastroesophageal reflux disease	Gastric bleeding, esophagitis
Angiotensin-converting enzyme (ACE) inhibitors, Angiotensin receptor blockers (ARBs)	Renal disease	Can decrease kidney function, especially in the elderly
Diuretics	Renal disease	Can decrease kidney function, especially in the elderly, especially if added to ACE inhibitors and ARBs
Methotrexate (MTX)	Rheumatoid arthritis, psoriasis, cancer	Potentiates MTX toxicity, bone marrow suppression*
Vitamin K deficiency	Alcoholism, liver disease	Bleeding
Warfarin	Myocardial infarction, atrial fibrillation, prosthetic heart valve	Aspirin contraindicated; bleeding; use NSAIDs with caution; they increase the anticoagulant effect of warfarin
Factor VIII	Hemophilia	Gastric bleeding
Probenecid*	Gout	Probenecid inhibits excretion of NSAIDs
Colchicine	Gout	More gastrointestinal adverse reactions
Allopurinol	Gout	No contraindications
None	Pregnancy	Use should be avoided during pregnancy, especially the third trimester
None	Glucose-6-phosphate dehydrogenase (G6PD) deficiency	Hemolysis
None	Hypoprothrombinemia	Bleeding
Acute viral illness	Dehydration	Decreased renal function

*Once-a-week dosing as for autoimmune diseases can be used with caution.

BOX 5.4 Patient Instructions for Use of Nonsteroidal Antiinflammatory Drugs (NSAIDs)

- Take with a full glass of water.
- Take with food to minimize gastrointestinal irritation.
- Use caution with driving because of possible drowsiness or dizziness.
- Do not use aspirin concurrently with this NSAID.
- If pain does not subside within 24 hours, call the dentist.
- Do not take over-the-counter (OTC) analgesics with prescription NSAIDs.

All NSAIDs are equally efficacious at equianalgesic doses. Fig. 5.6 shows the pain relief over time of several commonly used analgesics. Their relative effectiveness is discussed in the following paragraphs.

Specific Nonsteroidal Antiinflammatory Drugs
Ibuprofen
Ibuprofen (eye-byoo-PRO-fen; Advil, Motrin), the oldest member of the NSAIDs, has the most clinical experience. It is rapidly absorbed orally, and food decreases its rate but not its extent of absorption; antacids have no effect. The half-life is about 2 hours. Its onset of action is about half an hour, and its duration of action is 4 to 6 hours. It undergoes hepatic metabolism and is excreted by the kidney. It is an effective analgesic and has been studied in many dental situations. Ibuprofen is the drug of choice for treatment of dental pain when an NSAID is indicated. Only in rare cases or if new information becomes available are other NSAIDs indicated. When a longer-acting agent is desired for patient convenience, the naproxens can be used.

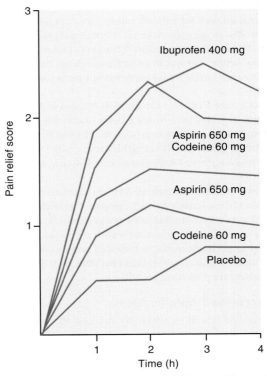

Fig. 5.6 Time-effect curves for placebo, codeine, aspirin, aspirin plus codeine, and ibuprofen. The mean pain relief scores are plotted against time in hours. (Adapted from Cooper SA, Engel J, Ladov M, Precheur H, Rosenheck A, Rauch D. Analgesic efficacy of an ibuprofen-codeine combination. *Pharmacotherapy.* 1982;2:162.)

The usual prescription analgesic dose of ibuprofen is 400 to 800 mg every 6 to 8 hours (maximum dose: 3200 mg/day) and the usual OTC analgesic dose is 200 to 400 mg every 4 to 6 hours (maximum dose: 1200 mg/day). The higher dosage range may have more antiinflammatory effects. Most studies can easily demonstrate that 400 mg of ibuprofen is better than any usual therapeutic dose of codeine.

Ibuprofen is available OTC in 200-mg tablets and by prescription in 400-, 600-, and 800-mg tablets. Side effects, such as CNS effects, are dose-dependent, so they occur more often at the higher end of the dosage range. Ibuprofen is also available OTC in suspension form for pediatric use and is often used for its fever-reducing effects.

Naproxen Sodium

> Drugs longer-acting than ibuprofen

Naproxen (na-PROX-en; Naprosyn), naproxen sodium (Anaprox), and naproxen sodium OTC (Aleve) are propionic acid NSAIDs that have slightly longer half-lives than ibuprofen and can be dosed on an 8- to 12-hour schedule. They should also be given with a loading dose (see Table 5.3). Aleve is dosed at 220 mg every 8 to 12 hours, not to exceed two tablets in the 8- to 12-hour period. The patient may take two tablets for the first dose for a total of three tablets in the first 24-hour time period. The pharmacologic effects, adverse reactions, and efficacy of naproxen are similar to those of ibuprofen. In addition to tablets, this product is available in suspension form. One should note that lithium blood levels rise when naproxen is given because it inhibits lithium clearance.

Other Nonsteroidal Antiinflammatory Drugs

Other NSAIDs (see Table 5.3), such as fenoprofen, ketorolac, and diflunisal, may be used for patients whose pain does not respond to either ibuprofen or naproxen sodium. Certain patients need an agent with which they are not familiar. "Shoppers" looking for scheduled drugs show better response to an unknown drug's name. Prescribing one of the new NSAIDs whose name has not yet become familiar may be effective.

Ketorolac (kee-TOE-role-ak; Toradol) is a newer NSAID. The use of this agent increased because it was being heavily advertised to dental professionals. It is equivalent in efficacy to the other NSAIDs; however, unlike other NSAIDs, it is also available parenterally. One should make sure that a new agent has some documented clinical advantage before it is prescribed.

Ketorolac is an NSAID indicated for the short-term (up to 5 days) management of moderately severe acute pain that requires analgesia at the opioid level. It is contraindicated as a prophylactic analgesic before any major surgery, when hemostasis is critical because of the increased risk of bleeding. Oral ketorolac is indicated only as continuation therapy to IV or intramuscular (IM) ketorolac (injectable must be used before the tablets are prescribed).

Cyclooxygenase II–Specific Agents

COX II-specific inhibitors selectively decrease the inflammatory effects of COX II while leaving the protective effects of COX I largely in place, leading to fewer adverse reactions than the older, nonselective NSAIDs. Celecoxib (Celebrex), a COX II-specific inhibitor, is indicated for arthritis. Celecoxib was thought to offer an advantage over nonselective NSAIDs because it was believed to be less irritating to the stomach. However, it has been found to be associated with a significantly higher incidence of serious GI adverse effects. Clinically, celecoxib is equivalent to nonselective NSAIDs. Because it offers no therapeutic advantage over nonselective NSAIDs it has no real use in dentistry.

ACETAMINOPHEN

Acetaminophen (a-seet-a-MEE-noe-fen) (paracetamol, *N*-acetyl *p*-aminophenol; Tylenol; APAP) is the only member of the *p*-aminophenols currently available for clinical use. Its exact mechanism and site of action are unknown. However, acetaminophen is thought to produce analgesia by elevating the pain threshold. Its potential mechanism of action may involve inhibiting the nitric oxide pathway, which is mediated by a variety of neurotransmitter receptors. Its antipyretic effects may be the result of inhibition of endogenous pyrogens on the heat-regulating centers of the brain by blockage of the formation and release of prostaglandins in the CNS.

Pharmacokinetics

Acetaminophen is rapidly and completely absorbed from the GI tract, achieving a peak plasma level in 1 to 3 hours. After therapeutic doses, it is excreted with a half-life of 1 to 4 hours. Acetaminophen is metabolized by the liver microsomal enzymes to the glucuronide conjugate, the sulfuric acid conjugate, and cysteine. When large doses are ingested, an intermediate metabolite is produced that is thought to be hepatotoxic and possibly nephrotoxic. Acetaminophen and aspirin are equally efficacious (kill the same degree of pain) and equally potent (same doses in milligrams needed for effect) as analgesics and antipyretics.

Pharmacologic Effects

> Alcoholics should avoid acetaminophen.

The analgesic and antipyretic effects of acetaminophen have approximately the same potency (on a milligram-for-milligram basis) as aspirin. This means that acetaminophen and aspirin are equally efficacious, and because virtually the same doses are used for each agent, they are equally potent. However, acetaminophen does not possess any clinically significant antiinflammatory effect; therefore it is less useful in the treatment of arthritis or any other type of inflammatory pain. Differences in degree of prostaglandin synthesis inhibition at different sites may account for this difference in action.

Therapeutic doses of acetaminophen have no effect on the CV or respiratory system. In contrast to aspirin, acetaminophen does not produce gastric bleeding or affect platelet adhesiveness or uric acid excretion.

Adverse Reactions

The principal toxic effects of acetaminophen are hepatic necrosis and nephrotoxicity.

Hepatic Effects

The toxic metabolite of acetaminophen that contributes to hepatic necrosis is *N*-acetyl-*p*-benzoquinoneimine. The minimum toxic dose of acetaminophen for a single ingestion is 7.5 to 10 g in adults and 150 mg/kg in children. The acute ingestion of more than 12 g of acetaminophen in single ingestion is considered a toxic dose and can pose a high risk for liver damage. In children, the acute ingestion of 250 mg/kg poses a high risk for liver damage, and the acute ingestion of 350 mg/kg can cause severe hepatotoxicity if not immediately treated. Children are more likely to experience accidental overdose with acetaminophen. This occurs because the wrong dose form is used (e.g., infant drops are given to older children or adult doses are given to children). Infant drops are concentrated, and doses for toddlers to 11-year-old children are not the same as those for infants. Parents may give the infant liquid to the older child and pour it in the measuring cup, not realizing that this would constitute an overdose. Also, normal doses over extended periods can lead to toxicity. Symptoms during the first 2 days after intoxication are minor. Nausea, vomiting, anorexia, and abdominal pain may occur. Liver injury becomes manifest on the second to third day, with alterations in plasma enzyme levels (elevations of transaminase and lactic hydrogenase), elevated bilirubin value, and prolongation of prothrombin time. Hepatotoxicity may progress to encephalopathy, coma, and death. If the patient recovers, no residual hepatic abnormalities persist. Patients with hepatic disease, such as those with a history of hepatitis, should avoid acetaminophen.

The FDA has recommended tighter dose controls and warnings with acetaminophen use, in the hope of preventing even more cases of accidental liver toxicity. The FDA advisory committee is recommending that people receive no more than 650 mg (2 regular-strength tablets [325 mg each] every 4 to 6 hours, and no more than 10 tablets in 1 day (24-hour time period) or 2 extra-strength tablets (500 mg or 650 mg each) every 6 hours, and no more than 6 tablets in 1 day. Doses of 1000 mg four times per day can, after only 1 or 2 days, lead to liver toxicity. This change would include decreasing the amount of acetaminophen that is often used in combination with opioid analgesics.

Alcohol stimulates the oxidizing enzymes that metabolize acetaminophen to its toxic metabolite. Depending on the amount of alcoholic beverages ingested, the maximum dose of acetaminophen varies. The normal maximum dose of acetaminophen (4 g) may be used in patients who usually do not drink. The dose should be restricted to 2 g if a patient is a moderate drinker (less than three alcohol beverages daily). People who consume three or more alcohol beverages every day should not take acetaminophen (Table 5.6).

Treatment of toxicity. The treatment of acetaminophen overdose toxicity should begin with gastric lavage if the drug has recently been ingested. The administration of activated charcoal should follow. The administration of sulfhydryl groups in the form of oral *N*-acetylcysteine reduces or even prevents liver damage if given soon enough after ingestion.

Nephrotoxicity

Nephrotoxicity has been associated with long-term consumption of acetaminophen. The primary lesion appears to be a papillary necrosis with secondary interstitial nephritis. Although no single agent can be identified, prolonged consumption of analgesics can lead to kidney disease. Because analgesics are used in dental practice on a short-term basis, the possibility of nephrotoxicity does not present a significant problem in dental therapy. Concurrent chronic use of the combination of acetaminophen and aspirin or NSAIDs increases the risk of analgesic nephropathy, renal papillary necrosis, end-stage renal disease, and cancer of the kidney or urinary bladder.

Skin Reactions

Acetaminophen now carries a safety warning because of the risk of three rare but potentially fatal skin reactions: Stevens-Johnson syndrome, toxic epidermal necrolysis, and acute generalized exanthematous pustulosis. This warning advises that anyone who experiences a skin reaction, such as rash or blister, while taking acetaminophen should stop taking it and seek immediate medical care. This warning was made on the basis of a review of the medical literature and reports of adverse reactions to the FDA Adverse Event Reporting System database.

Drug Interactions

Acetaminophen is remarkably free of drug interactions at its usual therapeutic doses. The hepatotoxicity of acetaminophen can be potentiated by administration of agents that induce hepatic microsomal enzymes, such as barbiturates, carbamazepine, phenytoin, and rifampin. Long-term ingestion of large doses of alcohol can increase the toxicity of acetaminophen.

Uses

Acetaminophen is used as an analgesic and antipyretic. It is especially useful in patients who have aspirin hypersensitivity or in whom aspirin-induced gastric irritation would present a problem. In young children, the use of acetaminophen as an antipyretic has replaced that of aspirin because of aspirin's association with Reye syndrome. It is not known to what degree the long-term use of therapeutic doses of acetaminophen might produce renal lesions. It has a greater propensity for causing hepatic necrosis when a large acute dose (overdose) is ingested. Box 5.5 lists the patient instructions for acetaminophen.

Doses and Preparations

Acetaminophen is available in many different dose forms. The usual adult dose is two 325-mg (regular-strength) tablets every 4 to 6 hours, two 650-mg (extra-strength) tablets every 6 hours, or two 500 mg caplets (extra-strength) every 6 hours. No more than 10 regular-strength tablets or 6 extra-strength tablets should be ingested by adults in 24 hours. Various suspensions and meltaway and chewable tablets that are convenient for administration to children are available. Acetaminophen infant and children's dosage forms have been reformulated so that both are available in an oral suspension in a concentration of 160 mg/5 mL (per teaspoon). This was done in an effort to reduce the incidence of overdose. The infant suspension comes with a calibrated syringe, and the oral suspension with a calibrated measuring cup. The infant suspension should be given only on the advice of the child's prescribing practitioner. The children's oral suspension is for those children older than 2 years. The meltaway tablets are now available only as 60-mg tablets (junior-strength for children 6–11 years of age) in order to avoid confusion. Acetaminophen should not be administered to a child more than five times in 24 hours. The dosing of acetaminophen in children can be determined using Table 5.7.

TABLE 5.6 Maximum Acetaminophen (APAP) Dose Related to Alcohol Use	
Alcohol Habitually Consumed (number of drinks per day)	Maximum Daily Dose of APAP
None	4 g
≥2 oz	<3 g
≥3 oz	None, consult with your physician.

BOX 5.5   Patient Instructions for Use of Acetaminophen

- Follow the specific directions regarding the dose of acetaminophen.
- Do not increase the dose or take more than is recommended in a 24-hour period because of the risk of liver toxicity.
- Give children the correct dose form and dose because of the risk of liver toxicity.
- If the pain does not subside within 24 hours, call the dentist.

TABLE 5.7 Dosing Chart for Pediatric Acetaminophen

Weight (lb)	Age (yr)	Milligrams	Suspension* 160 mg/5 mL (tsp)
24	<2	Consult	Consult with a physician
24–35	2–3	160	5 mL (1 tsp)
36–47	4–5	240	7.5 mL (1.5 tsp)
48–59	6–8	320	10 mL (2 tsp)
60–71	9–10	400	12.5 mL (2.5 tsp)
72–95	11	480	15 mL (3 tsp)

*CAUTION: Preparations with different concentrations are available; number of teaspoons given only for this concentration; infants' concentrated drops use much less volume.
Obtain the child's weight in pounds; check weight column and determine applicable row; read the dose (mg) column to determine dose; identify preparation parent has or will purchase; determine the volume or number of tablets needed for the dose and product.

DRUGS USED TO TREAT GOUT

Gout is an inherited disease occurring primarily in men, with an on-set that usually involves one joint, often the big toe or knee. Both hyperuricemia and urate crystals, or tophi, may be found in the joints or other tissues. The excess uric acid may be the result of excessive production or reduced excretion of uric acid (two types of gout). The disease responds to colchicine.

Both the NSAIDs and colchicine are used to treat acute attacks of gout. Other agents, such as probenecid and allopurinol (al-oh-PURE-i-nole), are available to prevent gout. These are briefly mentioned here although they are not analgesics per se.

Colchicine

Colchicine (KOL-chi-seen) has only one indication: the treatment of an acute attack of gout. It is so specific in its action on gouty attacks that it is sometimes used to diagnose the disease. Colchicine is taken hourly at the onset of the attack or until side effects, such as nausea and vomiting, are intolerable. Its mechanism is complex, but it appears to inhibit the chemotactic property of leukocytosis and to interfere with the inflammatory response to urate crystals. Colchicine possesses many side effects, but GI toxicity—including nausea, vomiting, and diarrhea—occurs often (in up to 80% of people). Bone marrow depression and hypersensitivity have also been reported.

Febuxostat

Febuxostat (Uloric) is a xanthine oxidase inhibitor that reduces the amount of uric acid in the body. It is used to treat chronic gout and hyperuricemia. Side effects include an initial flareup of gout when first starting the drug, nausea, diarrhea, arthralgias, headache, rash, and increased hepatic serum enzyme levels. It should not be used with azathioprine or 6-mercaptopurine. There have been reports of heart attack and stroke during clinical trials with febuxostat.

Allopurinol

Allopurinol (Zyloprim) is a xanthine oxidase inhibitor that inhibits the synthesis of uric acid. It is used to prevent the formation of excessive uric acid. It is also used in patients undergoing either chemotherapy or irradiation for malignancy because the death of many cells causes a release of large amounts of uric acid precursors. The side effects associated with allopurinol include hepatotoxicity of a hypersensitivity type. If a pruritic rash should occur, the drug should be discontinued promptly because fatalities have been reported in patients with this reaction. This drug is not indicated for asymptomatic hyperuricemia.

Probenecid

The other approach to the prevention of gout is to increase the excretion of uric acid by the administration of a uricosuric agent such as probenecid (Benemid). By blocking the tubular reabsorption of filtered urate, probenecid prevents new tophi from forming and mobilizes those present. Increasing frequency or severity of acute gouty attacks is an indication for administration of a uricosuric agent.

GI side effects and hypersensitivity may occur with probenecid use. Headaches and sore gums have also been reported. Concurrent administration of aspirin can interfere with the uricosuric action of probenecid. Diabetic tests using the copper sulfate urine test (Clinitest) may have false-positive results. Occasionally probenecid and colchicine are combined, with the colchicine preventing acute attacks and the probenecid enhancing the excretion of uric acid. Probably a more rational approach is to administer each drug separately as needed each day. Maintenance of adequate urinary output (2L per day) is important to minimize the precipitation of uric acid in the urinary tract.

Probenecid increases the plasma levels of NSAIDs and penicillin. In the latter case, this effect can be used therapeutically (see discussion of penicillin in Chapter 7). For the prevention of acute gout, either probenecid or allopurinol can be used. Acute gout is normally treated with NSAIDs and colchicine.

Other Drugs

For mild-to-moderate pain associated with gout, the drug of choice is either acetaminophen or aspirin in adults. Aspirin provides an antiinflammatory effect but is contraindicated in children and adolescents. If both aspirin and acetaminophen provide inadequate pain relief, then ibuprofen can be used. Its analgesic efficacy parallels that of many products combining nonopioids with opioids, such as aspirin with codeine (Empirin #3).

DRUGS USED TO TREAT ARTHRITIS

RA is an autoimmune disorder characterized by chronic inflammation of the body's joints, including the hands and feet. It affects joint linings, causing painful inflammation and swelling. Over time, this can lead to bone erosion and joint deformity. NSAIDs are often prescribed first for treating RA because they can treat join inflammation. However, NSAIDs only reduce the pain associated with RA and do not slow disease progression. The more common side effects of these drugs are GI and include stomach upset, nausea, vomiting, and diarrhea.

Disease-Modifying Antirheumatic Drugs

Disease-modifying antirheumatic drugs (DMARDs) slow and can stop the progression of RA. These drugs work by suppressing the body's overactive immune and inflammatory systems thereby slowing disease progression.

Immunosuppressives. Immunosuppressive drugs interfere with the formation of immune cells by damaging the RNA and DNA necessary for cell replication. They may also block immune system response to autoantibodies. The most commonly used DMARDs include azathioprine (Imuran), methotrexate, cyclophosphamide, auranofin (Ridaura), hydroxychloroquine (Plaquenil), leflunomide (Arava), and sulfasalazine (Azulfidine). DMARDs target the immune system, which puts the patient at a higher risk for developing infections.

Tumor Necrosis Factor (TNF)-α Inhibitors. TFN is a cytokine that is released by cells when body senses a foreign invader. High levels of TFN are found in the synovial fluid of persons with RA. TNF-α inhibitors are genetically engineered drugs that block the inflammatory process associated with the release of high concentrations of TNF-α. These drugs are referred to as monoclonal antibodies and include adalimumab (Humira), certolizumab (Cimzia), golimumab (Simponi), and infliximab (Remicade). Etanercept (Enbrel) is a fusion protein that inhibits TNF-α. All TNF-α inhibitors increase the risk for opportunistic infections including tuberculosis and fungal infections.

Biologic Response Modifiers

Biologic response modifiers work by inhibiting or modifying the body's immune system response. They inhibit the release of cells that mobilize to attack healthy cells that they recognize as a harmful invaders and inhibit the release of cytokines, leukocytes, B cells, and T cells. Rituximab (Rituxan) is a monoclonal antibody that reduces circulating B cells and tocilizumab (Actemra) inhibits interleukin-6. Both reduce inflammation by reducing mediators of the inflammatory response. Abatacept (Orencia) is a fusion protein that also inhibits TNF-α and works by blocking T-cell activation. Tofacitinib (Xeljanz) is a Janus kinase inhibitor (JAK). These drugs are also associated with an increased risk for infection.

DENTAL HYGIENE CONSIDERATIONS

- If nonopioid analgesics are necessary, the dental hygienist should conduct a thorough medication/health history in order to determine whether the patient has any contraindications to these drugs or risks potential drug interactions.
- Information regarding salicylates, NSAIDs, and acetaminophen should include warnings to not exceed the manufacturer's recommended daily dose over a 24-hour period.
- *The dental hygienist should encourage patients to check the OTC labels for any overlapping ingredients.* Often, these products contain ibuprofen, aspirin, acetaminophen, or any combination of the three with antihistamines and decongestants.
- The dental hygienist should also be aware of the fact that many opioid analgesics are combined with nonopioid analgesics. Remind the patient to not supplement with an OTC analgesic if a combination nonopioid/opioid analgesic is prescribed.
- Warnings about significant side effects associated with OTC nonopioid analgesics (such as bleeding) should be given to the patient along with instructions to call the dental practice if an adverse reaction occurs.
- NSAIDs should be avoided in persons with asthma.
- If patients complain of GI adverse effects, they may require a semisupine chair position during dental treatment.
- Review the information in Boxes 5.3–5.5.
- Patients taking DMARDs and biologic response modifiers should be carefully assessed for signs of infection since these drugs weaken the immune system.

ACADEMIC SKILLS ASSESSMENT

1. What is the rationale for using acetaminophen in a patient with an ulcer?
2. What dose and duration of therapy should be recommended for an adult male patient?
3. What are the adverse reactions to acetaminophen?
4. Are nephrotoxicity and hepatotoxicity associated only with toxic doses of acetaminophen?
5. What would increase the risk of development of nephrotoxicity with acetaminophen?
6. What are the pharmacologic effects of acetaminophen?
7. Compare and contrast acetaminophen with aspirin in terms of pharmacologic and therapeutic effects.
8. Does acetaminophen have any potential drug interactions? If so, what are they and how can they be avoided?
9. Are there any dental concerns associated with taking one baby aspirin each day?
10. Should a patient taking high blood pressure medication take a drug like ibuprofen? Why or why not?
11. Compare and contrast the OTC NSAIDs.
12. When would a prescription NSAID be appropriate?
13. Are there interactions between NSAIDs and antihypertensive drugs?
14. The dentist recommends a short course of OTC ibuprofen. What should a patient be told about this drug?
15. Can aspirin be used in children less than age 18? Why or why not?
16. Why is it especially important to use the correct dose form of acetaminophen in children?

CLINICAL CASE STUDY

James Smith, 45 years old, is new to your practice. This is your first meeting with him, and you would like to ask him some questions regarding his medication/health history. During the course of your conversation you learn that he has a history of coronary heart disease and is currently taking a baby aspirin each day. He takes acetaminophen for general aches and pains. He also likes to have a glass of wine with dinner each night and does not mind a few beers when he is watching football. During the course of his examination you and the dentist find two cavities, which are filled that day. Mr. Smith is experiencing some mild pain after the procedure.

1. What is the rationale for using acetaminophen instead of an NSAID to treat Mr. Smith's pain?
2. What dose and duration of therapy should be recommended for Mr. Smith?
3. At what doses does hepatotoxicity occur with acetaminophen?
4. How can Mr. Smith avoid acetaminophen toxicity?
5. Compare and contrast acetaminophen to aspirin in terms of pharmacology, adverse effects, and therapeutic effects.
6. What is the role of aspirin in the prevention of heart attack or stroke?
7. Are any dental concerns associated with low-dose aspirin therapy?
8. Can Mr. Smith take a drug like ibuprofen?
9. What should be said to Mr. Smith during a counseling session regarding acetaminophen?

Opioid (Narcotic) Analgesics and Antagonists

http://evolve.elsevier.com/Haveles/pharmacology

LEARNING OBJECTIVES

1. Explain the classification, mechanism of action, and pharmacokinetics of opioids.
2. List and describe the pharmacologic effects and potential adverse reactions of opioids.
3. Discuss the addiction potential of opioids, including treatment.
4. Name and explain the analgesic actions of the most common opioid agonists.
5. Discuss the actions of and provide examples of the mixed opioids.
6. Summarize the mechanism of action and adverse reactions of tramadol.
7. Apply the use of opioids to dentistry.

The opioid analgesics are often used to manage dental pain in patients in whom nonsteroidal antiinflammatory drugs (NSAIDs) are contraindicated. The dental hygienist and the dentist should be aware of the opioid groups, side effects, relative potency, and proper place in the management of dental pain.

HISTORY

Opium is the dried juice from the unripe seed capsules of the opium poppy. As early as 4000 BC, many cultures had recognized the euphoric effect of the poppy plant. In the early 1800s, morphine and codeine were isolated from opium. Until about 1920, patent medicines (medicines whose efficacy and safety were questionable) containing opium were promoted for numerous uses. When these agents, used orally, became unlawful, narcotic (opioid) abuse by injection began and has continued until the present.

CLASSIFICATION

The clinically useful opioids may be divided in several different ways. One way is by their mechanism of action at the receptor sites: agonists, mixed opioids, and antagonists. Table 6.1 shows the classifications.

MECHANISM OF ACTION

> Important opioid receptors are mu (μ), kappa (κ), and delta (δ).

The opioids bind to receptors located in both the central nervous system (CNS) and the spinal cord, producing an altered perception of reaction to pain. Receptors that mediate specific pharmacologic effects and adverse reactions are stimulated to varying degrees by individual opioids.

The discovery of three groups of endogenous substances with opioid-like action, the enkephalins, endorphins, and dynorphins, has helped explain the presence of these receptors. These naturally occurring peptides possess analgesic action and have addiction potential. They probably function as neurotransmitters, but their exact function has not been elucidated. They may be involved in the analgesic action of a placebo and the enhancement of well-being that occurs with running (an increase in β-endorphins).

Table 6.2 describes the pharmacologic effects of selected opioid receptors and the effect of some opioids on these receptors. Opioids may be complete agonists, partial agonists, agonist-antagonists, or antagonists. The three opioid receptors that have been characterized in more detail and that are stimulated by the opioids are the mu (μ), kappa (κ), and delta (δ) receptors. Differences in affinity for and action of different opioids in tolerance to pain might even be the result of variations in the endogenous levels of the neurotransmitters. Differences in affinity for and action of different opioids at these and other specific receptors explain some of the distinctions among the different opioids' adverse reactions. For example, stimulation of μ-receptors produces analgesia. The κ-receptor is responsible for dysphoria. Pentazocine, a κ-receptor agonist, produces dysphoria; morphine has little effect on the κ-receptor and causes less dysphoria than pentazocine. Naloxone is an antagonist at the three receptor sites (Fig. 6.1). Other opioid receptors include sigma (σ) and epsilon (ε). The stimulation of σ-receptors is associated with autonomic stimulation, dysphoria, hallucinations, nightmares, and anxiety. It is thought that the stimulation of ε-receptors may result in analgesia. More opioid receptors are sure to be identified and characterized. As more subreceptor types are elucidated, it will be possible to further separate beneficial (analgesic) effects of the opioids from their side effects (e.g., respiratory depression, constipation, and drug dependence).

PHARMACOKINETICS

> First-pass metabolism reduces bioavailability.

ADME, which is an acronym formed from the first letters of the components of drug handling, refers to absorption, distribution, metabolism, and excretion:

Absorption: Most opioid analgesic agents are absorbed well when taken orally; absorption occurs from the lungs and from the nasal and oral mucosa. Absorption occurs through the mucous membranes of the nose and the intact skin.

TABLE 6.1 Classification of the Opioids by Receptor Action

Group	Subgroup	Example
Agonists		Morphine, codeine
Mixed opioids	Agonist antagonists	Pentazocine
	Partial agonists	Buprenorphine
Antagonists		Naloxone

TABLE 6.2 Opioid Receptors, Effects, and Stimulation by Various Opioids

	μ (mu)	δ (Delta)	κ (Kappa)
Effects	Supraspinal and spinal analgesia, sedation, miosis (pruritus) respiratory depression, euphoria, physical dependence, constipation	Analgesia (emotion, seizures)	Analgesia (spinal, supraspinal), sedation, miosis (micturition, diuresis), dysphoria
Opioid Agonists			
Morphine	Ag	wk Ag	wk Ag
Codeine	wk Ag	wk Ag	
Fentanyl	Ag	Ag	Ag
Mixed Opioids			
Pentazocine	wk Ant, pAg		Ag
Buprenorphine	pAg		Ant
Butorphanol	wk pAg		Ag
Nalbuphine	Ant		Ag
Dezocine	pAnt		Ag
Opioid Antagonists			
Naloxone	Ant	wk Ant	Ant
Nalmefene	Ant	?Ant	?Ant
Naltrexone	Ant	?Ant	?Ant

Ag, Agonist; *Ant,* competitive antagonist; *pAg,* partial agonist; *pAnt,* partial antagonist; *wk,* weak; *?,* unknown.

Distribution: After absorption, the opioids undergo variable first-pass metabolism in the liver or intestinal cell wall, reducing their bioavailability. The opioids are bound to plasma proteins to varying degrees and distributed throughout the body.

Metabolism: The major route of metabolism for the opioids is conjugation with glucuronic acid in the liver. Given orally, most opioids have a similar duration of action for analgesia—4 to 6 hours.

Excretion: Metabolized opioids are excreted by glomerular filtration as their metabolites. The metabolites and the unchanged drug are excreted in the urine.

The dosing intervals and usual doses of some opioids are listed in Table 6.3. In general, onset occurs within 1 hour and duration necessitates dosing every 4 to 6 hours.

PHARMACOLOGIC EFFECTS

Although the pharmacologic effects and adverse reactions of the opioids are closely related, they are discussed separately. A pharmacologic effect may also be an adverse reaction, depending on the clinical use of the agent. In general, the severity of the side effects is proportional to the agent's efficacy (strength).

Analgesia

Efficacy is variable among opioids.

The opioid analgesics provide varying degrees of analgesia, depending on the strength of the agent. Fig. 6.2 shows the relative analgesic efficacies of selected opioids. Morphine is the opioid agonist by which other opioids are measured. The strongest opioids can reduce even the most severe pain; the weaker agents mixed with nonopioids are equivalent to the NSAIDs in their ability to relieve pain; and the analgesic potency of the weakest agent (codeine) is low (see Table 6.3).

Codeine raises the pain threshold and affects the cerebral cortex to depress the reaction to pain. Both μ-receptors and κ-receptors are involved in producing analgesia. The opioids alter the patient's reaction to painful stimuli, possibly by altering the release of certain central neurotransmitters.

Sedation and Euphoria

In the usual therapeutic doses, the opioid analgesics generally produce sedation by κ-receptor stimulation, which may potentiate their analgesic effect and relieve anxiety. This effect is additive with other CNS depressants such as alcohol. With larger doses, or if the pain is suddenly removed, euphoria can result. CNS excitation rarely occurs.

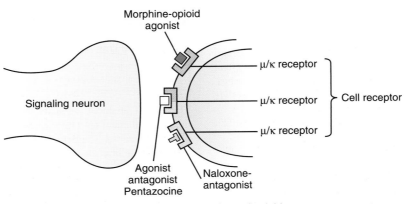

Fig. 6.1 Receptor actions of opioids.

TABLE 6.3   Selected Opioid Analgesics by Efficacy, Dosing Interval, Usual Doses, and Schedule

Drug Name	Dosing Interval (hr)	Usual Dose (PO, mg)*	Comments	Schedule for Controlled Substances
Strongest				
Morphine	4	10–30	Standard agent; prototype	II
Methadone (Dolophine)	8–12	2.5–10	Used PO for "methadone maintenance"	II
Meperidine (Demerol)	3–4	50	Abused by professionals	II
Hydromorphone (Dilaudid)	6–8	2	Most potent on an mg-for-mg basis	II
Intermediate in Strength				
Oxycodone (in Percodan, Percocet, Tylox, Roxiprin, Roxicet)	4–6	5–15	Popular with addicts "shopping" for opioids	II
Pentazocine (in Talwin NX)	3–4	50–100	Has antagonist properties	IV
Weakest				
Hydrocodone (in Vicodin, Lortab, Lorcet)	4–6	5–10	—	II
Codeine (in Tylenol #3, Empirin #3)	4–6	15–60	#2 = 15 mg; #3 = 30 mg; #4 = 60 mg	III
Dihydrocodeine (in Synalgos-DC)	4–6	30	16 mg per dose	III

*Average dose.
HCl, Hydrochloride; *PO,* by mouth.

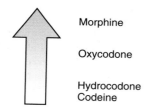

Morphine

Oxycodone

Hydrocodone
Codeine

Fig. 6.2 Comparing strengths of opioids. Opioids vary in efficacy (maximal effect attained) from codeine (low) to morphine (high).

Cough Suppression

The opioids exert their antitussive action by depressing the cough center, located in the medulla. The dose that produces the antitussive effect is much lower than that required for analgesia, so the least potent agents are effective (e.g., codeine). Related compounds, such as dextromethorphan, are often used as antitussives.

Gastrointestinal Effects

The opioids increase the smooth muscle tone of the intestinal tract and markedly decrease its propulsive contractions and motility. This effect has made opioids useful in the symptomatic treatment of diarrhea. Opioid-like agents without analgesic properties, such as diphenoxylate (in Lomotil), are used to treat diarrhea.

ADVERSE REACTIONS

Unlike the adverse reactions to many other drugs, the reactions to the opioids are not related to a direct damaging effect on hepatic, renal, or hematologic tissues but instead are an extension of their pharmacologic effects. Like the pharmacologic effects, the adverse reactions to the

TABLE 6.4   Contraindications to and Cautions for the Use of Opioids

Condition	Comment
Alcoholism or addiction	Greater potential for abuse
Head injury	Can increase intracranial pressure
Chronic pain	Addiction potential limits (e.g., temporomandibular disease) duration
Respiratory disease	Respiratory depression can occur
Pregnancy	Respiratory depression near term (fetus)
Nursing	No problem: watch infant
Nausea	Additive nausea
Constipation	Exacerbates or produces constipation

opioid analgesics are proportional to their analgesic strength. Table 6.4 lists contraindications to and cautions for the use of opioids.

Respiratory Depression

> Not a problem with usual doses in normal patients.

The opioid analgesic agonists depress the respiratory center in a dose-related manner. This depression is usually the cause of death with an overdose. The depression is related to a decrease in the sensitivity of the brainstem to carbon dioxide. Both the rate and depth of breathing are reduced. In elderly or debilitated patients, the usual therapeutic dose of morphine can significantly decrease pulmonary ventilation. Reduced ventilation produces vasodilation, which results in an increase in intracranial pressure. Opioids should not be used in patients with head injuries. Opioids may also mask CNS diagnostic symptoms. Patients with hyperthyroidism are more tolerant of the depression, whereas patients with hypothyroidism are more sensitive to it. Children less than 12 years of age and children less than 18 years of age post-tonsillectomy or -adenoidectomy should not receive codeine or tramadol because of the increased risk for respiratory depression.

Nausea and Emesis

Analgesic doses of opioid analgesics often cause nausea and vomiting. This is the result of their direct stimulation of the chemoreceptor trigger zone (CTZ), located in the medulla. This side effect is reduced if the patient does not ambulate. Administration of repeated, regular doses of an opioid can prevent vomiting by depressing the vomiting center (VC), another area in the CNS distinct from the CTZ.

Constipation

The opioids produce constipation by causing a tonic contraction of the gastrointestinal tract. Small doses of even weak opioids often have this effect, and their duration outlasts their analgesic effect. Even with continued administration, tolerance does not develop to this effect.

Miosis

The opioid analgesics cause miosis, an important sign (pinpoint pupils) in diagnosing an opioid overdose or identifying an addict. Tolerance does not develop to this effect.

Urinary Retention

The opioids increase the smooth muscle tone in the urinary tract, thereby causing urinary retention. They also have an antidiuretic effect through stimulation of the release of antidiuretic hormone (ADH) from the pituitary gland. This reaction may pose a problem in patients with prostatic hypertrophy.

Central Nervous System Effects

Occasionally, opioids may produce CNS stimulation, exhibited as anxiety, restlessness, or nervousness. Dysphoria can also occur from the opioids.

Cardiovascular Effects

The opioids may depress the vasomotor center and stimulate the vagus nerve. With high doses, postural hypotension, bradycardia, and even syncope may result.

Biliary Tract Constriction

In high doses, the opioids may constrict the biliary duct, resulting in biliary colic (pain associated with gallstones). This effect is important in patients passing gallstones who are being treated with opioids.

Histamine Release

Because the opioids can stimulate the release of histamine, itching and urticaria can result from their administration. This effect can occur at the site of intramuscular injection or at remote sites (e.g., itchy nose).

Pregnancy and Nursing Considerations

Opioids have not been shown to be teratogenic, although they may prolong labor or depress fetal respiration if given near term. The infant born to a mother using high-dose opioids, such as an addict, can have marked depressed respiration and experience withdrawal symptoms. The amount of opioid excreted in the mother's milk when therapeutic doses are given to the mother would pose no problem to the normal infant. Morphine and codeine are classified as US Food and Drug Administration (FDA) pregnancy category C. Acetaminophen is a pregnancy category B drug. Caution is urged because acetaminophen is often combined with opioid analgesics.

Addiction

Opioid addiction is a disease of the brain that involves both a physical dependence and a psychologic dependence on the drug. The two major signs of opioid addiction are cravings—an intense and overwhelming desire for the drug—and a loss of control of the ability to stop using the drug or to control the amount, which leads to a total loss of control. Both signs adversely affect the person's life. Long-term administration of opioid analgesics can lead to tolerance, habituation, and dependence. Tolerance is normally not a problem for those who take opioid analgesics for no more than 1 to 3 days, as is the case in managing dental-related pain. Because the duration of use in dentistry is usually short, addiction does not often pose a problem for the dentist. NSAIDs should be used to control dental pain in the addict.

The degree of addiction potential of an opioid is proportional to its analgesic strength. This fact limits the usefulness of the strongest of these agents. It also depends on the drug's ability to produce euphoria and reduce anxiety. Dependence is also related to the length of administration. An addict develops tolerance to the effects of the opioids, except for miosis and constipation. The rate of development of tolerance is related to the strength of the opioid and its frequency of use.

Overdose

The major symptom of opioid overdose is respiratory depression. In addition to pinpoint pupils and coma, this symptom is characteristic of opioid overdose. Opioid overdose is treated with an antagonist, naloxone, discussed later in this chapter.

Withdrawal

After abrupt discontinuation of an opioid, a withdrawal syndrome occurs. The symptoms include yawning, lacrimation, perspiration, rhinorrhea, gooseflesh, or goosebumps ("cold turkey"), irritability, nausea, vomiting, tachycardia, tremors, and chills. The name *cold turkey* comes from the symptom piloerection (which also occurs when a person is cold); this reaction reminded addicts of the way a plucked turkey looks (little bumps in its skin).

Identification of an Addict

"Shoppers" are addicts who try to find a physician or dentist who will prescribe their drug of choice. There have even been organized groups of shoppers headed by an individual. The members of the groups are directed to physicians and dentists with complaints whose symptoms are taught to them. Prescriptions for controlled substances that are given to these "patients" are returned to the leader, and the "patients" are paid for their time. New dentist offices are often targets for "shopping." If a prescription for a controlled substance is obtained, more addicts will contact the office. This is not the type of "practice builder" that any dental office needs. Dental practitioners should become suspicious if any of the following "shopper" symptoms are present in a patient:

- Requests a certain drug and says it is better; he or she may stumble over the name
- Claims many allergies and says lots of pain medications do not work
- Cancels dental appointments because he or she claims to be going out of town on business
- Experiences pain for days after scaling and root planing
- Moves from dental office to dental office because "others do not understand"
- Claims a "low pain threshold"

- Calls with a request for an opioid analgesic just as the office is closing, or after hours with the promise of coming in for an examination the next day
- Needs refills several days after a dental procedure without complications

Treatment

> Methadone maintenance is one method.

The following four general methods are used for treating opioid addiction:

- Substituting the equivalent amount of an oral opioid (usually methadone) for the injectable form that the addict had been using (e.g., heroin) and then gradually withdrawing that oral form.
- Having the patient go cold turkey by abruptly withdrawing the opioid and using adjunctive medication to alleviate the symptoms of withdrawal, such as phenothiazines, clonidine, or benzodiazepines.
- Maintaining a patient on high doses of methadone, termed *methadone maintenance*. With this method, the patient takes supervised large oral doses of methadone on a daily basis. Because the patient develops a tolerance for the effects of the opioids, a block is produced that prevents heroin-like agents from producing the "rush" feeling after injection.
- Administering an orally effective, long-acting antagonist, naltrexone (Trexan). Naltrexone blocks the action of usual doses of opioids administered illicitly.
- No treatment for opioid addiction is successful in all patients.

Allergic Reactions

> True opioid allergy is uncommon.

The most common type of true allergic reaction to the opioids is dermatologic in nature, including skin rashes and urticaria. Reports of gastrointestinal side effects of opioids are often reported as allergies but are truly just side effects. Contact dermatitis can occur with topical exposure. These allergic reactions must be differentiated from the symptoms related to the histamine-releasing properties of the opioids. If a patient gives a history of a true allergic reaction to an opioid, an opioid from a different chemical class should be chosen (Box 6.1). Fig. 6.3 shows choices of analgesics for the patient allergic to codeine. Some brands of opioid-analgesic combinations are formulated with sodium bisulfite. In patients with sulfite hypersensitivity, reference sources should be consulted to determine which brand contains sulfites.

BOX 6.1 Alternative Analgesics for Opioid Allergies

Severe Pain
- Allergies to Morphine and Codeine—Use meperidine or fentanyl, methadone or levorphanol can also be used

Mild to Moderate Pain
- Acetaminophen or nonsteroidal antiinflammatory drugs

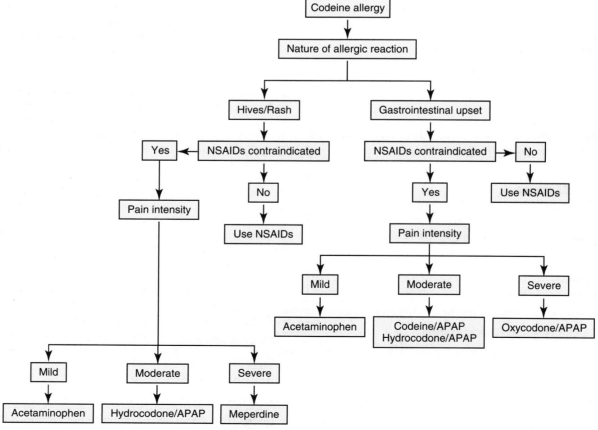

Fig. 6.3 Codeine allergy decision tree. Use this decision tree to choose an analgesic for patients with a history of codeine allergy. *APAP,* Acetaminophen; *NSAIDs,* nonsteroidal antiinflammatory drugs.

Drug Interactions

Some of the drug interactions of the opioids are listed in Table 6.5. The most common outcome is sedation.

The respiratory depression produced by the opioids is additive with that produced by other CNS depressants. Alcohol or sedative-hypnotic agents can potentiate the opioids' respiratory depressant effect. When promethazine or hydroxyzine (antihistamines) is added to an opioid regimen, the opioid dose should be reduced.

All opioids can interact with the monoamine oxidase inhibitors (MAOIs), a group of drugs used to treat depression. CNS excitation, hypertension, and hypotension have been reported. The accumulation of a metabolite of meperidine, normeperidine, may be responsible for the increased effect of meperidine in the presence of the antipsychotic agents such as chlorpromazine.

SPECIFIC OPIOIDS

Opioid Agonists

The analgesic action of the most commonly used opioids (agonists) is related to their action on the μ-receptors and κ-receptors (see morphine information in Table 6.3). These agonist opioids are discussed first (Table 6.6).

Morphine

Morphine (MORE-feen) is considered to be the prototype opioid agonist against which other opioids are measured. An equivalent number of milligrams of each opioid is compared with 10 mg of morphine. Morphine is used parenterally to control postoperative pain in hospitalized patients. It is also used orally, primarily in the treatment of terminal illnesses. Sustained-release morphine tablets are the most commonly used form of morphine for outpatient use in the terminally ill. Few, if any, sustained-release analgesics are useful in dentistry because the patient needs immediate relief, not future relief. The usual oral dosing interval and route of administration are listed in Table 6.3.

Oxycodone

Oxycodone (ox-i-KOE-done) is used alone or combined with either aspirin (in Percodan) or acetaminophen (in Percocet and Tylox) to provide relief of moderate-to-severe pain (see Table 6.6). Combining an opioid with a nonopioid analgesic has an additive analgesic effect with fewer adverse reactions. Oxycodone retains about two thirds of its action when given orally. It bridges the gap between codeine and morphine in terms of strength of analgesic action. The long-acting formulation is commonly used to treat chronic pain associated with cancer.

Oxymorphone

Oxymorphone is a metabolite of oxycodone that is available as parenteral and short- and long-acting oral dose forms. It is three times more potent than oral morphine and provides adequate pain relief in cancer patients that have been switched from long-acting morphine or oxycodone.

Hydrocodone

Hydrocodone is a synthetic opioid that is metabolized to hydromorphone after oral administration. Immediate-release hydrocodone is a Schedule II drug. The intent of this classification is to limit hydrocodone abuse and reduce the number of opioid deaths. Immediate-release hydrocodone is available only in combination with either ibuprofen or acetaminophen. New formulations of the brand name products are now available in combinations of doses of hydrocodone ranging from 5 to 10 mg and only 300 mg of acetaminophen. Generic versions of this combination will offer the same doses of hydrocodone but will have 325 mg of acetaminophen. Acetaminophen doses have been lowered because of the risk of hepatotoxicity. Also, as with any opioid product containing acetaminophen, the total dose of acetaminophen should not exceed 4 g (see Chapter 5).

Extended-Release Hydrocodone

Hydrocodone is now available as an extended-release oral dose form that is indicated for the management of severe pain that requires opioid analgesics and has not responded to other treatment options. Hydrocodone is a Schedule II drug because of its risk for abuse, addiction, and misuse even at recommended doses.

Codeine

Codeine (KOE-deen) is the most commonly used opioid in dentistry, and it is combined with acetaminophen (Tylenol #3) for oral administration. Codeine has a relatively weak analgesic action in comparison with morphine, hydromorphone, hydrocodone, or even oxycodone. Some commonly used codeine-analgesic combinations are listed in Table 6.6.

Because of codeine's weak analgesic efficacy, prescription doses of NSAIDs often produce better results in the management of dental pain. When codeine is combined with nonopioid analgesics, there is additive analgesic activity. In the combination products, lower doses of each analgesic may be used, and there is a potential for a reduction in adverse reactions.

Meperidine

Meperidine (me-PAIR-i-deen) (Demerol) is intended for the acute management (first 24–48 hours) of moderate-to-severe pain. It requires 100 mg to equal about 10 mg of morphine. It has a more rapid onset of action than morphine but it is short-acting. The drug interactions between meperidine and both the MAOIs and phenothiazines must be considered before meperidine is used.

Hydromorphone

An orally effective opioid, hydromorphone (hye-droe-MORE-fone) (Dilaudid) is reserved for the management of severe pain. It is more potent than morphine and better absorbed orally, but it tends to produce similar adverse reactions. Its use in dentistry should be limited to rare

TABLE 6.5	Drug Interactions of the Opioids	
	Medical Drug	**Potential Outcome**
General opioids	Alcohol Barbiturates	Additive CNS depression
Specific Opioids		
Propoxyphene	Carbamazepine	Carbamazepine toxicity
Meperidine	Barbiturates Chlorpromazine, neuroleptics Monoamine oxidase inhibitors	Toxicity of meperidine ↑BP, leading to central nervous system depression Severe reactions, excitation, rigidity, ↑BP
Methadone	Barbiturates Phenytoin Rifampin	↓Methadone levels ↓Methadone levels; withdrawal

BP, Blood pressure; ↑, increased; ↓, decreased.

TABLE 6.6   Make-Up of Common Opioid Analgesic Products

Trade or Generic	Opioid (mg)	Efficacy (+ to ++++)	Other Ingredients (mg)
Full Agonists			
Generic	Codeine (15, 30, 60; tablets)	++	None
Tylenol #2–#4*	Codeine #2 (15) #3 (30) #4 (60)	++	Acetaminophen (300) Sodium metabisulfite (trade name); generic also available
Tylenol with codeine elixir	Codeine (12 mg/5 mL)	++	Acetaminophen (120) Alcohol (7%) Sucrose Generic also available
Empirin #3–#4	Codeine (30, 60)	++	Aspirin (325)
Fiorinal #3	Codeine (30)	++	Aspirin (325) Butalbital (50) Caffeine (40)
Fioricet with codeine	Codeine (30)	++	Acetaminophen (325) Butalbital (50) Caffeine (40)
Zohydro ER	Hydrocodone extended-release (10, 15, 20, 30, 40, 50)	+++	None
Hydrocodone, Generic formulations	Hydrocodone (5, 7.5)	++	Acetaminophen (325)
Lortab	Hydrocodone (5, 7.5, 10)	++	Acetaminophen (325)
Lorcet	Hydrocodone (5, 7.5, 10)	++	Acetaminophen (325)
Vicodin	Hydrocodone (5, 7.5, 10)	++	Acetaminophen (300)
Vicoprofen	Hydrocodone (7.5)	++	Ibuprofen (200)
Percodan, Roxiprin, Endodan*	Oxycodone (≈5)	+++	Aspirin (325)
Percocet, Roxicet, Endocet, Oxycocet	Oxycodone (2.5, 5, 7.5, 10)	+++	Acetaminophen (325)
Tylox	Oxycodone (5)	+++	Acetaminophen (500)
Oxecta	Oxycodone 5, 7.5	+++	None
OxyContin† (extended release dose form)	Oxycodone (10, 15, 20, 30, 40, 60, 80)	+++	None
Opana	Oxymorphone (5, 10)	+++	None
Opana ER	Oxymorphone extended-release (5, 7.5, 10, 15, 20, 30, 40)	+++	None
Demerol	Meperidine (50, 100)	+++	None
Dilaudid	Hydromorphone (2, 4, 8)	++++	None
Agonist/Reuptake Inhibitors			
Nucynta	Tapentadol (50, 75, 100)	++	
Nucynta ER	Tapentadol (50, 100, 150, 200, 250)		
Ultram	Tramadol (50)	++ to +++	
Rybix	Tramadol orally disintegrating tablets (50)		
Ultram ER	Tramadol (100, 200, 300)		
ConZip	Tramadol extended-release tablets (100, 200, 300) Tramadol extended-release capsules (100, 150, 200, 300)		

*Most commonly prescribed.
†Sustained-release product; not for acute pain.
APAP, Acetaminophen; *ER*, extended release.

situations, the correct and lowest dose possible and careful monitoring. It is a favorite of the addict because of its strength (see Table 6.6).

Methadone

Methadone (METH-e-done) (Dolophine) is used primarily in the treatment of opioid addicts. It is used either to withdraw the patient gradually or for maintenance. Because it has a longer duration of action, withdrawal from methadone is easier than that from heroin. However, because methadone is an opioid analgesic, the risk for dependence still exists. Lately, methadone has been used as an analgesic in the treatment of chronic pain because it can be dosed less frequently than short-acting opioids such as morphine and hydrocodone. It also has a long half-life, has good bioavailability, and is cost-effective. The downside to methadone use is the risk of death and life-threatening changes in breathing and heart rates. These problems have been reported in persons newly starting methadone or in persons switching to methadone after using stronger opioid analgesics. As a result, only low doses should be prescribed for pain.

Fentanyl Family

Fentanyl (FEN-ta-nil) (Duragesic, Sublimaze), sufentanil (sue-FEN-ta-nil) (Sufenta), and alfentanil (al-FEN-ta-nil) (Alfenta) are short-acting, parenterally administered agonist opioid analgesics that are used perioperatively or during general anesthesia. They provide analgesia during and immediately after general anesthesia. Fentanyl is also available as a patch (Fentanyl [Duragesic] Transdermal System) for application to the skin every 3 days. The patches provide constant pain relief for the terminally ill.

Abuse-Deterrent Opioids

The FDA has approved several new abuse-deterrent opioid analgesics which have been formulated to help deter against substance abuse (Table 6.7). These new formulations have one or more properties that make intentional nontherapeutic use of the opioid more difficult, less attractive and less rewarding. Initial post-marketing surveillance data has seen a reduction in the prescription sales, abuse, and diversion. It has also reduced doctor shopping for *Oxycontin* and the number of reported cases of overdose and poisoning from *Oxycontin* had decreased as well.

Mixed Opioids

Mixed opioids include the agonist-antagonist opioid analgesics and the partial agonists. The only mixed opioid available for oral use is the agonist-antagonist pentazocine. Butorphanol (Stadol), available as a nasal spray for the management of pain and as transdermal patch (Butrans) for the treatment of chronic pain, is also in this group. At present, the place of these agents in dental therapeutics is unclear.

Agonist-Antagonist Opioids

The only agonist-antagonist opioid available in oral form is pentazocine (pen-TAZ-oh-seen) (Talwin). It has CNS effects not unlike those of the opioid agonists, including analgesia, sedation, and respiratory depression. The type of analgesia pentazocine produces is somewhat different from that produced by the agonist opioids. This may be the result of its agonist action at the κ-receptors and δ-receptors and its antagonist action at the μ-receptor. (References differ in attributing the dysphoric and psychomimetic adverse reactions—some say δ, and others say σ.)

Pentazocine is available as tablets containing 50 mg of pentazocine and 0.5 mg of naloxone, a pure opioid antagonist (Talwin-NX). Naloxone, a Schedule IV opioid, was added to pentazocine to reduce its addiction potential. How does it do so? First, naloxone, a pure antagonist, is effective parenterally but not orally because it is inactivated. Second, if the tablet is taken by the intended oral route, the naloxone will not affect the analgesic potency because it is rapidly inactivated when taken orally. Third, if the contents of the tablet are injected parenterally, the active naloxone will counteract the action of pentazocine, reducing its positive effects. This combination tablet is more difficult to abuse than Talwin, and the street value of Talwin-NX is half that of Talwin. (One cannot say that drug addicts do not know their pharmacology.)

Partial Agonists

The first and only available partial agonist is buprenorphine (byoo-pre-NOR-feen) (Buprenex, Subutex). It is a partial μ-receptor agonist but has no δ-receptor action. In abstinent morphine-dependent patients, buprenorphine suppresses withdrawal; in stabilized opioid-dependent patients, it precipitates withdrawal. Its abuse potential appears to be moderate, and it is classified as a Schedule III drug. It is available for oral and parenteral use.

Opioid Antagonists
Naloxone

> Naloxone reverses opioid overdose.

Naloxone (nal-OX-zone) (Narcan) is an essentially pure opioid antagonist that is active parenterally. It antagonizes the μ-receptors, δκ-receptors, and δ-receptors. When given alone, it has few pharmacologic effects in the usual therapeutic doses. Naloxone is the drug of choice for treating agonist or mixed opioid overdoses. It will reverse opioid-induced respiratory depression. If another agent, such as a barbiturate, is responsible for the depression, naloxone does not add to the respiratory depression. If naloxone is administered to an addict who has taken an overdose of an opioid, small doses must be carefully titrated to avoid opioid withdrawal. It also serves as a useful tool in research to determine the role of the opioid receptors in hypnosis, acupuncture, and the placebo effect.

A number of jurisdictions have passed naloxone access laws that make naloxone available to first responders, family member and close friends of persons taking or abusing opioids. Many of these laws grant civil and criminal immunity to laypeople who carry or administer naloxone, to healthcare professionals who prescribe or dispense it to laypeople, and to persons who call for emergency medical services in good faith to reverse an overdose. It also provides civil and criminal immunity to the person that is being treated for the overdose. Several state departments of health have issued standing prescription orders to all pharmacies for naloxone to treat opioid overdose. Naloxone use in the dental practice will be further discussed in Chapter 23.

TABLE 6.7 Selected US Food and Drug Administration-Approved Abuse-Deterrent Opioid Analgesics

Opioid	Abuse Deterrent Mechanism
Hydrocodone ER Hysingla ER Vantrela ER	Resist crushing and breaking; tablets form a viscous gel when dissolved
Morphine ER Morphabond Arymo ER	Resist crushing and breaking; tablets form a viscous gel when dissolved
Oxycodone IR Roxybond	Resists crushing and breaking; tablets resist extraction in solvents and form a viscous gel when dissolved
Oxycodone ER Oxycontin Xtampza	Resist crushing and breaking; tablets form a viscous gel when dissolved Microspheres resist effects of crushing and chewing; contents of melted or dissolved capsules are difficult to inject
Morphine ER/Naltrexone Embeda	Contains a sequestered opioid antagonist, which is released when the capsule is crushed or dissolved
Oxycodone ER/Naltrexone Targiniq ER Troxyca	Contains a sequestered opioid antagonist, which is released when the capsule is crushed or dissolved

ER, Extended release; *IR*, immediate release.

Nalmefene

> Nalmefene reverses opioid overdose.

Nalmefene (NAL-me-feen) (Revex) is another parenteral opioid antagonist used to reverse opioid overdose.

Naltrexone

> Naltrexone is used to prevent opioid and alcohol use in addicts.

A long-acting, orally effective opioid antagonist, naltrexone (nal-TREKS-zone) (ReVia, Vivitrol) is indicated for the maintenance of the opioid-free state in detoxified, formerly opioid-dependent patients. It should not be administered until the patient has remained opioid free for at least 1 week and has tested negative on a naloxone challenge. It is also used in the management of alcohol abstinence. Its adverse reactions include insomnia, nervousness, headache, abdominal cramping, nausea, vomiting, and arthralgia. Acute hepatitis and liver failure have been associated with naltrexone. It is administered daily or, in some instances, three times weekly. Patients taking naltrexone should not be given opioid analgesic agents for management of dental pain.

Full Agonist/Reuptake Inhibitors

Tapentadol

Tapentadol (Nucynta) is an oral opioid receptor agonist and a norepinephrine reuptake inhibitor. Its extended-release formulation appears to be similar in efficacy to extended-release oxycodone for osteoarthritis and low back pain. It does not appear to have serotonergic activity, but the drug's labeling carries a warning for the possibility of serotonergic syndrome when tapentadol is used with serotonergic drugs. It should not be taken within 14 days of an MAOI because of its adrenergic effects.

Tramadol

> Analgesic efficacy unimpressive; lack of addiction potential questionable.

Tramadol (Ultram) is a unique analgesic with an interesting mechanism of action. It has μ-opioid agonist action and inhibits the reuptake of norepinephrine and serotonin (modifies the ascending pain pathways). It has some but not all the properties of an opioid (like codeine and hydrocodone) because of its μ-agonist activity, and it does not affect the other two opioid receptors, kappa and delta. Tramadol's other mechanism involves the inhibition of reuptake of norepinephrine and serotonin, similar to the mechanism of the antidepressants. Its effectiveness in combination with acetaminophen is comparable to that of codeine with acetaminophen or oxycodone.

Adverse reactions of tramadol include CNS effects such as dizziness, somnolence, headache, and stimulation. Gastrointestinal tract side effects include nausea, diarrhea, constipation, and vomiting. Palpitations, diaphoresis, and seizures have been reported in patients taking tramadol. Package labeling also warns of the possible risk of suicide in patients who are suicidal, emotionally disturbed, or prone to addiction. Tramadol use is associated with physical dependency and withdrawal symptoms. This drug causes typical opiate withdrawal symptoms and atypical symptoms, including anxiety, palpitations, and anguish. One should watch for signs of addiction. In August 2014, the US Drug Enforcement Agency made tramadol a Schedule IV controlled substance.

DENTAL USE OF OPIOIDS

Although often overlooked as a source of opioid analgesics, dentists are frequent prescribers of opioid analgesics. In 2012, pharmacies (retail and mail order) and long-term care facilities dispensed 4.2 billion prescriptions, of which 289 million (60.8%) were for opioid analgesics. In 2011, more than 137 million prescriptions were written for hydrocodone alone. The number of prescriptions of hydrocodone dropped to 97 million in 2015 with the advent of its change to controlled substance II drug. Despite attempts to monitor prescribing of controlled substances, it has been reported that up to 15% of all prescription opioids are diverted and sold on the streets. In fact, one third of drugs that are sold illegally are prescription drugs. In a 2012 report, dentists ranked fourth among medical specialists in prescribing opioid analgesics at a rate of 28.9%. It should be noted that dentists were second only to family practice physicians as the practitioners prescribing the highest number of immediate-release opioids in the United States, amounting to 12.2% of all immediate-release opioids prescribed. Dentists alone were responsible for prescribing between 1 and 1.5 billion immediate-release opioid analgesics annually. Analgesics are the most common reason for dental visits for patients aged 18 to 30 and account for 40.2% of prescriptions written by dentists for this population. It has also been reported that analgesics are prescribed at a rate second only to that for antibiotics in a dental practice.

There are many reasons why the number of opioid analgesic prescriptions has risen in both dental and medical practices. Opioid analgesics are often necessary to treat acute dental pain, especially in patients who cannot tolerate NSAIDs or whose pain truly does not respond to NSAID therapy. However, the number of opioid tablets dispensed per prescription has been found to be in excess of what is actually necessary. Patients do not normally use all of their prescription opioids and just put the remaining opioids aside. As a result, the leftover opioids are often abused by family members or the patient, or are sold on the streets. Opioid analgesics are often prescribed because of the dentists' experience with their patients, or often out of habit, depending on the procedure and anticipated postprocedure pain. There is the misconception that limited opioid analgesic use for acute pain does not lead to addiction. However, that is not the case, and the potential for abuse remains high.

The advent of the NSAIDs has changed the use of the opioids in dental practice. Most dental pain can be better managed by NSAIDs. In the patient in whom NSAIDs are contraindicated, the dentist has a wide range of opioids from which to choose. By beginning with codeine or hydrocodone combinations and progressing to oxycodone combinations, one can manage almost all dental pain. Only in rare cases and for very short periods (1–2 days) should stronger opioids be prescribed for dental pain. The number of tablets of an opioid prescribed should also be limited. Box 6.2 lists the patient instructions for opioid analgesics.

BOX 6.2 Patient Instructions for Use of Opioid Analgesics

- Take with a full glass of water.
- Take with food to minimize gastrointestinal irritation.
- Use caution about driving because of the likelihood of dizziness and drowsiness.
- Avoid any situations that require thought or concentration because of the likelihood of sedation.
- These drugs can cause xerostomia. Drink plenty of water and avoid caffeinated beverages, juices, and sodas.

CHRONIC DENTAL PAIN AND OPIOID USE

Over the past 30 years, there has been much research in the area of chronic orofacial pain. In the United States, more than 3 million patients annually seek treatment for chronic orofacial pain. Because orofacial pain can negatively impact the patient's quality of life, it must be appropriately treated. In some instances, this type of pain may need to be treated with opioid analgesics. Once the patient has been correctly diagnosed with chronic orofacial pain, the dentist should initiate therapy with an NSAID. If this fails, opioids should be considered. Only a dentist who is comfortable with prescribing long-term opioid therapy should treat a patient with chronic orofacial pain. If not, the patient should be referred to a pain center or to a dentist who treats chronic pain. The dentist should assess the patient for signs of current drug abuse problems as well as monitor for potential signs of abuse once the patient has started therapy. Patients should also be monitored for pain relief.

New patients with a complaint of pain should be seen in the dental office, and definitive treatment rendered. Opioid prescriptions should be given only for small amounts without refills and only if dental treatment has been performed. If dental pain persists, the patient should be seen in the dental office for evaluation and local treatment. If the patient demands opioids repeatedly, the patient should be referred to a pain clinic for evaluation. Temporomandibular disease (TMD), formerly called temporomandibular joint (TMJ) disease, often causes chronic pain. In one study, 39% of patients assessed for chronic dental pain had at least one symptom associated with TMD and 16% of these patients experienced pain. Another study found that up to 40% of patients treated for TMD in a tertiary care setting can be refractory to treatment. When pain becomes chronic, the mechanisms producing the pain differ from those that produce acute pain. Treatment of TMD should include NSAIDs and possibly muscle relaxants and tricyclic antidepressants.

Patient Concerns Regarding Opioid Use

The fear of addiction or being thought of as an addict prohibits some patients from taking opioid analgesics and properly managing their pain. Once such patients stop adhering to prescribed therapy because of these fears, they can no longer adequately treat their pain, possibly complicating their recovery. The dental hygienist should remind patients that short-term use should not cause problems with addiction or dependence and that the proper use of the opioid analgesic will provide needed pain management.

DENTAL HYGIENE CONSIDERATIONS

- If opioid analgesics are necessary, the dental hygienist should conduct a thorough medication/health history of the patient to determine whether there are any contraindications or drug interactions.
- The dental hygienist should be aware that many opioid analgesics are combined with nonopioid analgesics. Remind patients to not supplement with over-the-counter (OTC) analgesics if a combination nonopioid/opioid analgesic is prescribed.
- The most common side effect of the opioid analgesics is sedation. Other sedating drugs should be avoided or used with caution if they are essential.
- Patients should avoid anything that requires thought or concentration while taking an opioid analgesic.
- If patients complain of gastrointestinal adverse effects, they may require a semisupine chair position during dental treatment.
- The dental hygienist should be aware of the signs of opioid addiction and how to identify an addict.
- Consult Box 6.2 for patient instructions regarding opioid analgesics.

ACADEMIC SKILLS ASSESSMENT

1. What are some red flags associated with opioid addiction?
2. Is any opioid more addicting than another? If so, what is this difference based on?
3. Is there a need for concern about opioid addiction for patients taking these drugs to treat or manage dental pain? Why or why not?
4. What is hydrocodone, and how effective is it in treating or managing dental pain?
5. Compare and contrast hydrocodone with ibuprofen.
6. What are the adverse reactions associated with hydrocodone?
7. Are there drug interactions with hydrocodone?
8. What are the dental concerns associated with hydrocodone?
9. What should patients be told about hydrocodone?
10. Can tramadol be used instead of hydrocodone?

CLINICAL CASE STUDIES

Paula Barnes is a 32-year-old woman with a history of poor teeth despite the use of fluoride toothpaste, brushing, and flossing. Her medication/health history reveals a healthy woman whose only medications include oral contraceptives and occasional over-the-counter analgesics and cough and cold products. She is in your office today for a root canal and a new crown. Ms. Barnes experienced a lot of pain with her last root canal. Ibuprofen did not help with the pain, and she required something stronger. The dentist decides to give Ms. Barnes a prescription for acetaminophen with codeine (Tylenol #3).

1. What is codeine, and how effective is it in treating or managing dental pain?
2. Compare and contrast codeine with ibuprofen.
3. What are the adverse effects associated with codeine?
4. Are there any drug interactions that Ms. Barnes should be aware of?
5. What are the dental concerns associated with codeine?
6. What should Ms. Barnes be told about this medication (include information regarding acetaminophen, too)?

Antiinfective Agents

LEARNING OBJECTIVES

1. Outline the history and basic principles of infection and its relevance to dentistry, including
   - Define the terms pertinent to a discussion about infection.
   - Identify the factors that determine the likelihood of an infection.
   - Describe the importance of cultures and sensitivity in relation to infections.
   - Discuss the reasons and understanding of "resistance" as important with regard to infections.
2. Summarize the principal indications for the use of antimicrobial agents.
3. Name and describe the major adverse reactions and disadvantages associated with the use of antiinfective agents.
4. Discuss penicillins, cephalosporins, macrolides, tetracyclines—their chemical makeup, properties, mechanisms of action, uses,

and potential adverse reactions—and name several specific types of each.
5. Name and describe two other types of antibiotics and antiinfectives, including their chemical makeup, properties, mechanism of action, potential adverse reactions, and uses.
6. Discuss the rationale for the use of antiinfective agents in dentistry.
7. Discuss antimicrobial agents for nondental uses including their pharmacokinetics, mechanism of action, adverse reactions, and spectrum of use.
8. Describe the drugs used to treat tuberculosis and the difficulties this disease presents.
9. Discuss the use of topical antibiotics in dentistry.
10. Summarize the concept and practice of antibiotic prophylaxis in dentistry.

Antiinfective agents play an important role in dentistry because infection, after pain management, is the dental problem for which drugs are most often prescribed. As the knowledge about the etiology of dental diseases is continually increasing and the involvement of microorganisms is becoming better understood, dental hygienists continue to better understand the proper place of antibiotics and their effect on microorganisms.

Dental infections can be divided into several types, as follows:
- *Caries:* Caries, produced by *Streptococcus mutans,* is the first important dental infection of the newly erupting teeth of the young patient. The treatment of choice is prevention and involves the use of fluoridated water, local physical removal of bacterial plaque from teeth on a regular basis (good oral hygiene, dental prophylaxis), and appropriately placed sealants.
- *Periodontal disease:* In the adult patient, the dental hygienist's biggest dental problem is periodontal disease. With an increase in knowledge about antiinfective agents, dental hygienists and dentists will be better able to understand and properly administer the appropriate drug therapy. Because it is now known that microorganisms, such as *Aggregatibacter actinomycetemcomitans,* black-pigmented bacteroides, motile rods, and spirochetes, are involved in periodontal disease, development of a more rational approach to treatment of periodontal disease may be possible.
- *Localized dental infections:* Most localized dental infections are extensions that arise from either periodontically or endodontically related sources. For most localized dental infections, if adequate drainage can be obtained, antiinfective agents are not indicated unless the patient is immunocompromised (Box 7.1). In the occasional situation in which antibiotics are indicated, the antibiotic of choice is determined by the organisms likely to be present.

- *Systemic infections:* Systemic dental infections can be identified because they produce systemic symptoms, such as fever, malaise, and tachycardia. Lesions associated with infections producing these types of symptoms should be drained, but if drainage is not possible, antibiotics should be given. The duration of therapy should be calculated as the number of days for the signs and symptoms to be totally gone plus 2 or 3 days. If the dental infection has systemic symptoms, the use of anti-infective agents is indicated and may even be critical.

DENTAL INFECTION "EVOLUTION"

Dental infections often follow similar pathways of evolution from beginning to end. In the beginning, the organisms responsible for a dental infection are primarily gram-positive cocci, such as *Streptococcus viridans,* or β-hemolytic streptococci. After a short time, the gram-positive infection begins to include a variety of both gram-positive and gram-negative anaerobic organisms, such as *Peptostreptococcus (Peptococcus)* and *Bacteroides (Porphyromonas* and *Prevotella* species). At this point, the infection is termed a *mixed* infection. Over time, the proportion of organisms that are anaerobic increases. With additional time and no treatment, the infection progresses until it consists of predominantly anaerobic flora. At this point, the anaerobic organisms coalesce into an abscess, often visible on radiograph (x-ray).

The choice of antibiotics for a dental patient's infection depends on where it is in its evolution. If the infection is just beginning, the organisms most likely to be present are gram-positive cocci. Penicillin is the drug of choice, unless the patient has a penicillin allergy. Amoxicillin is most often used because it is less irritating to the stomach and can be taken with food or milk. In patients

BOX 7.1 Diseases, Conditions, and Drugs that Decrease Resistance to Infection

Diseases/Conditions
Addison's disease
Acquired immunodeficiency syndrome (AIDS)–related complex
Human immunodeficiency virus
Alcoholism
Blood dyscrasias
Cancer
Cirrhosis of the liver
Diabetes mellitus
Down syndrome
Immunoglobulin deficiency
Leukemia
Malnutrition
Splenectomy

Drugs
Immunosuppressive drugs, such as:
  Azathioprine (Imuran)
  Cyclophosphamide (Cytoxan)
  Cyclosporine (Sandimmune)
  Methotrexate (Rheumatrex)
  Glucocorticosteroids

allergic to penicillin, alternatives include a macrolide antibiotic and clindamycin. When the infection is at the mixed stage, agents effective against both gram-positive organisms and anaerobic organisms may be successful. Treating gram-positive organisms is easier, and the drug of choice is penicillin/amoxicillin or, in the patient with a penicillin allergy, a macrolide antibiotic. For anaerobic organisms, metronidazole is effective. Eradicating one group of organisms alters the balance between the two types of organisms, and the body can then resolve the infection. Clindamycin affects both gram-positive cocci and gram-positive and gram-negative anaerobes. To treat a dental infection, it is critical to know what organism(s) are likely to be involved and the sensitivity of those organisms to antibiotics. Decisions are based on the likelihood of certain infections and their sensitivities.

DEFINITIONS

A discussion of individual antimicrobial agents is preceded by definitions of the following terms:
- *Antiinfective agents:* Substances that act against or destroy infections.
- *Antibacterial agents:* Substances that destroy or suppress the growth or multiplication of bacteria.
- *Antibiotic agents:* Chemical substances produced by microorganisms that have the capacity, in dilute solutions, to destroy or suppress the growth or multiplication of organisms or prevent their action.

The difference among the terms *antibiotic, antiinfective,* and *antibacterial* is that antibiotics are produced by microorganisms, whereas the other agents may be developed in a chemistry laboratory (not from a living organism). *Antibacterial* refers to a substance from any source that inhibits or kills bacteria. The term *antiinfective* refers to a substance from any source that inhibits or kills organisms that can produce infection, such as bacteria, protozoa, and viruses. This difference is largely ignored in general conversation, and antiinfectives are often referred to as "antibiotics."

- *Antimicrobial agents:* Substances that destroy or suppress the growth or multiplication of microorganisms.
- *Antifungal agents:* Substances that destroy or suppress the growth or multiplication of fungi.
- *Antiviral agents:* Substances that destroy or suppress the growth or multiplication of viruses.
The following are definitions of commonly used terms:
- *Bactericidal:* The ability to kill bacteria. This effect is irreversible; that is, if the bacteria are removed from contact with the drug, they do not live.
- *Bacteriostatic:* The ability to inhibit or retard the multiplication or growth of bacteria. This is a reversible process because if the bacteria are removed from contact with the agent, they are able to grow and multiply.

Whether an antibacterial agent is labeled bactericidal or bacteriostatic depends on variables such as the dose used and the organism being treated. Box 7.2 lists the most common antimicrobial agents and classifies them as bacteriostatic or bactericidal.

INFECTION

The factors that determine the likelihood that a microorganism will cause an infection are the following:
- Disease-producing power of the microorganism (virulence)
- Number of organisms present (inoculum)
- Resistance of the host (immunologic response): Host resistance should be regarded as having both local and systemic components. Systemically, both drugs (steroids and antineoplastic agents) and diseases (acquired immunodeficiency syndrome [AIDS] and diabetes mellitus) may reduce a patient's immunity (see Box 7.1) and increase the chance of an infection. Sleep deprivation and anxiety can also reduce a patient's immunologic response to infection.

RESISTANCE

There are a reported two million cases of antibiotic-resistant infections in the United States each year with approximately 23,000 reported deaths from these infections. It should also be noted that the presence of antibiotic-resistant bacteria is greatest during the month after completion of antibiotic therapy and can remain for up to 12 months after therapy.

BOX 7.2 Classification of Antiinfective Agents: Bactericidal or Bacteriostatic

Bactericidal
Aminoglycosides
Cephalosporins
Metronidazole
Macrolides*
Penicillins
Quinolones
Rifampin
Vancomycin

Bacteriostatic
Chloramphenicol
Clindamycin*
Macrolides*
Sulfonamides
Tetracyclines
Trimethoprim

*May be bactericidal against some organisms at higher blood levels.

Resistance (related to antibiotics) is the natural or acquired ability of an organism to be immune to or to withstand the effects of an antiinfective agent. Natural resistance occurs when an organism has always been resistant to an antimicrobial agent because of the bacteria's normal properties, such as lipid structures in the cell wall. Acquired resistance occurs when an organism that was previously sensitive to an antimicrobial agent becomes resistant. This can occur by natural selection of a spontaneous mutation ("survival of the fittest"). An increase in the use of an antibiotic in a given population (e.g., a hospital) increases the proportion of resistant organisms in that population. Conversely, a decrease in the use of an antibiotic decreases the proportion of organisms resistant to that antibiotic in that given population. Another method by which resistance develops is by the transfer of DNA (deoxyribonucleic acid) genetic material from one organism to another via transduction, transformation, or bacterial conjugation. The first organism, which is resistant to one or more antibiotics, transfers its genetic material to a second organism. The second organism, which was not previously resistant, thus becomes resistant to the same antibiotic as the first organism without ever having been exposed to that antibiotic. This transfer of genetic material from one organism to another may occur among very different microorganisms, including transfer from nonpathogenic bacteria to pathogenic bacteria. The three most common mechanisms of acquired resistance are a decrease in bacterial permeability, the production of bacterial enzymes, and an alteration in the target site.

The misuse of antibiotics has contributed to one of the United States' most pressing public health problems, antibiotic resistance. The number of antibiotic-resistant bacteria has increased dramatically over the past 10 years, and many bacterial infections are becoming resistant to some of the most commonly prescribed antibiotics. Every time a person uses an antibiotic, sensitive bacteria are killed off but resistant bacteria can thrive. Repeated and improper uses of antibiotics have jeopardized the usefulness of essential drugs. As a result of antibiotic resistance, some patients are experiencing longer-lasting illnesses, more doctor visits or hospital stays, and the need for more expensive antibiotic therapy.

Reducing the incidence of antibiotic-resistant bacteria can be achieved by reducing the number of prescriptions written annually as well as educating the patient and health professional about antibiotic-resistant bacteria. Health care professionals, including dentists and dental hygienists, can help reduce the incidence of resistance by prescribing antibiotics only when absolutely necessary. The correct antibiotic, with the correct dose and duration, should be prescribed. Only one antibiotic should be prescribed, and a second should be added only if it is clearly necessary. Patients should be educated about the correct use of antibiotics to include taking the antibiotic as prescribed and completing therapy. They should also be advised about the adverse effects of the antibiotic. If possible, the infection should be cultured and the continued need for antibiotic therapy should be assessed once the results of the culture are known. As always, patient education is the key.

INDICATIONS FOR ANTIMICROBIAL AGENTS

Considerable controversy exists regarding the need for antimicrobial agents in various situations. The two categories of indications are prophylactic and therapeutic.

Therapeutic Indications

Although there is no simple rule to determine whether antimicrobial therapy is needed in dentistry, many infections do not require it. Most patients who do not have immune function deficiencies and in whom drainage can be used need no antibiotics to manage their dental infections. Table 7.1 lists the indications for treatment of dental infections along with the antibiotics of choice and their alternatives. If local resistance patterns vary from those found in the table, antibiotic choice should be based on that information. However, before a decision is made, several factors must be considered.

Patient

The best defense against a pathogen is the host response. A properly functioning defense mechanism is of primary importance. When this defense is lacking, the need for antimicrobial agents is more pressing.

Infection

The virulence and invasiveness of the microorganism are important in determining the acuteness, severity, and spreading tendency of an infection. An acute, severe, rapidly spreading infection should generally be treated with antimicrobial agents, whereas a mild, localized infection in which drainage can be established need not be treated. If the periodontal pocket (site) remains active despite repeated root planing, then the use of antibiotics to alter the flora may be considered.

When antimicrobial agents are to be used in the treatment of dental infections, the organisms likely to produce the infection and their susceptibility to antimicrobial agents must be considered. Table 7.1 lists the antimicrobials of choice for various dental situations (when culture and sensitivity testing are unavailable) and alternatives if the drug of choice cannot be used.

Prophylactic Indications

Few situations arise for which a definite indication for prophylactic antibiotic coverage exists. One clear-cut use of antibiotics for prophylaxis before a dental procedure (recommended by the American Heart Association [AHA] and the American Dental Association [ADA]) is a history of infective endocarditis, presence of a heart valve prosthesis, or specific types of congenital heart disease. The most current guidelines regarding antibiotic prophylaxis are discussed in detail at the end of this chapter.

GENERAL ADVERSE REACTIONS AND DISADVANTAGES ASSOCIATED WITH ANTIINFECTIVE AGENTS

Superinfection (Suprainfection)

All antiinfective agents can produce an overgrowth of an organism that is different from the original infecting organism and resistant to the agent being used. The wider the spectrum of the antiinfective agent and the longer the agent is administered, the greater the chance that superinfection will occur. This side effect can be minimized by use of the most specific antiinfective agent, the shortest effective course of therapy, and adequate doses.

Allergic Reactions

Like all drugs, all antiinfective agents have the potential to produce a variety of allergic reactions, ranging from a mild rash to fatal anaphylaxis. Some antiinfective agents, such as the penicillins and the cephalosporins, are more allergenic than other agents. Many antiinfective agents, such as erythromycin and clindamycin, have a low allergenic potential.

Drug Interactions

Antiinfective agents can interact with oral contraceptives, oral anticoagulants, and other antiinfectives (a bacteriostatic agent interferes with a bactericidal agent).

TABLE 7.1   Antimicrobial Use in Dentistry*

Infection Situation	Drug(s) of Choice
Periodontal Disease	
Acute necrotizing ulcerative gingivitis[†]	Amoxicillin Metronidazole Penicillin VK Tetracycline
Abscess (periodontal)	Amoxicillin Penicillin VK Tetracycline
Localized aggressive periodontitis	Amoxicillin + metronidazole Amoxicillin + clavulanate (Augmentin) Azithromycin Doxycycline Tetracycline
Adult periodontitis[†]	Not usually treated with drugs Clindamycin if necessary
Generalized aggressive periodontitis	Amoxicillin + metronidazole Ciprofloxacin + metronidazole Doxycycline or minocycline Tetracycline Azithromycin Clindamycin
Oral Infections	
Soft tissue infections (abscess, cellulitis, postsurgical, pericoronitis)	Penicillin VK Amoxicillin Doxycycline Clindamycin Cephalosporins Tetracycline
Osteomyelitis	Penicillin VK Amoxicillin Clindamycin Cephalosporins
Mixed Infections Insensitive to Penicillin	
Aerobes	Amoxicillin Cephalosporins Sulfonamides Tetracycline
Anaerobes and chronic infections	Metronidazole Clindamycin Cephalosporins Amoxicillin + clavulanate (Augmentin) Tetracycline Metronidazole + penicillin
Prophylaxis for Infective Endocarditis	

Prosthetic heart valve[‡]	No penicillin allergy:
	    Amoxicillin[§]
	Penicillin allergy:
	    Clarithromycin
	    Azithromycin
	    Clindamycin

*Clinical conditions may alter drug therapy.
[†]No antimicrobial agents are usually required for these conditions.
[‡]See Table 7.3.
[§]See Table 7.2.

Oral Contraceptives

Some antibiotics have been found to decrease the efficacy of oral contraceptives by increasing their clearance from the body. This drug interaction, although unlikely, should be discussed with the patient whenever a patient using oral contraceptives receives a prescription for an antibiotic. Of those antibiotics used in dentistry, ampicillin and the tetracyclines are the most likely to have this effect. In certain patients, additional birth control measures should be used during antibiotic therapy.

Oral Anticoagulants

Antiinfective agents can potentiate the effect of oral anticoagulants. Oral anticoagulants are vitamin K inhibitors, so interfering with the production of vitamin K could increase the anticoagulant effect. Bacterial flora in the intestine produce most of the vitamin K in human bodies. Antiinfective agents (e.g., tetracycline) reduce the bacterial flora that produce vitamin K. With the vitamin K reduced, the oral anticoagulant's effect is increased. Erythromycin and azithromycin inhibit the enzymes that metabolize warfarin, leading to an increase in warfarin levels. Prolongation of the international normalized ratio (INR) leading to bleeding or hemorrhage may result. The INR should be monitored more closely in patients on antiinfective therapy. Antiinfective agents interact with warfarin to varying degrees, depending on the specific agent.

Gastrointestinal Complaints

All antiinfective drugs can produce a variety of gastrointestinal (GI) complaints. The complaints include stomach pain, increased motility, and diarrhea. The incidence varies greatly, depending on the particular agent used, the dose of the agent, and whether the patient takes the drug with food. Erythromycin has the highest incidence of GI complaints of any of the antibiotics. More serious GI complaints, such as pseudomembranous colitis (PMC), which has been historically linked with clindamycin, are now known to occur not only with a wide variety of antiinfective agents (cephalosporins, amoxicillin) but also in the absence of antimicrobial therapy.

Pregnancy Considerations

The antimicrobial agents that can be used during pregnancy to treat infections are limited. Although the risk-to-benefit ratio must be considered whenever pregnant women are given any medications, penicillin and erythromycin have not been associated with teratogenicity and are often used. The use of clindamycin is probably also acceptable, but before any antibiotics are used in the pregnant dental patient, the patient's obstetrician should be contacted (this procedure also helps prevent medical-legal problems). Metronidazole is not usually used during pregnancy, but exceptions exist. The tetracyclines are contraindicated during pregnancy because of their effect on developing teeth and skeleton.

Dose Forms

Common adult dose forms of antibiotics are tablets and capsules. Children's dose forms, including liquid and chewable antibiotic dose forms, contain sugar as the sweetening agent. After the dentition has erupted, the dental hygienist should encourage the parent or child to brush the child's teeth after the use of these agents. The chewable tablets can stick to the teeth, especially in the pits. Long-term administration of antibiotics could increase the child's caries rate.

Cost

Cost is an important factor in choosing an antibiotic for a patient. If the perfect antibiotic is chosen and prescribed but the patient does not purchase the medication because it is too expensive, then poor results

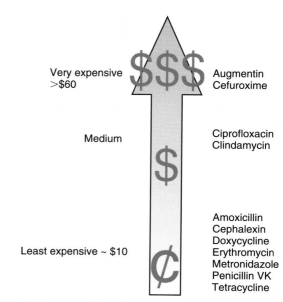

Fig. 7.1 Relative cost of dentally useful antibiotic agents.

are likely. The best inexpensive antibiotic will be more effective than an expensive one that cannot be purchased. Fig. 7.1 compares the costs of various antiinfective agents.

PENICILLINS

The penicillins (pen-i-SILL-ins) belong to the group of antibiotics known as β-lactam antibiotics. They are so named because of the β-lactam ring that is common to the molecular structure in all antibiotics in this group (Fig. 7.2). The penicillins can be divided into four major groups (Table 7.2). The first group contains penicillin G and V, the second group is composed of the penicillinase-resistant penicillins, the third group contains amoxicillin, and the fourth group consists of extended-spectrum penicillins. Because the penicillins have many properties in common, their similarities are discussed first. In dentistry, the first and third groups are commonly used.

Pharmacokinetics

Penicillin tubular secretion in the kidney; half-life = {1/2} hour.

Penicillin can be administered either orally or parenterally but should not be applied topically because its allergenicity is greatest by that route. When penicillin is administered orally, the amount absorbed depends on the type of penicillin. The percentage can vary from 0% to more than 90% (see Table 7.2) and when its absorption from the oral route is too low, then it is only available via injection. Penicillin V is better absorbed orally than penicillin G, so penicillin V is used for administration of oral penicillin.

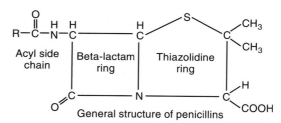

Fig. 7.2 β-Lactam ring.

TABLE 7.2 Penicillins

Drug Name*	Route(s)	Penicillinase-Resistant	Acid-Stable	Absorbed Orally (%)	Protein Bound (%)
Penicillin G and V					
Penicillin G potassium, generic	IM, IV	No	No	15–30	60
Penicillin G procaine, generic	IM	No	No	—	60
Penicillin G benzathine, generic	IM	No	No	—	60
Penicillin V (PC Pen VK, Pen-V)	PO	No	Yes	60–75	75–80
Penicillinase-Resistant					
Nafcillin generic	IM, IV	Yes	Yes	10–15	90
Oxacillin (Bactocill, generic)	PO, IM, IV	Yes	Yes	20–30	95
Ampicillins					
Ampicillin (Principen, Omnipen, generic)	PO, IM, IV	No	Yes	30–40	20
Ampicillin/sulbactam	IV, IM	No	Yes		28
Amoxicillin (Amoxil, generic)	PO	No	Yes	75–90	20
Amoxicillin + clavulanate (Augmentin)	PO	Yes	Yes	Very good	20
Extended-Spectrum					
Ticarcillin/clavulanic acid (Timentin)	IM, IV	No			45
Piperacillin/tazobactam (Zosyn, generic)	IM, IV	No			30

*__Bold type__ indicates drugs most used in dentistry.
IM, Intramuscular; *IV*, intravenous; *PO*, by mouth.

The oral route provides the advantages of convenience and less likelihood of a life-threatening allergic reaction. The disadvantages of using the oral rather than the parenteral route are that the blood levels rise more slowly, the blood levels are less predictable because of variable absorption or lack of patient compliance (biggest problem), and some penicillins are degraded by gastric acid. The highest blood levels are obtained if the patient takes the penicillin orally at least 1 hour before or 2 hours after meals, but penicillin V and amoxicillin can be taken without regard to meals.

After absorption, penicillin is distributed throughout the body, with the exception of cerebrospinal fluid, bone, and abscesses. This distribution includes the tissue, saliva, and kidneys. Penicillin crosses the placenta and appears in breast milk.

Penicillin is metabolized by hydrolysis in the liver and undergoes tubular secretion in the kidney. The elimination half-life for both penicillin G and penicillin V is about 0.5 hour. In five half-lives, about 2.5 hours, these penicillins are virtually eliminated from the body.

Mechanism of Action

Penicillin is a very potent bactericidal agent that attaches to penicillin-binding proteins (PBPs) on the bacterial cell membrane. The PBPs are enzymes that are involved in the synthesis of the cell wall and the maintenance of the cell's structural integrity. Penicillin acts as the structural analog of acyl-D-alanyl-D-alanine, inhibiting the formation of cross-linkages (transpeptidases). This destroys cell wall integrity and leads to lysis. The penicillins are more effective against rapidly growing organisms. Table 7.2 summarizes the types, routes of ingestion, and other properties of penicillins.

Spectrum

Penicillin G and V's narrow spectrum of activity includes gram-positive cocci, such as *Staphylococcus aureus*, *Staphylococcus pneumoniae*, *Streptococcus pyogenes*, *S. viridans*, and certain gram-negative cocci, such as *Neisseria gonorrhoeae* (produces gonorrhea) and *Neisseria meningitidis*. Penicillin is also effective against spirochetes and anaerobes such as *Actinomyces*, *Peptococcus*, *Peptostreptococcus*, *Bacteroides*,

Corynebacterium, and *Clostridium* species. The spectrum of activity of the penicillins matches the microbes responsible for many periodontal conditions. The other penicillins have somewhat different activity spectra that are discussed in each section.

Resistance

Resistance to penicillin can occur by several different mechanisms. Penicillinase-producing staphylococci are resistant because their enzymes destroy some penicillins. These penicillinases inactivate the penicillin moiety by cleaving the β-lactam ring.

In hospital environments, more than 95% of the population of staphylococci are penicillinase-producing organisms. Clavulanic acid serves as an inhibitor, which allows the use of amoxicillin to treat penicillinase-producing organisms. Certain bacteria have an outer cell membrane that prevents penicillin from reaching the PBPs.

Although most oral strains of *S. viridans* are sensitive to penicillin, an increasing number of strains are becoming resistant. The amount of bacterial resistance is proportional to the clinical use of the antibiotic; frequent use leads to increased resistance (and rarer use to decreased resistance).

Adverse Reactions

The untoward reactions to the penicillins can be divided into toxic reactions and allergic or hypersensitivity reactions. The penicillins are the most common cause of drug allergies.

Toxicity

Because penicillin's toxicity is almost nonexistent, large doses have been tolerated without adverse effects. For this reason, there is a large margin of safety when penicillin is administered. With massive intravenous (IV) doses, direct central nervous system (CNS) irritation can result in convulsions. Large doses of penicillin G have been associated with renal damage manifested as fever, eosinophilia, rashes, albuminuria, and a rise in blood urea nitrogen (BUN). Hemolytic anemia and bone marrow depression have also been produced by penicillin. The penicillinase-resistant penicillins are significantly more toxic than penicillin G. GI irritation can manifest as nausea with or without vomiting. The irritation caused by injection of penicillin can produce sterile abscesses if given intramuscularly (IM) or thrombophlebitis if given intravenously.

Allergy and Hypersensitivity

Allergic reactions to penicillin always should be considered when penicillin is prescribed. Some studies indicate that 5% to 10% of patients receiving penicillin will have a reaction. Allergic reactions to oral penicillin are less common than to parenteral penicillin. Anaphylactic reactions are more frequent in patients first treated with β-blockers and subsequently given oral penicillin. Anaphylactic reactions in these patients have been reported to be difficult to treat.

The following are types of allergic reactions associated with the penicillins:

Anaphylactic reactions: Anaphylactic shock, an acute allergic reaction, occurs within minutes of the administration of penicillin and presents the most serious danger to patients. It is characterized by smooth muscle contraction (e.g., bronchoconstriction), capillary dilation (shock), and urticaria caused by the release of histamine and bradykinin. If treatment does not begin immediately, death can result. The treatment of anaphylaxis is the immediate administration of parenteral epinephrine.

Rash: All types of rashes have been reported in association with the administration of penicillin. This type of reaction accounts for 80% to 90% of allergic reactions to the penicillins. These rashes are usually mild and self-limiting but can occasionally be severe. Even contact dermatitis has occurred as a result of topical exposure, for example, in a person preparing an injectable solution.

Delayed serum sickness: Serum sickness manifests as fever, rash, and eosinophilia or, when severe, as arthritis, purpura, lymphadenopathy, splenomegaly, mental changes, abnormal electrocardiographic findings, and edema. It usually takes at least 6 days to develop and can occur during treatment or up to 2 weeks after treatment has ceased.

Oral lesions: Delayed reactions to penicillin can exhibit themselves in the oral cavity. They include severe stomatitis, furred tongue, black tongue, acute glossitis, and cheilosis. These oral lesions can occur most commonly with topical application but have been reported with penicillin by other routes.

Other reactions: Interstitial nephritis, hemolytic anemia, and eosinophilia are types of allergic reactions occasionally reported during penicillin therapy.

When reactions to penicillin occur, the consequences are often serious. It is estimated that an anaphylactic reaction occurs in up to 0.05% of penicillin-treated patients, with a mortality of 5% to 10%. It is estimated that 400 deaths occur annually in the United States because of an allergic reaction to penicillin. Although the chance of a serious allergic reaction to penicillin is greater after parenteral administration, anaphylactic shock and death after oral use have also been reported. Patients who have a history of any allergy are more likely to be allergic to penicillin.

Allergic reactions to penicillin of any type may be followed by more serious allergic reactions on subsequent exposure. Any history of an allergic reaction to penicillin contraindicates its use, and another antibiotic should be substituted. However, a history negative for penicillin allergy does not guarantee its lack. If a penicillin is prescribed and any question of a reaction remains, one should make sure that, after the first dose is taken, the patient is somewhere where help can be summoned if necessary.

Uses

Penicillin is an important antibiotic in medical and dental practice. Its use in dentistry results from its bactericidal potency, lack of toxicity, and spectrum of activity, which includes many oral flora. It is often used for the treatment of dental infections. Table 7.1 demonstrates the dental infections for which penicillin is the drug of choice if patients are not allergic to it. Amoxicillin, a close penicillin relative, is also used for specific prophylactic indications. It is the agent of choice for the prophylaxis of infective endocarditis in nonallergic patients who have cardiac conditions associated with the highest risk of adverse outcomes from endocarditis (see the discussion on antibiotic prophylaxis of infective endocarditis at the end of this chapter). Penicillin's effectiveness in the treatment of dental infections is explained by its effectiveness against many aerobic and anaerobic bacteria.

Specific Penicillins

Penicillin G

Penicillin G, the prototype penicillin, is available as sodium, potassium, procaine, or benzathine salts. These salts differ in onset and duration of action and plasma level attained. One should note that the potassium salt given IV produces the most rapid and highest blood level, whereas the benzathine salt given IM produces the lowest and most sustained blood level. The potassium and procaine salts, given IM, produce intermediate blood levels and durations of action. The penicillin's duration of action is inversely proportional to the solubility of the penicillin form: The least soluble is the longest acting.

The sodium salts of penicillin should be avoided in patients with a limited sodium intake such as those with cardiovascular problems. Patients with renal disease should not be given potassium salts, because doing so could result in hyperkalemia. Patients may be allergic to the procaine moiety in procaine penicillin G. Both procaine and benzathine penicillins are suspensions given IM, from which the penicillin is slowly released.

Penicillin V

Penicillin V has a spectrum of activity very similar to that of penicillin G. The potassium salt of penicillin V (K penicillin V or penicillin VK) is more soluble than the free acid and therefore is better absorbed when taken orally. Table 7.1 lists some situations in which penicillin is the drug of first choice if the patient is not allergic to it. The usual adult dose is 250 to 500 mg three (tid) to four times a day (qid) for treatment of an infection for a minimum of 5 days and preferably 7 to 10 days.

Penicillinase-Resistant Penicillins

Penicillinase-resistant penicillins should be reserved for use against penicillinase-producing staphylococci. Compared with penicillin G, the penicillinase-resistant penicillins are less effective against penicillin G–sensitive organisms. They also have more side effects, such as GI discomfort, bone marrow depression, and abnormal renal and hepatic function. Patients allergic to penicillin are also allergic to the penicillinase-resistant penicillins.

Because cloxacillin and dicloxacillin are better absorbed than the other penicillinase-resistant penicillins, they are the drugs of choice.

Ampicillins

Ampicillin (am-pi-SILL-in) and amoxicillin (a-mox-i-SILL-in) are most often used in medicine. These penicillinase-susceptible penicillins have a spectrum of activity that includes gram-positive cocci, *Haemophilus influenzae,* and enterococci such as *Escherichia coli, Proteus mirabilis,* and *Salmonella* and *Shigella* species.

Amoxicillin, a relative of ampicillin, is most often used to treat infections because it produces higher blood levels, is better absorbed, and requires less frequent dosing (three times daily vs. four times daily for penicillin VK or ampicillin), and its absorption is not impaired by food. Amoxicillin is the drug of choice for prophylaxis for infective endocarditis before a dental procedure. Amoxicillin is used to treat upper respiratory tract infections (*H. influenzae*), urinary tract infection (*E. coli*), and meningitis *(H. influenzae).* Otitis media in children is often treated with amoxicillin. Amoxicillin is also available mixed with clavulanic acid, a β-lactamase inhibitor (Augmentin). Clavulanic acid combines with and inhibits the β-lactamases produced by bacteria. Therefore, the amoxicillin is protected from enzymatic inactivation. This combination can be used with penicillin-producing organisms. It has had some use in the management of certain periodontal conditions (see Table 7.1).

Both ampicillin and amoxicillin can produce a variety of allergic reactions. Ampicillin is much more likely to cause rashes than other penicillins. There is strong evidence to suggest that the ampicillin rash is benign and not an allergic response. This unusual ampicillin-related rash is much more common in patients with mononucleosis (almost 100%) or those taking allopurinol. Cross-allergenicity between penicillin VK, amoxicillin, and ampicillin is complete (omitting the "weird" ampicillin rash).

Extended-Spectrum Penicillins

Ticarcillin and piperacillin have a wider spectrum of activity than penicillin G, with special activity against *Pseudomonas aeruginosa* and some strains of *Proteus.* They are not penicillinase resistant and are available parenterally to treat systemic infections.

CEPHALOSPORINS

> "Expensive cousins" of the penicillins.

The cephalosporin (sef-a-loe-SPOR-in) group of antibiotics is structurally related to the penicillins. Cephalosporins are active against a wide variety of both gram-positive and gram-negative organisms. The oral cephalosporin products, listed in Box 7.3, are divided into first-, second-, third-, and fourth-generation agents. Most third-generation cephalosporins are available for parenteral use. The orally active cephalosporins are discussed.

The source of the original cephalosporins was *Cephalosporium acremonium,* which was isolated from a sewer outlet near Sardinia in Italy. Because cephalosporins are true antibiotics, they were originally produced by organisms. Those available for oral use are relatively acid stable and highly resistant to penicillinase, but they are destroyed by cephalosporinase, an enzyme elaborated by some microorganisms.

Pharmacokinetics

The cephalosporins can be administered orally, IM, or intravenously. The agents that cannot be used orally are too poorly absorbed to provide adequate blood levels. The cephalosporins used orally are well absorbed. They are bound to the plasma proteins in a proportion between 10% and 65% (see Box 7.3). After absorption, they are widely distributed throughout the tissues. Like penicillin, the cephalosporins are excreted by glomerular filtration and tubular secretion into the urine. Their half-lives vary between 50 and 240 minutes.

Spectrum

The cephalosporins, which are bactericidal, are active against most gram-positive cocci, penicillinase-producing staphylococci, and some gram-negative bacteria. They inhibit most *Salmonella* and *Klebsiella* organisms, some paracolon strains, and *E. coli. Serratia* and *Enterobacter* species, *H. influenzae,* indole-positive *Proteus,* methicillin-resistant staphylococci, and most *Pseudomonas* strains are unaffected. The generation of the cephalosporin (first, second, or third) designates the width of antimicrobial action; the first-generation width is narrower (gram-positive, few gram-negative) than the second-generation width (gram-positive, more gram-negative and anaerobes), and the third-generation agents (gram-positive weaker, many gram-negative and anaerobes) have the broadest spectrum of activity.

Mechanism of Action

The mechanism of action of the cephalosporins is like that of the penicillins: inhibition of cell wall synthesis. They bind to enzymes in the cell membrane involved in cell wall synthesis. The cephalosporin acts as an analog of acyl-D-alanyl-D-alanine to produce a deficiency in the cell walls, leading to lysis. They are more effective against rapidly growing organisms (which explains the potential drug interaction between bacteriostatic and bactericidal antibiotics).

Adverse Reactions

In general, the cephalosporins have a low incidence of adverse reactions (excluding allergic reactions) and are well tolerated. They have more adverse reactions than penicillin VK. The following adverse reactions may occur.

Gastrointestinal Effects

The most common adverse reaction associated with the cephalosporins is GI, including diarrhea, nausea, vomiting, abdominal pain, anorexia, dyspepsia, and stomatitis.

Nephrotoxicity

Evidence suggests that the cephalosporins may have nephrotoxic effects under certain conditions. Although some researchers have suggested that this is a toxic reaction, it may be an allergic reaction.

Superinfection

As with all antibiotics, especially those with a broader spectrum of activity, superinfection has been reported with the use of cephalosporins. Resistant gram-negative organisms are often the culprits.

Local Reaction

As with penicillin, the irritating nature of the cephalosporins can produce localized pain, induration, and swelling when given IM and abscess and thrombophlebitis when given intravenously.

Hemostasis and Disulfiram-Like Reaction

Certain parenteral cephalosporins can impair hemostasis or produce a disulfiram-like reaction. Dental health care workers do not use parenteral cephalosporins, and therefore this side effect is of no concern to dentistry.

Allergy

Various types of hypersensitivity reactions have been reported in approximately 5% of patients receiving cephalosporins. These reactions include fever, eosinophilia, serum sickness, rashes, and anaphylaxis.

BOX 7.3 Oral Cephalosporins

First-Generation
- Cephalexin (Keflex)
- Cefazolin (Ancef)

Second-Generation
- Cefaclor (Ceclor, Raniclor)
- Cefuroxime (Ceftin, Kefurox, Zinacef)

Third-Generation
- Cefixime (Suprax)
- Ceftriaxone (Rocephin)

Large doses often produce a direct positive Coombs reaction (immune mechanism is attacking the patient's own red blood cells). This can lead to a significant degree of hemolysis.

The cephalosporins and penicillin have similar structures; some cross-hypersensitivity can occur. Clinically, the incidence of hypersensitivity reactions to the cephalosporins is higher in patients with a history of penicillin allergy. The degree of cross-hypersensitivity reported is about 10%. Cephalosporins are often given to patients with a history of penicillin allergy, especially if the reaction was mild and in the distant past.

Patients who have experienced a nonsevere penicillin allergy, such as a minor, nonitchy rash, can receive a cephalosporin, especially if the documented allergy occurred more than 10 years ago. Cephalosporin use should be avoided in those persons who have experienced a severe allergy such as angioedema and anaphylaxis.

Uses

The cephalosporin antibiotics are indicated for the treatment of gram-positive organisms. They are indicated for infections that are sensitive to these agents but resistant to penicillin. They are especially useful in certain infections caused by gram-negative organisms such as *Klebsiella*. Their dental use includes prophylaxis for patients with at high risk for severe adverse outcomes from bacterial endocarditis who are undergoing dental procedures likely to produce bleeding. They are also used to treat infections with sensitive organisms when other agents are ineffective or cannot be used.

MACROLIDES

The macrolide antibiotics consist of erythromycin, clarithromycin, and azithromycin (Table 7.3).

Erythromycin
Mechanism and Spectrum

Erythromycin is usually bacteriostatic and interferes with protein synthesis by inhibiting the enzyme peptidyl transferase at the 50S ribosomal subunit. Its spectrum of activity closely resembles that of penicillin against gram-positive bacteria. It is also the drug of choice for *Bordetella, Legionella,* and *Actinomyces* organisms, *Mycoplasma pneumoniae, Entamoeba histolytica,* some *Chlamydia* species, and diphtheria. It is also indicated for streptococcal and staphylococcal infections.

Pharmacokinetics

Erythromycin is administered orally as tablets and capsules, oral suspensions in IV and IM forms, and in topical preparations. Because erythromycin is broken down in the gastric fluid, it is formulated as an enteric-coated tablet, capsule, or insoluble ester to reduce degradation by stomach acid. It should be administered 2 hours before or 2 hours after meals (Table 7.4). The peak blood level varies between 1 and 6 hours. Although food reduces the absorption of erythromycin, it may have to be taken with food to minimize its adverse GI effects. Its half-life is 2 hours.

Adverse Reactions

With usual therapeutic doses of erythromycin, side effects other than GI are usually minimal. Allergic reactions to erythromycin are uncommon.

Gastrointestinal effects. The side effects most often associated with erythromycin administration are GI and include stomatitis, abdominal cramps, nausea, vomiting, and diarrhea.

Cholestatic jaundice. Cholestatic jaundice has been reported primarily with the estolate form but has also been reported with the ethylsuccinate form. Erythromycin base has not been associated with this reaction. Symptoms include nausea, vomiting, and abdominal cramps followed by jaundice and elevated liver enzyme levels. Patients with a history of hepatitis should be given erythromycin base or stearate. The mechanism of this adverse effect is believed to be a hypersensitivity reaction.

Drug Interactions

Erythromycin can increase the serum concentrations of theophylline, digoxin, triazolam, warfarin, carbamazepine, and cyclosporine. This effect may produce toxicity, depending on the doses of each drug. The mechanism by which erythromycin produces these drug interactions may involve inhibition of hepatic metabolism of the drugs. Table 7.4 lists some drug interactions of the macrolides.

Uses

Because erythromycin is active against essentially the same aerobic microorganisms as penicillin, it is the drug of first choice against these infections in penicillin-allergic patients. Erythromycin is not effective against the anaerobic *Bacteroides* species implicated in many dental infections.

TABLE 7.3 Macrolides

Drug	Food	Metabolism/ Excretion	Dose
Erythromycin			
Base (E-Mycin, Ery-Tab, Eryc, PCE, various)	MT	Hepatic, in bile	250 mg q6h or 500 mg q12 hours
Stearate (Erythrocin)	MT	Hepatic, in bile	250 mg q6h or 500 mg q12 hours
Estolate (Ilosone)	OK	Hepatic, in bile	250 mg q6h or 500 mg q12 hours
Ethyl succinate (EES)	OK	Hepatic, in bile	400–800 mg q6h
Azithromycin (Zithromax, various)	MT	Unchanged in bile	500 mg stat, then 250 mg qd
Clarithromycin (Biaxin, various)	OK	Metabolized to active; renal	500 mg bid

bid, Twice a day; *MT,* take on an empty stomach (1 hour before or 2 hours after eating); *OK,* may take without regard to meals; *qd,* daily; *stat,* immediately.

TABLE 7.4 Erythromycin Drug Interactions

Interacting Drug	Mechanism	Management
Antibiotics (clindamycin, penicillin)	Interferes with action of other antibiotics	Choose one antibiotic for both purposes; stop one while administering the other
Carbamazepine (Tegretol)	Increased serum levels of carbamazepine	Monitor
Oral contraceptives (birth control pills)	Decreased effectiveness of some oral contraceptives	Use alternative method of birth control (e.g., condoms) until end of that cycle (rest of the month)
Warfarin (Coumadin)	Increased warfarin effect	Bleeding increased
Theophylline (Theo-Dur, Slo-bid)	Increased theophylline toxicity	OK to give two doses

Azithromycin and Clarithromycin

Both azithromycin (ay-ZITH-roe-my-sin) (Zithromax, Z-Pak) and clarithromycin (klare-ITH-roe-my-sin) (Biaxin) are macrolide antibiotics similar to erythromycin. They inhibit RNA-dependent protein synthesis by binding to the 50S ribosomal subunit They have activity against aerobic gram-positive cocci, such as *Staphylococcus* and *Streptococcus* organisms, and gram-negative aerobes. In contrast to erythromycin, azithromycin and clarithromycin have variable action against some anaerobes. They are bacteriostatic and can be taken without regard to meals.

The incidence of adverse reactions is lower with azithromycin and clarithromycin as compared to erythromycin. Adverse reactions relate to the GI tract, including dyspepsia, diarrhea, nausea, and abdominal pain. Azithromycin has been reported to elevate liver function test (LFT) results and should be used with caution in patients with hepatic impairment. Clarithromycin can produce an abnormal or metallic taste.

Several drug interactions can occur with both agents because of their reduction in the metabolism of certain drugs metabolized in the liver. Azithromycin can increase the levels of astemizole, loratadine, carbamazepine, digoxin, and triazolam but does not affect either warfarin or theophylline. The peak of azithromycin is reduced by cations, such as magnesium and aluminum, but the total drug absorbed is not affected. Clarithromycin increases the levels of drugs metabolized in liver, such as theophylline, carbamazepine, digoxin, omeprazole, and astemizole. Like the other macrolides, clarithromycin inhibits the cytochrome P-450 (CYP-450) liver microsomal enzymes.

Azithromycin and clarithromycin are indicated as alternative antibiotics in the treatment of common orofacial infections caused by aerobic gram-positive cocci and susceptible anaerobes. The dose for azithromycin consists of 5 days of therapy: first day, 500 mg as a single dose, and then 250 mg/day for 4 more days; for clarithromycin, the dose is 500 mg bid for 7 to 10 days. When amoxicillin and clindamycin cannot be used for the prophylaxis of endocarditis and prosthetic joint infections, these macrolides can be used as alternative antibiotics. The dose for prevention of infective endocarditis or joint prosthesis is 500 mg 1 hour before the dental procedure.

TETRACYCLINES

The tetracyclines (te-tra-SYE-kleens) are broad-spectrum antibiotics affecting a wide range of microorganisms (Table 7.5). Their adverse effects on developing teeth are well known.

The first tetracycline was isolated from a *Streptomyces* strain in 1948. Since then, other tetracyclines have been derived from different species of *Streptomyces,* and the rest have been produced semisynthetically. The tetracyclines are closely related chemically and clinically.

Pharmacokinetics

The tetracyclines are most commonly given by mouth (PO). Absorption after oral administration varies but is fairly rapid. There is wide tissue distribution, and tetracyclines are secreted in the saliva and in the milk of lactating mothers (at half the plasma concentration). Tetracyclines are concentrated by the liver and excreted into the intestines via the bile. Enterohepatic circulation prolongs the action of the tetracyclines after they have been discontinued. The tetracyclines are also stored in the dentin and enamel of unerupted teeth and are concentrated in the gingival crevicular fluid. The long-acting agents are concentrated to at least four times serum levels.

The various tetracyclines differ clinically in duration of action, percentage absorbed when taken orally, half-life, and mechanism of elimination. Doxycycline is excreted in the feces, whereas tetracycline is eliminated essentially unchanged by glomerular filtration, and minocycline (min-oh-SYE-kleen) is metabolized in the liver and excreted in the urine. Both doxycycline and minocycline may be given safely to patients with renal dysfunction. All tetracyclines cross the placenta and enter the fetal circulation.

Spectrum

The tetracyclines are bacteriostatic, interfering with the synthesis of bacterial protein by binding at the 30S subunit of bacterial ribosomes. As broad-spectrum antibiotics, they are effective against a wide variety of gram-positive and gram-negative bacteria (both aerobes and anaerobes), *Rickettsia*, spirochetes (*Treponema pallidum),* some protozoa (*E. histolytica),* and *Chlamydia* and *Mycoplasma* organisms.

Bacterial resistance to the tetracyclines develops slowly in a stepwise fashion. Cross-resistance among tetracyclines is probably complete. This resistance is caused by a decreased uptake of the tetracycline by the organism. In the study of sensitivity of organisms isolated from dental infections, one-fifth to three-fifths of *S. viridans* and one-fifth to two-fifths of *S. aureus* were found to be resistant to tetracycline. The advantage of penicillin over tetracycline in these aerobic gram-positive infections is clear.

Adverse Reactions

Although most adverse reactions to the tetracyclines occur infrequently, GI distress is not uncommon.

TABLE 7.5 Oral and Topical Tetracyclines

Drug Name/Form	Serum Protein Binding (%)	Normal Serum $t_{(1/2)}$ (h)	Usual Oral Adult Dosage	Lipid Solubility
Tetracycline* (Sumycin)	20–65	6–10	250–500 mg q6h	Intermediate
Doxycycline caps (Vibramycin)[†]:	60–90	14–25	50 q6h or 100 12h	High
Caps (Periostat)[†,‡]	—	—	20 mg bid	—
Gels (Atridox)[§]	—	—	—	—
Minocycline (Minocin)[†,¶]	55–75	11–20	100 mg q12h	High

bid, Twice a day.
*Avoid concomitant administration with food or divalent or trivalent cations.
[†]May be taken with food or milk but not high concentration of divalent or trivalent cations.
[‡]Systemic very low doses; effect from collagenase, not antibacterial action.
[§]Used topically in the sulcus.
[¶]Vestibular side effects, blue oral lesions.

Gastrointestinal Effects

The GI adverse effects include anorexia, nausea, vomiting, diarrhea, gastroenteritis, glossitis, stomatitis, xerostomia, and superinfection (moniliasis). The side effects are largely related to local irritation from alteration of the oral, gastric, and enteric flora.

If diarrhea occurs in a patient receiving tetracycline, the possibility of an infectious enteritis, such as staphylococcal enterocolitis, intestinal candidiasis, or PMC (secondary to *Clostridium difficile* overgrowth), must be ruled out. In some patients taking tetracyclines, a yellowish-brown discoloration of the tongue has developed. This can occur with either topical or systemic administration. Patients with dentures are at higher risk for developing candidiasis (moniliasis) caused by superinfection associated with the areas of the oral mucosa tissue where breakdown has occurred, and even with an intact oral mucosa.

Effects on Teeth and Bones

Tetracyclines are incorporated into calcifying structures. If they are used during the period of enamel calcification, they can produce permanent discoloration of the teeth and enamel hypoplasia (Fig. 7.3). Consequently, they should not be used during the last half of pregnancy or in children younger than 9 years. Tetracycline affects the primary teeth of a child whose mother is given the drug during the last half of pregnancy or who is given the drug during the first 4 to 6 months of life. If tetracycline is administered between 2 months and 7 or 8 years of age, the permanent teeth will be affected. The mechanism involves the deposition of tetracycline in the enamel of the forming teeth. These stains are permanent and darken with age and exposure to light. They begin as a yellow fluorescence and progress with time to brown. This process is accelerated by exposure to light. The permanent discoloration ranges from light gray to yellow to tan. With large doses of tetracyclines, a decrease in the growth rate of bones has been demonstrated in the fetus and infant.

Minocycline can cause black pigmentation of mandibular and maxillary alveolar bone and the hard palate. When viewed through the mucosa, the pigment appears bluish. Other cases of oral pigmentation have been said to involve the crowns of the permanent teeth (half of incisal surface) and the gingival mucosa. The incidence of this oral pigmentation in adults is 10% after 1 year and 20% after 4 years of therapy.

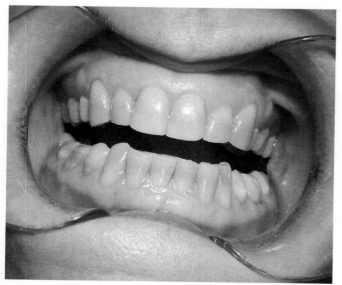

Fig. 7.3 Discoloration of teeth caused by tetracycline ingestion.

With discontinuation of minocycline, the pigmentation becomes less intense but is usually not completely reversible.

Hepatotoxicity

The incidence of liver damage increases with the IV use of tetracyclines. Deaths have occurred, especially in pregnant women. Renal impairment leads to accumulation of tetracycline and may increase the likelihood of hepatic damage.

Nephrotoxicity

Toxic renal effects with characteristic disorders of renal tubular function, producing Fanconi's syndrome, have been reported after the use of old (degraded) tetracycline. Old or outdated tetracycline should be discarded to prevent future use. Because the nephrotoxic effect of the tetracyclines is additive with that of other drugs, tetracyclines should not be used concomitantly with other nephrotoxic drugs.

Hematologic Effects

Although uncommon, the hematologic changes hemolytic anemia, leukocytosis, and thrombocytopenic purpura have been reported after tetracycline therapy.

Superinfection

With superinfection, resistant organisms multiply and may cause disease. One common situation, especially prevalent in the compromised host, is an overgrowth of *Candida albicans*. Oral or vaginal candidiasis can result from the administration of oral tetracycline.

Photosensitivity

Patients taking tetracyclines who are exposed to sunlight sometimes react with an exaggerated sunburn. Although the incidence seems to vary with the different tetracyclines, patients receiving a prescription for a tetracycline should be told to use a sunscreen before exposure to the sun.

Other Effects

Minocycline has been associated with CNS side effects, including lightheadedness, dizziness, and vertigo. Patients who will be driving a car should be warned about this reaction.

Allergy

Anaphylactic and various dermatologic reactions to the tetracyclines have occasionally occurred, but the overall allergenicity of these drugs is low. Glossitis and cheilosis have also been attributed to a hypersensitive reaction to tetracycline. A patient who is allergic to one tetracycline is almost certain to be allergic to all tetracyclines.

Drug Interactions

Cations

Divalent (Ca^{+2}, Mg^{+2}, Fe^{+2}, Zn^{+2}) and trivalent (Al^{+3}) cations reduce the intestinal absorption of tetracyclines by forming nonabsorbable chelates of tetracycline with, for example, calcium. Dairy products containing calcium, antacids (Ca^{+2}, Mg^{+2}, Al^{+3}), and mineral supplements (iron, calcium, zinc) or fortified foods should not be taken within 2 hours of ingesting tetracycline. Reasonable quantities of dairy products can be taken with doxycycline and minocycline because there is less interference with absorption, but concomitant administration with antacids or mineral supplements should be avoided.

Enhanced Effect of Other Drugs

Tetracycline enhances the effect of the oral sulfonylureas, potentially resulting in hypoglycemia. The effects of digoxin, lithium, and theophylline may also be enhanced, leading to toxicity from these agents with narrow therapeutic indices. Furosemide's toxicity may also be increased by tetracycline.

Reduced Doxycycline Effect

The barbiturates and phenytoin can reduce the action of doxycycline. The mechanism is stimulation of hepatic microsomal enzymes so that doxycycline is metabolized more rapidly.

General Antibiotic Interactions

Like all the antibiotics, tetracyclines may reduce the effectiveness of oral contraceptives or increase the effectiveness of oral anticoagulants. Also, in most instances, mixing a tetracycline with another antibiotic results in antagonism, especially if the other antibiotic is bactericidal.

Uses

Tetracyclines, including both tetracycline and doxycycline, have extensive medical and dental use.

Medical

Although active against a wide variety of microorganisms, tetracyclines are rarely the drugs of choice for a specific infection. Occasionally, they are alternative drugs to treat chlamydial and rickettsial infections. They are used to treat acne (topically and systemically), pulmonary infections in patients with chronic obstructive pulmonary disease (COPD), and traveler's diarrhea. Tetracyclines should not be used for prophylaxis against infective endocarditis except in one unusual situation in dentistry, which is discussed in the next section.

Dental

Tetracyclines are not drugs of choice or alternative drugs of choice for dental infections unrelated to periodontal disease. They are, however, often used for certain periodontal conditions. Conventional treatment with local measures should have failed before tetracycline therapy is initiated. A potential advantage of the tetracyclines in treatment of certain periodontal situations relates to their ability to concentrate in the gingival crevicular fluid. Because long-acting tetracyclines are concentrated to a greater extent in the gingival fluid and they require once-daily dosing, they may have some advantage over tetracycline itself.

CLINDAMYCIN

Clindamycin (klin-da-MYE-sin) (Cleocin) is a bacteriostatic antibiotic effective primarily against gram-positive organisms and anaerobic *Bacteroides* species. Clindamycin is produced by adding a -Cl group to lincomycin, which is elaborated by *Streptomyces lincolnensis,* found in a soil sample taken near Lincoln, Nebraska. Clindamycin is structurally unrelated to any antimicrobial agent other than lincomycin, which is not used.

Pharmacokinetics

Clindamycin may be administered orally, topically, IM, intravenously, or vaginally. Oral clindamycin is well absorbed, and food does not interfere with its absorption. It reaches its peak concentration in 45 minutes with a half-life of about 2.5 hours. Clindamycin is distributed throughout most body tissues, including bone, but not to the cerebrospinal fluid. Concentration in the bone can approximate that in the plasma. It crosses the placental barrier, and it is more than 90% bound to plasma proteins. Only about 10% of the active drug is eliminated in

the urine. The majority of clindamycin is excreted as inactive metabolites in the urine and feces (via the bile).

Spectrum

The antibacterial spectrum of clindamycin includes many gram-positive organisms and some gram-negative organisms. The antibacterial action results from interference with bacterial protein synthesis. Clindamycin is bacteriostatic in most cases, although occasionally it can be bactericidal at higher blood levels.

Like erythromycin's, clindamycin's activity includes *S. pyogenes* and *S. viridans,* pneumococci, and *S. aureus.* In contrast to erythromycin, clindamycin is very active against several anaerobes, including *Bacteroides fragilis* and *Bacteroides melaninogenicus, Fusobacterium* species, *Peptostreptococcus* (anaerobic streptococci) and *Peptococcus* species, and *Actinomyces israelii.*

Bacterial resistance to clindamycin develops in a slow, stepwise manner. It occurs by mutations in the bacterial ribosomes that result in a decrease in affinity and binding capacity of these drugs. Cross-resistance between clindamycin and erythromycin is often noted. An antagonistic relationship has been observed between clindamycin and erythromycin because of competition for the same binding site (50S subunit) on the bacteria.

Adverse Reactions

Gastrointestinal Effects

> Pseudomembranous colitis possible but not common.

The most commonly observed side effects of clindamycin are GI, including diarrhea, nausea, vomiting, enterocolitis, and abdominal cramps. Glossitis and stomatitis have also been reported with these agents. The incidence of diarrhea with clindamycin is approximately 10%.

The development of PMC, also known as *antibiotic-associated colitis (AAC),* has been a more serious consequence associated with clindamycin. It is characterized by severe, persistent diarrhea, and the passage of blood and mucus. This colitis, which can be fatal, is caused by a toxin produced by the bacterium *C.C. difficile.* It is associated not only with clindamycin but also with other antibiotics such as tetracycline, ampicillin, and the cephalosporins. Treatment of colitis includes discontinuation of the drug, vancomycin or cholestyramine administered orally, and fluid and electrolyte replacement. Systemically administered corticosteroids have sometimes proved helpful. Opioid-like agents, such as the combination of diphenoxylate and atropine (Lomotil), may exacerbate the condition and should not be used. PMC may occur during treatment, several weeks after cessation of antibiotic therapy, or without any antibiotic use.

Superinfection

As with other antibiotics, superinfection by *C. albicans* is sometimes associated with the use of clindamycin.

Other Effects

Adverse reactions affecting the formed elements in the blood include neutropenia, thrombocytopenia, and agranulocytosis. Abnormal LFT values and renal dysfunction have been noted.

Allergy

Morbilliform skin rashes occasionally occur in patients given clindamycin. Oral allergic manifestations include glossitis and stomatitis. More severe allergic reactions include urticaria, angioneurotic edema, erythema multiforme, serum sickness, and anaphylaxis.

Uses

Although clindamycin is effective against many gram-positive organisms, other agents are available that are at least as effective as clindamycin and do not usually cause PMC. The indications for treatment with clindamycin are limited to a number of infections caused by anaerobic organisms, especially *Bacteroides* species and some staphylococcal infections, in the patient allergic to penicillin.

Many oral infections have been shown to contain a predominance of anaerobic organisms. Many of these anaerobes, such as *Bacteroides oralis, Peptostreptococcus, Fusobacterium,* and *Veillonella* species and clostridia, are sensitive to oral penicillin V. Clindamycin is the drug of choice for some *Bacteroides* species and other anaerobes, endocarditis prophylaxis in the patient with penicillin allergy, and some pelvic infections.

Mixed gram-positive and gram-negative anaerobic infections may be treated with clindamycin. The use of clindamycin when anaerobic osteomyelitis is suspected is indicated if the organism is susceptible. It is important to emphasize that clindamycin should be used only when specifically indicated, not indiscriminately, and that the patient should be warned of the potential for PMC and informed about its symptoms (bloody diarrhea mixed with mucus). The usual adult dose of clindamycin for sinusitis is 150 to 300 mg q6h (qid).

METRONIDAZOLE

Metronidazole (me-troe-NI-da-zole) (Flagyl) is a synthetic nitroimidazole with trichomonacidal *(Trichomonas vaginalis)*, amebicidal *(E. histolytica)*, and bactericidal action. It has exceptional action against most obligate anaerobes, such as *Bacteroides* species. As with all antibiotics, resistance to this agent is increasing. It freely enters cells and is reduced into unknown polar compounds that do not contain the nitro group. This short-lived product is cytotoxic, but it causes DNA to lose its cyclic structure and inhibits nucleic acid synthesis, leading to death of the organisms. It affects cells whether they are or are not dividing.

In addition to its antiinfective effects, metronidazole also has antiinflammatory effects. It affects neutrophil motility, lymphocyte action, and cell-mediated immunity. What therapeutic purpose these actions might serve is yet to be identified.

Pharmacokinetics

Taken orally, metronidazole is well absorbed, with a peak level occurring between 1 and 2 hours after administration. Between 60% and 80% of a dose is excreted in the urine. Metabolites account for about 20% of the dose. The half-life averages 8 hours, but with alcoholic liver disease it averages 18 hours. Metronidazole is less than 20% protein bound. It is somewhat concentrated in the gingival crevicular fluid, producing concentrations that are bactericidal to pathogenic periodontal organisms. Metronidazole is distributed into the cerebrospinal fluid, saliva, and breast milk in levels approximating that in serum.

Spectrum

Metronidazole is bactericidal and penetrates all bacterial cells. Its spectrum of activity includes the protozoa *T. vaginalis* and *E. histolytica.* Metronidazole is active against obligate anaerobic bacteria such as *Bacteroides, Fusobacterium, Veillonella, Treponema, Clostridium, Peptococcus, Campylobacter,* and *Peptostreptococcus* organisms. The increased use of antibiotics is resulting in a continuing rise in the incidence of resistance. One should compare the spectrum of activity of metronidazole with that of the bacteria responsible for periodontal conditions and the concentration effective against those bacteria to minimize resistance.

Adverse Reactions

Gastrointestinal Effects

> Stomach distress is common.

Metronidazole's most common adverse reactions involve the GI tract. This side effect occurs in 12% of patients taking metronidazole. It includes nausea, anorexia, diarrhea, and vomiting. Epigastric distress and abdominal cramping have also been reported.

Central Nervous System Effects

Headache, dizziness, vertigo, and ataxia have been reported. Confusion, depression, weakness, insomnia, and serious convulsive seizures are rarely associated with metronidazole use.

Renal Toxicity

Cystitis, polyuria, dysuria, and incontinence can occur with metronidazole. Rarely, darkening of the urine as a result of a metabolite has been reported.

Oral Effects

> Xerostomia and unpleasant metallic taste.

Another effect that has been reported is a dry mouth. Often, an unpleasant or sharp metallic taste has also been reported. Altered taste of alcohol has been noted. Glossitis, stomatitis, and a black-furred tongue are side effects the dental health care worker might observe. These side effects may be related to monilial overgrowth. Appendix D discusses xerostomia in more detail.

Other Effects

Transient neutropenia in humans and carcinogenicity, mutagenicity, and tumorigenicity in lower life forms have been reported with use of metronidazole. This agent is in US Food and Drug Administration (FDA) pregnancy category B because its administration to pregnant mice caused fetal toxicity. Administration of metronidazole for dental infections during pregnancy is contraindicated. A nursing mother should not be given metronidazole unless she expresses and discards her breast milk beginning when she starts taking the drug and continuing for 48 hours after she stops taking it.

Drug Interactions

> No alcohol with metronidazole.

When alcohol is ingested with metronidazole, a disulfiram-like reaction can occur. Disulfiram (Antabuse) is a drug used to treat persons with alcohol problems (see Chapter 23). Symptoms include nausea, abdominal cramps, flushing, vomiting, and headache. Alcohol should be avoided during metronidazole administration and for 1 day after therapy has ceased. Products that contain alcohol, such as mouthwashes or elixirs, should not be used during this period.

Metronidazole can potentiate the effect of warfarin. The combination of metronidazole and disulfiram has led to confusion and should be avoided. Drugs that stimulate liver microsomal enzymes, such as phenobarbital and phenytoin, can reduce the plasma levels of metronidazole. Before metronidazole is administered to patients, the possibility of a drug interaction should be checked.

Uses

Metronidazole is used for the treatment of infections caused by susceptible organisms in both medical and dental conditions. It has special usefulness because of its anaerobic spectrum.

Medical

The medical uses of metronidazole include treatment of trichomoniasis, giardiasis, amebiasis, and susceptible anaerobic bacterial infections. It is effective against serious anaerobic infections of the abdomen, skeleton, and female genital tract. Endocarditis and lower respiratory tract infections caused by *Bacteroides* species are treated with metronidazole. It is available as oral tablets and capsules; vaginal cream and gel for vaginal infections; topical cream, gel, and lotions for the treatment of rosacea; and IV solution for anaerobic infections.

Dental

Because of its anaerobic efficacy, metronidazole is useful in the treatment of many periodontal infections. One notable exception is that it has no action against *A. actinomycetemcomitans*. One advantage of metronidazole is that when prescribed generically, it is inexpensive (see Fig. 7.1).

RATIONAL USE OF ANTIINFECTIVE AGENTS IN DENTISTRY

Stages of Infection

Most dental infections progress through stages. Stage 1 is primarily gram-positive organisms; the mixed stage, stage 2, has both aerobes and anaerobes; and the last stage, stage 3, is exclusively anaerobes. If incision and drainage are possible, most dental infections in patients with normal immunity, whether the infection is in stage 1, 2, or 3, do not need antiinfective agents.

Stage 1

Acute abscess and cellulitis are primarily the result of gram-positive organisms. The drug of choice in patients without a penicillin allergy is penicillin or amoxicillin. The patient must complete the full course of therapy to ensure that all of the bacteria are killed off and to help reduce to the chance for resistance. For those with an allergy to penicillin, erythromycin ethylsuccinate or clindamycin may be used (see Appendix C for a flowchart).

Stage 2

During stage 2, the infection is mixed. It can be handled by attacking either the gram-positive organisms or the anaerobes. The gram-positive organisms can be managed with the same drugs as in stage 1. To attack the anaerobes, an antiinfective with good anaerobic coverage is needed. The two antibiotics with the most anaerobic coverage are clindamycin and metronidazole. Penicillin V also has anaerobic coverage. If drainage can be established, antiinfective agents are not indicated in the immunocompetent patient.

Stage 3

In stage 3, the organisms have coalesced into one area and are almost solely anaerobic. Most often, incision and drainage are sufficient. In fact, drainage sometimes happens spontaneously and the patient is "cured" (in his or her mind because he or she does not have pain). If chronic infection persists or if the patient is immunocompromised, use of an antibiotic with anaerobic coverage is warranted.

Failure of Antiinfective Therapy

When a prescribed antiinfective is not effective, there may be several reasons for this outcome. If an antibiotic failure occurs, the patient must be reevaluated, with the following reasons why an antibiotic may be ineffective taken into account:

Patient adherence: The patient may not be taking the antibiotic, because he or she

- *Did not get the prescription filled:* Was the patient informed about the benefit that the medicine would have? Was the patient informed about the risk of not taking the medicine? Consequences?
- *Tried and failed to get the prescription filled:* There was a long wait at the pharmacy. The children have to be picked up from school. The checkbook was forgotten. When the patient was told the price of the prescription, he or she could not afford it. The patient was told that antibiotics can interfere with the effectiveness of birth control pills and she did not want to get pregnant.
- *Got prescription filled but …:* The patient noticed that the tablets "smelled bad" or were "hard to swallow," or he or she "decided to take an herbal product."
- *Did not complete prescription:* Patients often state that they "began to feel better," "forgot to take some pills," "took a few but then quit," "saved them for the next time I have a toothache," and so on.

Ineffective antibiotic: The antibiotic chosen may not be effective against the organism producing the infection. If there is no response to an antibiotic after 2 or 3 days, consideration should be given to changing the agent (check compliance first).

Poor débridement: Dead tissue, purulent exudate, or foreign bodies were not completely removed from the site of infection.

Resistant organism: The antibiotic may not be effective because the organism is resistant to it. Knowledge about the resistance patterns in the dental area is important to consider before an antibiotic is prescribed.

Failure of antibiotic concentration to reach site of infection: There are several mechanisms by which an adequate concentration of the antibiotic does not reach the site of the infection. Lack of penetration may occur because of decreased vascularity, an isolated location or "walled-off" area, or a drug interaction inactivating the antibiotic before absorption. Microvascular disease, often seen in diabetic patients, further reduces the blood flow and the amount of antibiotic sent to the area.

Inadequate host defenses: The ability of the host's immune system to fight the infection is very important in ridding the body of the infection.

ANTIMICROBIAL AGENTS FOR NONDENTAL USE

Vancomycin

> Used intravenous for systemic effect; used by PO for local effect.

Vancomycin (van-koe-MYE-sin) (Vancocin) is an antibiotic elaborated by *Streptomyces orientalis,* an actinomycete found in soil samples from India and Indonesia. It is unrelated to any other antibiotic currently marketed. Because it has very poor GI absorption and causes irritation when used IM, it is usually administered only intravenously for a systemic effect. When given PO, it is being used to eradicate organisms within the GI tract.

Spectrum

Vancomycin is bactericidal and has a narrow spectrum of activity against many gram-positive cocci, including both staphylococci and streptococci.

It acts by inhibition of bacterial cell wall synthesis. In the past, resistance to this agent did not develop readily, but vancomycin-resistant organisms have now appeared. When resistance was uncommon, vancomycin was rarely used. After resistance to other organisms increased, the use of vancomycin increased. This led, predictably, to an increase in resistance to vancomycin. Cross-resistance with other antibiotics is not believed to occur because vancomycin differs in structure from other antibiotics.

Adverse Reactions

Except when vancomycin is given in large doses, significant toxic reactions are infrequent. With oral use, nausea, vomiting, and a bitter taste may be experienced. With IV use, an erythematous rash on the face and upper body has been reported (red man syndrome). Hypotension accompanied by flushing, chills, and drug fever is also associated with vancomycin.

Aminoglycosides

As the name implies, the *aminoglycoside* (a-mee-noe-GLYE- koe-side) antibiotics are made up of amino sugars in glycosidic linkage. In 1943, a strain *of Streptomyces griseus* was isolated that elaborated streptomycin. Further strains of *Streptomyces* species furnished neomycin, kanamycin, tobramycin, and amikacin, and *Micromonospora* organisms produced gentamicin and netilmicin. They are bactericidal and appear to inhibit protein synthesis and to act directly on the 30S subunit of the ribosome. The amino glycosides are as follows:
- Neomycin (Neo-Fradin, Neo-Rx)
- Gentamicin (Garamycin)
- Tobramycin (AKTob, TOBI, Tobrex)
- Amikacin (Amikin)

Pharmacokinetics

Because aminoglycosides are poorly absorbed after oral administration, they must be administered IM or intravenously for a systemic effect. Aminoglycosides are used orally for their local effect within the intestines. Before GI surgery, aminoglycosides reduce the intestinal bacterial flora.

Spectrum

The aminoglycosides are bactericidal and have a broad antibacterial spectrum. They are used primarily to treat aerobic gram-negative infections when other agents are ineffective. They have little activity against gram-positive anaerobic or facultative bacteria.

Adverse Reactions

The adverse reactions of the aminoglycoside antibiotics seriously limit their use in clinical practice. Their major adverse effects include the following.

Ototoxicity. The aminoglycosides are toxic to the eighth cranial nerve, which can lead to auditory and vestibular (in ear) disturbances, or ototoxicity. Patients may have difficulty maintaining equilibrium and can experience vertigo. Hearing impairment and deafness, which can be permanent, have resulted from the administration of these agents. This side effect is more common in patients with renal failure because the drug accumulates in the body. Elderly patients are also more susceptible.

Nephrotoxicity. The aminoglycosides can cause kidney damage by concentrating in the renal cortex. The blood levels and total amount of drug given correlate with the incidence of nephrotoxicity.

Uses

The aminoglycosides are indicated for the treatment of serious gram-negative infections in hospitalized patients with. Topical aminoglycosides are used to treat certain eye infections and skin infections.

Sulfonamides

Sulfonamides were the first antibiotics, paving the way for the antibiotic revolution.

Mechanism of Action

> *p*-Aminobenzoic acid analog inhibits synthesis of folic acid.

The structural similarity between the sulfonamide agents and *p*-aminobenzoic acid (PABA) is the basis for most of their antibacterial activity. Unlike humans, many bacteria are unable to use preformed folic acid, which is essential for their growth. They must synthesize folic acid from PABA. Because of their structural similarity to PABA, the sulfonamides competitively inhibit dihydropteroate synthetase, the bacterial enzyme that incorporates PABA into dihydrofolic acid, an immediate precursor of folic acid (Fig. 7.4). Drugs that are metabolized to PABA (e.g., ester local anesthetics) could theoretically interfere with the action of the sulfonamides.

Spectrum

The sulfonamides are bacteriostatic against many gram-positive and some gram-negative bacteria. They are often used in medicine to treat acute otitis media in children *(H. influenzae),* acute exacerbations of chronic bronchitis in adults *(S. pneumoniae),* and urinary tract infections *(Klebsiella* and *Enterobacter* organisms and *E. coli).* They are ineffective against *S. viridans* but are active against some *Chlamydia* organisms. Sulfonamides are also used for prophylaxis of *Pneumocystis carinii* pneumonitis and for traveler's diarrhea caused by enterotoxigenic *E. coli* or *Cyclospora* organisms.

The readily absorbed sulfonamides are used for their systemic effects and are distributed throughout the body. Some poorly soluble sulfonamides, when given orally, act locally in the treatment of ulcerative colitis or before surgical procedures on the bowel.

Adverse Reactions

> Drink plenty of water.

The most common adverse reaction to the sulfonamides is an allergic skin reaction. Patients with an allergy to "sulfa" drugs may exhibit some cross-hypersensitivity with thiazide diuretics and the sulfonylureas (used orally to treat diabetes). There is no cross-hypersensitivity between sulfa drugs and sulfites, sulfates, or sulfur.

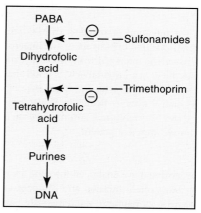

Fig. 7.4 Location of action of sulfonamides and trimethoprim. They inhibit the synthesis of folic acid at two different locations. *PABA, p*-Aminobenzoic acid.

The allergic reactions may manifest as rash, urticaria, pruritus, fever, a fatal exfoliative dermatitis, or periarteritis nodosa (serious blood vessel disease in which small and medium-sized arteries become swollen and damaged). Other cutaneous allergic reactions are erythema nodosum, erythema multiforme, Stevens-Johnson syndrome, and epidermal necrolysis.

Other relatively common side effects include nausea, vomiting, abdominal discomfort, headache, and dizziness. Liver damage, depressed renal function, blood dyscrasias (agranulocytosis, thrombocytopenia, aplastic and hemolytic anemias), and precipitation of lupus erythematosus are seen less often.

Patients with human immunodeficiency virus (HIV) are much more likely to exhibit adverse effects (65%), such as rash, fever, and leukopenia, and to discontinue therapy. In patients with HIV, the sulfisoxazole-trimethoprim combination is used prophylactically to prevent *P. carinii* pneumonia.

The possibility of renal crystallization (crystalluria) must always be kept in mind with the sulfonamides. The earlier sulfonamides had low solubility in the urine, and there was danger of crystallization in the kidney. The new sulfonamides are more soluble and therefore less likely to precipitate in the kidney. This is the reason patients taking sulfonamides are encouraged to drink plenty of water.

Uses

These agents have no use in dentistry.

Sulfamethoxazole-Trimethoprim

Trimethoprim (trye-METH-oh-prim), an antibacterial and antimalarial agent, and sulfamethoxazole (sul-fa-meth-OX-a-zole), a sulfonamide, are commonly used in combination (SMX-TMP, co-trimoxazole, Bactrim, Septra). Because sulfamethoxazole (SMX) inhibits the incorporation of PABA into folic acid and trimethoprim (TMP) inhibits the reduction of dihydrofolate to tetrahydrofolate, this combination inhibits two separate steps in the essential metabolic pathway of the bacteria, thus delaying resistance and having a synergistic effect.

SMX-TMP is bacteriostatic against a wide variety of gram-positive bacteria and some gram-negative bacteria. Its adverse effects are similar to those of the sulfonamides. Approximately 75% of the adverse reactions associated with this combination involve skin disorders.

SMX-TMP is indicated in the treatment of selected urinary tract infections and selected respiratory and GI infections. It is used extensively to treat acute otitis media in children, which is often caused by *H. influenzae*. A combination of erythromycin and sulfisoxazole (Pediazole) is also used to treat otitis media in children. SMX-TMP is used prophylactically to prevent *P. carinii* pneumonia in patients with AIDS, *Serratia* sepsis, and systemic *Salmonella* (ampicillin-resistant) and *Shigella* infections. SMX-TMP has no documented use in dentistry, but pediatric patients coming to the dental office may be taking it prophylactically for prevention of chronic ear infections.

Nitrofurantoin

Nitrofurantoin (nye-troe-fyoor-AN-toyn) (Macrodantin) possesses a wide antibacterial spectrum including both gram-positive and gram-negative bacteria. It is bacteriostatic against many common urinary tract pathogens, including *E. coli*. Many strains of *Klebsiella* and *Enterobacter* and all strains of *P. aeruginosa* are resistant to it. The most common adverse reactions are nausea, vomiting, and diarrhea, but taking the drug with food decreases them. Nitrofurantoin can also cause a brownish discoloration of urine. Many hypersensitivity reactions are associated with nitrofurantoin. Nitrofurantoin is used in the treatment or prophylaxis of certain urinary tract infections.

Quinolones (Fluoroquinolones)

> Orally effective and active against *Pseudomonas* organisms.

A group of orally effective antibacterial agents called the *quinolones* (KWIN-a-lones) are chemically related to nalidixic (nal-i-DIX-ik) acid (NegGram). This group may have potential use in dentistry because of its spectrum of activity. As with all antibiotics, their overuse produces resistance. They are bactericidal against most gram-negative organisms and many gram-positive organisms. They are the first orally active agents against certain *Pseudomonas* species. There is no cross-resistance with other antimicrobial agents.

The mechanism of action of the quinolones is unique and involves antagonism of the A subunit of DNA gyrase, which is an enzyme involved in DNA synthesis. The interference with DNA gyrase results in cell death, and resistance is not transferred from a resistant bacteria to an unexposed bacteria. Examples of the fluoroquinolones are listed in Box 7.4. The discussion concentrates on ciprofloxacin (sip-roe-FLOKS-a-sin) (Cipro), a prototype of the quinolones.

Pharmacokinetics

Ciprofloxacin is well absorbed orally and is eliminated with a half-life of 4 hours. Both antacids and probenecid interfere with ciprofloxacin's absorption and serum concentration. Patients should be well hydrated to prevent any possibility of crystalluria (drink water while taking it).

Spectrum

Ciprofloxacin is bactericidal against a wide range of gram-negative organisms, including *Klebsiella* and *Enterobacter* species, *E. coli, P. aeruginosa,* and gram-positive organisms such as *S. aureus*. It is especially effective against *Pseudomonas* organisms. Unlike with other antiinfective agents, an additive action may result when ciprofloxacin is combined with other antimicrobial agents. The emergence of organisms resistant to the fluoroquinolones and the cross-resistance among the fluoroquinolones is increasing. Use of fluoroquinolones in chickens may be partially responsible for increasing resistance.

Adverse Reactions

Gastrointestinal effects. Nausea, diarrhea, vomiting, painful oral mucosa, bad taste, and oral candidiasis have been reported. PMC has been seen in patients taking quinolones.

Central nervous system effects. CNS adverse reactions with quinolones include headache, restlessness, lightheadedness, and insomnia. CNS stimulation has been noted.

Hypersensitivity. Rash, pruritus, urticaria, hyperpigmentation, and edema of the lips have been noted. Fluoroquinolones are associated with photosensitivity reactions when patients are exposed to the sun. Patients taking these drugs should be advised to use sunscreen or to wear clothes that cover the whole body. A few anaphylactic reactions have been reported.

Other effects. An unusual reaction affecting the Achilles tendon has become fairly common in patients taking quinolones. These agents can

---

BOX 7.4 Examples of Fluoroquinolones

Ciprofloxacin (Cipro)
Gemifloxacin (Factive)
Levofloxacin (Levaquin)
Moxifloxacin (Avelox)
Norfloxacin (Noroxin)
Ofloxacin (Floxin)

cause tendinitis or tendon rupture in the Achilles tendon. In 2008, the FDA issued a boxed warning ("black box" warning) for these drugs, alerting physicians and patients to the serious risk of tendon damage and rupture. In 2013, the FDA strengthened its warning regarding the risk for sudden, serious, and potentially permanent peripheral neuropathy, which has been listed as a side effect of fluoroquinolones antibiotics since 2004.

Pregnancy and nursing considerations. Ciprofloxacin is contraindicated in the pregnant or nursing woman.

Uses

Ciprofloxacin is indicated for lower respiratory tract, skin, bone and joint, and urinary tract infections caused by susceptible organisms. Because of the spectrum of the quinolones, future use may include dental periodontal disease. In summary, the quinolones have an advantage over other antimicrobial agents because of their unique mechanism of action, making the development and transfer of resistance more difficult. Their gram-negative spectrum coupled with their oral efficacy and bactericidal action makes these agents a welcome addition to the antimicrobial armamentarium. However, because of the serious potentially permanent adverse effects associated with the quinolones, the FDA recommends that they should only be used when all other options have been exhausted.

ANTITUBERCULOSIS AGENTS

The treatment of TB, a disease caused by the acid-fast bacterium *Mycobacterium tuberculosis,* is difficult for several reasons.
- Patients with TB often have inadequate defense mechanisms (e.g., because of AIDS).
- Tubercle bacilli develop resistant strains easily and possess unusual metabolic characteristics, including long periods of inactivity (they become dormant) when they are resistant to treatment.
- Most of the drugs available are not bactericidal and because of their toxicity often cannot be used in sufficient doses.
- People using antituberculosis agents often do not take them as prescribed.

For these reasons, the development of multidrug-resistant TB (MDR TB) has continued to increase because of its spread among patients with HIV or other immunocompromising illness, among the homeless, and in other countries. Treatment of TB relies almost entirely on chemotherapy (Table 7.6). Because of the problem of resistance, at least three drugs are administered concurrently in all active cases. Isoniazid (INH), rifampin, ethambutol, and pyrazinamide are combined for the treatment of pulmonary TB. INH and rifampin are continued every day for 9 to 12 months. Pyrazinamide and ethambutol are only used during the first 2 months of therapy. With susceptible organisms, a patient compliant with therapy usually becomes noninfective within 2 to 3 weeks. Compliance presents a problem, however, because patients often stop taking their medication before the designated time.

The Centers for Disease Control and Prevention (CDC) recommends that the following patients receive INH because they are at risk for development of TB: close contacts of recently diagnosed patients, patients with a positive skin test result and radiographic findings consistent with nonprogressive TB, patients whose skin test result has become positive (converted), and immunosuppressed patients. If patients have been vaccinated against TB (with **bacillus Calmette-Guérin [BCG]**), results of skin tests (purified protein derivative [PPD]) will always be positive, and chest radiographs are required for screening. Because many people have TB, it is not unlikely that a TB-positive person may come in and request treatment. If a person with active TB seeks oral health care, contact that person's physician and delay health care until the disease is no longer in the active state.

Isoniazid

Isoniazid (eye-soe-NYE-a-zid) (Laniazid), or INH, is bactericidal only against actively growing tubercle bacilli. The mechanism of action may relate to inhibition of mycolic acid synthesis, which results in disruption of the bacterial cell wall. "Resting" bacilli exposed to the drug are able to resume normal growth when the drug is removed. Within a few weeks after the start of therapy, resistant strains develop.

TABLE 7.6 Antituberculosis Agents

Drug Name	Dose	Side Effects	Comments
Isoniazid (INH, Laniazid)	300 mg/day; 900 mg 2 × wk	Hepatitis (acetaminophen, alcohol exacerbates); peripheral neuropathy, give pyridoxine (vitamin B_6); CNS toxicity; GI	Alone for conversion or prophylaxis; combined with other TB drugs for treatment
Rifampin (Rifadin, Rimactane) Rifapentine (Priftin)* Rifabutin (Mycobutin)	600 mg/day 600 mg; 600 mg 1 × wk 300 mg/day	GI (nausea, vomiting, anorexia, pseudomembranous colitis); rash; renal (hematuria, pyuria, or proteinuria); hepatitis (alcohol exacerbates); CNS (mood changes, fatigue); blood dyscrasias	Reddish orange to reddish brown discoloration of urine, feces, saliva, sputum, sweat, and tears (permanent discoloration of contact lenses); induces enzymes
PZA	50–70 mg/kg 2 × wk	Hepatotoxicity; nausea, vomiting; hyperuricemia (gouty attack)	Used with ciprofloxacin for multidrug-resistant TB
Rifater (Isoniazid + rifampin + PZA)		All those of isoniazid, rifampin, and PZA	
Ethambutol (Myambutol)	15 mg/kg/day	Retrobulbar optic neuritis (eye examination for visual fields and acuity and red-green discrimination); peripheral neuritis; gouty arthritis; GI symptoms; CNS (confusion)	
Streptomycin	15 mg/kg/day; max 1 g	Ototoxicity (vertigo), nephrotoxicity	Given by IM injection; dose adjusted according to renal function

*Cyclopentyl rifamycin.

CNS, Central nervous system; *GI,* gastrointestinal; *IM,* intramuscular; *INH,* isonicotinyl hydrazine; *PZA,* pyrazinamide; *TB,* tuberculosis, *wk,* week.

Pharmacokinetics

INH is readily absorbed from the GI tract and is distributed throughout the body. Its metabolism varies by race. Most Eskimos and Japanese are fast acetylators, which means that their bodies quickly metabolize drugs, whereas whites and blacks in the United States are split 50-50 between fast and slow acetylators. The ability to acetylate rapidly is inherited as an autosomal dominant trait. Whether this ability to metabolize INH rapidly is related to the chance of development of INH-induced hepatitis is unknown. The half-life in fast acetylators is 1.5 hours and in slow acetylators is 3 hours.

Adverse Reactions

The incidence of all adverse reactions to INH is approximately 5%. The most common adverse reaction, occurring in about 20% of patients, involves the nervous system and may be a result of vitamin B$_6$ depletion by INH. Peripheral and optic neuritis, muscle twitching, toxic encephalopathy, insomnia, restlessness, sedation, incoordination, convulsions, and even psychoses have been reported. These neurotoxic symptoms can be prevented by coadministration of pyridoxine (vitamin B$_6$).

The other major adverse effect of INH is hepatotoxicity. Approximately 1% of patients taking INH exhibit clinical hepatitis and up to 10% have abnormal LFTs. Some cases of hepatitis have been fatal. Other side effects include hematologic effects, GI effects, dryness of the mouth, and a lupus-like reaction or rheumatic syndrome with arthralgia. The choice of whether to use INH depends on many factors, such as patient age, presence of renal or hepatic deficiency, history of seizures, GI disturbances, alcoholism, and history of neurotoxicity.

INH is both an inhibitor and an inducer of cytochrome P-450 2E isoenzymes. The benzodiazepines that are oxidized in the liver, such as diazepam and midazolam, may have an increased effect in patients taking INH. Foods (e.g., cheese and fish) and drugs that are contraindicated with monoamine oxidase (MAO) inhibitors may also react with INH.

Uses

INH is used alone for prophylaxis or for "converters" (patients with a change to TB test results). It is used in combination with other antituberculosis agents. The usual adult dose is 300 mg daily.

Rifampin

Rifampin (RIF-am-pin) (Rifadin, Rimactane) is a semisynthetic derivative of rifamycin, an antibiotic produced by *Streptomyces mediterranei*. Its mechanism of action involves inhibition of DNA-dependent RNA polymerase, which then suppresses the initiation of chain formation. It is active against *M. tuberculosis* and many gram-positive and some gram-negative bacteria. Rifampin's spectrum of activity also includes *S. aureus, N. meningitidis, H. influenzae,* and *Legionella* species. In TB, resistance quickly develops to rifampin administered alone in a one-step process as a result of a change in the RNA polymerase. Administering rifampin with other antituberculosis agents reduces the development of resistance.

Pharmacokinetics

Rifampin is absorbed from the GI tract and eliminated in the bile. Its half-life is 1.5 to 5 hours and is increased in hepatic disease but unaltered by renal disease. The half-life is reduced by INH coadministration because of enzyme induction.

Adverse Reactions

The most common adverse reactions are GI, including anorexia, stomach distress, nausea, vomiting, abdominal cramps, and diarrhea. Occasionally, rashes, thrombocytopenia, nephritis, and impairment of liver function are seen. A flulike reaction can occur with infrequent administration. Rifampin gives a red-orange color to body fluids, including tears (affecting contact lenses), urine, feces, saliva, and sweat.

Uses

Rifampin is used in combination with other agents for treatment of TB. The adult dose is no more than 600 mg daily. It is used to treat meningococcal carriers prophylactically and children exposed to *H. influenzae* meningitis.

Pyrazinamide

Pyrazinamide (peer-a-ZIN-a-mide) (PZA), a relative of nicotinamide, is well absorbed and widely distributed throughout the body. It is hepatotoxic and can cause rash, hyperuricemia, and GI disturbances. The CDC currently recommends PZA for use during the first 2 months with INH, rifampin, and ethambutol, to treat TB. PZA, which used to be a tertiary drug, now plays a much more important role than it had in the past.

If a patient is compliant and the organisms are susceptible, he or she usually becomes noninfective within 2 to 3 weeks to 2 to 3 months. A negative sputum sample result is required to ensure that the patient is noninfective.

Ethambutol

Ethambutol (e-THAM-byoo-tole) (Myambutol) is a synthetic tuberculostatic agent effective against *M. tuberculosis*. Resistance among tubercle bacilli develops very rapidly when this drug is used alone.

The most important side effect is optic neuritis, which leads to a decrease in visual acuity and loss of the ability to perceive red and green. Periodic ophthalmologic examinations are recommended in patients taking ethambutol. Other side effects are rash, joint pain, GI upset, malaise, headache, and dizziness. Ethambutol is used during the first 2 months of therapy with INH, rifampin, and PZA.

TOPICAL ANTIBIOTICS

In general, the use of topical antibiotics in dentistry is discouraged. Systemic administration is superior in most cases. If an agent is used topically, it should be one that cannot be used systemically. One old product and one newer product are mentioned briefly.

Neomycin, Polymyxin, and Bacitracin

The combination of an aminoglycoside, neomycin (nee-oh-MYE-sin), and two polypeptide antibiotics, polymyxin (pol-i-MIX-in) and bacitracin (bass-i-TRAY-sin), is available in ointment form (Neosporin, triple antibiotic ointment).

Neomycin affects gram-negative organisms, and polymyxin and bacitracin affect gram-positive organisms. This combination product is used topically on scratches; if the wound is infected, systemic antibiotics are indicated.

Mupirocin

Mupirocin (myoo-PEER-oh-sin) (Bactroban) is a topical antibacterial produced by *Pseudomonas fluorescens*. Mupirocin inhibits protein synthesis by binding to bacterial isoleucyl transfer–RNA synthetase. It shows no cross-resistance with other antibiotics. It is active against certain *Streptococcus* and *Staphylococcus* organisms and is indicated for the topical treatment of impetigo. Local itching and stinging have been reported. Mupirocin is as effective as the usual systemic treatments (penicillinase-resistant penicillins) and has fewer side effects.

In dentistry, mupirocin can be used to treat the bacterial infection with streptococci or staphylococci that is occasionally present with angular cheilitis (chronic inflammatory condition at the corners of the mouth). The secondary infection can be determined from its clinical presentation. Because angular cheilitis is most commonly a fungal infection, topical antifungal agents should be used first.

ANTIBIOTIC PROPHYLAXIS USED IN DENTISTRY

Infective endocarditis is caused by an infection of the heart valves or endocardium with an organism. Infective endocarditis often begins with sterile vegetative cardiac lesions consisting of amalgamations of platelets, fibrin, and bacteria. When bacteria are introduced into the bloodstream, they may infect the damaged valves. Infective endocarditis can also occur in patients without predisposing cardiac factors. The difficult question, to which there is currently no proven answer, is this: "Which factors will be predictive in identifying patients in whom appropriate antibiotics will prevent infective endocarditis when specific dental procedures are performed?"

Prevention of Infective Endocarditis

- Dental
- Cardiac
- Drug Therapy

Prophylaxis for infective endocarditis is based on the concept (which may not be true) that giving certain antibiotics to certain patients before certain procedures can keep these patients from having infective endocarditis. In January 2008, the *Journal of the American Dental Association (JADA)* published the most current guidelines from the AHA for antibiotic prophylaxis before dental procedures to prevent infective endocarditis. The newest guidelines recommend that only those people who are at highest risk for adverse outcomes from infective endocarditis receive short-term preventive antibiotics before select, common, and routine dental procedures.

According to the AHA, these newest guidelines are based on a comprehensive review of published studies suggesting that infective endocarditis is more likely to occur from bacteria entering the bloodstream as a result of daily activities than from a dental procedure. There was also no compelling evidence in the medical and dental literature that antibiotic prophylaxis before a dental procedure would prevent infective endocarditis in those at risk for its development. Also, the antibiotics used to prevent infective endocarditis carry risks, including adverse effects, risk of fatal allergic reactions, and the possibility of bacterial resistance.

For every situation in which it may be appropriate to use prophylactic antibiotics, the following factors should be considered:
- The specific dental procedure being performed
- The cardiac and medical condition of the patient
- Risk for bad outcomes from infective endocarditis
- The drug and the dose that may be needed

The updated guidelines also emphasize that maintaining optimal oral health and practicing daily oral hygiene are more important in reducing the risk for infective endocarditis than taking an antibiotic before a dental procedure.

Dental Procedures

When dental treatment is rendered (including periodontal probing), organisms are more likely to enter the blood supply, producing bacteremia. Bacteremia is also produced by eating potato chips, brushing teeth, or chewing wax. The organisms can then produce infective endocarditis.

According to the 2008 guidelines from the AHA regarding prophylactic antibiotic coverage, one should ask the following questions:
- Does the cardiac/medical condition warrant prophylaxis? Is the patient at highest risk for adverse outcomes from infective endocarditis?
- Will the dental procedure to be performed involve manipulation of gingival tissue or the periapical region of the teeth or perforation of the oral mucosa?

Only if both of these questions are answered in the affirmative would prophylaxis be indicated.

Depending on the dental procedure being performed, patients may or may not need prophylactic antibiotic coverage. Box 7.5 divides dental procedures into those procedures that involve manipulation of the gingival mucosa or the periapical region of the teeth or perforation of the oral mucosa, requiring prophylaxis, and those that do not and so do not require prophylaxis. Clinical judgment will determine whether antibiotic coverage is needed for each patient.

Cardiac Conditions

Patients with cardiac conditions can be divided into groups based on the cardiac condition (Box 7.6). The first group contains patients at highest risk for development of infective endocarditis (e.g., those with prosthetic cardiac valve, previous infective endocarditis) and who suffer the worst outcomes. Oral antibiotic prophylaxis is required for these patients if the dental procedure warrants it. The second cardiac group includes patients with conditions that do not require prophylactic antibiotic coverage (e.g., coronary bypass surgery after 6 months). Several new additions to the second group include patients with mitral valve prolapse and rheumatic heart disease. Although such patients still have a lifelong risk of infective endocarditis, they have a much higher risk from a random bloodborne bacterial infection from day-to-day activities than from a dental or medical procedure. These changes were made on the basis of the most current recommended guidelines from the AHA for preventing infective endocarditis.

Antibiotic Regimens for Dental Procedures

Table 7.7 lists the antibiotic regimens for prophylaxis of endocarditis before dental procedures. These situations include treating those patients with no allergies and those patients allergic to penicillin antibiotics or ampicillin.

When a patient's physician is contacted about the patient, the current medical condition of the patient should be explored. On the basis

---

BOX 7.5   Dental Procedures for Which Endocarditis Prophylaxis Is Reasonable for Patients With Specific Cardiac Conditions

Prophylaxis Is Considered Reasonable for
All dental procedures that involve manipulation of gingival tissue or the periapical region of the teeth or perforation of the oral mucosa

No Prophylaxis Is Necessary for
Routine anesthetic injections through noninfected tissues
Oral radiographs
Placement of removable prosthodontic or orthodontic appliances
Adjustment of orthodontic appliances
Placement of orthodontic brackets
Shedding of deciduous teeth
Bleeding from trauma to the lips or oral mucosa

Reprinted with permission *Circulation*. 2007;116:1736–1754 ©2007 American Heart Association, Inc.

BOX 7.6 Cardiac Conditions Associated With the Highest Risk of Adverse Outcomes from Endocarditis

Prophylaxis Reasonable

- Prosthetic cardiac valve
- Previous infective endocarditis
- Congenital heart disease (CHD):
  - Unrepaired cyanotic CHD, including palliative shunts and conduits
  - Completely repaired congenital heart defect with prosthetic material or device, whether placed by surgery or by catheter intervention, during the first 6 months after the procedure
  - Repaired CHD with residual defects at the site or adjacent to the site of a prosthetic patch or device (which inhibits endothelialization)
  - Cardiac transplant recipients in whom cardiac valvulopathy develops

No Prophylaxis Necessary

- With the exception of the cardiac conditions listed above, antibiotic prophylaxis is no longer recommended for any other form of CHD.
- Mitral valve prolapse
- Rheumatic heart disease
- Bicuspid valve disease
- Calcified aortic stenosis
- Congenital heart conditions:
  - Ventricular septal defect
  - Atrial septal defect
  - Hypertrophic cardiomyopathy

Reprinted with permission *Circulation*. 2007;116:1736–1754 ©2007 American Heart Association, Inc.

of the patient's medical status and the current recommendations, the dental health care worker determines whether antibiotics are indicated. The dental hygienist or dentist should explain to the medical provider that the choice of therapy will be determined by the patient's medical condition and the dental treatment being rendered. An agreement between the dentist and medical provider should be reached, but the dentist should not agree to practice outside the recommendation guidelines. This approach will minimize suggestions of inappropriate antibiotics or regimens. When no recommendations exist and the literature is contradictory, the choice should be based on a consensus between the dental health care worker and the patient's physician. If the patient is at highest risk for bad outcomes from infective endocarditis, then the usual regimens should be administered before dental treatment is provided.

If the patient is already taking the same antibiotic used for prophylaxis for another medical condition, the dental practitioner should prescribe an antibiotic from a different chemical class (i.e., if the patient is taking amoxicillin, clindamycin or azithromycin or clarithromycin should be prescribed as prophylaxis). Another concern associated with antibiotic prophylaxis is the fact that the antibiotic should be taken 1 hour prior to the procedure. Some patients often forget to take their antibiotic at the correct time. Patients can now be instructed that they can take their antibiotic up to 2 hours after the procedure if they forget to premedicate.

Prosthetic Joint Prophylaxis

The most recent recommendation of the American Dental Association (ADA) and the American Academy of Orthopedic Surgeons (AAOS) is that dental practitioners limit antibiotic prophylaxis in patients with joint replacement. An extensive review of the literature by the American

TABLE 7.7 Prophylactic Antibiotic Drug Regimens for Dental Procedures

Situation	Drug	Oral Dose (1 h before Procedure)		Parenteral Dose (Single Dose Administered 30 min Prior to Procedure)	
		Adult (mg)	Child (mg/kg)	Adult (mg)	Child (mg/kg)
No allergies to penicillin or amoxicillin (oral)	Amoxicillin	2000	50		
Patient unable to take oral medications but has no penicillins or ampicillin allergies	Ampicillin (IM/IV)			2000	50
	or				
	Cefazolin (IM/IV)			1000	50
	or				
	Ceftriaxone (IM/IV)			1000	50
Patient allergic to penicillins or ampicillin and can take oral medications	Cephalexin*,†	2000	50		
	or				
	Clindamycin	600	20		
	or				
	Azithromycin	500	15		
	or				
	Clarithromycin	500	15		
Patient allergic to penicillins or ampicillin and cannot take oral medication	Cefazolin† (IM/IV)			1000	50
	or				
	Ceftriaxone† (IM/IV)			1000	50
	or				
	Clindamycin (IM/IV)			600	20

*Or other first- or second-generation cephalosporins in equivalent adult or pediatric doses.
†Cephalosporins should not be used in individuals with a history of anaphylaxis, angioedema, or urticaria with penicillins or ampicillin.
Modified from Wilson W, Taubert KA, Gewitz M, et al: Prevention of infective endocarditis: Guidelines from the American Heart Association, *J Am Dent Assoc*, Volume 138, Issue 6, June 2007, Pages 739–745, 747–760.
IM, Intramuscular; *IV*, intravenous.

Dental Association Council on Scientific Affairs demonstrated that the benefits of antibiotic prophylaxis to prevent prosthetic joint infection do not outweigh the potential for harm in most patients. Although some dental procedures can cause a transient increase in bacteria in the blood, brushing teeth can cause transient bacteremia too.

Both the ADA and the AAOS recommend not routinely prescribing antibiotic prophylaxis in patients with joint replacements. However, people with joint replacement and a weakened immune system should speak with their dental practitioner or orthopedist about the necessity for antibiotic joint replacement. Medically compromised patients who require dental procedures such as gingival manipulation or mucosal inclusion should consider antibiotic prophylaxis only after talking to their orthopedist. Patients with serious medical conditions, such as those with serious immunocompromising diseases, may also require antibiotic prophylaxis. Ultimately, the new recommendations encourage dialogue between the patient and dentist and dental hygienist regarding the risk of joint infection and the need for prophylaxis with an antibiotic prior to a dental appointment.

Noncardiac Medical Conditions

Patients with noncardiac medical conditions may also require prophylactic antibiotic coverage before dental procedures, but lack of agreement among practitioners for these situations causes confusion. For some conditions in this group, there is consensus either that antibiotics are indicated or that antibiotics are not indicated. For other conditions, there is little consensus. One should consult with the most current guidelines established by the AHA to determine whether antibiotic prophylaxis is necessary in a particular patient.

DENTAL HYGIENE CONSIDERATIONS

- Establish a clear indication for antiinfective therapy.
- Determine the patient's health status.
- Select the appropriate antibiotic. Choose the antibiotic with the narrowest spectrum of activity and the lowest toxicity.
- Establish a dose regimen, duration of therapy, and route of administration. Review this information with the patient.
- Remind the patient that antibiotics should be taken on an empty stomach and with a full glass of water.
- Counsel the patient about the side effects, potential allergic reactions, drug interactions, and food interactions associated with the prescribed antibiotic therapy.

- Advise the patient to notify the dentist if adverse effects develop.
- Advise the patient to stop taking the drug and seek medical help if he or she begins to experience an allergic reaction with the antibiotic.
- Explain the importance of taking the antibiotic as prescribed and completing the full course of therapy.
- Monitor the patient for compliance with antibiotic prophylaxis.

ACADEMIC SKILLS ASSESSMENT

1. Under what conditions is antibiotic prophylaxis necessary?
2. Should antibiotic prophylaxis be given to a patient with a prosthetic joint before dental procedures? Describe the factors, if any, that would influence the decision.
3. What antibiotic dose and dosing regimen should be used?
4. What should a patient be told about an antibiotic?
5. What are the adverse reactions associated with penicillin? What should a patient be told about them?
6. What are some reasons that a patient might be noncompliant with drug therapy?
7. A patient has called and complained of nausea, itching, and a rash after taking a prescription for penicillin. What is happening to this patient?
8. What should the patient in question 7 do?
9. Is nausea caused by an allergic reaction or is it a side effect of penicillin?
10. Can a patient allergic to penicillin receive other types of penicillin antibiotics?

11. What is the role of tetracycline antibiotics in the treatment of periodontitis?
12. What are the different dose forms of tetracycline available, and how do they differ from one another?
13. What are the adverse reactions associated with tetracycline, and what should a patient be told about them?
14. What groups of patients should not receive tetracycline therapy? Why is it contraindicated in these patients?
15. What is the role of metronidazole in dentistry, and what are its adverse effects? Are there any drug/food interactions?
16. Compare and contrast antituberculosis drugs in terms of mechanism of action and adverse effects.
17. What are the dental concerns associated with tuberculosis and when is it okay to perform dental procedures on a person with tuberculosis?

CLINICAL CASE STUDY

Kathleen Fitzpatrick is 55 years old and has been coming to your practice for many years. She is married, has three children, and works as the secretary at her church. She runs to keep in shape. She takes no medication except for occasional cough and cold products and acetaminophen and naproxen for aches and pains. Mrs. Fitzpatrick had a hip replacement 7 months ago. She is scheduled to come in tomorrow for her regular oral health maintenance examination.

1. Would you recommend antibiotic prophylaxis for Mrs. Fitzpatrick? Why or why not?
2. Under what conditions is antibiotic prophylaxis recommended?

3. What antibiotics and doses are used for patients who require antibiotic prophylaxis?
4. What should patients be told about the antibiotics that may be prescribed for prophylaxis?
5. What are some reasons that Mrs. Fitzpatrick could be noncompliant with her medication?
6. Mrs. Patrick took warfarin for 4 weeks after hip replacement surgery. She is also taking a very-low-dose oral contraceptive for the symptoms of menopause. Are there any drug interactions with warfarin and antibiotics or oral contraceptives and antibiotics? What should be done for patients who may be taking either one of these combinations?

BIBLIOGRAPHY

American Dental Association, American Academy of Orthopaedic Surgeons. *Prevention of orthopaedic implant infections in patients undergoing dental procedures. Evidence-based guidelines and evidence report. AAOS Clinical Practice Guideline Unit*; 2012.

American Dental Association, American Academy of Orthopaedic Surgeons. Advisory statement: Antibiotic prophylaxis for dental patients with total joint replacements. *J Am Dent Assoc.* 2003;134:895.

Hatzenbuehler J, Pulling TJ. Diagnosis and management of osteomyelitis. *Am Fam Physician.* 2011;84:1027–1033.

Prakasam A, Elavarasu SS, Natarajan RV. Antibiotics in the treatment of aggressive periodontitis. *J Pharm Allied Biosci.* 2012;4(Suppl 2):S252–S255.

Roshna T, Nandakumar K. Generalized aggressive periodontitis and its treatment options: case reports and review of the literature. *Case Rep Med.* 2012;1–17.

Sollecito TP, Abt E, Lockhart PB, et al. The use of prophylactic antibiotics prior to dental procedures in patients with prosthetic joints: evidence-based clinical practice guideline for dental practitioners—a report of the American Dental Association Councilon Scientific Affairs. *J Am Dent Assoc.* 2015;146:11–16.

Stevens DL, Bisno AL, Chambers HF, et al. Practice guidelines for the diagnosis and management of skin and soft tissue infections. *Clin Infect Dis.* 2005;41:1373–1406.

Wilson W, Taubert KA, Gewitz M, et al. Prevention of infective endocarditis: guidelines from the American Heart Association. *J Am Dent Assoc.* 2008;139:3S–24S.

8

Antifungal and Antiviral Agents

 http://evolve.elsevier.com/Haveles/pharmacology

LEARNING OBJECTIVES

1. Name several types of antifungal agents and discuss their indications in dentistry and potential adverse reactions.
2. Discuss the use of antiviral agents in the treatment of herpes simplex.
3. Describe the various drugs and drug combinations used to treat acquired immunodeficiency syndrome.
4. Describe the various drugs used to treat chronic hepatitis.

This chapter discusses treatment and management of fungal and viral infections commonly encountered in the dental office: the fungus *Candida albicans* (candidiasis or thrush) and the herpes simplex virus. The viral infection acquired immunodeficiency syndrome (AIDS) and the different types of hepatitis (B, C) are discussed with reference to factors that might affect dental treatment.

ANTIFUNGAL AGENTS

> *Candida albicans:* Most common oral fungus.

Fungal infections are not often encountered in dental practice, but when they are present, they are often difficult to treat. In comparison with bacterial infections, fungal infections are more insidious. Fungal infections are more likely to occur in patients who are immunocompromised, and these infections can become chronic. Fungal infections can be divided into those that affect primarily the skin or mucosa (mucocutaneous) and those that affect the whole body (systemic). The dental hygienist usually treats skin or mucosal lesions, most commonly within the mouth. These mucosal lesions may be treated with a topical or systemic antifungal agent.

Although there are different groups of fungi, two common groups are candida-like and tinea. Dental hygienists manage oral candidal infections, primarily caused by *C. albicans,* with nystatin, clotrimazole, ketoconazole, or fluconazole (Table 8.1). Fig. 8.1 reviews where these drugs work on the fungal cell.

Nystatin

Nystatin (nye-STAT-in) (Mycostatin, Nilstat) is a prescription antifungal agent that is produced by *Streptomyces noursei.* Its mechanism of action involves binding to sterols in the fungal cell membrane. This binding produces an increase in membrane permeability and allows leakage of potassium and other essential cellular constituents.

Nystatin is not absorbed from the mucous membranes or through intact skin; taken orally, it is poorly absorbed from the gastrointestinal tract. In usual therapeutic doses, its blood levels are not detectable. When administered orally, it is not absorbed but is excreted unchanged in the feces. Nystatin is fungicidal and fungistatic against a variety of yeasts and fungi. In vitro, nystatin inhibits *C. albicans* and some other species of *Candida.*

The adverse reactions associated with nystatin are minor and infrequent. Applied topically or taken orally (through the gastrointestinal tract), there is little if any absorption. When higher doses have been used, nausea, vomiting, and diarrhea have occasionally occurred. Rarely, hypersensitivity reactions have been reported.

Nystatin is used for both the treatment and the prevention of oral candidiasis in susceptible patients. Although *C. albicans* is a frequent inhabitant of the oral cavity, only under unusual conditions does it produce disease. Often, patients affected are immunocompromised.

For the treatment of oral candidiasis, nystatin is available (see Table 8.1) in the form of an aqueous suspension (100,000 U/mL) containing 50% sucrose. The aqueous suspension should be used as a rinse and expectorated. The aqueous suspension can also be frozen and used as a popsicle. Swallowing the suspension will not cause harm because it is not absorbed by the gastrointestinal tract and it will not eradicate pharyngeal candidiasis either. If diabetic patients swallow the suspension, they must take the sugar content into account (2.5 g sucrose per tsp) when planning their meals and insulin use.

Nystatin pastilles are licorice flavored, are rubbery, and also contain sugar. The advantage of this preparation is that it takes 15 minutes for the lozenge to dissolve in the mouth, thus bathing lesions in the antifungal agent for a longer period than with the aqueous solution. It is dissolved in the mouth four times daily. The dental hygienist must discuss patients' oral health habits, especially when patients are ingesting these cariogenic agents over the long term.

Table 8.2 reviews the dosing instructions for the different nystatin preparations. Denture stomatitis can be treated by applying a thin layer of nystatin cream to the tissue side of the denture. Patients should be instructed to use the nystatin product for 10 to 14 days, depending on the severity of the infection, or for 48 hours after the signs and symptoms of the infection have been eradicated.

Imidazoles

Imidazoles useful in dentistry include clotrimazole, miconazole, and ketoconazole.

90

TABLE 8.1 Dentally Useful Antifungal Agents for Oral Candidiasis

Drug Name	Dentally Useful Dose Forms	Comments	Dose	Dose (g)
Nystatin (Mycostatin, Nilstat, others)	Aqueous suspension, cream, ointment, pastilles	Side effects uncommon	*Suspension:* 4–6 mL qid *Pastilles:* 1–2, 3–5 times/day	2.5* (50%)
Clotrimazole (Mycelex)	Troches (lozenges)	Nausea	*Troches:* Dissolve 1 troche 5 times/day	0.9† (90%)
Ketoconazole (Nizoral)	Oral tablets (200 mg), cream	Hepatoxicity, anaphylaxis, teratogenic, drug interactions	*Tablet:* 1 tablet daily *Cream:* apply once or twice daily	N/A N/A
Fluconazole (Diflucan)	Oral tablets (50, 100, 150, 200 mg)		200 mg first day; then 100 mg daily	N/A

*Sucrose.
†Glucose.
N/A, Not available; *qid,* four times a day.

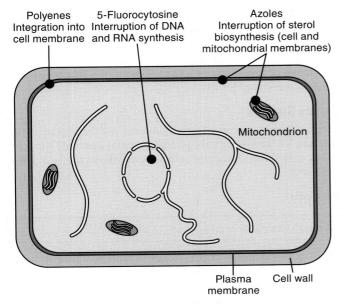

Polyenes
Integration into
cell membrane

5-Fluorocytosine
Interruption of DNA
and RNA synthesis

Azoles
Interruption of sterol
biosynthesis (cell and
mitochondrial membranes)

Mitochondrion

Plasma membrane   Cell wall

Fig. 8.1 Antifungal drugs' mechanism of action.

TABLE 8.2 Nystatin Dose Forms

Dose Form	Instructions for Use
Aqueous suspension (100,000/mL)	*Children and adults:* Swish, swirl (hold in mouth for 5 min), expectorate or swallow 4–6 mL 4–5 times daily. Freeze 2.5 mL into popsicle form. Place in the mouth and allow to completely dissolve. This should be done 5 times a day. *Infants:* Administer 2 mL 4 times daily; place one half dose in each side of the mouth. Avoid feeding infants for 5–10 min afterward.
Pastille	Suck on 1–2 tablets 4–5 times daily.
Cream	Apply to affected area (including the tissue area surrounding dentures). Insert denture.

Clotrimazole

Clotrimazole (kloe-TRIM-a-zole) (Mycelex) is a synthetic antifungal agent available in the form of a slowly dissolving, sugar-containing lozenge for oral use. It is also available as an over-the-counter (OTC) cream for topical application to the skin or vaginal canal.

Clotrimazole's mechanism of action involves alteration of cell membrane permeability. It binds with the phospholipids in the cell membrane of the fungus. As a result of the alteration in permeability, the cell membrane loses its function and the cellular constituents are lost.

Clotrimazole troches: 1 box = 70 lozenges.

Clotrimazole oral lozenges or troches dissolve in approximately 15 to 30 minutes. Patients with xerostomia may have difficulty dissolving this product. Saliva drug concentrations that are sufficient to inhibit most *Candida* species are maintained in the mouth for approximately 3 hours. The drug is bound to the oral mucosa, from which it is slowly released. The amount of clotrimazole absorbed systemically by this route is unknown, but some absorption occurs. Each lozenge also contains 0.9 g of glucose. The spectrum of activity of clotrimazole is primarily against the *Candida* species.

The most common adverse reactions associated with clotrimazole involve the gastrointestinal tract, including abdominal pain, diarrhea, and nausea. Clotrimazole has been reported to produce elevated liver enzyme (aspartate aminotransferase) values in approximately 15% of patients. It is not recommended for use in pregnant women or in children younger than 3 years.

Clotrimazole is indicated for the local treatment of oropharyngeal candidiasis. Patients should be instructed to dissolve the lozenge in the mouth slowly, like a cough drop, to minimize gastrointestinal discomfort. They should also be told to take all of the medication prescribed to minimize relapse. The usual adult dosage is 1 lozenge (10 mg) five times daily for 10 to 14 days (or longer for immunosuppressed patients) or for 48 hours after the symptoms have cleared. Clotrimazole can be used to treat denture stomatitis. A thin layer of clotrimazole cream should be applied as a thin layer to the tissue side of the denture base.

Ketoconazole

Ketoconazole (kee-toe-KON-a-zole) (Nizoral), another imidazole used in dentistry, alters cellular membranes and interferes with intracellular enzymes. By interfering with the synthesis of ergosterol, a cellular component of fungi, this agent alters membrane permeability and inhibits purine transport. The imidazoles inhibit the C-14 demethylation of lanosterol, an ergosterol precursor. It also inhibits sex steroid biosynthesis, including testosterone, perhaps by blocking several cytochrome P-450 (CYP-450) enzyme steps.

Ketoconazole is indicated in the treatment and management of mucocutaneous and oropharyngeal candidiasis (oral thrush). It can be used prophylactically in chronic mucocutaneous candidiasis. The most frequent adverse reactions (3%–10%) associated with ketoconazole are nausea and vomiting, which can be minimized by taking ketoconazole with food. The most serious adverse reaction associated with ketoconazole is hepatotoxicity. Its incidence is at least 1:10,000. It is usually reversible on discontinuation of the drug, but occasionally it has been fatal. It is thought to be an idiosyncratic reaction that can happen at any time. With extended use, the patient should have periodic liver function tests (LFTs). Patients taking other hepatotoxic agents, those with liver disease (e.g., alcoholic hepatitis), and those on prolonged therapy should be monitored closely because they may be more susceptible to this hepatotoxicity. Because of its adverse reaction profile, ketoconazole should be used only after topical antifungal agents have been ineffective or if there is reason to believe that they will be ineffective.

Ketoconazole has many drug interactions that have been reported in the literature. Because an acidic environment is required for dissolution and absorption of ketoconazole, agents that alter the amount of stomach acid could theoretically reduce the absorption of ketoconazole (H_2 receptor blockers, H^+-pump inhibitors, anticholinergic agents, and antacids). At least 2 hours should elapse between the ingestion of these agents and ketoconazole's administration. In addition, ketoconazole and the other imidazoles interact with the anticoagulant warfarin, which may increase warfarin blood levels and increase the risk for bleeding.

The usual adult dose of ketoconazole for the treatment of *Candida* species is 200 to 400 mg orally (PO) daily (qd). It should be used for at least 2 weeks, and 6 to 12 months may be required for chronic mucocutaneous candidiasis. Maintenance therapy may be necessary for certain patients.

> Systemic imidazole ketoconazole

Other Imidazoles

Other imidazoles, such as fluconazole (floo-KON-a-zole) (Diflucan), an oral triazole antifungal agent, are used to treat certain fungal infections. Fluconazole prevents the synthesis of ergosterol in the fungal cell membranes by inhibiting fungal CYP-450 enzymes. Phospholipids and unsaturated fatty acids accumulate in the fungal cells.

Fluconazole is indicated for treatment of oropharyngeal and esophageal candidiasis and serious systemic candidal infections. One tablet of fluconazole is now indicated to treat vaginal candidiasis. Fluconazole is used prophylactically against candidiasis in immunocompromised patients or for the treatment of candidal infections that do not respond to other agents.

ANTIVIRAL AGENTS

The search for drugs useful in the treatment of viral infections has posed the greatest problem of all infectious organisms. This is because viruses are obligate intracellular organisms that require cooperation from their host's cells. Therefore, to kill the virus, often the host's cell must also be harmed. The herpes virus, because of the location of the lesions around the oral cavity or in some cases on the dentist's or hygienist's finger (herpetic whitlow), has been of the most interest to the dental health care worker. Currently, with the symptoms of AIDS being seen clinically in the mouth, the treatment of this virus takes on more importance. Tables 8.3 and 8.4 list some antiviral agents along with their routes of administration and indications. Fig. 8.2 separates the antivirals into related groups.

Herpes Simplex

Herpes viruses are associated with "cold sores," and dental practitioners are asked for "something to help." Most antiviral agents are either purine or pyrimidine analogs that inhibit deoxyribonucleic acid (DNA) synthesis.

Acyclovir

> Acyclovir: Activated by herpes enzymes.

Acyclovir (ay-SYE-kloe-veer) (Zovirax) is a purine nucleoside that works by inhibiting DNA replication. It is much less toxic to normal uninfected cells because it is preferentially taken up by infected cells. In the host's cells, acyclovir is only minimally phosphorylated, explaining its excellent adverse reaction profile.

Pharmacokinetics. When acyclovir is taken orally, between 15% and 30% is absorbed. Peak concentrations occur within approximately 2 hours. Food does not affect the drug's absorption. Acyclovir is distributed widely throughout the body. Approximately 10% of a dose of acyclovir is metabolized in the liver.

TABLE 8.3	Antiviral Agents for the Treatment of Herpes Simplex Virus 1			
Drug Name	**Route(s)**	**Indication(s)**		**Comments**
Acyclovir (Zovirax)	Oral (PO), topical, intravenous (IV)	Primary and recurrent herpes in immunocompromised and immunocompetent patients		*Local:* burning *Oral:* nausea, central nervous system (CNS) effects
Famciclovir (Famvir)	PO	Primary and recurrent herpes in immunocompromised and immunocompetent patients		*Oral:* nausea, CNS effects
Valacyclovir (Valtrex)	PO	Primary and recurrent herpes in immunocompromised and immunocompetent patients		*Oral:* nausea, CNS effects
Penciclovir (Denavir)	Topical	Oral herpes simplex labialis (cold sores)		*Local:* Erythema at the site of application
Docosanol (Abreva)	Topical	Oral herpes simplex labialis		Available without a prescription (over-the-counter [OTC]) *Local:* Application site reactions, rash, pruritus

TABLE 8.4   Examples of Drugs Used to Treat Human Immunodeficiency Virus (HIV)

Drug Class	Drug Name	Comments
Nucleoside analogs or nucleoside/nucleotide reverse transcriptase inhibitors	Abacavir (Ziagen) Didanosine (Videx) Emtricitabine (Emtriva) Lamivudine (Epivir) Stavudine (Zerit) Tenofovir (Viread) Zalcitabine (Hivid) Zidovudine (Retrovir)	Monitor for adverse drug reactions Use caution to prevent instrument and needle sticks Antibiotic prophylaxis when polymorphonuclear leukocyte count (PMN) <500 PMNs/mm; delay elective treatments until normal Anticipate oral candidiasis Encourage meticulous oral hygiene Frequent oral maintenance therapy needed
Nonnucleoside analogs or nonnucleoside reverse transcriptase inhibitors	Delavirdine (Rescriptor) Efavirenz (Sustiva) Etravine (Intelence) Nevirapine (NVP) (Viramune) Rilpivirine (Edurant)	Encourage meticulous plaque control to minimize, prevent, and control inflammation Used in combination with other anti-HIV therapy
Protease inhibitors	Amprenavir (Agenerase) Atazanavir (Reyataz) Darunavir (Prezista) Fosamprenavir (Lexiva) Indinavir (Crixivan) Nelfinavir (Viracept) Tipranavir (Aptivus) Ritonavir (Norvir) Saquinavir (Invirase, Fortovase)	
Fusion/entry inhibitors	Enfuvirtide (Fuzeon) Maraviroc (Selzentry)	Used in combination with other anti-HIV therapy
Integrase inhibitors	Dolutegravir (Tivicay) Elvitegravir (Vitekta) Raltegravir (Isentress)	Used in combination with other antiretroviral agents
Pharmacokinetic enhancer	Cobicistat (Tybost)	Used in combination with other antiretroviral agents

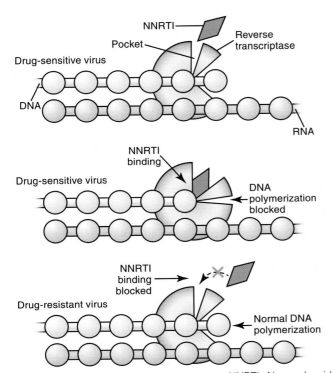

Fig. 8.2 Related groups of antiviral agents. *NNRTI,* Nonnucleoside reverse transcriptase inhibitor. (From Clavel F, Hance AJ. HIV drug resistance. *N Engl J Med.* 2004;350:1023–1035.)

Spectrum. The antiviral action of acyclovir includes various herpes viruses, including herpes simplex types 1 and 2 (HSV-1 and HSV-2), varicella-zoster, Epstein-Barr, *Herpesvirus simiae* (B virus), and cytomegalovirus. Several mechanisms of resistance to acyclovir have been found.

Adverse reactions. The type and extent of the adverse reactions experienced depend on the route of administration of acyclovir.

Topical administration. When administered topically, acyclovir produces burning, stinging, or mild pain in approximately a third of patients. Itching and rash have also been reported.

Oral administration. One of the most common adverse effects associated with oral acyclovir is headache (13%). Other central nervous system (CNS) effects include vertigo, dizziness, fatigue, insomnia, irritability, and mental depression. Oral acyclovir also commonly produces gastrointestinal adverse reactions, including nausea, vomiting, and diarrhea. Anorexia and a "funny taste" in the mouth have also been reported rarely. Other side effects associated with oral acyclovir include acne, accelerated hair loss, arthralgia, fever, menstrual abnormalities, sore throat, lymphadenopathy, thrombophlebitis, edema, muscle cramps, leg pain, and palpitation.

Dental uses

Topical. The indications for topical acyclovir include limited non–life-threatening initial and recurrent mucocutaneous herpes simplex (HSV-1) in immunocompromised patients. Topical acyclovir has not been effective in the treatment of herpes labialis infections in nonimmunocompromised patients. It does produce a limited shortening in the duration of viral shedding in males, by a few hours. It does not prevent the transmission of infection, and it does not prevent recurrence. Although available literature does not support the use of topical acyclovir for management of herpes labialis in dentistry, it is used extensively. No acyclovir products are approved for the treatment of recurrent herpes labialis in the immunocompetent patient.

Oral. In the treatment of herpes labialis, oral acyclovir has shown unimpressive results. Even with hundreds of patients in some studies, only a small difference in a few measured parameters is seen. However, in an immunocompetent individual, a dose of 200 mg five times daily, each dose q 4 hours, for 5 days and 400 mg every five times daily for 5 days, each dose q 4 hours, in an immunocompromised individual have been shown to be effective and is often used to treat HSV-1.

Docosanol 10%

Docosanol 10% (Abreva), available topically and without a prescription, has been shown to decrease healing time by approximately a half day in patients with recurrent orolabial herpes when started within 12 hours of the appearance of prodromal symptoms. The advantage of docosanol 10% is that it is available without a prescription.

Penciclovir

Penciclovir (pen-CY-klo-veer) (Denavir), available topically, has been shown to reduce both the duration of the lesion and the pain of the lesions on the lips and face associated with both primary and recurrent herpes simplex. The advantages of penciclovir over acyclovir are that it can achieve a higher concentration within the cell and that the drug remains in the cells longer.

Famciclovir

Famciclovir (fam-CY-klo-veer) and valacyclovir (val-a-CY-klo-veer) are prodrugs converted to penciclovir and acyclovir, respectively, as they pass through the intestinal wall. They are indicated in the treatment of recurrent episodes of genital herpes. They have not been studied for use in herpes labialis. Organisms that have resistance to acyclovir often have cross-resistance with these other agents. Famciclovir and valacyclovir are indicated for acute localized varicella-zoster infections. Intravenous ganciclovir is indicated for serious cytomegalovirus retinitis in immunocompromised patients.

Acquired Immunodeficiency Syndrome

AIDS is a chronic disease produced by infection with the retrovirus human immunodeficiency virus (HIV). Antiretroviral agents are used in combinations called "cocktails" to manage AIDS. Nucleoside reverse transcriptase inhibitors, nonnucleoside reverse transcriptase inhibitors, protease inhibitors, fusion/entry inhibitors, and integrase inhibitors are the groups discussed in this chapter (see Table 8.4). Opportunistic infections often occur in patients with AIDS, so they may be taking various antiinfective agents to prevent diseases such as tuberculosis, *Pneumocystis jirovecii* pneumonia, herpes infections, and candidiasis (Table 8.5).

Nucleoside/Nucleotide Reverse Transcriptase Inhibitors

The nucleoside reverse transcriptase inhibitors are the first class of drugs developed to treat HIV (see Table 8.5 and Fig. 8.3). Zidovudine (zye-DOE-vue-deen) (AZT, Retrovir), a thymidine analog, was the first in this group and is converted into zidovudine triphosphate by cellular enzymes. This AZT derivative is then integrated into DNA polymerase (reverse transcriptase) so that synthesis of viral DNA is terminated. The reverse transcriptase of HIV is 100 times more susceptible to inhibition than are normal human cells. The nucleoside

TABLE 8.5   Opportunistic Infections in Patients with Human Immunodeficiency Virus (HIV) and Drugs of Choice

Organism	Effect	Treatment
Cryptococcus neoformans	Meningitis	Amphotericin B
Candida	Esophagitis	Fluconazole, itraconazole, clotrimazole, ketoconazole
Pneumocystis jirovecii	Pneumonia	Atoquavone, clindamycin, dapsone, primaquine, trimethoprim-sulfamethoxazole (TMP-SMZ), pentamidine
Cytomegalovirus (CMV)	Lungs, pneumonitis	Ganciclovir, valganciclovir, foscarnet, cidofovir
Mycobacterium tuberculosis	Lungs	Isoniazid (INH) + rifampin or rifamycin + pyrazinamide + ethambutol
Toxoplasma gondii	Encephalitis	Pyrimethamine-sulfadiazine

antiretroviral analog or agents are converted into the nucleotide analog, which blocks viral replication and conversion into a form that can get into an uninfected host cell. The analog has no effect on cells already containing HIV. AZT is well absorbed orally, metabolized by the liver, and excreted by the kidneys with a half-life of approximately 1 hour. It is distributed to most body tissue, including cerebrospinal fluid. AZT inhibits HIV synthesis and reduces the morbidity and mortality from AIDS and AIDS-related complex. Opportunistic infections are reduced in both number and frequency with its use.

The toxicity of AZT is related to bone marrow depression, which can lead to anemia, granulocytopenia, and thrombocytopenia. Transfusions are often required. CNS effects include headache, agitation, and insomnia. Nausea occurs in almost half the patients. A causal relationship with AZT has not been established, but oral manifestations reported include altered sense of taste, edema of the tongue, bleeding gums, and mouth ulcers. Adverse reactions sometimes limit treatment with AZT.

Acetaminophen, indomethacin, and aspirin can inhibit AZT's metabolism and potentiate the toxicity of both drugs. Other nonsteroidal antiinflammatory agents have not been implicated, but current literature should be consulted. A higher incidence of granulocytopenia was reported when acetaminophen was used with AZT.

Nonnucleoside Reverse Transcriptase Inhibitors

Nevirapine (ne-VYE-ra-peen) (NVP, Viramune), a nonnucleoside reverse transcriptase inhibitor, is specific for HIV-1. HIV-2 is different from HIV-1 in that it is transmitted only from a woman to her child while the child is in the womb. This particular form of the virus appears to be centralized in western Africa. HIV-1 is transmitted via sexual intercourse, sharing of bodily fluids, and intravenous substance abuse and during pregnancy and childbirth. These agents inhibit the same enzymes as the nucleoside analogs, but they do not require bioactivation (see Table 8.4). Adverse reactions include CNS effects (headache, drowsiness), rash, gastrointestinal effects (diarrhea, nausea), and elevated LFT values. When these agents are used alone, resistance to them develops quickly, so this group is often combined with the nucleoside analogs and the protease inhibitors.

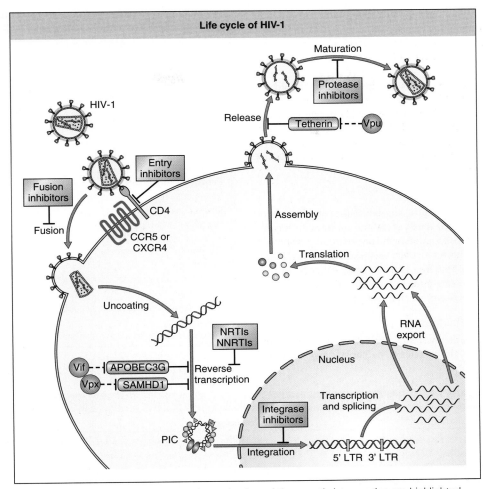

Fig. 8.3 Life cycle of HIV-1. Accessory proteins and points of therapeutic intervention are highlighted. (Modified from Barre-Sinoussi, et al. *Nat Rev Microbiol* 2013; 11: 877–883.)

Protease Inhibitors

Saquinavir (sa-KWIN-a-veer) (Invirase), the first protease inhibitor, prevents the cleavage of viral protein precursors needed to generate functional structural proteins in and modulation of reverse transcriptase activity, preventing the maturation of HIV-infected cells (see Table 8.4). The difference between the protease inhibitors and the other two groups is that the former can interfere with the action of HIV-infected cells. Saquinavir's adverse reactions include rash, hyperglycemia, and paresthesias. Gastrointestinal adverse reactions include pain, diarrhea, and vomiting. Oral adverse reactions involve buccal mucosal ulceration. Ketoconazole significantly increases the blood levels of saquinavir. Patients taking saquinavir should take it 2 hours after a full meal and should avoid sunlight. Although adverse reactions can occur, they are generally less serious than with the older agents. The discovery of the protease inhibitors has made a substantial difference in both the mortality and morbidity of AIDS patients.

Fusion/Entry Inhibitors

Entry or fusion inhibitors are used in combination with other antiretroviral drugs for the treatment of HIV infection (see Table 8.4). These drugs work by interfering with binding and fusion entry of an HIV virion into a human cell. These agents halt the progression from HIV infection to AIDs by blocking this step in the HIV replication cycle. Common side effects associated with enfuvirtide include skin itchiness, swelling, and pain at the site of injection. Common side effects associated with maraviroc include cough, fever, dizziness, nausea, and headache.

Integrase Inhibitors

Integrase inhibitors are designed to block or inhibit the action of integrase, which is a viral enzyme that inserts the viral genome into the DNA of the host cell (see Table 8.4). Because integration is an important process of the retroviral replication process, blocking it can halt further spread of the virus.

Pharmacokinetic Enhancers

Pharmacokinetic enhancers are designed to boost the effects of certain antiretroviral medications and prolong their effects (see Table 8.4). The pharmacokinetic enhancer blocks the metabolism of the antiretroviral drug.

Highly Active Antiretroviral Therapy

In the management of HIV and AIDS, drugs are combined for improved effect. Highly active antiretroviral therapy (HAART) is the combination of several different classes of antiretroviral drugs that slow the rate in which HIV replicates in the body. The combinations of drugs, called "cocktails," used to manage HIV or AIDS are changing constantly. Rapid changes in retroviral drug therapy make it impossible to predict what specific agents will be used in a few years. Within each group, the agents chosen are often the newest ones, which have quickly been brought to the market. Because the drugs that patients with AIDS take are the newest agents, it is important to obtain information about the drugs before planning dental treatment in such a patient. Normally, patients with HIV take three drugs: a nucleoside, a nonnucleoside reverse transcriptase inhibitor, and a protease inhibitor. An example of this combination is lamivudine, nevirapine, and saquinavir. Box 8.1 lists available combination products of anti-HIV drugs.

Postexposure Prophylaxis

Dental hygienists and other oral health care practitioners should begin occupational postexposure prophylaxis for HIV within 72 hours of exposure to the virus, usually via a needle or other instrument stick. The sooner the individual is treated, the better. Current guidelines recommend Truvada (tenofovir and emtricitabine) plus raltegravir (Isentress; RAL) 400 mg by mouth twice daily or dolutegravir (Tivicay) 50 mg PO once daily for 28 days.

Chronic Hepatitis

Hepatitis B and hepatitis C are the most common causes of chronic hepatitis, accounting for almost two-thirds of all cases of hepatitis. People with hepatitis C are most at risk for development of chronic hepatitis. In recent years, hepatitis B has become a treatable disease. Hepatitis is characterized by inflammation of the liver and can cause either no or very few symptoms. However, it often leads to jaundice, anorexia, and malaise. Hepatitis is considered chronic when it lasts more than 6 months.

Nucleoside/Nucleotide Analogs

Currently, five oral nucleoside/nucleotide analogs are available for the treatment of chronic hepatitis B (Table 8.6). These drugs are better

---

BOX 8.1   Combination Antiviral

Nucleoside/Nucleotide Reverse Transcriptase Inhibitors
Atripla (efavirenz, emtricitabine, and tenofovir disoproxil fumarate)
Complera (emtricitabine, rilpivirine, and tenofovir disoproxil fumarate)
Combivir (zidovudine + lamivudine)
Epzicom (abacavir + lamivudine)
Descovy (emtricitabine and tenofovir alafenamide)
Odefsey (emtricitabine, rilpivirine, and tenofovir alafenamide)
Trizivir (abacavir + zidovudine + lamivudine)
Truvada (tenofovir + emtricitabine)

Protease Inhibitors
Evotaz (atazanavir and cobicistat)
Kaletra (lopinavir + ritinavir)
Prezcobix (darunavir and cobicistat)

Nucleoside/Nucleotide Reverse Transcriptase/Integrase Inhibitors
Genvoya (elvitegravir, cobicistat, emtricitabine, and tenofovir alafenamide fumarate)
Stribild (elvitegravir, cobicistat, emtricitabine, and tenofovir disoproxil fumarate)
Triumeq (abacavir, dolutegravir, and lamivudine)

TABLE 8.6   Drugs for Treating Chronic Hepatitis

Clinical Use	Classification	Comments

Chronic hepatitis B	Oral nucleoside/nucleotide analogs:
	  Tenofovir (Viread)
	  Entecavir (Baraclude)
	  Telbivudine (Tyzeka)
	  Adefovir (Hepsera)
	  Lamivudine (Epivir HBV)
	  Emtricitabine (Emtriva)
	Interferons:
	  Interferon alfa-2b (Intron A)
	  Peginterferon alfa-2a (Pegasys)
		Hepatitis is highly contagious; use universal precautions all the time
		Acetaminophen may be contraindicated
		Generally well tolerated

Chronic hepatitis C	Protease inhibitors:
	  Simeprevir (Olysio)
	  HCV Polymerase Inhibitors
	    Sofosbuvir (Sovaldi)
	    HCV NS5A Inhibitors
	    Daclatasvir (Daklinza)
	Antivirals:
	  Ribavirin (Rebetol)
	Interferons:
	  Peginterferon alfa-2a (Pegasys)
	  Peginterferon alfa-2b (PegIntron)
	Combination Products
	  Elbasvir-Grazoprevir (Zepatier)
	  Glecaprevir-Pibrentasvir (Mavyret)
	  Ledipasvir-Sofosbuvir (Harvoni)
	  Ombitasvir-Paritaprevir-Ritonavir (Technivie)
	  Ombitasvir-Paritaprevir-Ritonavir and Dasabuvir (Viekira Pak)
	  Sofosbuvir-Velpatasvir (Epclusa)
	  Sofosbuvir-Velpatasvir-Voxilaprevir (Vosevi)
		Used in combination with peginterferon and ribavirin
		
		Used in combination with peginterferon and the protease inhibitors
		
		Used in combination with ribavirin and the protease inhibitors
		
		HCV NS5A inhibitor/HCV NS3/4A protease inhibitor
		NS3/4A protease inhibitor/HCV NS5A inhibitor,
		HCV NS5A protein inhibitor/HCV NSB5B RNA-dependent RNA polymerase inhibitor
		NS3/4A serine protease inhibitor/NS3/4A serine protease inhibitor/protease inhibitor
		NS3/4A serine protease inhibitor/NS3/4A serine protease inhibitor/protease inhibitor/nonnucleoside NS5B RNA-dependent polymerase inhibitor
		HCV nucleotide analog NS5B polymerase inhibitor/HCV NS5A inhibitor
		HCV nucleotide analog NS5B polymerase inhibitor/HCV NS5A inhibitor/HCV NS3/4A protease inhibitor

HCV, Hepatitis C virus; *NS*, nonstructural protein; *RNA*, Ribonucleic acid.

tolerated, and most have better rates of virologic suppression than the interferons. The optimal duration of therapy is unknown. However, many patients are treated for at least 5 years, and some are treated indefinitely. Sudden discontinuation of these drugs can lead to a rapid increase in hepatitis B virus DNA levels, which results in a severe flare-up of the disease that can be fatal. These drugs are generally well tolerated. The more commonly reported adverse effects are headache, nausea, vomiting, and diarrhea.

Interferons

The interferons (in-ter-FEER-ons) are a large group of endogenous proteins that have antiviral, cytotoxic, and immunomodulating action. The US Food and Drug Administration (FDA) has approved interferon-α for the treatments of chronic hepatitis B and hepatitis C.

Interferons are used parenterally, and injection site reactions, such as necrosis, can occur. The interferons interact with cells through cell surface receptors. Activation of these receptors has the following effects: induction of gene transcription, inhibition of cellular growth, alteration of the state of cellular differentiation, and interference with oncogene expression. Other effects are altering cell surface antigen expression, increasing phagocytic activity of macrophages, and augmenting the cytotoxicity of lymphocytes. Adverse reactions vary, depending on the interferon, but some can be serious and even require discontinuation of the drug. A flulike syndrome, consisting of myalgias, fatigue, headache, and arthralgia, occurs in many patients. Other side effects include CNS effects (fatigue, fever, headache, depression, and chills), gastrointestinal tract effects (nausea, vomiting, and diarrhea), and rash. Oral effects include taste changes, reactivation of herpes labialis, and excessive salivation.

Protease Inhibitors

Both boceprevir and telaprevir were approved by the FDA for use in combination with peginterferon alfa-2b and ribavirin for the treatment of chronic hepatitis C genotype 1 infection. The addition of either boceprevir or telaprevir to peginterferon alfa-2b and ribavirin increases sustained virologic response (SVR) rates and is now the standard treatment for this indication. Adverse effects include fatigue, anemia, nausea, and rash.

DENTAL HYGIENE CONSIDERATIONS

- Counsel the patient as to the proper application of the antiviral or antifungal drug.
- Make sure that the patient knows how to take or apply the drug and understands the importance of completing drug therapy.
- Counsel the patient on the correct use of oral dose forms of antifungal drugs. Encourage the patient to brush his or her teeth, rinse, and swallow after using an antifungal drug such as nystatin or clotrimazole. Both products contain sugar.
- Counsel the patient on the appropriate application of topical antiviral drugs.
- Be aware of drug interactions and the clinical implications of taking drugs to treat hepatitis or HIV.

ACADEMIC SKILLS ASSESSMENT

1. Discuss the use of the antifungal agent nystatin in the treatment of oral candidiasis. State three dose forms useful in dentistry and describe their pros and cons.
2. Discuss the use of clotrimazole and ketoconazole in the treatment of oral candidiasis. State one problem with each agent. Explain when administration of each is appropriate.
3. Describe the reason for the difficulty associated with the treatment of herpes simplex labialis with antiviral agents. Describe any useful clinically proven effect of either topical or systemic agents in dentistry.
4. Describe the mechanism of action of nucleoside reverse transcriptase inhibitors and their role in treating HIV.
5. Compare and contrast nonnucleoside reverse transcriptase inhibitors.
6. Describe the serious adverse reactions associated with zidovudine.
7. Describe how drug combinations are used to manage HIV.
8. Describe the role of interferons in the treatment of chronic viral hepatitis.

CLINICAL CASE STUDY

Haley Rothstein is a 5-year-old girl who has been coming to your practice for the past 3 years. Her mother calls you today because she has noticed that Haley has a "sort of white milky discharge coming from her mouth." Haley had a bacterial infection last week and was treated with amoxicillin.

1. What is happening to Haley?
2. What is the "white milky discharge," and how should it be treated?
3. What are the different dose forms of nystatin, and which one would you recommend for Haley?
4. Is clotrimazole an option for Haley? If yes, include mechanism of action, adverse reactions, and dose forms. If not, why and what would you recommend?
5. Compare and contrast ketoconazole, fluconazole, and itraconazole. Can any one of these be given to Haley? Why or why not?

9

Local Anesthetics

http://evolve.elsevier.com/Haveles/pharmacology

LEARNING OBJECTIVES

1. Discuss the history and reasons for the use of local anesthetics in dentistry, including:
   - List the properties an ideal local anesthetic would possess.
   - Describe the importance of understanding the chemistry involved in local anesthetic agents.
2. Explain the mechanism of action, pharmacokinetics, pharmacologic effects, and adverse reactions of local anesthetics.
3. Describe the composition of each of the drugs used in local anesthetic solutions and summarize the factors involved in the choice of a local anesthetic.
4. Briefly discuss the use, types, and doses of topical anesthetics used in dentistry.

> Local anesthetics: most often used drugs in dentistry.

No drugs are used more often in the dental office than the local anesthetic agents. Because their use can become routine, it is easy to forget that these agents have a potential for systemic effects in addition to the desired local effects. Dentists and, in most states, dental hygienists are responsible for the administration of local anesthetic agents when necessary. With this duty comes the need for an in-depth knowledge of the local anesthetic agents.

HISTORY

> First local anesthetic: cocaine.

"Painless" dentistry, through the use of a local anesthetic, is a relatively recent development. It began with the observation that the indigenous people of the South American Andes chewed certain leaves that made them feel better. The active ingredient of the leaves was cocaine, isolated by Niemann in 1860. He noted that tasting this substance produced not only the loss of taste but also of the sensation of pain (Figs 9.1 and 9.2). In 1884, Koller noted that cocaine instilled in the eye produced complete anesthesia. Cocaine was immediately adopted for use in eye surgery. During this time, Sigmund Freud was also experimenting with cocaine and its effects on the central nervous system (CNS). CNS stimulation, toxicity, and the potential for abuse were quickly recognized as major problems with the widespread use of cocaine as a local anesthetic.

The search for a more acceptable local anesthetic for dentistry continued. Einhorn synthesized procaine in 1905, but it was not until many years later that its use in dentistry became common. In 1952, the amide lidocaine (Xylocaine) was approved by the US Food and Drug Administration (FDA), and mepivacaine (Carbocaine) was approved in 1960. More recently, bupivacaine (Marcaine) has been made available for dental use. The search for the perfect local anesthetic agent continues.

IDEAL LOCAL ANESTHETIC

Although local anesthesia can be produced by several different agents, many are not clinically acceptable. The ideal local anesthetic should possess certain properties (Box 9.1). No local anesthetic agent currently in use meets all of these requirements, although many acceptable agents are available.

CHEMISTRY

Local anesthetic agents are divided chemically into two major groups: the esters and the amides (Table 9.1). A few agents fall outside these two groups, such as dyclonine, and are called other. The clinical importance of this division is associated with potential allergic reactions. A patient who has an allergy to one group is more likely to exhibit a hypersensitivity reaction to other agents within the same group. Cross-hypersensitivity between the amides and the esters is unlikely. The structure of local anesthetics is composed of the following three parts:
- Aromatic nucleus (R)
- Linkage (either an ester or an amide, followed by an aliphatic chain, R). The Rs are normally numbered 1, 2, 3, etc. to differentiate between each other.
- Amino group

The aromatic nucleus *(R)* is lipophilic (lipid soluble), and the amino group is hydrophilic (water soluble). The esters are largely metabolized in the plasma and the amides in the liver.

MECHANISM OF ACTION

Action on Nerve Fibers

> Interfere with function of the neurons.

A resting nerve fiber has a large number of positive ions (cations) on the outside (electropositive) and a large number of negative ions (anions) on the inside (electronegative). The nerve action potential results in the opening of the sodium (Na^+) channels and an inward flux of sodium, resulting

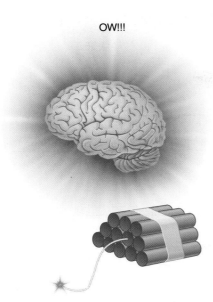

OW!!!

Fig. 9.1 The conduction of nerve impulses that lead a patient to experience pain can be compared with a fuse. The "fuse" is the nerve, and the "dynamite" is the brain. If the fuse is lit and the flame reaches the dynamite, an explosion occurs, and the patient experiences pain. (From Malamed SF. *Handbook of Local Anesthesia.* 6th ed. St. Louis: Mosby; 2013.)

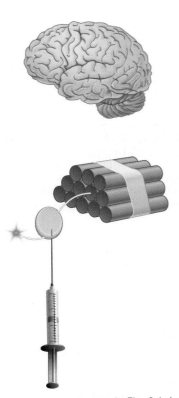

Fig. 9.2 Using the same comparison as in Fig. 9.1, local anesthetic is placed at some point between the pain stimulus ("fuse") and the brain ("dynamite"). The nerve impulse travels up to the point of the local anesthetic application and then "dies," never reaching the brain. Thus the patient does not experience pain. (From Malamed SF. *Handbook of Local Anesthesia.* 6th ed. St. Louis: Mosby; 2013.)

BOX 9.1 Properties of the Ideal Local Anesthetic

- Potent local anesthesia
- Reversible local anesthesia
- Absence of local reactions
- Absence of systemic reactions
- Absence of allergic reactions
- Rapid onset
- Satisfactory duration
- Adequate tissue penetration
- Low cost
- Stability in solution (long shelf life)
- Sterilization by autoclave
- Ease of metabolism and excretion

---

in a change from the -90-mV potential to a $+40$-mV potential (Fig. 9.3 and Box 9.2). The outward flow of potassium (K^+) ions repolarizes the membrane and closes the sodium channels. Local anesthetics attach themselves to specific receptors in the nerve membrane. After combining with the receptor, the local anesthetics block conduction of nerve impulses (thus the term **nerve block**) by decreasing the permeability of the nerve cell membrane to sodium ions. This then decreases the rate of depolarization of the nerve membrane, increases the threshold for excitability, and prevents the propagation of the action potential. Local anesthetics may reduce permeability by competing with **calcium (Ca^{++})** for the membrane binding sites and by preventing the onset of nerve conduction.

Ionization Factors

> Ionization equilibrium depends on pH and pK_a.

The local anesthetic agents are weak bases occurring in equilibrium between their two forms, which are the fat-soluble (lipophilic) free base and the water-soluble (hydrophilic) hydrochloride salt (Fig. 9.4). Table 9.2 provides an overview of the characteristics of the lipophilic free base and water-soluble hydrochloride salt forms of the local anesthetics. The proportion of drug in each form is determined by the pK_a—the pH at which half is in each form (salt and base equal)—of the local anesthetic and the pH of the environment. Local anesthetics without a vasoconstrictor range in pH from 5 to 6. Local anesthetics with a vasoconstrictor range in pH from approximately 3 to 5 because of the addition of the preservative sodium bisulfate. In the acidic pH of the dental cartridge (4.5), the proportion of the drug in the ionized form rises, thereby increasing solubility. Once injected into the tissues (pH 7.4), the amount of local anesthetic in the free-base form increases. This provides for greater tissue (lipid) penetration (Fig. 9.5). In the presence of an acidic environment, such as infection or inflammation (pH lower), the amount of free base is reduced (more in ionized form), one reason that dental anesthesia with a local anesthetic is more difficult when infection is present. Other reasons include dilution by fluid, inflammation, and vasodilation in the area. Although the free-base form is needed to penetrate the nerve membrane, it is the cationic form that exerts blocking action by binding to the specific receptor site.

PHARMACOKINETICS

Absorption

> Systemic absorption greater, especially with inflammation.

TABLE 9.1   Local Anesthetic Agents Grouped by Chemical Structure

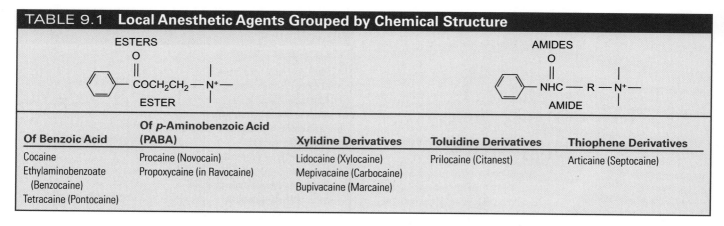

Of Benzoic Acid	Of *p*-Aminobenzoic Acid (PABA)	Xylidine Derivatives	Toluidine Derivatives	Thiophene Derivatives
Cocaine	Procaine (Novocain)	Lidocaine (Xylocaine)	Prilocaine (Citanest)	Articaine (Septocaine)
Ethylaminobenzoate (Benzocaine)	Propoxycaine (in Ravocaine)	Mepivacaine (Carbocaine)		
Tetracaine (Pontocaine)		Bupivacaine (Marcaine)		

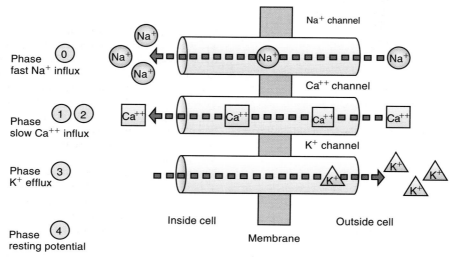

Fig. 9.3 An action potential involves opening both sodium (*Na$^+$*) and potassium (*K$^+$*) channels. *Ca^{++}*, Calcium.

BOX 9.2   Mechanism of Action = Blockade of Voltage-Gated Sodium Channels

1. Membrane potential = -90 to -60 mV
2. Excitatory impulse
3. Na$^+$ channels open
4. Na$^+$ flows in (depolarizes membrane [$+40$ mV])
5. Na$^+$ channels close
6. K$^+$ channels open
7. K$^+$ flows out
8. K$^+$ channels close
9. Na$^+$/K$^+$ exchange
10. Repolarizes membrane (-95 mV)

TABLE 9.2   Properties of Base and Salt Forms of Local Anesthetics

Free Base	Salt
Viscid liquids or amorphous solids	Crystalline solids
Fat soluble (lipophilic)	Water soluble (hydrophilic)
Unstable	Stable
Alkaline	Acidic
Uncharged, nonionized	Charged, cation (ionized)
Penetrates nerve tissue	Active form at site of action
Form present in tissue (pH 7.4)	Form present in dental cartridge (pH 4.5–6.0)

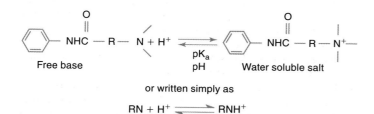

Fig. 9.4 Properties of base and salt forms of local anesthetics.

The absorption of a local anesthetic depends on its route. When it is injected into the tissues, the rate of absorption depends on the vascularity of the tissues. This is a function of the degree of inflammation present, the vasodilating properties of the local anesthetic agent, the presence of heat, and the use of massage. It is important to reduce the systemic absorption of a local anesthetic when it is used in dentistry. With lower systemic absorption, the chance of systemic toxicity is reduced. To reduce absorption, a vasoconstrictor is added to the local anesthetic. The vasoconstrictor reduces the blood supply to the area, limits systemic absorption, and reduces systemic toxicity.

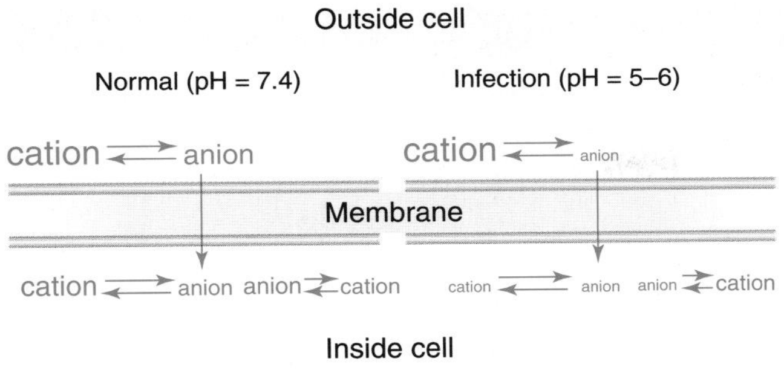

Outside cell

Normal (pH = 7.4)   Infection (pH = 5–6)

cation ⇌ anion   cation ⇌ anion

Membrane

cation ⇌ anion anion ⇌ cation   cation ⇌ anion anion ⇌ cation

Inside cell

Fig. 9.5 Effect of hydrogen ion concentration (pH) on local anesthetic drug action. In the normal extracellular environment (pH 7.4, *left* side of diagram), the anion form of the local anesthetic drug exists in sufficient numbers to make anesthesia possible. In infection (pH 5.6, *right* side of diagram), the lower pH reduces the number of anesthetic anions available to penetrate the nerve membrane, and the number of these base molecules needed for anesthesia may not be sufficient to be rendered effective. (Modified from Daniel S, Harfst S, Wilder R, et al. *Dental Hygiene Concepts, Cases and Competencies.* 2nd ed. St. Louis: Mosby; 2008.)

With topical application, especially on the mucous membranes or if the surface is denuded, absorption can approximate that produced by intravenous (IV) injection. Absorption is also determined by the proportion of the agent present in the free-base form (nonionized).

Distribution

After absorption, local anesthetics are distributed throughout the body. Highly vascular organs have higher concentrations of anesthetics. Local anesthetics cross the placenta and blood-brain barrier. The lipid solubility of a particular anesthetic affects the potency of the agent. For example, bupivacaine, used as a 0.5% solution, is approximately 10 times more lipid soluble than lidocaine used as a 2% solution.

Metabolism

Metabolism:
    Esters: plasma.
    Amides: liver.

The local anesthetic agents are metabolized differently, depending on whether they are amides or esters. Esters are hydrolyzed by plasma pseudocholinesterases and liver esterases. Procaine is hydrolyzed to *p*-aminobenzoic acid (PABA), a metabolite that may be responsible for its allergic reactions. Some patients who have an atypical form of pseudocholinesterase that does not allow them to hydrolyze these esters may exhibit an increase in systemic toxicity if given an ester.

Amide local anesthetics are metabolized primarily by the liver. In severe liver disease or with alcoholism, amides may accumulate and produce systemic toxicity. A small amount of prilocaine is metabolized to orthotoluidine, which can produce methemoglobinemia if given in very large doses. By reducing hepatic blood flow, cimetidine can interfere with the metabolism of the amides. (This is usually unimportant in dentistry because only one dose is given. No accumulation can result if repeated doses are not administered.)

Excretion

The metabolites and some unchanged drug of both esters and amides are excreted by the kidneys. With end-stage renal disease, both the parent drug and its metabolites can accumulate.

BOX 9.3 Common Order of Nerve Function Loss

1. Autonomic
2. Cold
3. Warmth
4. Pain
5. Touch
6. Pressure
7. Vibration
8. Proprioception
9. Motor

PHARMACOLOGIC EFFECTS

Peripheral Nerve Conduction (Blocker)

The main clinical effect of the local anesthetics is reversible blockage of peripheral nerve conduction. These agents inhibit the movement of the nerve impulse along the fibers, at sensory endings, at myoneural junctions, and at synapses. Therefore they may have wide-reaching effects on many kinds of nerves. Because they do not penetrate the myelin sheath, they affect the myelinated fibers only at the nodes of Ranvier. The local anesthetics affect the small, unmyelinated fibers first and the large, heavily myelinated fibers last. This pattern is probably related to the ability of these agents to penetrate to their sites of action.

The losses of nerve function are listed in Box 9.3. The list is in the order in which the senses are typically lost, but some individual variation occurs among patients. In some patients the pain sensation is lost before the cold sensation. The functions of the individual nerves return in reverse order.

Antiarrhythmic

Local anesthetics have a direct effect on the cardiac muscle by blocking cardiac sodium channels and depressing abnormal cardiac pacemaker activity, excitability, and conduction. They also depress the strength of cardiac contraction and produce arteriolar dilation, leading to hypotension. These properties make them useful to be given intravenously in the treatment of arrhythmias.

ADVERSE REACTIONS

The adverse reactions and toxicity of the local anesthetics are directly related to the plasma level of drug.

Considering the widespread use of these agents, their potential for danger must be minimal. Deaths from local anesthetics are difficult to document, but dental treatment–related mortality is even rarer. Table 9.3 lists the maximal safe doses for common local anesthetics. Factors that influence toxicity include the following:

- *Drug:* Both the inherent toxicity of the particular local anesthetic and the amount of vasodilation it produces can contribute to toxicity.
- *Concentration:* The higher the concentration injected, the higher the amount of drug entering the systemic circulation.
- *Route of administration:* Inadvertent IV injection can produce extremely high blood levels. Even topical administration can produce high blood levels and lead to toxicity.
- *Rate of injection:* The faster the injection is made, the lower the chance that the local area can accept the volume injected. The operator, who has control over this variable, may find that counting the seconds during injection is helpful.

TABLE 9.3   Maximum Safe Dose of Local Anesthetics

Local Anesthetic (Concentration)	Epinephrine	Dose (mg/lb)	ABSOLUTE MAXIMUM	
			mg	No. of Cartridges
Lidocaine 2%	1:50,000	3.2	500	5.5
	1:100,000	3.2	500	11.1
	1:200,000	3.2	500	11.1
Mepivacaine 3%	None (plain)	3	400	7.4
Mepivacaine 2%	1:20,000[a]	3	400	11.1
Prilocaine 4%	None (plain) and 1:200,000	4	600	8.3
Bupivacaine 0.5%	1:200,000	0.9	90	10
Articaine 4%	1:100,000	3.2	[b]	[b]
	1:200,000	3.2	[b]	[b]

[a]Vasoconstrictor—levonordefrin.
[b]no maximum dose provided but the lowest, most effective dose possible should be used. This dose is determined by body weight.

- *Vascularity:* The presence of inflammation, infection, or vasodilation produced by the agent will increase the vascularity and therefore the systemic toxicity.
- *Patient's weight:* The same dose administered to a child and an adult produces different blood levels because of their differences in weight.
- *Rate of metabolism and excretion:* Amides may accumulate with liver disease; both amides and their metabolites and ester metabolites may accumulate in renal disease.

Children, elderly individuals, and debilitated persons are more susceptible to the adverse reactions of the local anesthetic agents. The symptoms of an overdose of the local anesthetic agents are directly proportional to the blood level attained.

Toxicity

The two main systems affected by local anesthetic toxicity are the CNS and the cardiovascular system.

Central Nervous System Effects

CNS stimulation may occur before CNS depression. CNS stimulation due to depression of the inhibitory fibers results in restlessness, tremors, and convulsions. CNS depression due to depression of both the inhibitory and facilitative fibers results in respiratory and cardiovascular depression, and coma follows.

Cardiovascular Effects

The local anesthetic agents can produce myocardial depression and cardiac arrest with peripheral vasodilation. The usual concentrations that are achieved with administration of dental anesthesia would not be expected to result in any of these adverse reactions, although deaths have been reported with the use of lower doses of anesthetic. It is postulated that the effect of these agents on heart conduction may cause a fatal arrhythmia.

Local Effects

Local effects can occur with the administration of local anesthetic agents. This is most commonly the result of physical injury caused by the injection technique or the administration of an excessive volume too quickly to be accepted by the tissues. Occasionally, a hematoma may result.

Malignant Hyperthermia

Malignant hyperthermia not related to amides.

Malignant hyperthermia is an inherited disease that is transmitted as an autosomal dominant gene with reduced penetration and variable expression. Its symptoms include an acute rise in calcium, which leads to muscular rigidity, metabolic acidosis, and extremely high fever. The mortality rate of malignant hyperthermia is approximately 50%. Treatment includes supportive measures and the administration of dantrolene (Dantrium). In the past, it was thought that the amide local anesthetics might precipitate malignant hyperthermia, but currently they are no longer implicated. Patients with a family history of malignant hyperthermia can be given amide local anesthetic agents. Halothane, the inhalation anesthetic, and succinylcholine, the neuromuscular blocking agent, are the agents that most commonly precipitate malignant hyperthermia.

Pregnancy and Nursing Considerations

Elective dental treatment should be rendered before a patient becomes pregnant. However, if dental treatment is needed, most sources suggest that lidocaine may be administered to a pregnant woman. Fetal bradycardia has been reported when larger doses are administered to the mother near term. Both lidocaine and prilocaine are FDA pregnancy category B, whereas mepivacaine, articaine, and bupivacaine are category C drugs.

If a local anesthetic is needed, lidocaine in the smallest effective dose should be used. Usual doses of local anesthetics given to nursing mothers will not affect the health of normal nursing infants.

Allergy

Probably no allergies to amides.

Allergic reactions that result from local anesthetics have been reported, and they range from rash to anaphylactic shock. An allergy history should be elicited from each patient before a local anesthetic agent is chosen. Esters have a much greater allergic potential; in fact, there is some question about whether amides can cause allergic reactions at all. Cross-allergenicity exists between the esters but does not seem to occur between the amides in the xylidine and toluidine groups.

Local anesthetics with vasoconstrictors also contain a sulfite that serves as an antioxidant. In sulfite-sensitive patients, the sulfites may cause a hypersensitivity reaction that exhibits itself as an acute asthmatic attack. This reaction is the same as the "salad bar" syndrome, a hypersensitivity reaction to sulfites: In the past, certain restaurant foods offered at salad bars, such as lettuce, contained sulfites to prevent browning. Sulfites were used to help the lettuce and other greens retain their green color. Some restaurant menus still describe salad bars as "sulfite free." Deaths of hypersensitive asthmatic people who ate in restaurants have been reported. The nature of the reaction involves bronchoconstriction and anaphylactic reactions. A patient with an allergy to "sulfa" drugs does not exhibit cross-hypersensitivity with sulfites. Appendix C discusses the implications of a sulfite hypersensitivity in more detail.

COMPOSITION OF LOCAL ANESTHETIC SOLUTIONS

In addition to the local anesthetic agent, local anesthetic solutions usually contain several other ingredients, such as the following:

Vasoconstrictor: A vasoconstrictor, such as epinephrine, is added to local anesthetic solutions to retard absorption, reduce systemic toxicity, and prolong duration of action.

> Sulfites: asthmatic hypersensitivity reaction.

Antioxidant: An antioxidant (sodium metabisulfite, sodium bisulfite, or acetone sodium bisulfite) is included in local anesthetic solutions to retard oxidation of the epinephrine. The antioxidants, such as sodium bisulfite or metabisulfite, prolong shelf life. Asthmatic dental patients who are given local anesthetic agents with a vasoconstrictor, which also contains a sulfite agent, should be watched for symptoms of wheezing or chest tightness.

Sodium hydroxide: Sodium hydroxide alkalinizes the solution, or adjust, its pH to between 6 and 7.

Sodium chloride: Sodium chloride makes the injectable solution isotonic.

Propylparaben: Prevents bacterial growth. These are not used in single-dose cartridges, which is how dental cartridges come.

LOCAL ANESTHETIC AGENTS

Many local anesthetic agents are available with similar pharmacologic and clinical effects and systemic toxicity. Commonly used local anesthetics are discussed next, and dental issues associated with local anesthetics are listed in Box 9.4. Table 9.4 lists the local anesthetics available in dental cartridges. In 2003 the American Dental Association (ADA) Council on Scientific Affairs implemented a color-coding system as part of the labeling for all injectable local anesthetics that carried the ADA Seal of Acceptance. This system was developed because of the different colors used by different manufactures for the same local anesthetic which led to confusion. The ADA worked with the manufacturers to come up with a uniform color system the cartridges of each local anesthetic agent. Box 9.5 shows the color codes.

BOX 9.4 Instructions for Patients Receiving Local Anesthetics

- Patients should be advised to tell the dental practitioner if they are feeling anxious or nervous or if they are having heart palpitations.
- Most of these symptoms can be avoided by lowering the dose or switching to another local anesthetic.
- Some local anesthetics may cause drowsiness.
- Patients should use caution if an opioid analgesic or antianxiety drug is also prescribed.
- Patients should avoid driving or doing anything that requires thought or concentration.
- Patients should avoid eating or drinking very hot or cold foods or drinks. The local anesthetic may make it difficult to detect temperature changes.

TABLE 9.4 Local Anesthetic Combinations Available in Dental Cartridges

Local Anesthetic	%	Vasoconstrictor	Concentration
Lidocaine (Xylocaine, Octocaine)	2	Epinephrine	1:50,000 1:200,000
	2	Epinephrine	1:100,000
Mepivacaine (Carbocaine, Isocaine)	3	Plain	—
	2	Levonordefrin	1:20,000
Prilocaine (Citanest)	4	Plain	—
Prilocaine (Citanest Forte)	4	Epinephrine	1:200,000
Bupivacaine (Marcaine)	0.5	Epinephrine	1:200,000
Articaine (Septocaine)	4	Epinephrine	1:100,000 1:200,000

BOX 9.5 Local Anesthetic Cartridge Color Codes

Local anesthetic cartridge color codes
Mandated uniform system for local anesthetic cartridges bearing the ADA Seal of Acceptance.*

Product	Color
Lidocaine 2% with epinephrine 1:100,000	
Lidocaine 2% with epinephrine 1:50,000	
Mepivacaine 2% with levonordefrin 1:20,000	
Mepivacaine 3% plain	
Prilocaine 4% with epinephrine 1:200,000	
Prilocaine 4% plain	
Bupivacaine 1.5% with epinephrine	
Articaine 4% with epinephrine 1:100,000	
Articaine 4% with epinephrine 1:200,000	

Amides

The amide local anesthetic agents are the only class of anesthetics used parenterally. Esters are occasionally used topically. The relative lack of allergenicity of the amides is probably responsible for this use.

Lidocaine

> Lidocaine with epinephrine is good for almost all dentistry.

An amide derivative of xylidine introduced in 1948, lidocaine (LYE-doe-kane) (Xylocaine, Octocaine) quickly became an anesthetic standard against which other local anesthetics were compared. It has a rapid onset, which is related to its tendency to spread well through the tissues. Lidocaine 2% with vasoconstrictor provides profound anesthesia of medium duration. It is the local anesthetic solution most commonly used in dental offices.

No cross-allergenicity between the amide lidocaine and either other available amides or esters has been documented. Some patients appear to experience some sedation with lidocaine, and in toxic reactions one is likely to observe CNS depression initially rather than the CNS stimulation characteristic of other local anesthetics (Fig. 9.6).

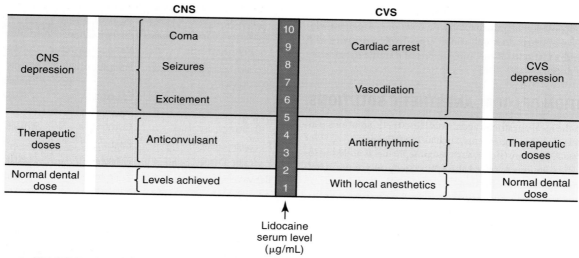

Fig. 9.6 Relationship between levels of local anesthesia in serum and the pharmacologic and adverse effects. *CNS,* Central nervous system; *CVS,* cardiovascular system.

Adverse reactions include hypotension, positional headache, and shivering. Lidocaine is used for topical, infiltration, block, spinal, epidural, and caudal anesthesia. It is also used intravenously to treat cardiac arrhythmias during surgery.

In dentistry, lidocaine 2% with 1:100,000 epinephrine is used for infiltration and block anesthesia. Lidocaine is used for topical anesthesia as a 5% ointment, a 10% spray, and a 2% viscous solution. When it is used topically, its onset is rapid (2–3 minutes). Lidocaine with epinephrine 1:100,000 provides a 1- to 1.5-hour duration of pulpal anesthesia. Soft tissue anesthesia is maintained for 3 to 4 hours. Lidocaine with epinephrine 1:50,000 is used for hemostasis during surgical procedures. Rebound vasodilation (β-adrenergic effect) can be expected after the α-adrenergic effect (vasoconstriction) has occurred.

Mepivacaine

> To avoid vasoconstrictors, one should use mepivacaine plain.

Another amide derivative of xylidine is mepivacaine (me-PIV-a-kane) (Carbocaine, Polocaine, Isocaine). Introduced in 1960, this agent is similar to lidocaine in rate of onset, duration, potency, and toxicity. No cross-allergenicity between the amide mepivacaine and other currently available amides or the esters has been documented.

Mepivacaine is not effective topically; however, it is used for infiltration, block, spinal, epidural, and caudal anesthesia. The usual dose form in dentistry is a 2% solution with the addition of 1:20,000 levonordefrin (Neo-Cobefrin) as the vasoconstrictor. Because mepivacaine produces less vasodilation than lidocaine, it can be used as a 3% solution without a vasoconstrictor (called *plain*). It can be used for short procedures when a vasoconstrictor is contraindicated (not often). Caution should be exercised in the use of increased concentrations of the local anesthetic without a vasoconstrictor because systemic toxicity is more likely. Except in unusual cases, the benefit of a shorter duration does not warrant eliminating the vasoconstrictor, especially when the concentration of the drug is increased.

Prilocaine

> *Ortho*-toluidine can induce methemoglobinemia.

Prilocaine (PRILL-loh-kane) (Citanest, Citanest Forte) is related chemically and pharmacologically to both lidocaine and mepivacaine. Chemically, lidocaine and mepivacaine are xylidine derivatives, whereas prilocaine is a toluidine derivative. Prilocaine appears to be less potent and less toxic than lidocaine and has a slightly longer duration of action. It has been shown to produce satisfactory local anesthesia when used with low concentrations of epinephrine and without epinephrine.

Although toxicity of prilocaine is 60% of that occurring with lidocaine, several cases of methemoglobinemia have been reported after its use. Prilocaine is metabolized to *ortho*-toluidine and, in large doses, can induce some methemoglobinemia. A very large dose (greater than the maximum safe dose) would be required to cause clinical symptoms: cyanosis of the lips and mucous membranes and occasionally respiratory or circulatory distress. Although the small doses required in dental practice are not likely to present a problem in healthy, nonpregnant adults, prilocaine should not be administered to patients with any condition in which problems of oxygenation may be especially critical. Drugs that affect the hemoglobin, such as acetaminophen, may exacerbate the adverse reaction. Methemoglobinemia can be reversed by IV methylene blue.

Prilocaine is used for infiltration, block, epidural, and caudal anesthesia. It is available in dental cartridges as a 4% concentration both with and without 1:200,000 epinephrine.

Prilocaine's niche in dentistry involves situations in which the desired duration of action is somewhat longer than that obtained with mepivacaine (without and with a vasoconstrictor). Prilocaine plain has a duration of action slightly longer than mepivacaine plain, and prilocaine with epinephrine has a duration of action slightly longer than lidocaine with epinephrine. The other potential advantage of prilocaine is that the concentration of epinephrine (1:200,000) is lower than in other local anesthetic amide combinations. Therefore use of prilocaine with epinephrine would expose the patient to half of the amount of epinephrine that would be in a solution of lidocaine with epinephrine 1:100,000.

Bupivacaine

> Bupivacaine: prolonged duration.

Bupivacaine (byoo-PIV-a-kane) (Marcaine) is an amide type of local anesthetic related to lidocaine and mepivacaine. It is more potent and toxic than the other amides. The major advantage of bupivacaine is its greatly prolonged duration of action. It is indicated for lengthy dental procedures in which pulpal anesthesia longer than 1.5 hours is needed or when postoperative pain is expected (e.g., endodontics, periodontics, or oral surgery). After sensation begins to return, a period of reduced or altered sensation (analgesia) may last several hours. Compared with lidocaine with epinephrine, the onset of bupivacaine with epinephrine is slightly longer, but its duration is at least twice that of lidocaine. It is available in dental cartridges as a 0.5% solution with 1:200,000 epinephrine. It should not be used in patients prone to self-mutilation (mental patients or children younger than 12 years). During its early use in anesthesiology and obstetrics, fatal unresuscitable cardiac arrests occurred. The doses used in obstetrics were much higher than those used in dentistry. After the maximal doses for obstetrics were lowered, these cardiac arrests essentially disappeared. Because much lower maximal doses are recommended for dental procedures, these adverse reactions are very unlikely to occur in dental practice. Bupivacaine has been used for infiltration, block, and peridural anesthesia.

Articaine

Articaine (Septocaine) was approved for use in the United States in 2000 and has been used in Europe since the mid-1970s.

Articaine differs from other amide local anesthetics in that it is derived from thiophene. This difference allows for greater lipid solubility and ability to cross lipid barriers such as nerve membranes. It has been suggested that this mechanism may account for articaine's enhanced action in comparison with other local anesthetics. Articaine also differs from other amide local anesthetics in that it has an extra ester linkage. This extra linkage causes articaine to be hydrolyzed by plasma esterase. Only 5% to 10% of articaine is metabolized by the liver, the other 90% to 95% being metabolized in the blood. The major metabolite is articainic acid, and it is unclear how active this metabolite is.

Articaine is excreted by the kidneys, 40% to 70% as articainic acid, 2% to 5% unchanged, and 4% to 15% as articainic acid glucuronide, which also appears to be inactive. The half-life of articaine is much shorter than that of lidocaine, approximately 20 minutes compared with approximately 90 minutes. The shorter half-life is the result of metabolism by plasma esterases. Other amides are metabolized by the liver and have much longer half-lives. Because of its rapid metabolism, articaine may be a safer drug to reinject later during a dental visit.

Despite its short half-life and apparent safety, articaine is a 4% solution with a toxic dose of 7 mg/kg for the average healthy adult. Because lidocaine is only a 2% solution with the same maximal dose, the average patient can tolerate twice as much lidocaine as articaine before the maximum safe dose is reached. In addition, like prilocaine, articaine in very high doses may cause methemoglobinemia. It should be noted that no reported cases of methemoglobinemia have been reported with articaine in doses recommended for dental local anesthesia. However, since its introduction in 2000, there have been many reports of paresthesia when the 4% solution is used. *Paresthesia* is defined as a persistent anesthesia beyond the expected duration of the local anesthetic's action. The patient can experience tingling or burning for an extended period. Articaine is used for local, infiltrative, and conductive anesthesia. It is available as a 4% concentration with 1:100,000 epinephrine in a 1.7-mL dental cartridge, rather than the more common 1.8-mL dental cartridge. In 2006 a solution of articaine 4% 1:200,000 was approved for dental use. Its duration and pulpal effectiveness are similar to those of the 1:100,000 formulation. Articaine has become the most widely used local anesthetic in just about every country in which it has been introduced. Its relative lack of significant active metabolites, which lowers the risk for toxicity, makes it more desirable in patients who may need to be reinjected.

Esters

There are currently no esters available in a dental cartridge. Esters, such as benzocaine, are commonly used topically.

Procaine

Procaine (PROE-kane) (Novocain) is a PABA ester. Procaine is used as an antiarrhythmic agent (procainamide) and is combined with penicillin to form procaine penicillin G. Procaine is not currently used in dentistry because of the high rate of allergic reaction. The allergic reaction is usually a result of PABA, not procaine.

Tetracaine

Tetracaine (TET-ra-kane) (Pontocaine), an ester of PABA, has a slow onset and long duration and is generally estimated to have at least 10 times the potency and toxicity of procaine. In view of this drug's high toxicity and the rapidity with which it is absorbed from mucosal surfaces, great care must be exercised if it is used for topical anesthesia. Dermatologic reactions include contact dermatitis, burning, stinging, and angioedema. A maximal absorbed dose of 20 mg is recommended for topical administration. Tetracaine is available in various sprays, solutions, and ointments for topical application. The concentration of tetracaine in most topical preparations is 2%.

Other Local Anesthetics

Dyclonine

Dyclonine (DYE-kloe-neen) (Dyclone) is a topical local anesthetic that is neither an ester nor an amide. Its side effects involving the cardiovascular system and CNS are similar to those of the other local anesthetics. Dyclonine may produce slight irritation and stinging when applied. Patients can exhibit allergic reactions to dyclonine, but cross-allergenicity with other local anesthetics would not be expected because of its unique structure. The onset of local anesthesia is 2 to 10 minutes, and its duration is 30 to 60 minutes. The solution and topical product are available as 0.5% and 1% concentrations.

VASOCONSTRICTORS

Overview

> Vasoconstriction keeps anesthetic in area injected.

The vasoconstricting agents are included in local anesthetic solutions for many reasons (Box 9.6).

The vasoconstrictors are members of the autonomic nervous system drugs called the *adrenergic agonists* or *sympathomimetics* (see Chapter 4).

BOX 9.6 Reasons for Use of Vasoconstricting Agents in Local Anesthetics

Vasoconstricting agents in local anesthetics are used because they:
- Prolong the duration of action.
- Increase the depth of anesthesia.
- Delay systemic absorption.
- Reduce the toxic effect in the systemic circulation.

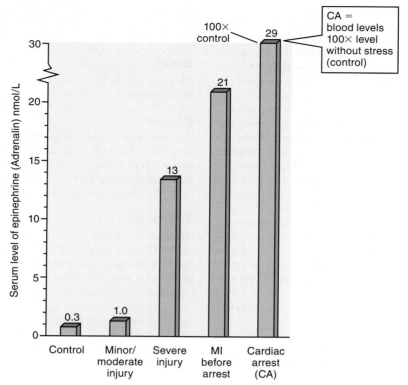

Fig. 9.7 Blood levels of endogenous epinephrine during rest; with minor, moderate, or severe injury; myocardial infarction *(MI)* before arrest; and cardiac arrest.

When a local anesthetic solution does not contain a vasoconstrictor, the anesthetic drug is more quickly removed from the injection site and distributed into systemic circulation than when the solution does contain a vasoconstrictor. Plain (without vasoconstrictor) anesthetics exhibit a shorter duration of action and result in a more rapid buildup of a systemic blood level. Therefore any anesthetics given without vasoconstrictors are more likely to be toxic than those given with vasoconstrictors. Any advantage gained by eliminating the vasoconstrictor (shorter duration and increased possible systemic effect of the vasoconstrictor) must be weighed against the potential for adverse effects of the epinephrine.

The decision about whether epinephrine should be used in a patient is made by weighing the risks and the benefits. Fig. 9.7 shows the amount of epinephrine at rest and during mild-to-severe stress and Fig. 9.8 compares the doses for anaphylaxis and dental use.

A sufficient concentration must be used to keep the local anesthetic localized at its site of action and provide adequate depth and duration of anesthesia and low systemic toxicity. The 1:100,000 and 1:200,000 concentrations have been shown to produce about the same amount of vasoconstriction and the same distribution of the local anesthetics. No justification exists for the use of epinephrine in a concentration greater than 1:200,000, except in cases in which local hemostasis is needed (1:50,000 is used). Lidocaine is available with 1:100,000 epinephrine, although the weaker concentration has been shown to have similar results.

In the 1940s, the literature stated that dental local anesthetics containing vasoconstrictors should not be used in patients with cardiovascular disease. This recommendation stemmed from the fear that the vasoconstrictor would elevate the blood pressure too much. It is now known that a patient can produce endogenous epinephrine far in excess of that administered in dentistry in the presence of inadequate anesthesia, which sometimes occurs when vasoconstrictors are avoided.

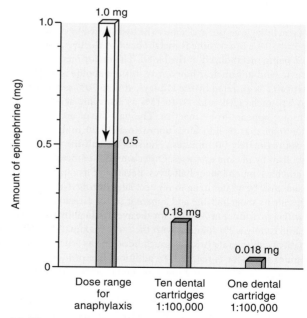

Fig. 9.8 Histogram showing the dose range of epinephrine for anaphylaxis and the doses provided in dental cartridges.

Patients with uncontrolled high blood pressure, hyperthyroidism, angina pectoris, and cardiac arrhythmias and those who have had a myocardial infarction or cerebrovascular accident in the past 6 months should make an appointment for elective dental treatment after their medical condition is under control. For patients who have had a myocardial infarction or cerebrovascular accident, that would be 6 months

TABLE 9.5 Vasoconstrictors: Maximum Safe Dose in Normal and Cardiac Patients

Drug	Concentration	Relative Pressor Potency	Normal Adult		Cardiac Patient		Approximate % of (α/β) Activity
			mg	No. of Cartridges	mg	No. of Cartridges	
Epinephrine	1:50,000	1	0.2	5.5	0.04	1.1	50/50
	1:100,000	1	0.2	11.1	0.04	2.2	50/50
	1:200,000	1	0.2	22.2	0.04	4.4	50/50
Levonordefrin (Neo-Cobefrin)	1:20,000	1/5	1.0	11.1	0.2 or 1.0*	2.2 or 11.1*	75/25

*Data from Logothetis DD. Local Anesthesia for the Dental Hygienist, 2nd ed. St. Louis, Elsevier, 2017.

after the cardiovascular or cerebrovascular event. Those undergoing general anesthesia with a halogenated hydrocarbon inhalation anesthetic should be monitored for arrhythmias if epinephrine (including epinephrine-soaked retraction cords) is used for its hemostatic effect (used commonly with halothane). If arrhythmias occur, antiarrhythmic agents are administered.

> Epinephrine cardiac dose: 0.04 mg.

Patients with cardiovascular disease who are able to withstand elective dental treatment can receive epinephrine-containing local anesthetic agents. The anesthetic should be administered in the lowest possible dose by the best technique, including aspiration and a very slow injection rate to minimize systemic absorption. Maximal cardiac doses should not be exceeded in patients with severe cardiovascular disease. Table 9.5 lists the maximum safe doses of epinephrine for the healthy patient (0.2 mg) and the cardiac patient (0.04 mg); the number of cartridges each of these doses represents is included. For example, the cardiac patient could be given two cartridges of 1:100,000 epinephrine without exceeding the cardiac dose.

Drug Interactions

> Significant drug interactions with epinephrine: tricyclic antidepressants and nonselective β-blockers.

Selected drug interactions of epinephrine are listed in Table 9.6. Of the most important drug interactions with epinephrine, two are clinically significant and two are not. The two epinephrine drug interactions that are most likely to be clinically significant are those with tricyclic antidepressants and nonselective β-blockers. In patients taking tricyclic antidepressants, administration of epinephrine may cause an exaggerated increase in pressor response (increased blood pressure). In those taking nonselective β-blockers, hypertension and reflex bradycardia may be exhibited. These are not absolute contraindications to the use of epinephrine, but patients taking these agents should be monitored for symptoms of alterations in blood pressure. The two drug interactions that are commonly mentioned but are not usually clinically significant are with monoamine oxidase inhibitors (MAOIs) and phenothiazines. Epinephrine can be given to patients taking MAOIs because epinephrine is eliminated primarily by reuptake and secondarily by catechol O-methyltransferase (COMT) rather than by monoamine oxidase (MAO). If any small interaction

TABLE 9.6 Drug Interactions of Epinephrine

Medical Drug Group	Examples	Potential Outcomes
Tricyclic antidepressants	Amitriptyline (Elavil) Imipramine (Tofranil)	Pressor response to intravenous EPI markedly enhanced
β-Blockers, nonselective	Pindolol (Visken) Propranolol (Inderal) Timolol (Blocadren)	Hypertension and reflex bradycardia
Antidiabetics	Tolbutamide (Orinase) Chlorpropamide (Diabinese)	Blood glucose increased
Interactions Not Significant in Dentistry		
Phenothiazines	Chlorpromazine (Thorazine)	Reverse pressor response of EPI; avoid using EPI to raise blood pressure
MAOIs	Phenelzine (Nardil) Tranylcypromine (Parnate)	EPI not inactivated by MAO

EPI, Epinephrine; *MAOIs*, monoamine oxidase inhibitors; MAO, monoamine oxidase.

exists, it would be the result of "denervation hypersensitivity." In contrast to epinephrine, the indirect-acting sympathomimetic agents (e.g., pseudoephedrine) should be avoided in patients taking MAOIs because they are inactivated in significant amounts by MAO. The drug interaction between epinephrine and phenothiazines occurs because the phenothiazines are α-blockers, and when an α and β agonist (epinephrine) is given, the β-adrenergic effects (vasodilation) predominate. Therefore if epinephrine is used for its vasopressor effect (to raise the blood pressure), the blood pressure is likely to decrease. When epinephrine is used in a local anesthetic solution, it is not being given for its vasopressor effect, so this interaction is not clinically significant.

CHOICE OF LOCAL ANESTHETIC

> One should choose two local anesthetic solutions.

Practitioners should choose a few local anesthetic solutions to use, depending on the duration of local anesthesia desired and the side effects that must be avoided. Box 9.7 lists the local anesthetics by their durations of action, including both pulpal and soft

BOX 9.7 Categories of Duration of Action of Local Anesthetic Agents—Plain (Without) and With a Vasoconstrictor

General Categories

Short-Duration (Pulpal Anesthesia 30 min)
Lidocaine plain (without) (No longer available in North America)
Mepivacaine plain (without)
Prilocaine plain (infiltration)

Intermediate-Duration (Pulpal Anesthesia 60 min)
Lidocaine with
Mepivacaine with
Prilocaine plain (block) (without)
Prilocaine with
Articaine with

Long-Duration (Pulpal >90 min)
Bupivacaine with

Pulpal and Soft Tissue Anesthesia

Agent	Pulpal Anesthesia (min)	Soft Tissue Anesthesia (h)
Lidocaine with	60	3–5
Mepivacaine plain (without)	20 (Supraperiosteal) 40 (Nerve Block)	2–3
Mepivacaine with	60	3–5
Prilocaine plain (without)	10–15 (Supraperiosteal) 40–60 (Nerve Block)	1.5–2 (Supraperiosteal) 2–4 (Nerve Block)
Prilocaine with	60–90	3–8
Bupivacaine with	90–180	4–9 (up to 12)
Articaine with 1:100,000	60–75	3–6
Articaine with 1:200,000	45–60	2–5

tissue anesthesia. Figs. 9.9 and 9.10 illustrate the durations of action of local anesthetic agents for soft tissue and pulpal anesthetics, respectively. Several properties of local anesthetic agents determine their differences in pharmacokinetics. Table 9.7 lists these physical properties for some local anesthetics. For example, the pK_a is related to the onset of action. With a lower pK_a, the local anesthetic is distributed more in the base form and so is better absorbed. The duration of action of the local anesthetic is primarily related to its protein-binding capacity. Its lipid solubility may also play some part. The duration is unrelated to the local anesthetic's half-life because its action is terminated when the drug is removed from the receptor. The lipid solubility determines the potency of a local anesthetic agent. The vasodilating property of a local anesthetic can affect both the potency and the duration of action. One should note that the vasodilating effect of lidocaine (1) is more than that of mepivacaine (0.8) and prilocaine (0.5). Because mepivacaine and prilocaine have less vasodilating effect, they can be used without vasoconstrictor. In contrast, lidocaine (1) and bupivacaine (2.5) produce too much vasodilation to be used without a vasoconstrictor. The dental hygienist should become familiar with a short-, an intermediate-, and a long-acting agent. The duration of the procedure and any patient-specific information will determine the anesthetic of choice. Table 9.8 lists some common contraindications to the use of local anesthetic agents.

TOPICAL ANESTHETICS

Benzocaine, an ester, is the most commonly used topical anesthetic; lidocaine, an amide, is the second most commonly used. Some topical anesthetics are listed in Table 9.9. Comparison among the agents should take into account their onset, duration of action, and allergenic potential. The patient should be instructed to avoid eating for 1 hour after application to oral mucosa so that the gag reflex can become fully functional.

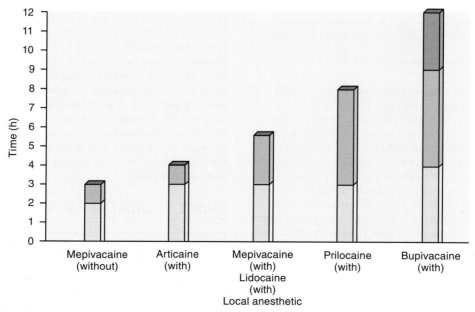

Fig. 9.9 Duration of anesthesia in soft tissue after a nerve block. *With,* With vasoconstriction; *without,* without vasoconstriction.

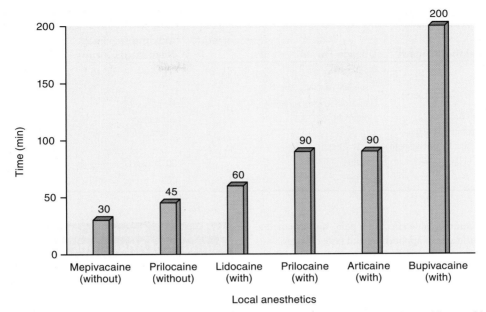

Fig. 9.10 Duration of pulpal anesthesia after a nerve block. *With,* With vasoconstriction; *without,* without vasoconstriction.

TABLE 9.7   Physical Properties of Local Anesthetics

Local Anesthetic	pKa*	Vasodilating†	t_{1/2}‡	Lipid Solubility§	Protein Binding‖(%)
Lidocaine	7.7	1	90	2.9	65
Mepivacaine	7.7	0.8	90¶	0.8	75
Prilocaine	7.7	0.5	80	0.9	55
Bupivacaine	8.1	2.5	76	27.5	95
Articaine	7.8	Uncertain	20	1.5	54

*pKa, Dissociation constant; rate of onset.
†Vasodilating lidocaine given value of 1.
‡Half-life (min).
§Lipid solubility oil/water solubility; intrinsic potency, increased penetrability.
‖Protein binding duration of action.
¶Estimated.

TABLE 9.8   Contraindications to the Use of Local Anesthetic Combinations

Categories	Situation	Preferred Anesthetic
History of allergy	To amides (very unlikely)	Amides, with informed consent
	To esters	Amide
	Sulfa	Any
	Sulfite hypersensitivity (asthma)	Any without vasoconstrictor
Choice of local anesthetic agent	Pregnancy	Lidocaine
	Congenital cholinesterase deficiency	Amides
	Malignant hyperthermia	Any amide
	Methemoglobinemia	Any but prilocaine
	Severe renal disease	Any, but limit dose
	Severe liver disease	Any, but limit dose
Vasoconstrictor limits	Very severe cardiovascular disease	Limit to cardiac dose
	Untreated (or drug-treated) hyperthyroidism	Limit to cardiac dose
	Tricyclic antidepressants	Limit to cardiac dose
	β-Blockers, nonselective	Limit to cardiac dose

Amides

Lidocaine

Lidocaine (Xylocaine) is available as the base or hydrochloride salt. The base is preferred when large areas of the mucosal surfaces are ulcerated, abraded, denuded, or erythematous. The hydrochloride salt is water soluble and penetrates the tissue better. Therefore its propensity for systemic absorption is greater than that of the base. Lidocaine base is available as a jelly and an oral topical solution, and hydrochloride is available as an ointment, an oral topical, and an oral aerosol. Concentration of the creams ranges from 2% to 5%. Viscous lidocaine (2%) is available for oral rinse to manage aphthous lesions or reduce gagging.

Lidocaine and Prilocaine (Injection-Free Local Anesthesia)

More often than not, the fear of injection prevents many people from seeking necessary dental treatment. Either the thought of the injection or the injection itself can be painful and upsetting. The combination of lidocaine and prilocaine gel (Oraqix) applied into the periodontal pocket offers pain relief during scaling and root planing procedures. The combination of lidocaine and prilocaine, in the gel form, provides a duration of action of approximately 20 minutes. Its onset of action is approximately 30 seconds after application. Lidocaine provides rapid anesthesia, and prilocaine has a slower onset of action. The combination appears to be

TABLE 9.9 Selected Topical Local Anesthetics

	Local Anesthetic Agent	Dosage Forms	Concentration (%)	Maximum Dose (mg)	Peak (min)	Duration (min)	Chemical Group
Lidocaine	Xylocaine	Spray, ointment, solution, viscous, jelly	2 or 5	200	2–5	15–45	Amides
Benzocaine	Hurricaine Orajel Mouth-Aid Anbesol Maximum Strength Americaine Anesthetic Lubricant	Liquid, gel, cream, spray, ointment	6–20	No published maximum dose.	2	15–15	Esters
Tetracaine	Pontocaine; in Cetacaine	Solution	2	20	3–8	45	Esters
Dyclonine	Dyclone	Solution	0.5–1	200	<10	<60	Ketone

well tolerated. The more common side effects are pain, soreness, irritation, edema or redness at the area of application, and taste changes.

Esters

Benzocaine

Benzocaine (BEN-zoe-kane) (Hurricaine, Anbesol, Benzodent, Orabase-B), an ester of PABA, cannot be converted to a water-soluble form for injection. Because it is poorly soluble, it is poorly absorbed and lacks significant systemic toxicity. Local reactions reported include burning and stinging. Dermatologic reactions have included angioedema and contact dermatitis, which can occur if the operator does not wear gloves (an unacceptable practice nowadays). Benzocaine is available in dental products and in many over-the-counter (OTC) products for teething, sunburn, hemorrhoids, or insect bites (up to 20% for many but not all). Benzocaine is used in many dental offices, although a hypersensitivity reaction is possible.

Precautions in Topical Anesthesia

Some local anesthetics are absorbed rapidly when applied topically to mucous membranes. To avoid toxic reactions from surface anesthesia, the dental health care provider should consider many factors (Box 9.8).

DOSES OF LOCAL ANESTHETIC AND VASOCONSTRICTOR

Some regional local anesthesia board examinations now require candidates to calculate local anesthetic doses on the basis of the labeled amount of solution, 1.8 mL or 1.7 mL depending on the manufacturer. The amounts of local anesthetic and vasoconstrictor contained in a certain volume of solution can be calculated from the concentration of that solution. The local anesthetic percentage, for example, 2%, may be expressed as seen in Box 9.9. Box 9.10 shows how to calculate the amount of epinephrine. Box 9.11 shows how to calculate the dose of a local anesthetic on the basis of the patient's weight.

BOX 9.8 How to Prevent Toxic Reactions from Surface Anesthesia

1. Know the relative toxicity of the drug being used.
2. Know the concentration of the drug being used.
3. Use the smallest volume.
4. Use the lowest concentration.
5. Use the least toxic drug to satisfy clinical requirements.
6. Limit the area of application (avoid sprays).

BOX 9.9 Sample Calculation to Determine Amount of Anesthetic in 2% Solution

Amount of local anesthetic in a 2% solution:
2% solution = 2 gm/100 mL, so 2% = 2000 mg/100 mL = 20 mg/mL
Amount in one cartridge:
20 mg/mL × 1.8 mL/cartridge = 36 mg/cartridge

BOX 9.10 Sample Calculation for Amount of Epinephrine per Cartridge

Amount of epinephrine in a milliliter of a 1:100,000 local anesthetic:
1000 mg/100,000 mL = 1 mg/100 mL = 0.01 mg/1 mL of solution
Amount of epinephrine in one cartridge:
0.1 mg/mL × 1.8 mL = 0.018 mg/cartridge

BOX 9.11 Sample Calculation of the Maximum Recommended Dose (in milligrams), Number of Cartridges, and Milliliters of Solution for a 2% Solution of a Local Anesthetic for a 150-Pound Patient

Step 1: Determine the number of mg in one cartridge of solution (see Box 9.9):
2% solution = 2 × 10 mg/mL = 20 mg/mL × 1.8 mL/cartridge = 36 mg in one cartridge
Step 2: Calculate the maximum recommended dose (mg/lb; 2 mg/lb) (see Table 9.3):
150 × 2 = 300 mg
Step 3. Determine the maximum number of cartridges:
300/36 = 8.3 cartridges

The dental hygienist should be able to determine the number of milligrams of both local anesthetic and vasoconstrictor given in any clinical situation. The maximum safe dose for each component should not be exceeded.

Each dose should be recorded in the patient's chart as soon as possible after the injection. The information placed in the chart should include the strength of both ingredients and the volume of solution used or the number of milligrams of each given. For example, if a patient were given one cartridge of lidocaine 2% with 1:100,000 epinephrine, the chart would read "lidocaine 2% with epinephrine 1:100,000 1.8 mL" or "lidocaine 36 mg with epinephrine 0.018 mg."

One reason for including this information in the chart is to minimize questions that might arise later if the patient or a future practitioner has concerns about the treatment. Because of the rising incidence of lawsuits against dentists and hygienists, maintaining a complete chart to prevent any ambiguity is extremely important.

DENTAL HYGIENE CONSIDERATIONS

Injectable Local Anesthetics

- Select the local anesthetic on the basis of the patient's medication/health history.
- Use the maximum safe dose of local anesthetic and vasoconstrictor according to the patient's physical health and medication history.
- Record the local anesthetic concentration, vasoconstrictor concentration, and number of cartridges used.
- See Boxes 9.4, 9.6, and 9.8.

Topical Anesthetic Agents

- Limit the area of application.
- Select the topical anesthetic on the basis of the patient's medication/health history.
- Avoid using spray formulations.

ACADEMIC SKILLS ASSESSMENT

1. Name the properties of the ideal local anesthetic.
2. Differentiate between the two major chemical groups of local anesthetic agents.
3. Contrast the allergenicity and metabolism of the ester and amide local anesthetics.
4. List the systemic adverse reactions to the local anesthetics.
5. List five injectable local anesthetic agents and give their compositions.
6. Explain the presence in a dental cartridge of agents other than the local anesthetic.
7. State the rationale for the inclusion of vasoconstricting agents in local anesthetic solutions.
8. State the maximum safe dose of the two vasoconstrictors used in dentistry for both the normal patient and the cardiac patient.
9. Explain the rationale for use of Oraqix in a dental practice.

CLINICAL CASE STUDY

Frank Castinelli is 55 years old, is slightly overweight, and has been coming to your practice for close to 10 years. He has a somewhat stressful job that takes up quite a bit of his time. His medications include nitroglycerin sublingual tablets for angina, ibuprofen for aches and pains, and antacids for heartburn. Mr. Castinelli comes in today for a scheduled oral health maintenance examination and tells you that he suffered a heart attack and was diagnosed with hypertension approximately 4 months ago. He is now taking an angiotensin-converting enzyme (ACE) inhibitor to treat high blood pressure, simvastatin for high cholesterol, and an aspirin a day to prevent a second heart attack. Unfortunately, you find two cavities during your examination of Mr. Castinelli that need to be addressed.

1. Would you and the dentist recommend that Mr. Castinelli have his cavities filled within the next 2 weeks? Why or why not?
2. If not, when should Mr. Castinelli have his cavities filled?
3. Can you use a local anesthetic with a vasoconstrictor in a patient with hypertension?
4. What is the relationship between vasoconstrictors and cardiovascular disease?
5. What are the adverse effects associated with vasoconstrictors?
6. What would be an appropriate cardiac dose of a vasoconstrictor?
7. Mr. Castinelli weighs 170 pounds. Please calculate the appropriate dose for him using a 2% lidocaine anesthetic solution. How many cartridges will you need? What is the maximum number of cartridges allowed?

10

General Anesthetics

http://evolve.elsevier.com/Haveles/pharmacology

LEARNING OBJECTIVES

1. Summarize the history of general anesthesia in dentistry.
2. Describe how general anesthesia works and the stages and planes involved, as well as possible adverse reactions associated with its use.
3. Compare and contrast the classifications of general anesthesia.
4. Discuss the use of nitrous oxide in dentistry, including how it works, the pharmacologic effects, adverse reactions, and contraindications.
5. Name and describe several types of halogenated hydrocarbons.
6. List the goals of surgical anesthesia and the importance of using balanced general anesthesia.

Reversible loss of consciousness and insensibility to painful stimuli.

Contemporary general anesthetic techniques use *balanced anesthesia*, which employs a combination of drugs to produce a reversible loss of consciousness and insensibility to painful stimuli while minimizing adverse reactions, taking into account the patient's physical status and preanesthetic and postanesthetic needs.

Hospital: General anesthesia.
Dental office: Conscious sedation.

In oral health care, oral and maxillofacial surgeons use general anesthetic drugs in their offices. General dentists use nitrous oxide to provide conscious sedation and pain control. Although dental hygienists are not generally involved with the administration of general anesthesia, many states allow them to monitor and/or administer nitrous oxide for conscious sedation. In today's practice, the dental hygienist should have an understanding of the principles of general anesthesia because it is an indispensable tool used to meet the needs of special patients and for extensive oral and maxillofacial surgery.

HISTORY

The original methods of producing general anesthesia involved either strangulation or cerebral concussion. Later, opium, belladonna, hemp, and alcohol were used to render patients unconscious. During this time, the operations were "quick and dirty." Nitrous oxide was discovered in 1776, and 20 years later Sir Humphrey Davy suggested that the administration of nitrous oxide might be useful in surgery. About the middle of the 1800s, true general anesthetics were discovered in the United States. In 1846, surgically related mortality dropped dramatically with the introduction of ether. Today, anesthesiologists use a combination of inhaled and intravenous general anesthetics and adjuvant drugs to produce a generalized, reversible depression of the central nervous system (CNS) that results in a loss of consciousness, amnesia, and immobility but not necessarily complete analgesia.

MECHANISM OF ACTION

Overview

Many theories have been proposed to explain the mechanism of action of the various general anesthetic agents, but unfortunately no theory does so completely. It may seem relatively simple to say that these drugs are CNS depressants. However, the way in which they depress the normal functions of the CNS is complicated by the lack of knowledge of the physiologic and biochemical events of arousal and unconsciousness. Proposed mechanisms for the action of different general anesthetics involve an increase in the threshold for firing, facilitation of inhibitory γ-aminobutyric acid (GABA), and a decrease in the duration of opening of nicotinic receptor-activated cation channels. The increase in the threshold or hyperpolarization is a result of the activation of the potassium channels.

Stages and Planes of Anesthesia

Guedel described four stages and planes of anesthesia.

The extent of CNS depression produced by general anesthetics must be carefully titrated to avoid excessive cardiorespiratory depression. In 1920, Guedel described a system of stages and planes to describe the effects of anesthetics (Table 10.1). Although Guedel's classification applied to the effects produced by ether during the open drop method of administration, modern anesthetic techniques seldom show these exact stages. However, the four stages are briefly described here because Guedel's terminology is still used to describe the depth of anesthesia.

Induction is the term used to refer to the quick change in the patient's state of consciousness from stage I to stage III, as follows:

Stage I analgesia is characterized by the development of analgesia or reduced sensation to pain. The patient is conscious and can still respond to command. Reflexes are present, and respiration remains regular. Some amnesia may also be evident. Nitrous oxide, as used in the dental office, keeps the patient in stage I. The end of this stage is marked by the loss of consciousness.

TABLE 10.1	Stages and Planes of Anesthesia
Stage and Plane	**Patient Response**
Stage I: Analgesia	Patient is unresponsive Reduced sensation to pain Can still respond to commands Reflexes are present Regular respiration Some amnesia Loss of consciousness (end of stage)
Stage II: Delirium or excitement	Unconsciousness Amnesia Involuntary movement and excitement Irregular respiration Increased muscle tone Sympathetic stimulation: tachycardia, mydriasis, hypertension
Stage III: Surgical anesthesia	Return to regular respiration, muscle relaxation, and normal heart and pulse rates Divided into four planes
Stage IV: Respiratory or medullary paralysis	Cessation of respiration Subsequent circulatory failure Respiration must be artificially maintained

Copyright 1996 Elena Bablenis Haveles.

Stage II delirium or excitement begins with unconsciousness and is associated with involuntary movement and excitement. Respiration becomes irregular, and muscle tone increases. Sympathetic stimulation produces tachycardia, mydriasis, and hypertension. This can be an uncomfortable time for the patient because emesis and incontinence can occur. As the depth of anesthesia increases, the patient begins to relax and proceeds to stage III. To ensure the patient's comfort and safety, it is important to have a smooth and rapid induction. The ultrashort-acting barbiturates accomplish this readily. When balanced anesthesia is used, the patient does not pass through each stage as listed. Adjunct drugs reduce the side effects of each of the drugs used during surgery.

Stage III surgical anesthesia is the stage in which most major surgery is performed. This stage is further divided into four planes that are differentiated on the basis of eye movements, depth of respiration, and muscle relaxation. The onset of stage III (planes I and II) is typically characterized by the return of regular respiratory movements, muscle relaxation, and normal heart and pulse rates. Reflexes associated with the eye disappear during planes I and II. Vomiting reflex stops during stage II, but swallowing reflex is maintained until stage III, plane I. Plane III is associated with decreased skeletal muscle tone, dilated pupils, tachycardia, and hypotension. Beginning in plane III and progressing to plane IV, stage III is characterized by intercostal muscle paralysis (diaphragmatic breathing remains), absence of all reflexes, and extreme muscle flaccidity. If the depth of anesthesia is allowed to increase, the patient will rapidly progress to the last stage, with cessation of all respiration.

Stage IV respiratory or medullary paralysis is characterized by complete cessation of all respiration (diaphragmatic respiration is the last to go) and subsequent circulatory failure. At this point, pupils are maximally dilated and blood pressure falls rapidly. If this stage is not reversed immediately, the patient will die. Respiration must be artificially maintained.

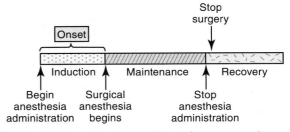

Fig. 10.1 Levels of anesthesia: induction, maintenance, and recovery.

Modern anesthetic techniques now use more rapidly acting agents than those associated with the four stages described by Guedel. Flagg's approach, used to describe the levels of anesthesia (Fig. 10.1), uses the following categories:

Induction: The induction phase encompasses all the preparation and medication necessary for a patient up to the time the operation begins, including preoperative medications, adjunctive drugs for anesthesia, and anesthetics required for induction.

Maintenance: The maintenance phase begins with the patient at a depth of anesthesia sufficient to allow surgical manipulation and continues until completion of the procedure.

Recovery: The recovery phase begins with the termination of the surgical procedure and continues through the postoperative period until the patient is fully responsive to the environment.

ADVERSE REACTIONS

> Risk of general anesthesia must always be compared with the benefit of surgery.

The goals of surgical anesthesia are good patient control, adequate muscle relaxation, and pain relief. To produce anesthesia, potent CNS depressants are given in relatively high doses, and many combinations of drugs are used in balanced anesthesia. The hazards encountered with the administration of general anesthetics are summarized in Table 10.2.

GENERAL ANESTHETICS

Classification of Anesthetic Agents

The general anesthetic agents can be classified according to their chemical structures or routes of administration. Table 10.3 categorizes the agents according to their routes of administration.

Induction Anesthesia
Intravenous Anesthetics

The intravenously administered general anesthetics are a diverse group of CNS depressants that include the opioids, the ultrashort-acting barbiturates, and the benzodiazepines. Although most injectable general anesthetics are administered intravenously, one agent, ketamine, can also be given intramuscularly. These drugs find their greatest utility in induction of general anesthesia but may occasionally be used as single agents for short procedures. Although they offer the advantage of convenience, the depth and duration of anesthesia are less easily controlled with them than with the inhalation agents.

Ultrashort-Acting Barbiturates

The ultrashort-acting barbiturates used include methohexital (meth-oh-HEX-i-tal) sodium (Brevital), thiopental (thye-oh-PEN-tal) sodium (Pentothal), and thiamylal (thye-AM-i-lal) sodium (Surital). These ultrashort-acting agents have a rapid onset of action (about 30–40 seconds) when given intravenously. They are highly

TABLE 10.2 Adverse Reactions to General Anesthetics

System	Effect/Comment*
Cardiovascular system	Cardiovascular collapse Cardiac arrest
Arrhythmias	Ventricular fibrillation with halogenated hydrocarbons
Blood pressure	Hypertension (stage II) Hypotension
Respiration	Depressed respiration (stage III) Respiratory arrest (stage IV) Laryngospasm with ultrashort-acting barbiturates "Boardlike" chest with neuroleptanalgesia
Explosions/flammability	Cyclopropane Ether
Teratogenicity (either male or female exposure)	Chronic exposure fetal abnormalities Spontaneous abortions
Hepatotoxicity (repeated exposure)	Operating room personnel Halogenated hydrocarbons
Other	Headache, fatigue, irritability, addicting

*Stage refers to Guedel's stage of anesthesia.

TABLE 10.3 Classification of General Anesthetics by Route of Administration

INHALATION AGENTS		
Gases	**Volatile Liquids**	**Intravenous agents**
Nitrous oxide	Halogenated hydrocarbons: • Halothane (Fluothane) Halogenated ethers: • Methoxyflurane (Penthrane) • Enflurane (Ethrane) • Isoflurane (Forane) Ethers: • Diethyl ether (ether)*	Barbiturates: • Methohexital (Brevital) • Thiamylal (Surital) • Thiopental (Pentothal) Dissociative: • Ketamine (Ketalar) Opioids: • Morphine • Fentanyl (Sublimaze) • Sufentanil (Sufenta) • Alfentanil (Alfenta) Benzodiazepines: • Diazepam (Valium) • Midazolam (Versed) Others: • Etomidate (Amidate) • Propofol (Diprivan)

*Of historic interest only.

lipid soluble, and repeated dosing during anesthesia can result in a prolonged recovery period. However, blood and brain levels of these agents quickly decrease as the drugs redistribute to lean tissues (skeletal muscle).

Other complications with ultrashort-acting barbiturates include laryngospasm and bronchospasm. In some patients, hiccups, increased muscle activity, and delirium occur on recovery. Premedication with atropine or opioids has proved reasonably effective in reducing these recovery problems. Like all barbiturates, these drugs can cause cardiovascular and respiratory adverse effects.

Etomidate

Etomidate is a short-acting intravenous anesthetic agent that is used for the induction of general anesthesia and for sedation. It is used for conscious sedation and as part of the sequence of rapid general anesthesia induction. Etomidate has a rapid onset of action and a safe cardiovascular profile. It is metabolized by the liver. This agent can cause adrenal suppression, especially after repeated dosing.

Propofol

> Patient feels good; used for day surgery.

One of the general anesthetics unrelated to any other general anesthetic is propofol (PROE-po-fole) (Diprivan). It is an intravenous (IV) anesthetic that produces an onset of anesthesia in 30 seconds (similar to the barbiturates) and a duration of action of about 5 minutes. During recovery, patients "feel better" and begin ambulation sooner than with other agents. Propofol produces little vomiting and may have antiemetic effects. It is also used for IV sedation. Propofol can be used for induction and for maintenance of balanced anesthesia. It can cause cardiovascular and respiratory depression. It is metabolized by the liver.

Ketamine

> Chemically related to phencyclidine (PCP); produces dissociative anesthesia.

The anesthetic ketamine (KEET-a-meen) (Ketalar) is related chemically to phencyclidine (PCP), a hallucinogen. The anesthetic state that ketamine produces has been given the name *dissociative anesthesia* because the drug appears to disrupt association pathways in the brain. Under ketamine anesthesia, the patient appears to be catatonic and has amnesia; ketamine produces analgesia without actual loss of consciousness.

Ketamine may be given intravenously or intramuscularly, with a rapid (1–2 minutes) onset of action occurring with either route. It is distributed first to lipid tissues then to more vascular areas. Pharyngeal and laryngeal reflexes remain active, and there is little respiratory change. Ketamine increases cerebral blood flow and stimulates the heart to increase cardiac output. Because excessive salivation is a common finding with ketamine, atropine is a necessary premedication. Muscle tone may increase during its use. Ketamine has some sympathomimetic properties and can stimulate the cardiovascular system. It is safe when used correctly. Ketamine is used primarily by oral surgeons and is not used in general dentistry.

Opioids

The opioids (OH-pee-oyds) have long been used as adjunctive drugs to general anesthesia in preanesthetic medication and to provide analgesia during and after a surgical procedure. The opioids used include morphine, fentanyl (Sublimaze), sufentanil (Sufenta), and alfentanil (Alfenta). These drugs do not significantly alter cardiovascular function or peripheral resistance. Prolonged respiratory depression is the major disadvantage and requires careful attention to ventilatory function throughout the anesthesia period. Reversal of this depression can be accomplished with the opioid antagonist naloxone.

Benzodiazepines

The anxiolytic benzodiazepines have been an integral part of conscious sedation and preanesthetic medication for years. Diazepam

(Valium) has been used intravenously for many years. Midazolam (Versed), which is water soluble, does not need a solvent for solution, so one of diazepam's major side effects, thrombophlebitis, can be avoided. Other advantages include a shorter duration of action and production of more amnesia than diazepam. They are discussed in detail in Chapter 11.

Induction and Maintenance Anesthesia

Inhalation Anesthetics

Inhalation agents can be divided into gases and volatile liquids. The liquids are vaporized and carried to the patient in the form of gas. The inhalation agents are often used in combination, oxygen being a carrier gas.

> Volatile anesthetics: liquids that easily evaporate.

The volatile general anesthetics are liquids that evaporate easily at room temperature because of their low boiling points. They are classified chemically as halogenated hydrocarbons because they contain fluorine, chlorine, or bromine in their structures. These are potent agents with limited solubility in body tissues, and they have successfully replaced ether in anesthesia. Both methoxyflurane and halothane are used infrequently; enflurane and isoflurane are the more popular volatile liquids in current use.

Physical Factors

The concentration of anesthetic in the inspired mixture is proportional to its partial pressure or tension. The depth of anesthesia produced is a function of the tension (partial pressure) of the anesthetic agent in the brain. The most important physical factors influencing brain anesthetic tension are the tension of the anesthetics in the inspired gases, the rate and volume of delivery of anesthetics to the lungs, and the anesthetic's solubility in body tissues. Induction can be hastened with high initial anesthetic concentrations and hyperventilation. As anesthesia depth develops, both the concentration and rate of delivery are reduced to maintenance levels.

Table 10.4 gives the physical properties of some of the anesthetics. The solubility in blood is expressed by the blood/gas partition coefficient. The less soluble the anesthetic is in body tissues, the more rapid the onset and recovery. The low solubility of nitrous oxide (0.47) correlates well with its rapid onset and recovery. This physical factor allows the anesthesiologist to quickly adjust the desired level of anesthesia. In contrast, halothane, with its higher solubility (2.30), has a longer induction and recovery, and changes in level of anesthesia occur more slowly.

TABLE 10.4   Physical Properties of Selected Inhalation General Anesthetics

Anesthetic	Blood/Gas Partition Coefficient* and Implications	Comments
Nitrous oxide	(0.47); very low solubility in blood; quick onset	Incomplete anesthetic, rapid onset and recovery
Halothane	(2.3); longer induction and recovery	Intermediate onset and recovery
Methoxyflurane	(12); high solubility in blood; slow onset	Slow onset and recovery

*Partition coefficient (relative distribution by area; blood, brain, gas).

Nitrous Oxide

Nitrous (NYE-trus) oxide (N_2O) is a colorless gas with little or no odor and is the least soluble in blood of all the inhalation anesthetics. It has little potency and is used in clinical outpatient dentistry as an inhaled agent that results in conscious sedation. Although nitrous oxide is a good analgesic, it is only a weak general anesthetic.

> Provides anxiety relief.

Administration of nitrous oxide-oxygen (N_2O-O_2) has become a primary part of anxiety reduction procedures in the dental office. When nitrous oxide is properly administered, the patient remains conscious with the protective reflexes intact. Nitrous oxide provides anxiety relief coupled with analgesia.

> Onset rapid: a few minutes.

The N_2O-O_2 sedation technique involves increasing the concentration of nitrous oxide to bring the patient to a desired level of sedation. Starting with 100% oxygen for 2 to 3 minutes, nitrous oxide is gradually added in 5% to 10% increments until the patient response indicates that the desired level of sedation has been achieved. Once the nitrous oxide is added, onset occurs rapidly, within 3 to 5 minutes. Table 10.5 shows the typical responses observed with increasing concentrations of nitrous oxide. The percentage of nitrous oxide required for patient comfort is variable and may range from 10% to 50% (average 35%).

TABLE 10.5   Signs and Symptoms of the Response to Nitrous Oxide and Oxygen Conscious Sedation

Concentration of Nitrous Oxide (N_2O) (%)	Response
10–20	Body warmth Tingling of hands and feet
20–30	Circumoral numbness Numbness of thighs
20–40	Numbness of tongue Numbness of hands and feet Droning sounds present Hearing distinct but distant Dissociation begins and reaches peak Mild sleepiness Analgesia (maximum concentration of 30%) Euphoria Feeling of heaviness or lightness of body
30–50	Sweating Nausea Amnesia Increased sleepiness
40–60	Dreaming, laughing, giddiness Further increased sleepiness, tending toward unconsciousness Increased nausea and vomiting
50 and over	Unconsciousness and light general anesthesia

From Clark M, Brunick A. *Handbook of Nitrous Oxide and Oxygen Sedation.* 3rd ed. St. Louis: Mosby; 2008.

At the termination of an N_2O-O_2 sedation procedure, the patient should be placed on 100% oxygen for at least 5 minutes. Recovery occurs rapidly as nitrous oxide is quickly removed from the tissues. If the mask is removed without the oxygen recovery period and the patient is allowed to breathe room air, a phenomenon known as *diffusion hypoxia* may result. This occurs because of the rapid outward flow of nitrous oxide accompanied by oxygen and carbon dioxide. The loss of carbon dioxide, a stimulant to respiratory drive, could decrease ventilation, with resultant hypoxia. Patients may complain of headache or other side effects if this occurs. Recovery with 100% oxygen avoids this problem.

As has been implied, the N_2O-O_2 technique has sufficient advantages to recommend its consideration in many dental procedures. Among its advantages are rapid onset and recovery, easy administration, and close patient control or monitoring. Patient response to questions is a good indication of the level of sedation (see Table 10.5). The patient's time frame is also distorted by nitrous oxide, so the patient assumes that the procedure was much shorter than it actually was. This impression may be due to the amnestic qualities of nitrous oxide. Nitrous oxide is a valuable adjunct in managing some apprehensive children before dental care. However, it cannot be used when a child's behavior is openly defiant or hysterical, and it is not a substitute for good behavioral management techniques. The N_2O-O_2 technique not only will offer comfort to the patient and increase the acceptance of dental procedures but also will afford more relaxed treatment—that is, the dental team should be less tense and fatigued at the end of the office day.

Pharmacologic Effects

Nitrous oxide produces predictable, dose-related effects on the CNS, resulting in sedation, analgesia, and amnesia.

Pharmacokinetics

Nitrous oxide has a very rapid onset of action as a result of its absorption from pulmonary alveoli into the circulatory system. Nitrous oxide has low solubility in the blood and tissues which allows for the equilibrium between the inhaled N_2O-O_2 mixture in body tissues to be reached within minutes.

Adverse Reactions

> Be smart; think; monitor the patient.

Invariably, complications that have occurred with the use of N_2O-O_2 techniques have been the result of misuse or to faulty installation of equipment.

> O_2: Green tank.
> N_2O: Blue tank.

All cylinders are now colored in a standardized manner. Nitrous oxide cylinders are blue, and oxygen cylinders are green. The cylinders are also "pin coded" (their connectors are different) to prevent inadvertent mixing of cylinders and lines.

Equipment with built-in safety features is now available. Modern equipment has built-in features that allow no more than 70% of N_2O to be dispensed. Oxygen, in the gaseous mixture, must be dispensed at concentrations of 30% or higher during the sedation period. The inhalation administration equipment in every dentist's office should automatically limit the percentage of nitrous oxide that can be administered and should have a failsafe system that shuts down the nitrous oxide if the oxygen runs out.

Other adverse effects are nausea and vomiting. The dental hygienist should advise the patient to eat a light meal prior to the appointment and to avoid eating a large meal within 3 hours after the appointment.

Chronic use or misuse of nitrous oxide has been shown to reduce the activity of methionine synthetase, the enzyme involved with the function of vitamin B_{12}. Extreme cases of megaloblastic anemia have also been reported with chronic use or misuse of nitrous oxide. This problem does not appear to happen in the dental patient undergoing routine procedures in which the agent is used.

Contraindications and Dental Issues

Respiratory obstruction. Because the nasal passages are used for gaseous exchange, upper respiratory obstruction or a stuffy nose is an absolute contraindication to this technique. Other respiratory diseases must also be carefully evaluated.

Chronic obstructive pulmonary disease. Patients with chronic obstructive pulmonary disease (COPD), particularly emphysema, have respirations that are driven by a lack of oxygen and not by elevated carbon dioxide levels. These patients would have a great difficulty if they received more oxygen than they normally breathe.

Emotional Instability. Because patients may experience euphoria with nitrous oxide analgesia, a patient's emotional instability is a relative contraindication to its use. Patients taking psychotherapeutic medication must be carefully evaluated before nitrous oxide is used. Fanciful dreams occurring during a procedure may be interpreted upon recovery as actually occurring events; therefore a female staff member must be in attendance when a female patient is being treated by a male dentist or dental hygienist and nitrous oxide is used. Aberrant sensations may lead to unfounded accusations unless this requirement is strictly enforced. This practice is required to minimize legal liability (record in chart).

Pregnancy considerations

> Pregnant dental practitioners should determine levels in dental operatory before exposure.

Safety of the use of nitrous oxide in pregnant patients or administration by pregnant operators is in question. Although no direct correlation has yet been found, several epidemiologic studies cast doubt on the safety of exposure to nitrous oxide during pregnancy. The incidence of spontaneous abortion or miscarriages is higher in female operating personnel with long-term exposure to anesthetic agents and in wives of male operators. Women exposed to high levels of nitrous oxide (>5 hours/week) were significantly less fertile than unexposed women. This issue is especially important to female dentists and dental hygienists because dental operatories have been found to have higher concentrations of gases than even hospital operating rooms (poorer ventilation).

Dental health care workers should be aware of the concentration of nitrous oxide present in the dental operatories in which they practice. Machines are available that monitor the concentration of nitrous oxide. Scavenger systems that can retrieve much of the expired gas can be installed, and turnover of the room air can be improved. Checking of the nitrous oxide concentration in the dental operatory should be repeated, especially if the use changes or personnel are pregnant.

Misuse. The dental team should be knowledgeable about the potential hazards associated with the misuse of nitrous oxide. Symptoms include numbness and paresthesia of the hands or legs that progresses to more severe neurologic symptoms with continued misuse (**neuropathy**). Liver and kidney problems have also been mentioned in association with nitrous oxide misuse.

Situations that determine that misuse has begun include self-using nitrous oxide, using nitrous oxide for anything other than dental anxiety, using nitrous oxide during lunch or after work, sneaking nitrous oxide use, missing appointments, not keeping promises, and having problems with family or money.

Halogenated Hydrocarbons
Halothane
Halothane (HA-loe-thane) (Fluothane) has a fruity, pleasant odor and is nonflammable and nonexplosive. Both induction and recovery are relatively rapid with this agent. Because halothane is nonirritating to bronchial mucous membranes, it is considered safe for use in asthmatic patients. As with the other volatile agents, the halothane dose must be carefully regulated to prevent overt respiratory depression.

Halothane can cause hypotension and cardiac depression. It sensitizes the heart to catecholamines such as epinephrine and norepinephrine, leading to serious cardiac arrhythmias such as ventricular fibrillation. It is eliminated primarily through the lungs, and approximately 15% of the drug is metabolized by the liver. Its metabolites are thought to cause hepatotoxicity.

Enflurane
Enflurane (EN-floo-rane) (Ethrane) is a halogenated ether anesthetic with a pleasant smell. Induction of and recovery from anesthesia with this agent are rapid because of its low tissue solubility. The heart is depressed, and blood pressure is reduced. Myocardial sensitization to catecholamines is less than that associated with halothane.

Enflurane is metabolized less than other volatile agents, possibly accounting for the absence of hepatotoxicity. Enflurane also produces a transient depression of renal function.

Isoflurane
A drug chemically related to enflurane is isoflurane (eye-soe-FLURE-ane) (Forane). Its low tissue solubility allows for rapid induction and recovery. Isoflurane has a slightly pungent smell, limiting the induction concentration, which otherwise could provoke coughing. The pharmacologic effects of isoflurane are similar to those of the other halogenated ethers and include respiratory depression, reduced blood pressure, and muscle relaxation. Only a small amount of isoflurane undergoes metabolism, and liver toxicity does not seem to be a problem. It causes limited, if any, myocardial sensitization to catecholamines. Nausea, vomiting, and shivering on recovery from isoflurane anesthesia are comparable to responses to the use of other anesthetic agents. The most undesirable side effect is respiratory acidosis, which is associated with deeper levels of anesthesia.

Desflurane and Sevoflurane

> Desflurane requires a special vaporizer.

Desflurane and sevoflurane have the advantage of having low blood/gas partition coefficient so that they have a more rapid onset and a shorter duration of action than the other halogenated hydrocarbon anesthetics. Unfortunately, they have other difficulties. Desflurane's low volatility requires a special vaporizer. Because it induces cough and laryngospasm, it cannot be used for induction. Recovery from anesthesia with desflurane, despite its physical properties, does not appear to be faster than that with older agents. Sevoflurane is chemically unstable when exposed to carbon dioxide absorbents, producing a potentially nephrotoxic compound. Because it releases fluoride (F^-) when metabolized, renal damage may occur.

BALANCED GENERAL ANESTHESIA
The goals of surgical anesthesia are good patient control, adequate muscle relaxation, and pain relief. Many agents can produce general anesthesia. Each drug has its own adverse reaction profile. The many specific steps in Guedel's classification were developed to describe the effects when ether was used alone. When balanced anesthesia is used, the patient readily passes from stage I to stage III (surgical anesthesia), skipping over the signs of stage II. The ultrashort-acting IV barbiturates accomplish this process readily. These barbiturates are combined with the N_2O-O_2, which are then administered along with a volatile inhalation anesthetic (e.g., halogenated hydrocarbons). If local anesthetic blocks are administered before oral surgery procedures, the depth of general anesthesia can be lighter.

DENTAL HYGIENE CONSIDERATIONS
- Review the patient's medication/health history for evidence of contraindications to nitrous oxide, such as medical conditions and medications.
- Check equipment before use to ensure that it works properly.
- Several states now allow dental hygienists to administer nitrous oxide. Table 10.5 reviews patient response at different concentrations of nitrous oxide.
- Patient response is the best indicator of the level of sedation.
- Make sure that the patient's blood pressure and pulse are always within normal limits.
- Encourage the patient to refrain from making any major decisions while still feeling sedated from any of the anesthetics.

ACADEMIC SKILLS ASSESSMENT
1. Name and describe the four stages of anesthesia.
2. State the pharmacologic effects of the general anesthetics.
3. Describe the effects observed with varying concentrations of nitrous oxide.
4. What adverse reactions are associated with nitrous oxide?
5. List the contraindications to the use of nitrous oxide.
6. State the potential hazards associated with the general anesthetic agents.
7. Describe which general anesthetics would be useful in the following situations:
   a. A patient with anxiety.
   b. A patient requiring oral surgery.
8. Explain the rationale for the use of several agents during general anesthesia.

CLINICAL CASE STUDY

Tiesha Wilkins is a 23-year-old newly licensed dental hygienist who has recently started working with the local dental practice. She is engaged and will be married in 6 months. Ms. Wilkins has some general concerns regarding the use of general anesthesia in this office practice, especially because dental hygienists can administer nitrous oxide in the state where she currently practices. Also, Ms. Wilkins and her fiancé would like to start a family someday.

1. What are some of Ms. Wilkin's concerns regarding nitrous oxide and pregnancy?

2. Nitrous oxide is a general anesthetic that is used to induce conscious sedation in dental patients who may require sedation during a procedure. What are the contraindications to the use of nitrous oxide?

3. Nitrous oxide can cause a miscarriage in the pregnant patient. Who else is at risk for miscarriage and how can it be avoided?

4. What should pregnant women be told about the risk of miscarriage with nitrous oxide?

5. What are some of the other side effects associated with the abrupt discontinuation of nitrous oxide-oxygen combination?

6. How can the side effects in question 5 be treated and even avoided?

Antianxiety Agents

LEARNING OBJECTIVES

1. Discuss the value of patient relaxation in dentistry.
2. Describe the pharmacokinetics, mechanism of action, pharmacologic effects, adverse reactions, drug interactions, medical uses, and dental relevance of the benzodiazepines and barbiturates.
3. Name and briefly describe the mechanism of action of the nonbenzodiazepine-nonbarbiturate sedative-hypnotics and the nonbenzodiazepine-nonbarbiturate receptor agonists.
4. Name a melatonin receptor agonist and summarize its actions.
5. Explain the workings of the centrally acting muscle relaxants and how they are used.
6. Name and briefly describe a few of the miscellaneous muscle relaxant agents that can be used.
7. Discuss some general precautions about which the dental practitioner should be aware with the use of antianxiety agents.

> Dental professionals often do not recognize or relate to a patient's stress level while treatment is being provided.

Many patients who require dental care never go to the dental office because of fear and apprehension. Almost 20% of Americans seek oral health care only when absolutely necessary, whereas approximately 7% refuse to seek any care because they are afraid. Those patients who avoid maintenance oral health care examinations and those who come in only when in severe pain further raise their levels of anxiety. Patients who delay treatment are now faced with longer appointments that may require oral injections; all of these factors lead to increased anxiety levels (Fig. 11.1).

Both the dental hygienist and the dentist recognize the value of a relaxed patient. Often, patient anxiety is sufficiently reduced by a calm, patient, confident, and understanding attitude on the part of the dental health care team. However, individual responses to dental treatment vary widely, ranging from total relaxation and even sleeping to severe apprehension and the inability to approach the dental office, much less the dental chair. Each dental patient should be provided with the most pleasant experience possible within the limits of safety. When the patient is relaxed, appointments can be more productive, and the dentist, hygienist, and patient all benefit.

Dental hygienists and dentists can help a patient overcome his or her fears by meeting with the patient in the office and not in the treatment chair. They should discuss the procedure and all concerns that the patient may have and let the patient get to know them. Some patients are fearful of the instruments and their noises. If possible, allow the patient to hold the instruments and encourage the patient to bring in ear plugs or music to listen to during the appointment. Other patients may feel uncomfortable lying completely back during an oral examination. In this instance, simply putting the patient in a semireclined position may alleviate the fears. Ask the patient's opinion, allowing the patient to feel in control of the situation. All of these actions helps the dental health care team develop empathy toward the patient and provide for a much more stress-free visit.

The appropriate use of antianxiety agents might encourage more patients to seek needed dental treatment. It is necessary to objectively assess each patient's anxiety on both the first and subsequent visits. A patient who is clutching the dental chair arms and has white knuckles is not in a relaxed state (Fig. 11.2). By questioning and observing the patient, the dental care team can determine the need for antianxiety agents. Thus the patient can feel comfortable and relaxed during subsequent dental appointments. The dental health professional should remember that whatever procedure is performed, he or she has performed it many times. However, for many patients, this may be the first experience with the procedure, and their reactions may be altered by their interpretation of what is happening (e.g., "that sharp, pointy thing is going to hurt!" or "What are those gunlike things?").

As there are many different drugs available to treat anxiety, the dental practitioners should become familiar with one or two drugs and use them repeatedly. In the long run, this practice will produce greater benefits than changing from drug to drug. The dose of a particular antianxiety agent that is effective for a particular patient is vastly variable, involving both intrapatient and interpatient variations. Predicting the correct dose is a guess at best. The amount needed is poorly related to the patient's anxiety level or the dental procedure to be performed. The normal sedative dose (calms normal patient without dental appointment) is not expected to produce calmness in a dental patient, but the hypnotic dose (induces sleep in the normal patient) can often achieve the desired degree of sedation before dental treatment.

DEFINITIONS

The sedative-hypnotic agents can produce varying degrees of central nervous system (CNS) depression, depending on the dose administered. A small dose causes mild CNS depression described as sedation (reduction of activity and simple anxiety). This level of CNS depression has some anxiolytic effects. A larger dose of the same drug, the hypnotic dose (inducing sleep), produces greater CNS depression. Thus the same drug may be either a sedative or a hypnotic, depending on the dose administered.

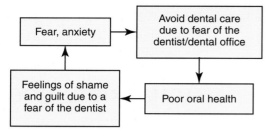

Fig. 11.1 Cycle of oral health care anxiety.

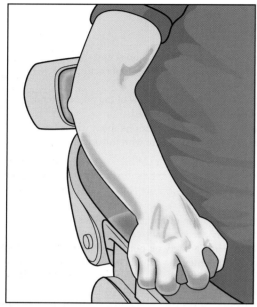

Fig. 11.2 White-knuckle syndrome indicates that a patient is not in a relaxed state. (From Clark MS, Brunick A. *Handbook of Nitrous Oxide and Oxygen Sedation*. 4th ed. St. Louis: Mosby; 2015.)

This chapter discusses the benzodiazepines, the barbiturates, and the nonbenzodiazepine-nonbarbiturate sedative-hypnotics. The benzodiazepines are discussed first because they are used most often.

BENZODIAZEPINES

The benzodiazepines (ben-zoe-dye-AZ-e-peens) are the most commonly prescribed antianxiety drugs. The members of this group differ mainly in onset and duration of action, dose, and dose forms available (Table 11.1).

Chemistry

These drugs are named benzodiazepines because of their structure: a 1,4-benzodiazepine nucleus.

Pharmacokinetics

The benzodiazepines are well absorbed when administered by the oral route. The rapid onset of action of the benzodiazepines is related to their lipid solubility. Diazepam, which is highly lipid soluble, has a quick onset and is concentrated in the adipose tissue. Storage in adipose tissue prolongs the action of lipid-soluble benzodiazepines. The benzodiazepines are available in the following dose forms: tablets, capsules, oral solution, rectal gel, and injectable forms. The intramuscular (IM) route, for benzodiazepines other than midazolam, gives slow, erratic, and unpredictable results. In contrast, the intravenous (IV) route, for those available in parenteral form, produces a rapid, predictable

Generic Drug Name (Trade Name)	FDA* INDICATIONS AND DOSE (mg/day) Insomnia	Anxiety	Onset of Action (min)
Benzodiazepines			
Alprazolam		1–4	45–60
Chlordiazepoxide (Librium)		15–100	15–45
Clorazepate (Tranxene)		15–60	30–60
Diazepam (Valium)†		4–40	15–45
Estazolam (ProSom)	1–2		
Flurazepam (Dalmane)	15–30		15–45
Lorazepam (Ativan)‡	2–4	1–10	15–45
Midazolam (Versed)‡,§		Titrate	IV 1–5
Oxazepam (Serax)		30–120	45–90
Quazepam (Doral)	7.5–15		
Temazepam (Restoril)	7.5–30		25–60
Triazolam (Halcion)	0.125–0.5		15–30
Nonbenzodiazepine-Benzodiazepine Receptor Agonists			
Zolpidem (Ambien)	Men: 5 or 10 Women: 5		<30
Zolpidem (Ambien CR)	Men: 6.25 or 12.5 Women: 6.25		30
Sublingual Zolpidem (Edluar)	Men: 5 or 10 Women: 5		30
Zolpidem (Intermezzo)	Men: 3.5 Women: 1.75		20
Oral Spray Zolpidem (Zolpimist)	Men: 10 Women: 5		20
Zaleplon (Sonata)	5–20		15–30
Eszopiclone (Lunesta)	1–3		15–30
Melatonin Receptor Agonist			
Ramelteon (Rozerem)	8		15–30
Orexin Receptor Antagonist			
Suvorexant (Belsomra)	10–20		30

*Food and Drug Administration.
†Injectable form contains propylene glycol—can produce thrombophlebitis.
‡Available parenterally.
§Midazolam administered intravenously in United States.
IV, Intravenous; *PO*, orally.

response that makes them ideal for conscious sedation. Once a benzodiazepine is absorbed, the rate at which it crosses into the cerebrospinal fluid (CSF) through the blood-brain barrier depends on protein binding, lipid solubility, and the ionization constant of the compound. Most benzodiazepines are highly protein bound and are present in the un-ionized, lipid-soluble form. They easily cross the blood-brain and placental barriers to have effects in the CNS and adverse effects on the fetus (Chapter 22), where they can accumulate with repeated doses.

After absorption, the benzodiazepines are metabolized in the liver by either phase II metabolism or phase I followed by phase II metabolism. Phase I metabolism is decreased in the elderly, in patients taking certain drugs that inhibit hepatic metabolism, and in the presence of hepatic disease. Phase I metabolism results in active metabolites that, with repeated administration, can accumulate. Benzodiazepines that undergo only phase II metabolism are much less affected by drugs or hepatic disease. Age does not seem to affect phase II metabolism. However, one should still use caution when prescribing these drugs for elderly persons.

MECHANISM OF ACTION

> Benzodiazepines facilitate γ-aminobutyric acid (GABA)-mediated transmission.

Benzodiazepines enhance or facilitate the action of the neurotransmitter γ-aminobutyric acid (GABA), a major inhibitory transmitter in the CNS (Fig. 11.3). It acts at the limbic, thalamic, cortical, and hypothalamic levels of the CNS. Benzodiazepines act as agonists at the benzodiazepine receptor site, thereby reducing the symptoms of anxiety.

Pharmacologic Effects

The pharmacologic effects of the various benzodiazepines have qualitatively similar actions but vary in potency.

Behavioral Effects

The clinical effects of these agents in humans are anxiety and panic reduction at lower doses and production of drowsiness and sleep at higher doses. Repeated doses of benzodiazepines reduce rapid eye movement (REM) sleep. Usual doses cause a marked reduction in stages 3 and 4 sleep (deep sleep), which, after long-term use, can interfere with restorative sleep.

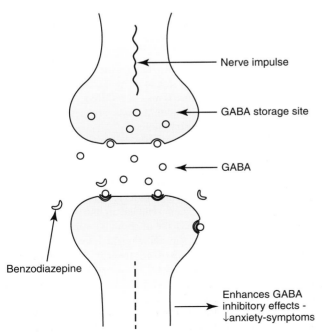

Fig. 11.3 Mechanism of action of benzodiazepines. *GABA,* γ-Aminobutyric acid.

- Nerve impulse
- GABA storage site
- GABA
- Benzodiazepine
- Enhances GABA inhibitory effects - ↓anxiety-symptoms

Antiseizure Effects

The benzodiazepines, such as diazepam, have antiseizure activity (i.e., they increase the seizure threshold). Diazepam, used parenterally, has been shown to be an effective antiseizure drug for the prevention of seizures associated with local anesthetic toxicity and for the treatment of status epilepticus. Clonazepam, an oral benzodiazepine, is used in combination with other antiseizure drugs to manage partial seizures. The benzodiazepines prevent the spread of seizures in tissues surrounding the anatomic seizure focus (when such a focus exists) but have little effect on the discharges at the focus itself.

Muscle Relaxation

Like all CNS depressants, benzodiazepines can produce relaxation of skeletal muscles. Some studies show benzodiazepines to be superior to other skeletal muscle relaxants for relief of musculoskeletal pain; other studies show the pain relief effect of benzodiazepines to be no better than that of aspirin or placebo. Benzodiazepines are effective for muscle spasticity secondary to pathologic states such as cerebral palsy and paraplegia.

Adverse Reactions

In general, benzodiazepines used alone have a wide margin of safety. They have similar adverse effects but differ in the frequency of these effects. Agents with long-elimination half-lives tend to accumulate and produce more side effects.

Central Nervous System Effects

The most common side effect attributed to benzodiazepines is CNS depression, manifested as fatigue, drowsiness, muscle weakness, and ataxia. These side effects are more likely to occur in elderly persons. The patient may also experience lightheadedness and dizziness. Tolerance to this effect occurs over time. Paradoxical CNS stimulation that produces talkativeness, anxiety, nightmares, tremulousness, hyperactivity, and increased muscle spasticity can occur. This reaction is more common in psychiatric patients, and benzodiazepines should be discontinued if this reaction occurs.

When benzodiazepines are used in dentistry to produce conscious sedation, the CNS depression, normally a side effect, is used as the primary effect. The amount of the benzodiazepine used to provide conscious sedation is titrated to the patient's response. The appearance of ptosis is used as an initial endpoint for the dose administered. These agents have a rapid onset of action and an initial effect of 45 minutes to 1 hour.

Diazepam was the benzodiazepine most commonly used parenterally until newer benzodiazepines were developed. Diazepam's long half-life and its metabolism to an active metabolite prolonged its duration of action. Its effect lasted past the dental appointment time and even into the next day.

Midazolam, a water-soluble benzodiazepine, is metabolized primarily to inactive metabolites. This feature is an advantage over diazepam for IV use in conscious sedation. Because these benzodiazepines are inactivated either directly by metabolism or indirectly by metabolism of their active metabolites, the duration and depth of sedation can be magnified by administration of drugs that inhibit the hepatic microsomal enzymes. Agents that inhibit these enzymes include cimetidine and erythromycin.

Anterograde Amnesia

It can be easily demonstrated that parenteral benzodiazepines, such as diazepam and midazolam, cause amnesia beginning when the drug is taken. This effect is used to therapeutic advantage in patients scheduled for an unpleasant dental procedure. Clinical use of several benzodiazepines has produced episodes of amnesia that can sometimes last several hours. Oral triazolam seems to have a greater likelihood to produce amnesia than other oral benzodiazepines. Patients should be warned not to sign important papers or make important decisions after benzodiazepines are administered. The mechanism of amnesia results from an impairment of consolidation processes that store the information in the brain.

Respiratory Effects

Usual doses of benzodiazepines have no adverse effect on respiration. However, doses of diazepam administered for outpatient dental procedures have been occasionally reported to cause respiratory depression. An isolated case of apnea after IV diazepam has also been observed. These respiratory effects are more common in elderly patients. The minimal respiratory depression can be exacerbated by opioids or alcohol.

Cardiovascular Effects

Therapeutic doses of benzodiazepines have no adverse effect on circulation. The relief of anxiety may result in drops in blood pressure and pulse rate. The pulse rate has also been reported to rise (tachycardia) and then return to normal after a few minutes.

Visual Effects

Benzodiazepines are contraindicated in angle-closure (narrow-angle) glaucoma and can produce other visual changes, such as diplopia, nystagmus, and blurred vision. They may be used in treatment of wide-angle glaucoma, which is the most common kind of glaucoma.

Dental Effects

The benzodiazepines have been reported to cause xerostomia, increased salivation (note that these are opposite effects), swollen tongue, and a bitter or metallic taste.

Thrombophlebitis

Parenteral diazepam can produce thrombophlebitis. Because diazepam is poorly soluble in water, the vehicle propylene glycol is used to solubilize it. The vehicle is responsible for the thrombophlebitis. The incidence is lower when the IV infusion is given in the antecubital space rather than the dorsum of the hand (more blood and faster blood flow). Because midazolam is soluble in water and propylene glycol is not used to solubilize it, it is much less likely to have this effect. With parenteral use of benzodiazepines, apnea, hypotension, bradycardia, and cardiac arrest have been reported. These are more frequent with rapid administration. Equipment for respiratory and cardiovascular assistance must be available if these agents are to be used parenterally (e.g., for conscious sedation in the dental office). Special training of the dental team administering benzodiazepines is required.

Other Effects

Benzodiazepines can affect the gastrointestinal tract, producing cramps or pain, and the genitourinary tract, causing difficulty in urination. They can also produce allergic reactions, including rash and itching.

Pregnancy and Lactation Considerations

An increased risk of congenital malformation in infants of mothers taking benzodiazepines in the first trimester has been reported. Rates of cleft lip, cleft palate, microencephaly, and gastrointestinal and cardiovascular abnormalities were greater in the group taking benzodiazepines in the study. Most of these agents are classified as FDA pregnancy category D drugs; triazolam and temazepam are in FDA pregnancy category X adversely effect the developing fetus. (see Chapter 22).

Near-term administration of benzodiazepines to the mother has resulted in floppy infant syndrome—consisting of hypoactivity, hypotonia, hypothermia, apnea, and feeding problems. Because these agents are seldom absolutely needed (except for treatment of epilepsy), they should be avoided in women who are or may become pregnant and in nursing mothers. Before a benzodiazepine is administered to a female dental patient, her pregnancy status should be determined. The first trimester, often before the patient knows that she is pregnant, is the time benzodiazepines are most likely to be teratogenic or to cause problems in the fetus.

Abuse and Tolerance
Overview

Benzodiazepines can be abused, and physical dependence and tolerance have been documented. Physiologic addiction can occur if large doses are taken over an extended period. However, their abuse and addiction potential is less than that of the other sedative-hypnotic agents such as the barbiturates.

Prolonged intake of large doses of benzodiazepines can result in a degree of CNS tolerance. Cross-tolerance also exists between the benzodiazepines and other CNS depressants. This may explain why benzodiazepines can be substituted for ethyl alcohol to relieve the symptoms of delirium tremens precipitated by acute alcohol withdrawal.

Very wide therapeutic index.

One advantage of benzodiazepines over barbiturates is the wider therapeutic index, or range of safe dose. Overdose poisoning with benzodiazepines has been rare and appears to be difficult to achieve when they are used alone, although apnea has rarely been reported. In most instances, excessively large doses must be ingested to produce respiratory or central vasomotor depression. Combining benzodiazepines with other CNS depressants can reduce their safety, so the combination can be lethal. The addition of alcohol can result in coma, respiratory depression, hypotension, or hypothermia.

Treatment of Overdose

Long-term use in insomnia is not recommended.

Rarely does the ingestion of a benzodiazepine alone result in severe symptoms. Supportive therapy should be undertaken if symptoms occur. With recent ingestion, emesis may be induced. Activated charcoal and a saline cathartic may be administered. The patient's respiration and blood pressure should be monitored.

To reverse some of the effects of a benzodiazepine, flumazenil (floo-MA-zee-nill) (Romazicon), a benzodiazepine antagonist available for IV administration, may be used. It has been shown to reverse the sedating and psychomotor effects, but its reversal of the respiratory depression produced by the benzodiazepines is incomplete. The amnesia is not consistently reversed. Flumazenil has an initial half-life of about 10 minutes and a terminal half-life of about 60 minutes. Side effects include pain at the injection site, agitation, and anxiety. The patient's pain level does not increase as this drug takes effect. (Some patients experience increased pain with anxiety.) Some patients have been found to have been resedated before the end of 3 hours when high doses of long-acting benzodiazepines were ingested (the antagonist wore off before the agonist had been metabolized and excreted). Administering flumazenil to benzodiazepine-dependent individuals could precipitate withdrawal symptoms (like the effect of naloxone in opioid-dependent patients).

Drug Interactions

All benzodiazepines now carry Black Box warnings regarding the concomitant use of benzodiazepines and either opioid analgesics, alcohol or other CNS depressant drugs (including street drugs). Patients should be warned that these combinations can lead to severe drowsiness, respiratory depression, coma and death. Like other antianxiety agents, benzodiazepines interact in an additive fashion with other CNS depressants, notably alcohol, barbiturates, anticonvulsants, and phenothiazines. Because diazepam and desmethyldiazepam are cytochrome P-450 2C enzyme substrates, enzyme inducers may increase their metabolism and enzyme stimulators may decrease their metabolism.

Smoking diminishes the effectiveness of the benzodiazepines. The tars produced by smoking cigarettes stimulate the hepatic microsomal enzymes in the liver. The greater number of liver enzymes raises the rate of metabolism of the benzodiazepines, so a higher dose of a benzodiazepine is required to have the same effect.

Drugs such as cimetidine, disulfiram, isoniazid, and omeprazole may increase the effects of benzodiazepines. Valproic acid may displace diazepam from binding sites, possibly resulting in an increase in sedative effects. Selective serotonin reuptake inhibitors (e.g., fluoxetine, sertraline, paroxetine) have greatly raised diazepam levels by altering its clearance. Benzodiazepines may reduce the effectiveness of levodopa, and parkinsonism has been exacerbated in patients with Parkinson disease. Benzodiazepines may augment the effect of digoxin, phenytoin, and probenecid.

Medical Uses

Benzodiazepines are useful in short-term treatment of anxiety, panic attacks, insomnia, and alcohol withdrawal. They are used for the acute treatment of seizures. Some neuromuscular diseases can be treated with the benzodiazepines. These agents are also used in conscious sedation, in general anesthesia, and during surgery.

Anxiety Control

Generalized anxiety disorder and panic disorder are common indications for use of benzodiazepines in general medicine. Their use is limited because of their potential for abuse and dependence. Most patients with generalized anxiety disorder and panic attacks are now treated with antidepressant drugs (Chapter 15). Anxiety produces a physiologic response resembling fear, with manifestations including restlessness, tension, tachycardia, and dyspnea. Benzodiazepines are effective and safe to use in patients being treated for social or situational anxiety, such as that caused by the thought of going to a dentist or fear of dental treatment. Most well-controlled clinical trials have shown that the antianxiety effects of benzodiazepines are better than those of placebo, barbiturates, and meprobamate for all types of anxiety and muscle strain. Benzodiazepines also cause less sedation and are safer than the classic sedative-hypnotic agents.

Conscious Sedation

Conscious sedation is used to help relax the anxious patient during a dental procedure. The patient is relaxed and somewhat sedated during the procedure. Though the patient is sedated, he or she can easily be awakened once the procedure is completed. Oral benzodiazepines can be used for this purpose and are usually administered to the patient 15 to 30 minutes prior to the dental procedure. Midazolam is the only intravenously administered benzodiazepine that is used in oral health care. Only those dentists trained in its administration can use it. IV sedation allows the dentist to regulate the level of sedation during the procedure.

Insomnia Management

> For dental anxiety.

If insomnia is a manifestation of anxiety, sleep usually improves when a benzodiazepine is prescribed to be taken at bedtime as an antianxiety drug. The benzodiazepines are preferable to the barbiturates as hypnotics because the risk of physical addiction or serious poisoning is much less. The occasional use of the benzodiazepines within controlled limits can be useful. The efficacy of the benzodiazepines in the treatment of chronic insomnia has not been demonstrated past 1 month.

Repeated use of a sedative-hypnotic leads to tolerance and a need for a higher dose to produce the same effect. Most agents become increasingly less effective with regular use. These agents can also alter sleep architecture (REM sleep).

The normal sleep cycle involves several stages. Latency is the time it takes to get to sleep. Sleeping is distributed between REM sleep (30%) and non-REM (NREM) sleep. NREM sleep has four stages.

Benzodiazepines reduce latency, REM sleep, and NREM sleep stages 3 and 4 while increasing NREM sleep stage 2. When benzodiazepines have been used long-term and are discontinued, rebound REM sleep often occurs, resulting in an increase in vivid dreams. Some patients continue to take benzodiazepines because they do not want to experience these scary dreams.

Underlying causes of insomnia, such as depression and alcoholism, should be identified and treated. Nonaddicting agents, such as trazodone, may be useful in the treatment of insomnia, and unlike the benzodiazepines, no tolerance or dependence is produced even with long-term use. Nonpharmacologic management of sleep disorders (Box 11.1) should be instituted before any benzodiazepine is prescribed.

If a patient is being treated for "dental appointment" insomnia, caused by a number of issues (i.e., fear, dental pain, poor oral hygiene), a benzodiazepine may be necessary. Once the patient comes in for treatment(s) and sees that there is no reason to fear the appointment, nonpharmacologic sleep measures should be tried prior to the next appointment.

Treatment of Epilepsy (Seizures)

Diazepam or lorazepam is the drug of choice for treatment of repetitive, intractable seizures (status epilepticus) that require IV therapy. They are also used for treatment of seizures caused by local anesthetic toxicity. Orally administered diazepam is of little value, even as a maintenance anticonvulsant. Oral clonazepam is used as an adjunct to other

---

BOX 11.1   Nonpharmacologic Management of Sleep Disorders

The following several habits should be developed to minimize insomnia:
- Have a regular bedtime regardless of whether sleepy.
- Remain in bed no more than 20 min without sleeping.
- Get up if not sleeping and perform a quiet activity.
- Awaken regularly at 6 a.m. even if sleep only began at 5 a.m.
- Limit sleeping to fewer hours, go to bed later, get up earlier.
- Exercise during the day (not within 3 hr of bedtime).
- Have a light snack (warm milk) at bedtime.
- Do not take naps during the day regardless of sleep problems.
- Avoid caffeine within 8 hr of bedtime (cola, sodas [check label for caffeine], coffee, and tea).
- Avoid smoking within 8 hr of bedtime.
- Get ready for bed by engaging in quiet activities such as reading and listening to music. Use "noise" to disguise noise by listening to white noise.

anticonvulsants for some difficult-to-control types of seizures. It is also used in the management of mood disorders.

Treatment of Alcoholism

The benzodiazepines are used in the treatment of the alcohol withdrawal syndrome. Administration of an adequate amount of a benzodiazepine can prevent the emergence of the signs and symptoms of acute alcohol withdrawal, such as agitation and tremor. It has not been shown, however, that these agents prevent hallucinations or delirium tremens.

Control of Muscle Spasms

Benzodiazepines are used to control the muscle spasticity that accompanies various diseases such as multiple sclerosis and cerebral palsy. They are used for the relief of pain and spasm of back strain. Studies have suggested that the benzodiazepines are more effective than other muscle relaxants, such as methocarbamol, carisoprodol, and chlorzoxazone.

Management of the Dental Patient Taking Benzodiazepines

The dental implications of the benzodiazepines are described in Box 11.2.

Dental Procedures

Ensure that the patient has a responsible driver before releasing.

Orally administered diazepam has been shown to be more effective than placebo in allaying apprehension in patients undergoing restorative procedures. It is used in combination with other agents, such as opioids and anticholinergic agents. If diazepam is used for the initial treatment of patients with dental anxiety, it is hoped that future appointments may be completed successfully without benzodiazepine increases. For preoperative dental anxiety, a benzodiazepine should be chosen that has a fast onset of action and a relatively short half-life. This choice reduces the patient's waiting time and allows resumption of normal functions as soon as possible. The dose used should be in the range of the usual hypnotic dose (see Table 11.1). The patient given either an oral or parenteral benzodiazepine should not be allowed to operate a motor vehicle, and the dental staff should ensure that a driver is present before dismissing the patient.

Premedication

The benzodiazepines have been used before surgical procedures to allay anxiety. They may be used orally or parenterally. The amnesia that occurs with parenteral administration is especially useful during stressful dental procedures. Diazepam is used as a premedication before general anesthesia, endoscopy, cardioversion, gastroscopy, sigmoidoscopy, and cystoscopy.

Conscious Sedation

Conscious sedation using the benzodiazepines is usually accomplished by IV administration. Diazepam, lorazepam, or midazolam, given intravenously, provides muscle relaxation and anterograde amnesia (amnesia occurs of events beginning immediately after the injection) during dental procedures. Although amnesia quickly follows the IV injection of diazepam and midazolam, it depends on several variables. Amnesia may be expected to persist for up to 45 minutes; therefore postoperative instructions should be provided in writing. Benzodiazepines available for parenteral administration (diazepam, midazolam, and lorazepam) are used for conscious sedation. The patient maintains reflexes, but time perception is lost and amnesia reduces the patient's memory. Because parenteral benzodiazepines have been associated with respiratory depression and arrest when used for conscious sedation, their use requires continuous monitoring of respiratory and cardiac function. Emergency drugs, equipment, and personnel must be available. Because some states and insurance companies are placing controls on the use of IV sedation in dentistry, dentists without additional training cannot use conscious sedation. Additional training is required before dentists can administer parenteral benzodiazepines.

BARBITURATES

Barbiturates (bar-BI-tyoo-rates), the original sedative-hypnotic agents, are chemically related and have similar pharmacologic effects. They differ from one another mainly in their onset and duration of action (Table 11.2). Because these agents have been used for years, the problems with their use have been well documented. Barbiturates have long been associated with a high rate of abuse and complete cardiovascular and respiratory depression with overdose. Because the benzodiazepines have a much more acceptable safety profile, they have almost completely replaced barbiturates in clinical use for treating anxiety and insomnia. Barbiturates are still used as anticonvulsants and to induce general anesthesia.

BOX 11.2 Management of the Dental Patient Taking Benzodiazepines

- Avoid additive central nervous system (CNS) depression with other CNS depressants (including alcohol).
- Avoid in addicts or women who could be pregnant (women 11–63 years of age).
- Keep track of exact number prescribed and usage rate in patient's chart.
- Use the glucuronidated type in elderly patients and in patients taking cimetidine.
- Warn the patient about sedation and amnesia.
- Match the agent's onset and duration of action with dental procedure requirements.
- Make sure the patient has arranged for transportation to and from dental appointment.

CNS, Central nervous system.

TABLE 11.2 Barbiturates

Barbiturate Group	Route of Administration	Onset*	Duration† of Action (hr)
Ultrashort-Acting			
Methohexital (Brevital)	IV	Immediate	Minutes
Thiopental sodium (Pentothal)	IV	Immediate	Minutes
Short-Acting			
Pentobarbital (Nembutal)	PO, IM, IV, rectal	10–15 min	3–4
Secobarbital (Seconal)	PO, IM, IV, rectal	10–15 min	3–4
Intermediate-Acting			
Amobarbital (Amytal)	PO, IM, IV, rectal	40–60 min	6–8
Butabarbital (Butisol)	PO	40–60 min	6–8
Long-Acting			
Phenobarbital (Luminal)	PO, IM, IV	30–60 min	10–16

*Onset = time until the drug's action begins.
†Duration = length of drug's action.
IM, Intramuscular; *IV,* intravenous; *PO,* orally.

Chemistry

The clinically useful barbiturates are formed by substitution of R groups (organic groups) on the barbiturate nucleus sites A and B. Another modification of the barbiturate nucleus involves replacing the oxygen atom with a sulfur atom site C. Compounds with the S-substitution are effective as IV agents, such as thiopental.

Pharmacokinetics

Barbiturates are well absorbed orally and rectally. Because the injectable solutions are highly irritating, the IM route is avoided and the drugs are used intravenously. The IV agents are inactivated mainly by redistribution from their site of action in the CNS to the muscles and finally to adipose tissue. The short- and intermediate-acting barbiturates are rapidly and almost completely metabolized by the liver. Long-acting barbiturates are largely excreted through the kidneys as the free drugs. Patients with liver damage may have an exaggerated response to short- and intermediate-acting agents, and patients with renal impairment may have an accumulation of the long-acting agents.

Mechanism of Action

Barbiturates produce their effect by enhancing GABA-receptor binding. They prolong the opening of the chloride channels. In higher doses, they may also act directly on the chloride channels without GABA presence. This mechanism is less specific than that of the benzodiazepines, a difference that may account for the ability of the barbiturates to induce surgical anesthesia and have pronounced generalized CNS depressant effects.

Pharmacologic Effects
Central Nervous System Depression

The principal effects of the barbiturates are on the CNS. When normal doses of these agents are administered, relaxation occurs. With larger doses, the inhibitory fibers of the CNS are depressed, resulting in disinhibition and euphoria. If excitation occurs at this point, it is a result of depression of the inhibitory pathways. Anxiety relief cannot be separated from the sedative effects. When higher doses are administered, hypnosis can be produced. The administration of even higher doses can result in anesthesia, with respiratory and cardiovascular depression and finally arrest. This progressive CNS depression parallels that caused by most CNS depressants, including general anesthetics (see Chapter 10).

The CNS depression produced by the barbiturates is additive with other agents that have this effect. For example, a patient who drinks an alcoholic beverage or is given an opioid analgesic will show additive CNS depression when given a barbiturate.

Analgesia

Barbiturates have no significant analgesic effects. Even doses that produce general anesthesia do not block the reflex response to pain. Patients in pain may become agitated and even delirious if barbiturates are administered without analgesic agents.

Anticonvulsant Effect

The barbiturates possess anticonvulsant action. The long-acting agents such as phenobarbital are used in the treatment of epilepsy (see Chapter 14).

Adverse Reactions
Sedative or Hypnotic Doses

In the usual therapeutic doses, barbiturates are relatively safe. However, one should be aware that CNS depression may be exaggerated in elderly and debilitated patients or in those with liver or kidney impairment. In some patients, especially the elderly, barbiturates can have an idiosyncratic effect, causing stimulation instead of sedation. Barbiturates can harm the fetus if administered to a pregnant woman.

Anesthetic Doses

With higher doses, barbiturate concentrations attained in the blood can be lethal. High concentrations are used for intubation or very short procedures. Coughing and laryngospasm have been reported with IV use of barbiturates. High doses may reversibly depress liver and kidney function, reduce gastrointestinal motility, and lower body temperature.

Acute Poisoning

When barbiturates are prescribed, the possibility that acute poisoning can occur must be considered. Although a lethal dose can only be approximated, severe poisoning follows the ingestion of 10 times the hypnotic dose, and life is seriously threatened when more than 15 times the hypnotic dose is consumed. The cause of death when an overdose occurs is respiratory failure. The treatment involves conservative management and therapy of specific symptoms.

Long-Term Use

Long-term use of barbiturates can lead to physical and psychological dependence, a state similar to alcohol intoxication. The barbiturate addict becomes progressively depressed and is unable to function. Tolerance develops to most effects of barbiturates but not to the lethal dose. Therefore a larger and larger dose must be used to have an effect, and this dose can approximate the lethal dose. Cross-tolerance occurs among barbiturates and between the barbiturates and nonbarbiturate sedative-hypnotic agents. Chapter 24 discusses the abuse of the barbiturates.

Contraindications

The use of barbiturates is absolutely contraindicated in patients with intermittent porphyria or a positive family history of porphyria. The reason is that barbiturates can stimulate and increase the synthesis of porphyrins, which are already at an excessive level in this metabolic disease. In fact, barbiturates have been reported to precipitate an acute attack of porphyria.

Drug Interactions

Because barbiturates are potent stimulators of liver microsomal enzyme production, they are involved in many drug interactions. These enzymes are responsible for the metabolism of many drugs, so an increase in the enzymes could raise the rate of drug destruction and shorten the duration of action. For example, if an epileptic patient who is currently receiving phenytoin (Dilantin) is subsequently given phenobarbital, the phenobarbital stimulates the liver microsomal enzymes that destroy the phenytoin and the phenobarbital more rapidly, possibly resulting in convulsions. This drug interaction requires repeated doses and is not significant with a single dose. Some barbiturate drug interactions are listed in Box 11.3.

Uses

The therapeutic uses of barbiturates are determined by their duration of action (see Table 11.2). The ultrashort-acting agents, such as thiopental (thye-oh-PEN-tal), are used intravenously for the induction of general anesthesia. For very brief procedures, they may be used alone. For more extensive procedures, they are used to induce stage III surgical anesthesia (see Chapter 10).

The short- and intermediate-acting agents have little medical use. Benzodiazepines have replaced them for insomnia and anxiety relief. The short-acting agents were popular agents of abuse because of their fast onset of action.

The long-acting barbiturates, such as phenobarbital (fee-noe-BAR-bi-tal), are used for the treatment of epilepsy.

BOX 11.3 Barbiturate Drug Interactions

Barbiturates Reduce These Drugs' Effects
Acetaminophen
β-Blocker
Birth control pills
Chlorpromazine
Doxycycline
Estrogens
Griseofulvin
Phenytoin
Quinidine
Steroids
Tricyclic antidepressants
Warfarin

Barbiturates' Effects Enhanced by These Drugs
Disulfiram
Propoxyphene
Phenytoin

Drugs With Enhanced or Additive CNS Depressant Effect when Used With Barbiturates
Alcohol
CNS depressants
Opioid analgesics
Monoamine oxidase inhibitors

CNS, Central nervous system.

NONBENZODIAZEPINE-NONBARBITURATE SEDATIVE-HYPNOTICS

Buspirone

Buspirone (byoo-SPYE-rone) (BuSpar) is unique in structure and action. It is the only member of this anxiolytic group and is an azapirone. Its onset of action is about 1 week. It is discussed separately because of its unique structure and pharmacology. Its mechanism of action is unknown but is believed to be related to interactions with neurotransmitters in the CNS, including serotonin (5-hydroxytryptamine 1A [5-HT_{1A}]), dopamine (DA_2), and cholinergic and α-adrenergic receptors. Buspirone undergoes first-pass metabolism and has a half-life of 2 to 4 hours. It has no effect on GABA and lacks CNS depressant activity.

The pharmacologic effect of buspirone is called *anxioselective* because of its selective anxiolytic action without hypnotic, anticonvulsant, or muscle-relaxant properties. It produces much less CNS depression than other sedative-hypnotic agents and does not affect driving skills. Some patients experience nervousness or insomnia. Buspirone does not cause tolerance or dependence. It does not appear to be addicting, and there is no withdrawal syndrome.

NONBENZODIAZEPINE RECEPTOR HYPNOTICS

Zolpidem (Ambien), zaleplon (Sonata), and eszopiclone (Lunesta) are a class of drugs that are not benzodiazepines. They decrease sleep latency with little effect on sleep stages. All of these drugs have agonist effects on $GABA_A$ receptor. These drugs are used to treat insomnia only. They are controlled substance schedule IV and have the potential to cause both physical and psychologic dependence.

Zolpidem

Zolpidem (zole-PI-dem) is a hypnotic agent that is indicated for the short-term management of insomnia. Its structure is unlike that of the benzodiazepines. In contrast to some sedative-hypnotic agents that act at all benzodiazepine (BZ) receptors, zolpidem interacts with the $GABA_A$ receptor at the BZ_1 receptor. Although zolpidem retains its hypnotic and anxiolytic effects, its receptor specificity gives zolpidem fewer muscle relaxant and anticonvulsant effects. It may be less likely to produce depression of sleep stages 3 and 4. Side effects include headache, drowsiness, dizziness, and diarrhea. Myalgia, arthralgia, sinusitis, and pharyngitis have been reported. Amnesia may also occur. Withdrawal can occur if zolpidem therapy is abruptly stopped after 1 to 2 weeks of use. Rebound insomnia may be experienced. Its quicker onset of action makes it useful to initiate sleep. Because of its fast onset of action, it should be taken immediately before bedtime. Patients should not drive while taking this drug until they see what effect it has on them.

Zolpidem may be used in dentistry if the patient is having difficulty falling asleep the night before a dental appointment. This drug is usually used in persons with chronic insomnia.

Zolpidem is also available as Ambien CR, a controlled-release dose form. There have been reports of behavioral and emotional changes in patients taking Ambien CR. Patients have reported a decrease in inhibition similar to that seen with alcohol and other CNS depressant drugs. Amnesia, anxiety, and a worsening of depression have been reported in patients taking Ambien CR. Patients taking zolpidem immediate-release and controlled-release dose forms have experienced drowsy driving as well as driving at night while asleep or "sleep driving." There have also been reports of binge eating while sleeping in patients taking zolpidem. The doses of zolpidem immediate-release and controlled-release formulations have been reduced for both men and women to cut down on the incidence of daytime drowsiness, which could be a hazard during the performance of tasks that require thought or concentration, such as driving (see Table 11.1).

Zaleplon

Zaleplon is a rapid-acting hypnotic that is less potent and has a shorter duration of action than zolpidem. It does not appear to decrease premature awakenings or to lengthen total sleep time, but it seems to have a lower risk of next-day residual effects, even when used in the middle of the night. It also does not seem to affect driving the morning after nighttime use. Zaleplon can cause anterograde amnesia.

Eszopiclone

Eszopiclone is the newest agent of this class available in the United States. It has the longest half-life of the three, but comparative clinical data are lacking. A 6-month trial with eszopiclone found no development of tolerance. Anterograde amnesia has been reported with this drug. Some patients have reported an unpleasant taste while taking it. Because of its long half-life, eszopiclone could impair driving the morning after nighttime use.

MELATONIN RECEPTOR AGONIST

Ramelteon (Rozerem) has been approved by the FDA for the treatment of insomnia characterized by difficulty falling asleep. This drug is an indenofuran derivative that is highly selective for melatonin type 1 (MT_1) and melatonin type 2 (MT_2) receptors. Studies in animals indicate that the MT_1 receptor regulates sleep and the MT_2 receptor may mediate the phase-shifting effects of melatonin on a 24-hour biologic clock. In clinical trials, ramelteon produced small, statistically significant improvements in sleep latency but had little effect on sleep maintenance.

The most common adverse effects reported during clinical trials were somnolence, dizziness, fatigue, headache, and insomnia. It is not a controlled substance like the benzodiazepines and the nonbenzodiazepine receptor agonist hypnotics, and there have been no reports of tolerance, rebound insomnia, or withdrawal effects. The long-term safety of ramelteon is unknown.

MELATONIN

Melatonin is a naturally occurring hormone made by the pineal gland that is released as the day ends and darkness takes over, usually by about 9 p.m. Melatonin levels rise sharply, and the person begins to feel less alert and sleepy. Once daylight begins, melatonin levels drop dramatically. Melatonin is manufactured synthetically and is used to treat insomnia and jet lag. Melatonin is sold as a food supplement or natural product and is available without a prescription. It is sold as a dietary supplement because it occurs naturally in some foods. Melatonin can cause daytime sedation, morning grogginess, depression, headache, stomach cramps, and irritability. Several clinical trials have found that it shows no benefit over placebo.

OREXIN RECEPTOR ANTAGONIST

Suvorexant (Belsomra) is the first in a new class of drugs to treat insomnia. It works by blocking orexin neuropeptides from binding to their receptors. Orexin neurons are active during wakeful times and dormant during sleep time. Once orexin neuropeptides are signaled its neuropeptides maintain wakefulness. Narcolepsy has been associated with a loss of orexin signaling. The most common side effects associated with suvorexant therapy include next-day somnolence and cataplexy-like symptoms (leg weakness). Suvorexant can impair next-day performance of activities that require mental alertness and motor coordination.

CENTRALLY ACTING MUSCLE RELAXANTS

Drugs classified as centrally acting muscle relaxants (Table 11.3) exert their effects on the CNS to produce skeletal muscle relaxation.

TABLE 11.3 Centrally Acting Skeletal Muscle Relaxants

Drug	Comments	Dose (mg)
Carisoprodol (Soma)	Tachycardia, flushing, Schedule IV	250–350 tid-qid
Chlorzoxazone (Parafon Forte DSC)	GI distress, hypersensitivity, CNS depression	375–750 tid-qid
Methocarbamol (Robaxin)	CNS depression, GI distress, rash	1000–1500 qid
Orphenadrine (Norflex)	Xerostomia, GI tract, vision changes	100 bid extended release
Cyclobenzaprine (Flexeril)	Sedation (40%), xerostomia (30%)	5–10 tid
Diazepam (Valium)	Benzodiazepine	2–10 tid-qid

bid, Twice per day; *CNS*, central nervous system; *GI*, gastrointestinal; *qid*, 4 times per day; *tid*, 3 times per day.

Pharmacologic Effects

Some degree of sedative effect is exhibited by all the CNS muscle relaxants because they act on the CNS. Xerostomia is common with these agents.

Clinical tests have shown that the sedative effects of centrally acting muscle relaxants dominate over the "selective" muscle relaxant activity. When administered intravenously in humans, these agents have been shown to be useful in treating muscle spasm and producing muscle relaxation for certain orthopedic procedures. When these agents are given orally, they do not cause the flaccidity obtainable with IV administration. Thus until better studies are performed, the beneficial effects of these drugs can be logically ascribed to their sedative action. They are used for back and neck pain and in the patient with muscle spasms related to a car accident.

Individual Centrally Acting Muscle Relaxants

Centrally acting skeletal muscle relaxants exert their muscle-relaxing properties indirectly by producing CNS depression. They act in the CNS and have no direct effect on striated muscle, the motor endplate, or nerve fibers. They do not directly relax tense skeletal muscles.

As a group they have many common side effects, including gastrointestinal upset, sedation, and dizziness (results of CNS depression). All of the muscle relaxants have the potential to produce allergic reactions. Most of these agents can cause xerostomia, and the dental health care worker should question the patient about self-treatment for this adverse effect.

Structurally related to the tricyclic antidepressants, cyclobenzaprine (sye-kloe-BEN-za-preen) (Flexeril) is considered the strongest muscle relaxant. Because sedation occurs in about 40% of the patients taking cyclobenzaprine, it is the most sedating muscle relaxant. It is also most likely to cause xerostomia, with an incidence of 30%. (This fact demonstrates typical effects and adverse reactions of drugs: the more pharmacologic effect [wanted], the more adverse reactions [unwanted].)

A relative of meprobamate is carisoprodol (kar-eye-soe-PROE-dole) (Soma). Chlorzoxazone (klor-ZOX-a-zone) (Paraflex) may discolor the urine purple-red. The patient should be warned about this harmless property. Other muscle relaxants include methocarbamol (meth-oh-KAR-ba-mole) (Robaxin) and orphenadrine (or-FEN-a-dreen) (Norflex). Diazepam (Valium), a benzodiazepine, also possesses muscle-relaxant properties and is used for spastic muscles such as occurs in multiple sclerosis. Table 11.3 lists the muscle relaxants that function via the brain and their selected side effects and usual doses.

Use

The muscle relaxants are all indicated as adjuncts to rest and physical therapy for relief of muscle spasm associated with acute painful musculoskeletal conditions. Questions about their efficacy still linger in the literature. They are also used in the treatment of temporomandibular disorder (TMD) because relaxation of the muscles is helpful to the symptoms. The success of muscle relaxants in the management of TMD has not been documented.

MISCELLANEOUS AGENTS

Baclofen

Baclofen (BAK-loe-fen) (Lioresal) inhibits both monosynaptic and polysynaptic reflexes at the spinal level. It also inhibits GABA, but whether this feature is related to its action is unknown. The agent is indicated for spasticity from multiple sclerosis or from spinal cord injuries or diseases. Baclofen has been used to treat trigeminal neuralgia, although it is not approved by the FDA for this purpose. Drowsiness, weakness, headache, and insomnia have been reported. Nausea, dry mouth, taste disorder, and urinary frequency have been seen. Lowering of the seizure threshold and an increase in ovarian cysts in rats have also occurred.

Tizanidine

Tizanidine (tye-ZAN-i-deen) (Zanaflex) is a short-acting muscle relaxant. It is a centrally acting α-adrenergic receptor agonist, like clonidine, that increases presynaptic inhibition of motor neurons. Also like clonidine, tizanidine can produce sedation, drowsiness, hypotension, and xerostomia.

Dantrolene

Dantrolene (DAN-troe-leen) (Dantrium) affects the contractile response of the skeletal muscle by acting directly on the muscle itself. It dissociates the excitation-contraction coupling, probably by interfering with the release of calcium from the sarcoplasmic reticulum. It is indicated in the treatment of spasticity from upper motor neuron disorders such as spinal cord injury, cerebral palsy, and multiple sclerosis. It is also used orally to prevent and intravenously to treat malignant hyperthermia brought on by succinylcholine or inhalation of general anesthetics. The hepatotoxicity that dantrolene produces is more common with higher doses and in older female patients taking concomitant medications. This agent may cause drowsiness or photosensitivity.

GENERAL COMMENTS ABOUT ANTIANXIETY AGENTS

Analgesic-Sedative Combinations

The use of an analgesic and a sedative-hypnotic agent to provide concomitant sedation and analgesia is rational for several reasons (Box 11.4).

Both sedation and analgesia can be obtained from the opioid analgesics alone. However, it is not desirable to prescribe an opioid to add sedation to analgesia unless the analgesic potency is required. In cases in which anxiety is an important component of pain relief, either a nonopioid or opioid can be used concomitantly with a sedative. This combination may be prescribed separately, although a few fixed-dose products are available. A combination of a sedative with an analgesic is available in a butalbital compound (Fiorinal) and as butalbital/acetaminophen (Fioricet). If the patient's pain is more severe, then an opioid and a sedative-hypnotic agent can be prescribed. The previously mentioned agents are available mixed with codeine (#3 contains 30 mg codeine) to make Fiorinal #3. In a dental patient in whom anxiety is magnifying the pain reaction, the prescribing of a combination agent might be useful.

Special Considerations

> Psychological management must accompany use of antianxiety agents.

Certain generalizations should be kept in mind in a discussion of the use of the antianxiety agents. The dental practitioner plays an important role in helping the patient understand the possible effects of the drugs used to allay anxiety. The patient may raise questions about these agents, and their effects should be explained. Dental patients who are to use antianxiety agents should be driven to and from their dental appointments.

Drugs are not to be used as substitutes for patient management. The practitioner should not rely exclusively on drugs to provide a calm and cooperative patient. The dental team should exhibit a confident and

---

BOX 11.4 Rationale for Use of Analgesic-Sedative Combinations

Relief of both anxiety and pain is often required in one patient.
Sedatives potentiate analgesic agents.
Sedatives may induce excitation when given without an analgesic to patients with uncontrolled pain.
Anxiety can lower the pain threshold.

---

relaxed manner. A pleasant, soothing office atmosphere is of great importance in relaxing an anxious patient. Appropriate use of music of the patient's choice can reduce anxiety. Drugs should not be substituted for patient education or for the proper psychological approach to patient care.

When a drug is required for anxiety relief, the selection of the specific drug should be based on knowledge of the advantages and disadvantages of the agents available and an understanding of the needs and contraindications related to the case at hand.

Precautions

Regardless of the antianxiety agent selected, the following precautions pertain:

- Patients with impaired elimination may experience exaggerated effects of these medications. They include the young, the elderly, the debilitated, and patients with liver or kidney disease.
- Depression caused by all sedative-hypnotics will add to depression caused by other CNS depressants that the patient may be taking. The patient should be made aware of this effect, particularly in regard to alcohol; over-the-counter (OTC) sleep aids may also be a potential source of hazard.
- The patient should understand that the drug prescribed will make it unsafe to perform acts requiring full alertness and muscle coordination, such as driving a car. The patient should be accompanied to the appointment by a responsible adult who can drive the patient home. The patient should be warned against signing any important papers or documents for several hours after taking the drug or once they feel cognitively intact (varies from person to person). These cautions are particularly important if the patient has not taken the drug previously and consequently his or her response is less predictable.
- Psychic and physical dependence has been observed with almost all drugs used to allay anxiety. The dentist should realize that these drugs have abuse potential and should limit their use accordingly. This issue is particularly important in regard to the treatment of chronic conditions or of persons with a history of addiction or alcoholism.
- Suicide may be attempted by people taking sedative-hypnotic drugs. Consequently, the amount of drug prescribed should be limited to the minimum required to accomplish the therapeutic objective. With benzodiazepines, the therapeutic index is wide unless they are mixed with alcohol.
- These drugs should never be administered to pregnant women or those who may be pregnant unless the potential benefit to the mother outweighs the risk to the fetus.
- Sedatives do not provide analgesia. In fact, the use of a sedative without adequate pain control may cause the patient to become highly excited and act irrationally. However, sedatives may potentiate the effect of an analgesic taken concomitantly.

DENTAL HYGIENE CONSIDERATIONS

- Review the patient's medication/health history for any contraindications.
- These medications are sedating, so it is best to try to avoid other sedating medications. If this is not possible, counsel the patient about the increased risk for sedation.
- Encourage the patient to have someone drive him or her to and from the appointment.

- Encourage the patient to refrain from any activity that requires thought or concentration for at least several hours or the patient feels cognitively intact.
- Encourage the patient to go home, if possible, and rest until the remaining sedation clears up.
- Review Boxes 11.1, 11.2, and 11.4.

ACADEMIC SKILLS ASSESSMENT

1. What are some of the nonpharmacologic methods of helping a patient deal with his or her anxiety?
2. The dentist decides to prescribe diazepam, which is to be taken the night before the patient's appointment and approximately 1 hour before the appointment. What is the rationale for using benzodiazepines to treat anxiety?
3. What are the adverse reactions associated with benzodiazepines?
4. Is memory loss a problem with benzodiazepines? What should a patient be told?
5. Should a patient be concerned about becoming addicted to benzodiazepines? Why or why not?
6. What should a patient be told about diazepam?
7. Discuss the use of midazolam as conscious sedation in a patient with dental anxiety. Counsel the patient regarding midazolam.

8. Name two major pharmacologic effects of barbiturates.
9. Describe the major adverse reactions to barbiturates.
10. Name the one absolute contraindication to the use of barbiturates.
11. Describe the mechanism of the most important drug interaction of barbiturates.
12. State the potential advantages of the nonbenzodiazepine, benzodiazepine receptor agonists.
13. Describe the concerns associated with zolpidem use.
14. What was the rationale for reducing the dose of zolpidem?
15. What is the rationale for combining a sedative-hypnotic drug with an analgesic?

CLINICAL CASE STUDY

Leslie Fitzsimmons is a 33-year-old and has been coming to your practice for several years. She has always been somewhat anxious, and her dental appointments seem to intensify her level of anxiety. Her medications include the occasional use of lorazepam when her anxiety "gets the best of her." She does not like taking benzodiazepines because they make her tired and she cannot drive. She comes in today and tells you that her doctor has started her on buspirone for her anxiety. She also has questions regarding the use of Ambien the night prior to her appointment.

1. What is buspirone?
2. How does buspirone differ from the benzodiazepines?

3. Is buspirone appropriate for the treatment of dental anxiety?
4. What are the adverse effects associated with buspirone?
5. Would there be a problem if the dentist had to prescribe a sedating medication for or use one during treatment of Ms. Fitzsimmons while she was taking buspirone?
6. Would a benzodiazepine be the better choice? How can Ms. Fitzsimmons deal with the issues surrounding sedation and driving?
7. What is zolpidem?
8. What are some of the concerns regarding zolpidem therapy? How have these concerns been addressed by the manufacturer?

PART III

Drugs That May Alter Dental Treatment

Chapter 12
Drugs for the Treatment of Cardiovascular Diseases, 131

Chapter 13
Drugs for the Treatment of Gastrointestinal Disorders, 158

Chapter 14
Drugs for the Treatment of Seizure Disorders, 165

Chapter 15
Drugs for the Treatment of Central Nervous System Disorders, 174

Chapter 16
Adrenocorticosteroids, 184

Chapter 17
Drugs for the Treatment of Respiratory Disorders and Allergic Rhinitis, 192

Chapter 18
Drugs for the Treatment of Diabetes Mellitus, 204

Chapter 19
Drugs for the Treatment of Other Endocrine Disorders, 215

Chapter 20
Antineoplastic Drugs, 225

Drugs for the Treatment of Cardiovascular Diseases

http://evolve.elsevier.com/Haveles/pharmacology

LEARNING OBJECTIVES

1. Identify the dental implications of cardiovascular disease including the contraindications to treatment, vasoconstrictor use, and its relationship to periodontal disease.
2. Describe heart failure and identify drugs commonly used to treat it, including the mechanisms of action, pharmacologic effects, and adverse reactions.
3. Discuss the use of digoxin and the management of dental patients taking it.
4. Define arrhythmia and dysrhythmia and describe how the heart maintains its normal rhythm.
5. Describe the classifications, mechanisms of action, adverse reactions, and uses of antiarrhythmic agents and identify the issues to consider in dental treatment.
6. Define angina pectoris and describe the types of drugs used to treat it; identify the dental implications of these drugs.

7. Define hypertension, describe the categories it is divided into, and identify its treatment with the various types of antihypertensive agents, including
   - Describe the mechanisms of action, pharmacologic effects, adverse reactions, and uses of the various antihypertensive agents.
   - Identify potential drug interactions and the dental implications of these drugs.
   - Discuss the management of dental patients taking these drugs.
8. Define hyperlipidemia and hyperlipoproteinemia and summarize the types of drugs used to restore cholesterol homeostasis in the body including the dental implications of their use.
9. Describe the role of warfarin in blood coagulation and the potential adverse reactions and interactions associated with its use.
10. Identify several other drugs that affect blood coagulation.

Cardiovascular disease affects many dental patients.

The term *cardiovascular disease* refers to a variety of diseases of the heart and blood vessels. Examples of these diseases are hypertension, angina pectoris, coronary artery disease, arrhythmias, and heart failure (HF). Although cardiovascular disease is the leading cause of death in the United States, patients with cardiovascular disease are now living longer, more productive lives because of cardiac care units, comprehensive drug therapy, and intensive screening procedures. These developments explain why cardiovascular disease affects such a large proportion of the dental patient population.

The dental hygienist first identifies the patient with cardiovascular disease while taking the medical or drug history. It is common for such a patient to have several cardiovascular conditions, such as HF, hypertension, and hypercholesterolemia. For each disease, a patient may take one or more medications.

Because cardiovascular medications are often given for the patient's lifetime, knowledge of the actions, problems, and effects of these drugs on dental treatment is essential. Both the disease and the drugs used in its treatment can affect the management of a patient's dental care.

Before each group of drugs is discussed in this chapter, the disease for which the drugs are used is briefly described, beginning with general considerations concerning the dental treatment of patients with cardiovascular disease.

DENTAL IMPLICATIONS OF CARDIOVASCULAR DISEASE

Contraindications to Treatment

Although most patients with cardiovascular disease can be safely treated in the dental office, circumstances may arise in which dental treatment should be delayed until the patient's disease is under better control. Patients who have suffered a myocardial infarction (MI) should wait 6 months before receiving any type of oral health care to give the heart a chance to heal. Bacteria from the mouth can enter the bloodstream and weaken an already weakened heart. If oral health care is necessary before 6 months have elapsed, one should consult with the patient's cardiologist or general practitioner to determine whether or not the patient's heart has healed sufficiently.

Certain medical situations, listed in Box 12.1, are absolute contraindications to dental treatment until a consultation with the patient's provider has identified any special treatment alterations that might be warranted. These absolute contraindications apply only to uncontrolled or severe cardiovascular diseases. Examples of absolute contraindications to elective dental treatment include very high blood pressure and uncontrolled arrhythmias. Most patients with cardiovascular disease can be treated in the dental office. The type of procedure anticipated, the stress of the procedure, and the fact that many procedures are elective must be considered. Once a thorough health history is obtained, a determination can be made about whether the patient's provider should be consulted before dental treatment is begun. When the health care provider is contacted, it is important to explain the procedure(s) indicated for the patient.

Vasoconstrictor Limit

Cardiovascular patients should receive epinephrine.

When a local anesthetic containing a vasoconstrictor is used in the treatment of a patient with cardiovascular disease, the severity of the patient's disease must be considered. The majority of cardiovascular patients should benefit from the use of epinephrine in the local anesthetic agent. The amount and effect of the epinephrine administered must be weighed against the fact that poor pain management can produce the release of endogenous epinephrine. Limiting the dose of epinephrine to the cardiac dose may be warranted in a few severely affected patients (see Chapter 9 for a detailed discussion of vasoconstrictor limits).

Using a slow rate of injection and appropriate aspiration techniques to avoid intravascular injection reduces the chance of vasoconstrictor adverse reactions. A "fight-or-flight" reaction related to the patient's anxiety also results in the release of endogenous epinephrine indistinguishable in effect from that of the exogenous epinephrine. (So, being really scared feels exactly like epinephrine because one is making epinephrine.)

Periodontal Disease and Cardiovascular Disease

Researchers and government agencies continue to investigate the possible relationship between periodontal disease and cardiovascular disease. Studies both support and reject such a relationship. Researchers do agree that more studies are needed. Regardless of study outcomes, it is very important that patients maintain optimal oral health care by receiving oral health care twice a year, brushing teeth a minimum of twice a day, regularly flossing teeth, and making sure that dentures fit properly.

HEART FAILURE

Heart failure: Heart cannot pump efficiently.

The incidence of HF in the United States has remained relatively stable, at almost 650,000 cases diagnosed annually. Approximately 5.1 million Americans have clinical symptoms of HF, and its prevalence is expected to rise. The incidence of HF rises with age. The incidence in those 65 to 69 years is 20 per 1000, and in those older than 85 years, it is more than 80 per 1000 individuals.

The heart functions as a pump, ensuring adequate circulation of the blood to meet the oxygen needs of all the body's tissues. When oxygen needs are increased, as in exercise, the normal heart adjusts its output to meet them higher. If the heart is unable to keep up with the body's needs, it becomes a "failing" heart, and the pumping mechanism becomes inefficient. This occurs because the heart muscle has suffered an injury and cannot keep up its work. Some enlargement of the heart produces a more efficient heartbeat and cardiac output (Starling's law).

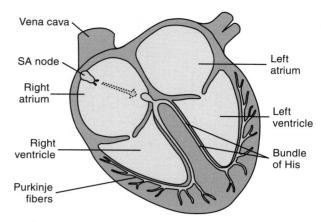

Fig. 12.1 Cross-section of heart with conduction tissues. *SA,* Sinoatrial.

However, over time, additional cardiac enlargement occurs (cardiac muscle stretched past its maximum effectiveness by the presence of excess blood that it cannot pump out), and the patient becomes tachycardic. This inefficient pumping mechanism results in an inadequate cardiac output and unsatisfactory circulation. Various forms of injury to the heart, such as MI (heart attack), arrhythmias, and valvular abnormalities from rheumatic heart disease, can contribute to a failing heart.

The heart has two sides: the right and the left (Fig. 12.1). In HF, the heart does not provide adequate cardiac output to provide for the oxygen needs of the body. Over time, the blood accumulates in the failing ventricle(s). The ventricle(s) enlarge(s) and finally become(s) ineffective as a pump.

One or both sides of the heart can fail. Usually, the left side fails first. If the left side of the heart fails, the blood backs up into the pulmonary circulation (lungs). Pulmonary edema results, producing **dyspnea** and **orthopnea**. Dental patients with left HF may need to be in a semireclined position to undergo dental treatment. If the right side of the heart fails, then the right ventricle is unable to remove all the blood from that side of the heart. Right-sided HF causes systemic congestion. Symptoms include peripheral edema with fluid accumulation evidenced by pitting edema (**pedal** edema). Over time, many patients experience failure of both sides of the heart, with symptoms of failure on both sides.

Treatment of Heart Failure

HF therapy is based on the American Heart Association (AHA) stage of HF and whether the patient has any comorbid conditions (Fig. 12.2). Once the patient has been evaluated, the physician can treat him or her with the drugs reviewed in this section. Many patients may require a combination of medications. The following discusses the role of the listed classes of medication and their role in treating HF. A detailed discussion of their pharmacologic effects can be found in the section on hypertension.

Diuretics

Most patients with HF have edema, or fluid retention. Diuretics are used in these patients to relieve the symptoms of HF. The American College of Cardiology (ACC) and AHA recommend that all patients who have evidence of fluid retention and most patients with a history of fluid retention be prescribed a diuretic. In clinical trials, patients taking a combination of a diuretic and other drugs used to treat HF had better survival. Loop diuretics, such as furosemide, appear to be more effective than thiazide diuretics, although some patients may show a more favorable response to other diuretics (i.e., bumetanide, torsemide) because of their increased oral bioavailability. Diuretics should be combined with angiotensin-converting enzyme inhibitors (ACEIs), angiotensin receptor antagonists or blockers, β-blockers, or aldosterone antagonists.

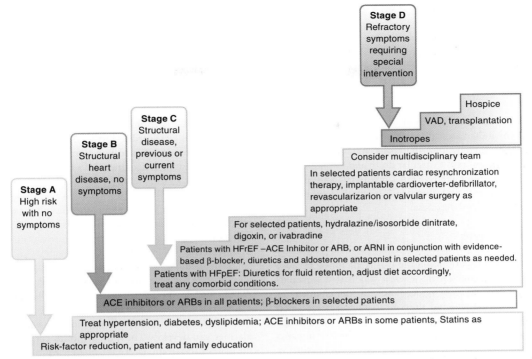

Fig. 12.2 Stages in the development of heart failure (*HF*) and recommended therapy by stage. *ACE*, angiotensin-converting enzyme inhibitor; *AF*, atrial fibrillation; *ARB*, angiotensin receptor blocker; *ARNI*, Angiotensin Receptor Neprilysin Inhibitor; *CAD*, coronary artery disease; *CRT*, cardiac resynchronization therapy; *DM*, diabetes mellitus; *EF*, ejection fraction; *GDMT*, guideline-directed medical therapy; HMG CoA Reductase Inhibitors, Stains; *HPpEF*, heart failure with preserved ejection fraction; *HFrEF*, heart failure with reduced ejection fraction; *HRQOL*, health-related quality of life; *HTN*, hypertension; *ICD*, implantable cardioverter-defibrillator; *LV*, left ventricular; *LVH*, left ventricular hypertrophy; *MCS*, mechanical circulatory support; *MI*, myocardial infarction; *VAD*, ventricular assist device. (Modified from Jessup M, Brozena S. (2003): Heart failure. *N Engl J Med.* 348(20):2007–18).

Angiotensin-Converting Enzyme Inhibitors

Current guidelines from the ACC and the AHA now recommend prescribing an ACEI for all patients with symptomatic (stage C) HF and for asymptomatic patients with a decreased left ventricular ejection fraction (LVEF) or a history of MI unless there are contraindications to an ACEI. ACEIs improve symptoms in patients with HF within a period of 4 to 12 weeks, decrease the incidence of hospitalization and MI, and prolong survival. ACEIs are now considered first-line therapy and are the cornerstone of HF therapy. Unless there are contraindications, an ACE inhibitor should be used in combination with a β-blocker.

Angiotensin Receptor Blockers

Angiotensin receptor blockers (ARBs) have also been shown to reduce mortality and symptoms. They are recommended for patients who cannot tolerate ACEIs and are also considered first-line therapy for HF. These drugs may be used as alternatives to ACEIs in the patient already taking an ARB for a comorbid condition such as hypertension.

β-Adrenergic Blockers

The ACC/AHA guidelines now recommend β-blockers for patients with symptoms of HF and for asymptomatic patients with decreased LVEF or a history of an MI unless otherwise contraindicated. Although it has been customary to start a β-blocker after an ACEI, the results of several clinical trials suggest that starting with a β-blocker may be equally, if not possibly more, effective. The ACC/AHA guidelines recommend bisoprolol, carvedilol, and sustained-release metoprolol for patients with current or prior symptoms of HF with decreased LVEF to reduce morbidity and mortality.

Aldosterone Antagonists

Aldosterone antagonists are recommended for patients with New York Heart Association (NYHA) class II through class IV HF with an LVEF of 35% or less to reduce morbidity and mortality. Unless contraindicated, aldosterone antagonists are also recommended for patients with a LVEF of 40% or less who have recently had an MI and are showing symptoms of HF or who have a history of diabetes mellitus. In one clinical trial, the addition of spironolactone to standard therapy reduced the risk of mortality and hospitalization. In another clinical trial, the addition of selective aldosterone antagonist eplerenone to standard therapy reduced both all-cause mortality and cardiovascular mortality in patients with acute MI complicated by left ventricular systolic dysfunction and HF.

Vasodilators

Hydralazine, an arterial vasodilator, lowers peripheral resistance through arterial vasodilation. With a reduction in the afterload, the work of the heart is decreased. Isosorbide dinitrate, a venous dilator, reduces the preload, in turn decreasing the work of the heart. With this combination of agents, the heart is pumping against less resistance and less blood is returning to it (some blood remains in the venous circulation). The heart's workload is reduced, and symptoms of HF subside. The addition of hydralazine and isosorbide dinitrate to standard therapy in black patients with class III to IV HF significantly lowered mortality and the rate of hospitalization and improved quality-of-life scores. Unless otherwise contraindicated, the same combination can be used in patients with current or prior symptomatic HF and LVEF reduction who cannot take an ACEI or ARB because of poor tolerance to the drug, hypotension, or renal insufficiency.

ANGIOTENSIN II RECEPTOR NEPRILYSIN INHIBITOR

Entresto is the first in a new class of drugs that combines sacubitril (neprilysin inhibitor) and valsartan (ARB). Neprilysin is an enzyme that is responsible for the degradation of atrial and brain natriuretic peptides, which lower blood pressure by primarily reducing blood volume.

The drug works by inhibiting neprilysin and blocking angiotensin II type-1 receptors which increases the levels of peptides that are broken down by neprilysin, thereby lowering blood pressure. It is FDA-approved to reduce the risk of cardiovascular death and hospitalization for HF in patients with chronic HF (NYHA Class II-IV) and reduced ejection fraction. Side effects include hypotension, cough, angioedema, hyperkalemia, renal failure, and dizziness.

I$_F$ CHANNEL INHIBITOR

Ivabradine (Corlanor) acts by inhibiting the If (f is for funny because of its seemingly unusual characteristic when it was first discovered) ion channel in the sinoatrial (SA) node. Blocking this channel reduces cardiac pacemaker activity and slows heart rate. It is indicated to reduce the risk of hospitalization for worsening HF in patients with stable, symptomatic chronic HF with LVEF ≤35%, who are in sinus rhythm with resting heart rate ≥70 bpm and either are on maximally tolerated doses of β-blockers or have a contraindication to β-blocker use. Common side effects include bradycardia, hypertension, and visual brightness.

CARDIAC GLYCOSIDES

Digitalis Glycosides

> Positive inotropic effect.

Digoxin was first described by William Withering in 1785. At first, he thought that cardiac glycosides affected the kidneys because they produced diuresis. Later, these substances were referred to as *cardiac* or *digitalis glycosides:* cardiac because they affect the heart and glycoside because of their chemical structure. Digoxin (di-JOX-in) (Lanoxin) is the most commonly used cardiac glycoside. Once the first-line agent for the treatment of HF, digoxin is now used only in selected patients with stage C HF and reduced LVEF.

Pharmacologic Effects

The major effect of digoxin on the failing heart is to increase the force and strength of contraction of the myocardium (positive inotropic effect). It allows the heart to do more work without increasing its oxygen use. When the contractile force of the heart is improved, the heart becomes a more efficient pump and the cardiac output increases. After the patient takes digoxin, the heart is reduced to a more efficient size and can function more effectively.

Digoxin also reduces the edema that occurs with HF. As a result of the improved pumping action, more blood circulates through the kidneys (increase in glomerular filtration rate), which mobilizes the edema from the tissues, producing diuresis. The diuresis is not a result of an effect on the kidneys; it is a result of digoxin's indirect effect in improving the heart's function. The size of the heart is reduced as the excess blood volume that has collected there is removed via the kidneys.

Digoxin can affect automaticity, conduction velocity, and refractory periods of different parts of the heart in different ways. It slows atrioventricular (AV) conduction, prolongs the refractory period of the AV node, and decreases the rate of the SA node. When the refractory period of the AV node is prolonged, fewer impulses are transmitted to the ventricle and the heart rate falls. These effects are useful in the treatment of certain arrhythmias.

Uses

The most common use of digoxin is in the treatment of HF. It is also used for atrial arrhythmias, including atrial fibrillation (AF) and paroxysmal atrial tachycardia (PAT). Patients with HF and normal sinus rhythm may not experience long-term benefit in terms of a lower mortality with the use of digoxin.

Adverse Reactions

Because of digoxin's narrow therapeutic index (see Chapter 3), toxic effects are not uncommon. Even slight changes in dose, absorption, or metabolism can trigger toxic symptoms. Toxicity is more likely to occur in the elderly.

Gastrointestinal effects. Early gastrointestinal signs of digoxin toxicity include anorexia, nausea and vomiting, and copious salivation. A reduction in the dosage of digoxin usually alleviates these adverse reactions.

Arrhythmias. If a sufficient overdose is given, severe cardiac irregularities can develop. These arrhythmias can progress to ventricular fibrillation and death. Diuretics, often used in the treatment of HF, can produce hypokalemia, which can predispose a patient to serious arrhythmias. One should note that digitalis is used to treat arrhythmias and that its toxicity can cause arrhythmias.

Neurologic effects. The neurologic signs of toxicity include headache, drowsiness, and visual disturbances (green and yellow vision, halo around lights). A pain in the lower face resembling that of trigeminal neuralgia has been reported as a neurologic symptom of digitalis toxicity. Weakness, faintness, and mental confusion have also been reported.

Oral effects. Increased salivation is associated with digoxin toxicity. An increase in the gagging reflex, which may interfere with taking a dental impression, has also been reported with this agent.

Dental Drug Interactions

With either increased or decreased blood digoxin levels, serious problems can occur when the digoxin interacts with other drugs. One drug interaction, between digoxin and a sympathomimetic, both of which can cause ectopic pacemaker activity, may increase the chance of arrhythmias if they are administered concomitantly.

For this reason, the vasoconstrictors added to local anesthetics, which are sympathomimetics, should be used with caution. In patients with severe cardiac disease, the epinephrine dose should be limited to the cardiac dose (see Chapter 9). Erythromycin and tetracycline can increase the toxicity of digoxin in some patients.

Management of the Dental Patient Taking Digoxin

Box 12.2 summarizes the management of the dental patient taking digoxin.

Gastrointestinal effects. If a patient complains of nausea or vomiting, special care must be taken to prevent emesis. These symptoms may be associated with digitalis toxicity, and the patient's physician should be consulted if the nausea and vomiting have been protracted.

Epinephrine administration. Because digoxin toxicity can sensitize the myocardium to arrhythmias, epinephrine should be used cautiously or limited to the cardiac dose in patients taking digitalis. Patients taking digitalis should be questioned about toxic symptoms before epinephrine is administered. Hypokalemia from diuretics can exacerbate this arrhythmogenic potential.

BOX 12.2 Management of the Dental Patient Taking Digoxin

Watch for overdose side effects such as nausea, vision changes, and copious salivation.

Use epinephrine with caution to minimize arrhythmias.

Monitor pulse to check for bradycardia.

Tetracycline and erythromycin can increase digoxin levels (in approximately 10% of patients).

Pulse monitoring. Because digitalis can cause bradycardia or arrhythmias, the patient's pulse should be checked before each dental appointment for a normal rate and a regular rhythm. An abnormally slow rate or an irregular rhythm should be reported to the patient's provider for evaluation.

ANTIARRHYTHMIC AGENTS

The terms arrhythmia (*ar*, insensibility; *rhythmos*, rhythm) and dysrhythmia (*dys*, bad; *rhythmos*, rhythm) are used interchangeably to mean "abnormal rhythm." Arrhythmias may result from abnormal impulse generation or abnormal impulse conduction. Cardiac diseases, such as myocardial anoxia, arteriosclerosis, and heart block, can cause arrhythmias. The antiarrhythmic agents are drugs that are used to prevent arrhythmias.

Automaticity

Cardiac tissue has inherent automaticity. (Each part has a different rate.)

The cells of the cardiac muscles, unlike those of skeletal muscles, have an intrinsic rhythm called *automaticity.* "Pacemaker" cells spontaneously produce action potentials as they undergo slow spontaneous depolarization during diastole (as they rest, they leak ions). If any heart muscle cell is left undisturbed and isolated from the rest of the heart with appropriate nutrients and oxygen, it will beat spontaneously at its own rate. Each type of cardiac cell differs in its automaticity, depending on the function of the particular cell. The cells that specialize in conduction functions have a faster rate of automaticity than other cardiac cells. This design ensures that the heart will beat in a coordinated manner.

The SA node has the fastest rate of depolarization and therefore directs all the other cells in the heart. It normally fires impulses approximately 80 times/min. The SA node is innervated by both the parasympathetic nervous system (PNS) and the sympathetic nervous system (SNS). The SA node sends a message (action potential) to the AV node via the atrial muscle. When the impulse arrives at the AV node there is a slight delay because the muscles beyond the AV node are thinner. The AV node sends the message via the bundle of His to the Purkinje fibers. The Purkinje fibers then send the message to the cardiac muscle cells, to the apex of the ventricles, directing them all to contract as they get the message. This system is repeated with each heartbeat.

In the normal patient, this system functions seamlessly. In the patient with cardiac arrhythmias, diseased parts of the heart can produce abnormal conduction pathways, which may result in arrhythmias.

Arrhythmias

The many types of arrhythmias produce various abnormalities of the heartbeat. These arrhythmias are usually divided into supraventricular (atrial) and ventricular types, depending on the location of the genesis of the arrhythmia. Abnormal arrhythmias may result in tachycardia or bradycardia of the supraventricular (atrial) or ventricular parts of the heart or from ectopic foci. The ectopic foci are "emergent leaders" that preempt the SA or AV nodal rate. The electrical impulses begin at the SA node and travel to the AV node. At the conduction level, different patterns of conduction include the normal pattern, bifurcation (conduction splits and goes two ways), reentry, unidirectional block (action potential is blocked from being stimulated from one side of the tissue but not from the other), and prolonged refractory period.

Several recent deaths of fit adolescents during athletic events have been linked to congenital presence of a prolonged QT interval (torsades de pointes, previously undiagnosed).

Antiarrhythmic Agents

Long-term effects of these drugs must be studied.

Antiarrhythmic agents are divided into four groups (Table 12.1). The specific actions of these agents are complicated. They work by depressing parts of the heart that are beating abnormally.

Antiarrhythmics may change the slope of depolarization, raise the threshold for depolarization, and alter the conduction velocity in different parts of the heart. For example, decreasing the slope of depolarization reduces the frequency of discharge, and the rate slows. If the threshold for producing an action potential is raised, extra beats may be suppressed. Examples of specific actions of these drugs are decrease in the velocity of depolarization, decrease in impulse propagation, and

TABLE 12.1 Classification and Mechanism of Action of the Antiarrhythmics

Class	Examples	Mechanism	Effect(s)	Comment
IA	Quinidine, procainamide, disopyramide	Na⁺ channel blocker (medium)	Blocks conduction	Prolongs the duration of the AP
IB	Lidocaine, phenytoin, mexiletine	Na⁺ channel blocker (fast)	Blocks conduction; decreases ERP	Shortens the AP
IC	Flecainide, encainide, propafenone	Na⁺ channel blocker (slow)	Blocks conduction; little effect on ERP	Slows conduction without affecting the AP
II	Propranolol, esmolol, acebutolol, sotalol, atenolol, timolol, metoprolol, bisoprolol	β-Blockers	Decreases SA node automaticity	Reduces sympathetic activity
III	Bretylium and *d*-sotalol (non-β-blocking enantiomer)	K⁺ channel blockers	Prolongs the AP	Prolongs phase 3 repolarization
	Amiodarone	K⁺ Blocker	Prolongs the AP	Prolongs phase 3 repolarization
	Dofelitide	K⁺ Blocker	Prolongs the AP	Prolongs phase 3 repolarization
IV	Verapamil, diltiazem	CCBs	Slows conduction velocity at AV node	Decreases the firing rate of the SA and AV nodes

AP, Action potential; *AV,* atrioventricular; *CCBs,* calcium channel blockers; *ERP,* effective refractory period; *K⁺,* potassium; *Na⁺,* sodium; *SA,* sinoatrial.

TABLE 12.2 Management of Dental Patients Taking Antiarrhythmics

Specific Antiarrhythmic(s)	Implications and Management
All	Check for abnormal or extra heart beats when taking patient's blood pressure and pulse. Record the type of arrhythmia and the drug therapy.
Atrial fibrillation	Patients taking warfarin—check international normalized ratio. Patients taking direct thrombin inhibitors and factor Xa Inhibitors—check for signs of bruising and bleeding.
Amiodarone	Liver toxicity, blue skin discoloration, photosensitivity—to dental light
Calcium channel blockers	Gingival enlargement (verapamil most reported)
Disopyramide	Anticholinergic xerostomia
Procainamide	Reversible lupus erythematosus–like syndrome, 25%–30%; central nervous system depression; xerostomia
Quinidine	Nausea, vomiting, diarrhea; cinchonism with large doses; atropine-like effect; xerostomia
Phenytoin	Gingival enlargement
β-Blockers, nonspecific	Drug interaction with epinephrine; limit to cardiac dose if patient's condition warrants.

CCBs, Calcium channel blockers; *CNS,* central nervous system; *INR,* international normalized ratio.

inhibition of aberrant impulse propagation. Tables 12.1 and 12.2 describe the classification and mechanisms of action of the antiarrhythmics, the dental-related adverse reactions, and the dental implications of the antiarrhythmics.

Digoxin

Although digoxin is not included in the antiarrhythmic groups, it is used to treat some arrhythmias. It shortens the refractory period of atrial and ventricular tissues while prolonging the refractory period and diminishing conduction velocity in the Purkinje fibers. Toxic doses of digoxin can result in ventricular arrhythmias.

ANTIANGINAL DRUGS

Angina Pectoris

Angina: insufficient oxygen for body's demand.

Angina pectoris is a common cardiovascular disease characterized by pain or discomfort in the chest radiating to the left arm and shoulder. Pain can also be reported radiating to the neck, back, and lower jaw. The lower jaw pain can be of such intensity that it may be confused with a toothache. Angina occurs when the coronary arteries do not supply a sufficient amount of oxygen to the myocardium for its current work. Anginal pain can be precipitated by the stress (increased workload on the heart) induced by physical exercise or by emotional states such as the anxiety and apprehension generated by a dental appointment.

According to the most current ACC/AHA guidelines regarding the treatment of chronic stable angina, the primary goals of therapy are to prevent MI and death and to completely or nearly completely eliminate ischemic symptoms. Goals also include treating both risk factors and comorbid disease states that can precipitate or worsen angina and increase the risk for cardiovascular problems. Fig. 12.3 reviews the most current recommendations.

The basic pharmacologic effect of drugs used to manage angina is reduction of the workload of the heart through a decrease in the cardiac output, the peripheral vascular resistance, or both. The oxygen requirement of the myocardium is in turn reduced, relieving the painful symptoms of angina. It is important, however, to keep in mind that these drugs are not curative, and the dental team should be alert to the fact that an anginal episode could occur at any time. Appropriate emergency procedures to manage an acute anginal attack should be reviewed before a patient with angina is treated in the dental office (see Chapter 21). Table 12.3 lists the major antianginal drugs and some of their more pertinent characteristics.

Nitroglycerin-Like Compounds

Nitroglycerin (nye-troe-GLI-ser-in) (NTG) is by far the nitrate most often used for the management of acute anginal episodes (see Table 12.3). In addition to the long-acting nitrates, NTG is also used to prevent anginal attacks induced by stress or exercise. Box 12.3 provides guidelines for managing the patient taking NTG-like compounds.

Mechanism

Releases nitric oxide: Vasodilator.

NTG is a vasodilator that produces relaxation of vascular smooth muscle throughout the body. Indirectly, the work of the heart is reduced by the effect on both the venous and the arterial sides of the circulation. The venous dilation decreases the amount of blood returning to the heart (preload) and thereby lowers the heart's workload. The arterial dilation reduces the resistance against which the heart must pump (afterload). By lowering the workload on the heart, NTG decreases the oxygen demand, with relief or reduction of angina pain. Tolerance to these effects occurs, unless a nitrate-free period is observed daily.

Sublingual (SL) NTG is used to treat acute anginal attacks. It has a rapid onset (a few minutes) by this route, and its effect can last up to 30 minutes. It is available as an SL tablet (Nitrostat), a spray used sublingually (Nitrolingual), or as a SL powder (GoNitro). GoNitro is supplied in single-use packets that contain 0.4 mg of NTG which should be stored at room temperature. One or two packets should be placed under the tongue at the onset of the angina attack and allowed to dissolve. The patient should be in a sitting position if possible and should keep their mouth closed for at least 5 minutes while the powder dissolves.

SL isosorbide dinitrate is also effective for an acute anginal attack. The dental office emergency kit should contain one of these products to manage acute anginal attacks. Dental patients with a history of angina should be asked to bring their NTG to each dental appointment.

Adverse Reactions

Most adverse reactions associated with NTG occur because of its effect on vascular smooth muscle. Severe headaches are often reported (vasodilation) after the use of NTG. Flushing, hypotension, lightheadedness, and syncope (fainting) can also result. Hypotension is enhanced by alcohol and hot weather. SL NTG can cause a localized burning or tingling at the site of administration. The presence of stinging is not indicative of the potency of the NTG.

Significant Drug Interactions and Contraindications

Phosphodiesterase 5 (PDE5) inhibitors are a class of drug used to treat erectile dysfunction. These drugs include sildenafil (Viagra), vardenafil (Levitra), and tadalafil (Cialis). The administration of any of these

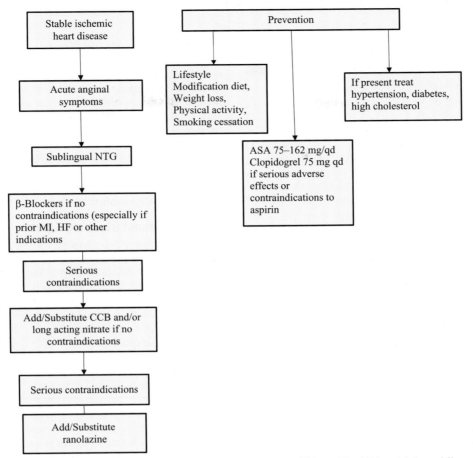

Fig. 12.3 Treatment of stable ischemic heart disease. *CCB,* Calcium channel blocker; *ASA,* aspirin; *HF,* heart failure; *MI,* myocardial infarction; *NTG,* nitroglycerin. (Modified from Fihn SD, Gardin JM, Abrams J, et al. ACCF/AHA/ACP/AATS/PCNA/SCAI/STS guideline for the diagnosis and management of patients with stable ischemic heart disease: a report of the American College of Cardiology Foundation/American Heart Association Task Force on Practice Guidelines, and the American College of Physicians, American Association for Thoracic Surgery, Preventive Cardiovascular Nurses Association, Society for Cardiovascular Angiography and Interventions, and Society of Thoracic Surgeons. *J Am Coll Cardiol.* 2012;60:e44–e167.)

TABLE 12.3 Antianginal Preparations

Drug	Route(s)	Onset of Action (min)	Duration of Action
Acute Attacks			
Nitrates			
Amyl nitrite	Inhalation	0.5	3–5 minutes
Short-Acting Nitrates			
Nitroglycerin (NTG, Nitrostat) (Nitrolingual)	Sublingual	1–3	30–60 minutes
	Oral spray		30–60 minutes
Isosorbide dinitrate	Sublingual	2–5	60–120 minutes
Prophylactic Use			
Long-Acting Nitrates			
Nitroglycerin (Nitro-Bid)	Sustained-release oral tablets	~60	10–14 Hours
(Nitro-Bid)	Ointment	15–30	2–12 Hours
(NITRO-DUR, Minitran)	Transdermal patches	30–60	to 24 Hours
Isosorbide dinitrate (Isordil, Sorbitrate-DSC)	Oral	20–40	4–6 Hours
Isosorbide mononitrate (Imdur, Ismo, Monoket)	Oral	60–120	6–8 Hours
β-Blockers*			
Propranolol	Oral	30	6–8 Hours
Calcium Channel Blockers*			
Verapamil (Calan, Isoptin)	Oral	30	6–8 Hours
Nifedipine (Procardia)	Oral, sublingual	20	3–6 Hours

*For a more complete listing, see Box 12.4.

drugs with either daily or intermittent doses of any nitrate is contraindicated. The combination of a PDE5 inhibitor with any type of nitrate can cause dangerously low blood pressure.

Storage

NTG is degraded by heat moisture and light. NTG should be stored in its original brown glass container and tightly closed because it can be adsorbed by plastic. It should not be refrigerated because condensation of the moisture in the air produces moisture that can reduce the drug's effectiveness.

If the original bottle is unopened, NTG is active until the expiration date printed on the bottle (assume average storage conditions). When the bottle is opened, the date opened should be written on the outside of the bottle. It should be discarded after 3 months or in accordance with the expiration date printed on the bottle (whichever date is earlier). The NTG spray is effective until its expiration date is reached because air does not enter the container with use

Various long-acting NTG-like products (see Table 12.3), such as isosorbide dinitrate (eye-soe-SOR-bide dye-NYE-trate) and isosorbide mononitrate, are available for the long-term prophylaxis of anginal attacks. The dose forms available include tablets (swallowed) and topical (ointment and patch) products. With long-term, regular use of such products, tolerance to this effect develops. In fact, no difference can be detected between a long-acting nitrate and placebo when taken without a daily "vacation." To prevent tolerance, prophylactic nitrates should be given with at least an 8- to 12-hour "vacation" every day (often during sleep, depending on symptom pattern). The mononitrate dose form requires a 7-hour "vacation" daily; the first dose is given in the morning, and the second dose is given 7 hours later.

β-Adrenergic Blocking Agents

β-Adrenergic blocking drugs (β-blockers) such as propranolol (proe-PRAN-oh-lole) (Inderal), metoprolol (me-TOE-proe-lole) (Lopressor), and atenolol (a-TEN-oh-lole) (Tenormin), are used in the treatment of angina pectoris as initial therapy, if not contraindicated, in patients with or without a prior MI. These drugs block the β-adrenergic receptor response to catecholamine stimulation, thereby reducing both the chronotropic and inotropic effects. The net result is a reduced myocardial oxygen demand. β-Blockers are effective in reducing both exercise- and stress-induced anginal episodes. They are also recommended because they can help prevent MI and death in patients with documented coronary artery disease. Adverse effects include bradycardia, HF, headache, dry mouth, blurred vision, and unpleasant dreams. β-Adrenergic blocking drugs are discussed in the section on hypertension and in Chapter 4 in the section on sympathetic blockers.

Calcium Channel Blocking Agents

Another group of drugs approved for use in angina pectoris is the calcium channel blockers (CCBs) (see discussion in the section on hypertension). CCBs can be used as initial therapy when β-blockers are contraindicated or their side effects are intolerable or in combination with β-blockers when the initial treatment with β-blockers is unsuccessful or side effects are not acceptable. A few examples are verapamil (ver-AP-a-mil) (Calan, Isoptin), diltiazem (dil-TYE-a-zem) (Cardizem), and nifedipine (nye-FED-i-peen) (Procardia, Adalat) (Table 12.4).

> Vasodilation decreases the work of the heart.

The mechanism of action of CCBs for the treatment of angina pectoris is related to the inhibition of the movement of calcium during the contraction of cardiac and vascular smooth muscle. Vasodilation and a decrease in peripheral resistance result, thereby reducing the work of the heart. Some CCBs decrease myocardial contractility (negative inotropic effect), resulting in reduced cardiac output. Others increase coronary vasodilation. CCBs reduce ischemia and relieve the symptoms of chronic stable angina. The choice of the specific CCB depends on the patient's cardiac disease. Short-acting dihydropyridine CCBs should be avoided.

Ranolazine

Ranolazine is indicated for the treatment of chronic angina alone or in combination with nitrates, β-blockers, CCBs, antiplatelet therapy, lipid-lowering therapy, ACEIs, or ARBs. It can be used alone in patients with contraindications to β-blockers and CCBs. Although it has several pharmacologic activities, its exact mechanism of action is unknown. It does not significantly alter heart rate or blood pressure. It does prolong the QT interval, and caution should be used when it is used in combination with other drugs that increase the QT interval. Ranolazine is generally well tolerated. Adverse effects include dizziness, headache, constipation, and nausea.

TABLE 12.4   Calcium Channel Blocker Subgroups

Subgroup	Example	Mechanism	% Autoregulation	Comments
Diphenylalkylamines	Verapamil (only)	Least selective; affects both cardiac and vascular smooth muscle, vasodilator; direct effect on the myocardium (SA and AV nodes)	10	Inhibits P-450 enzymes
Benzothiazepines	Diltiazem (only)	Less selective; affects both cardiac and vascular smooth muscle, vasodilator; direct effect on myocardium (depresses SA and AV nodes); less negative inotropic effect and better side effect profile than verapamil	2	Inhibits P-450 enzymes
Dihydropyridines	Nifedipine and all others	Selective for vascular smooth muscle myocardium, primarily vasodilation; reflex tachycardia	20	

AV, Atrioventricular; SA, sinoatrial.

Angiotensin-Converting Enzyme Inhibitors

ACEIs are recommended for all people with chronic stable angina who also have hypertension, diabetes mellitus, an LVEF less than 40%, chronic kidney disease, or other vascular disease. Evidence supports the concept that ACEIs have cardioprotective effects that can reduce the incidence of ischemia. ACEIs lower angiotensin II and raise bradykinin levels, possibly leading to reductions in LV and vascular hypertrophy, atherosclerotic progression, plaque rupture, and thrombosis. These hemodynamic changes result in improved myocardial oxygen supply/demand balance.

Angiotensin Receptor Blockers

ARBs are indicated for those patients with chronic stable angina who also have hypertension, diabetes mellitus, an LVEF less than 40%, or chronic kidney disease and who cannot tolerate ACEIs. These agents work much like ACEIs.

Dental Implications

Treatment of an Acute Anginal Attack

Before treating a patient with a history of angina, the dental team should be prepared to treat an acute anginal attack. Before administering NTG for such an attack, however, the dental team should make sure that the patient has not used a PDE5 inhibitor within the past 24 hours. If the patient has used one of these drugs, NTG cannot be given. The best course of action is to immediately contact 911. The patient's personal NTG tablets or spray should be available and placed on the bracket table in case of an acute attack. Long-acting nitrates and topical products are not useful for the treatment of an acute anginal attack. For acute emergencies, the dental office should have a supply of SL NTG (see previous discussion of storage). The patient should be in the seated position before ingesting the NTG. One tablet can be administered at once, followed in 5 minutes by another, and in another 5 minutes by a third tablet. If these tablets do not stop the anginal attack, the patient should be taken to the emergency room. If using the spray, one should make sure that the patient does not inhale while spraying.

Prevention of Anginal Attack

An acute attack of angina may be prevented through pretreatment with either an anxiolytic agent (e.g., benzodiazepine or nitrous oxide [N$_2$O]) or SL NTG. One should make sure that the patient has not used a PDE5 inhibitor within the past 24 hours. If he or she has, then SL NTG cannot be used as prophylaxis against an angina attack.

Anxiolytics. Because anxiety produces stress and causes the heart to work harder, an antianxiety agent, or anxiolytic (benzodiazepine), may be prescribed to allay anxiety and prevent an acute anginal attack. N$_2$O-oxygen (N$_2$O-O$_2$) can also relax an anxious dental patient, and N$_2$O itself produces vasodilation.

Nitroglycerin. Premedicating an anxious dental patient with SL NTG before an anxiety-provoking procedure can reduce the chance of an attack. For example, the patient can be given SL NTG a few minutes before a local anesthetic injection.

Because of NTG's instability, it must be properly stored in the dental office, as previously described, and the expiration date should be checked regularly.

Myocardial Infarction

A patient with symptoms of an anginal attack that is not relieved by SL NTG (1 SL tablet placed under the tongue every 5 minutes for a total of three doses) may be experiencing an MI. If the patient who has not been previously diagnosed as having angina experiences chest pain, he or she should be taken to an emergency room for diagnosis. Occasionally, an anginal attack can proceed to an acute MI. For this reason, the dental team should make sure any patient with an attack that is not relieved by NTG is accompanied by an employee to the hospital emergency room.

ANTIHYPERTENSIVE AGENTS

> The silent killer: hypertension.

Hypertension is the most common cardiovascular disease, affecting some 75 million Americans (34%) and more than 1 billion individuals worldwide. However, based upon the most recent recommendations of the American Heart Association, the percentage of Americans with hypertension will rise to 46%. The most current National Health and Nutrition Examinations Survey (NHANES) for 2011–14, based upon the most current recommendations, reported that the prevalence of hypertension continues to increase with age and is higher among women than men for those over 75 years of age (85% versus 79%). Overall, men have higher prevalence than women (48% versus 43%). The age-adjusted prevalence of hypertension was 45% in non-Hispanic blacks, 38% in non-Hispanics whites, 28% in non-Hispanic Asians, and 26% in Hispanics. Data from the Framingham Heart Study suggested that individuals with normal blood pressure at age 55 years have a 90% lifetime risk for development of hypertension. Statistically, it is likely that many dental patients have hypertension because only 68% of patients with diagnosed hypertension are being treated.

The rise in the number of Americans being diagnosed with hypertension is based upon new scientific guidelines. Anyone with a blood pressure of greater than 130/80 mm Hg is now considered to have hypertension. Previously published guidelines recommended a blood pressure goal of less than 140/90 mm Hg for patients with hypertension and less than 150/90 mm Hg for some patients older than 60 years of age, unless they have chronic kidney disease and/or diabetes. The most current recommendations by the AHA are a blood pressure goal of less than 130/80 mm Hg for all people with diagnosed hypertension regardless of age or presence or absence of chronic kidney disease or diabetes. Normal blood pressure is defined as a systolic pressure less than 120 mm Hg and a diastolic pressure less than 80 mm Hg (120/80 mm Hg). Although the number of people with hypertension will increase based upon the new guidelines, the actual number of patients that will need pharmacologic therapy will not increase significantly. Instead, the guidelines, published in the journal *Hypertension*, emphasize that practitioners need to focus on a healthier lifestyle for their patients.

Most commonly, no symptoms are associated with hypertension, which is therefore called the "silent killer." Complications of hypertension affect organs such as the heart, kidney, and brain as well as the retina. After some damage has occurred, symptoms of malfunction become noticeable.

Eventually, a sustained elevated blood pressure damages the body's organs, so untreated hypertensive patients are more likely to have kidney and heart disease and cardiovascular problems (MI, cerebrovascular accident). Likelihood of these complications is greatly increased with concomitant smoking.

Fortunately, early detection and treatment with drug therapy (Box 12.4) reduces the possibility of damage to vital organs (reduced morbidity) and extends the patient's lifetime (reduced mortality). Only about 50% of those with known hypertension are properly treated. If hypertensive patients are properly treated (blood pressure is normalized), their risk of complications is equal to that of patients without hypertension.

BOX 12.4   Antihypertensive Agents

Diuretics
Thiazide
Bendoflumethiazide (Aprinox)
Chlorothiazide (Diuril)
Hydrochlorothiazide (HCTZ, Esidrix)
Methyclothiazide (Enduron)

Thiazide-Like
Chlorthalidone (Hygroton)
Indapamide (Lozol)
Metolazone (Zaroxolyn, Mykrox)

Loop
Bumetanide (Bumex)
Ethacrynic aci (Edecrin)
Furosemide (Lasix)
Torsemide (Demadex)

Potassium-Sparing
Amiloride (Midamor)
Spironolactone (Aldactone)
Triamterene (Dyrenium)
Eplerenone (Inspra)

Angiotensin-Converting Enzyme Inhibitors (ACEIs)
Benazepril (Lotensin)
Captopril (Capoten)
Enalapril (Vasotec)
Fosinopril (Monopril)
Lisinopril (Zestril, Prinivil)
Moexipril (Univasc)
Perindopril (Aceon)
Quinapril (Accupril)
Ramipril (Altace)
Trandolapril (Mavik)

Angiotensin Receptor Blockers (ARBs)
Azilsartan (Edarbi)
Candesartan (Atacand)
Eprosartan (Teveten)
Irbesartan (Avapro)
Losartan (Cozaar)
Olmesartan (Benicar)
Telmisartan (Micardis)
Valsartan (Diovan)
Direct Renin Inhibitor
Aliskiren (Tekturna)

Calcium Channel Blockers (CCBs)
Diltiazem (Cardizem [SR], Dilacor [XR])
Verapamil (Isoptin [SR], Calan [SR])

Dihydropyridines
Amlodipine (Norvasc, generic)
Felodipine (Generic)
Isradipine (Generic)
Nicardipine (Generic)
Nifedipine Extended Release (Procardia XL, Adalat CC, Generic)
Nisoldipine (Sular)
Nondihydropyridines

Diltiazem, extended release (Cardizem LA, Matzim LA, Taztia XT, Tiazac, generic)
Diltiazem, continuous delivery (Cardizem CD, Cartia XT, generic)
Diltiazem, degradable (Dilt-XR, generic)
Verapamil (Calan, generic)
Verapamil, long acting (Calan SR)

β-Adrenergic Blocking Agents
Atenolol (Tenormin)
Betaxolol (Kerlone)
Bisoprolol (Zebeta)
Metoprolol (Lopressor)
Metoprolol (Toprol-XL)
Nadolol (Corgard)
Propranolol (Inderal [LA])
Timolol (Generic)

β-Blockers With Intrinsic Sympathomimetic Activity
Acebutolol (Sectral)
Penbutolol (Levatol)
Pindolol (Generic)

β-Blockers With α-Blocking Activity
Carvedilol (Coreg, generic)
Carvedilol, extended release (Coreg CR)
Labetalol (Generic)
β-Blocker With Nitric Oxide-Mediated Vasodilating Activity
Nebivolol (Bystolic)

α-Adrenergic Blocking Agents
Doxazosin (Cardura [XL])
Prazosin (Minipress)
Terazosin (Hytrin)

Central α-Adrenergic Agonists
Clonidine (Catapres [TTS])
Guanfacine (Tenex)
Methyldopa (Aldomet)

Vasodilators (Direct)
Hydralazine (Apresoline)
Minoxidil (Loniten)

Peripheral Adrenergic Neuron Antagonist
Reserpine

Selected Combinations
Thiazides + Potassium-Sparing Diuretics
Hydrochlorothiazide/spironolactone (Aldactazide)
Hydrochlorothiazide/triamterene (Dyazide, Maxzide)
Hydrochlorothiazide/amiloride (Moduretic)

β-Blockers + Diuretics
Metoprolol/hydrochlorothiazide (Lopressor HCT)
Nadolol/bendroflumethiazide (Corzide)

ACEIs + HCTZ
Benazepril/hydrochlorothiazide (Lotensin HCT)
Captopril/hydrochlorothiazide (Capozide)
Enalapril/hydrochlorothiazide (Vaseretic)
Fosinopril/hydrochlorothiazide (generic)

BOX 12.4   Antihypertensive Agents—cont'd

Lisinopril/hydrochlorothiazide (Prinzide, Zestoretic)
Moexipril/hydrochlorothiazide (Uniretic)
Quinapril/hydrochlorothiazide (Accuretic)

ARBs and Diuretics
Azilsartan/chlorthalidone (Edarbyclor)
Candesartan/hydrochlorothiazide (Atacand HCT)
Irbesartan/hydrochlorothiazide (Avalide)
Losartan/hydrochlorothiazide (Hyzaar)
Olmesartan/hydrochlorothiazide (Benicar HCT)
Telmisartan/hydrochlorothiazide (Micardis HCT)
Valsartan/hydrochlorothiazide (Diovan HCT)

Direct Renin Inhibitor and HCTZ
Aliskiren/hydrochlorothiazide (Tekurna HCT)

CCB + ACEIs
Amlodipine/benazepril (Lotrel)
Verapamil extended-release/trandolapril (Tarka)

CCB + ARBs
Amlodipine/telmisartan (Twynsta)
Amlodipine/valsartan (Exforge)
Amlodipine/olmesartan (Azor)

CCG + Direct Renin Inhibitor
Amlodipine/aliskiren (Tekamlo)

Direct Vasodilator + Diuretic
Hydralazine/hydrochlorothiazide (Hydra-Zide)
Central α-Adrenergic Agonist + Diuretic
Clonidine/chlorthalidone (Clorpres)

Triple-Drug Combinations
Aliskiren/amlodipine/hydrochlorothiazide (Amturnide)
Valsartan/amlodipine/hydrochlorothiazide (Exforge HCT)
Olmesartan/amlodipine/hydrochlorothiazide (Tribenzor)

Hypertension is generally divided into the following categories according to the cause or progression of the disease:

Essential hypertension: Approximately 90% to 95% of patients diagnosed with hypertension have essential, idiopathic, or primary hypertension, which tends to be familial and may be the result of the interaction between environmental and genetic factors. These terms all stand for hypertension from an unknown cause. Antihypertensive agents are used to control the hypertension in this group of patients. Essential hypertension is divided into stages, depending on the severity of the elevation of the blood pressure (Table 12.5). This is the form usually seen in the dental office.

Secondary hypertension (identifiable causes): In approximately 10% of hypertensive patients, the cause can be identified and associated with (secondary to) a specific disease process involving the endocrine or renal system. For example, renal hypertension can result from a narrowed renal artery. Drug therapy, such as with steroids, nonsteroidal antiinflammatory drugs (NSAIDs), birth control pills, decongestants, and tricyclic antidepressants, can also produce secondary hypertension. Secondary hypertension can be eliminated by removing the cause—that is, by surgically correcting the renal artery narrowing or discontinuing the offending drug.

Malignant hypertension: In the third group of hypertensive patients, those with malignant hypertension, blood pressures are very high or rapidly rising and there is usually evidence of retinal and renal damage. The small number of patients in this group must be treated aggressively with antihypertensive agents. Malignant hypertension can develop in about 5% of patients with primary or secondary hypertension.

Patient Evaluation

The evaluation of patients with hypertension has three objectives: to assess lifestyle and identify other cardiovascular risk factors or concomitant disorders that may affect prognosis and treatment, to reveal identifiable causes of hypertension, and to assess for the presence or absence of target-organ damage or cardiovascular disease.

Treatment of Hypertension

Pharmacologic management of hypertension involves a process shown in the algorithm in Fig. 12.4, as diastolic pressures become greater than 80 mm Hg. The principle of hypertension treatment is to treat blood

TABLE 12.5   Classification of Blood Pressure

Category	Systolic (mm Hg)		Diastolic (mm Hg)
Normal	<120	and	<80
Elevated blood pressure	120–129	and	<80
Hypertension:			
Stage 1	130–139	or	80–89
Stage 2	≥140	or	≥90

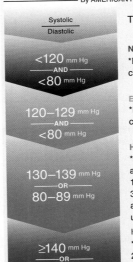

KNOW YOUR BLOOD PRESSURE
–AND WHAT TO DO ABOUT IT
— By AMERICAN HEART ASSOCIATION NEWS —

Systolic / Diastolic

<120 mm Hg —AND— **<80** mm Hg

120–129 mm Hg —AND— **<80** mm Hg

130–139 mm Hg —OR— **80–89** mm Hg

≥140 mm Hg —OR— **≥90** mm Hg

The newest guidelines for hypertension:

NORMAL BLOOD PRESSURE
*Recommendations: Healthy lifestyle choices and yearly checks.

ELEVATED BLOOD PRESSURE
*Recommendations: Healthy lifestyle changes, reassessed in 3–6 months.

HIGH BLOOD PRESSURE/ STAGE 1
*Recommendations: 10-year heart disease and stroke risk assessment. If less than 10% risk, lifestyle changes, reassessed in 3–6 months. If higher, lifestyle changes ane medication with monthly follow-ups until BP controlled.

HIGH BLOOD PRESSURE/ STAGE 2
*Recommendations: Lifestyle changes and 2 different classes of medicine, with monthly follow-ups until BP controlled.

*Individual recommendations need to come from your doctor.
Source: American Heart Association's Journal Hypertension
Published Nov. 13, 2017

Fig. 12.4 Guidelines for blood pressure and hypertension. Reprinted with permission Hypertension. 2017;HYP.0000000000000065 © 2017 American Heart Association, Inc.

pressures less than 130/80 mm Hg based upon the most current recommendations of the AHA regardless of the patient's age or the presence or absence of chronic kidney disease or diabetes.

Lifestyle modifications are the mainstay of prehypertension therapy and instituted for elevated blood pressure and both stage 1 and stage 2 hypertension. Lifestyle modifications are encouraged even if the patient's blood pressure is normal. Lifestyle modifications include weight reduction; aerobic physical activity; a diet rich in fruits, vegetables, and low-fat dairy products with reduced content of saturated and total fats; dietary sodium restriction; moderate alcohol consumption; and smoking cessation. If patients with prehypertension present with compelling indications, these indications must be treated.

Initial drug choices: Once the patient has been diagnosed with either stage 1 or stage 2 hypertension, he or she must be further evaluated for any compelling indications (Table 12.6). The choice of antihypertensive therapy is based on the stage of hypertension and the presence or absence of compelling indications (see Table 12.6 and Fig. 12.4). Many people require two drugs to control the blood pressure. With a combination of agents, the side effects of individual agents are less and the high blood pressure can be normalized. If compelling indications (for a different disease state) are present, they must be treated, and other antihypertensive drugs can be added as needed.

Table 12.7 lists some common antihypertensive agents and their mechanisms of action and side effects, whereas Fig. 12.5 reviews sites and mechanisms of action. The groups recommended for initial use include diuretics, β-blockers, ACEIs, CCBs, and ARBs (Box 12.5). Antihypertensive products may contain one drug or may be combinations of drugs (see Box 12.4). If the patient's blood pressure is not at goal, current drug dosages can be optimized or drugs can be added until goal pressure is achieved.

Regardless of medication use, the blood pressure of each hypertensive patient seen in the dental office should be measured and recorded. Only by recording successive blood pressures for an individual patient can the patient's blood pressure control be evaluated and any abnormality for a particular patient noted. In addition, because control of blood pressure is so important to patient health, patients should be questioned about compliance with antihypertensive medication. Abrupt discontinuation of some blood pressure medicines may result in rebound hypertension—the blood pressure rises to a higher level than it was before treatment. Concern for patient total health is based on the fact that it is of little use for a patient to have clean and perfectly restored teeth if the patient has a fatal MI resulting from untreated hypertension.

Diuretic Agents

The three major types of diuretics are thiazides (thiazide-like), loop, and potassium (K) sparing (Fig. 12.6).

Thiazide Diuretics

The thiazide diuretics are among the agents most commonly used for the treatment of hypertension. Hydrochlorothiazide (hye-droe-klor-oh-THYE-a-zide) (HCTZ) is the most commonly used thiazide. The thiazide-like agent chlorthalidone (klor-THAL-i-doan) (Hygroton), however, is 1.5 to 2 times more potent than HCTZ and has a longer duration of action; it continues through the night (these drugs are taken in the morning because they cause dieresis). Many patients with stage 1 hypertension are treated solely with HCTZ. When other antihypertensive drugs are used, they are often combined with thiazides. Although a large number of thiazide and thiazide-like diuretics are currently available, these agents all have essentially the same pharmacologic effects. Even thiazide-like agents, such as chlorthalidone, act by a similar mechanism, interfering with the sodium reabsorption in the distal tubule.

TABLE 12.6   Compelling Indications for Drug Classes

Compelling Indication	Angiotensin-Converting Enzyme Inhibitors	Diuretics (Thiazide)	Angiotensin Receptor Blockers	Calcium Channel Blockers	β-Blockers	Aldosterone Antagonists
Heart failure	×	×	×		×	×
Post-myocardial infarction	×		×		×	×
High cardiovascular risk	×	×	×	×	×	
Diabetes	×	×	×	×	×	
Chronic kidney disease	×		×			
Recurrent stroke prevention	×	×	×			

TABLE 12.7   Selected Antihypertensives: Mechanisms and Adverse Reactions

Group	Examples	Mechanism	Important Dental Comments
Thiazides	Hydrochlorothiazide	Inhibit the reabsorption of sodium in the distal convoluted tubules of the kidneys	Hypokalemia
Angiotensin-converting enzyme inhibitors (ACEIs)	Lisinopril	Block conversion of angiotensin I to II (inhibits ACEI activity)	Dry, hacking cough
Angiotensin receptor blockers	Candesartan Irbesartan	Lower blood pressure by blocking the angiotensin II receptor	Loss of taste
Calcium channel blockers	Verapamil Diltiazem Nifedipine	Inhibit calcium ion movement into the cell and lowers blood pressure	Gingival enlargement
β-Blockers	Atenolol Metoprolol	Reduce cardiac output, decreases sympathetic effect to blood vessels (blocks β stimulation), inhibits renin release	

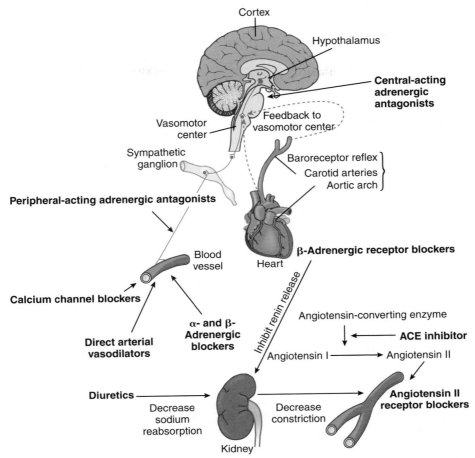

Fig. 12.5 Site and method of action of various antihypertensive drugs. *ACE,* Angiotensin-converting enzyme. (From US Department of Health and Human Services. *Seventh Report of the Joint National Committee on Prevention, Detection, Evaluation, and Treatment of High Blood Pressure* [JNC 7]. [NIH Publication No. 04-5230]. Washington, DC: National Institutes of Health; 2004.)

BOX 12.5 The Big Four Antihypertensive Groups

Diuretics
Angiotensin-converting enzyme inhibitors (ACEIs)
Angiotensin receptor blockers (ARBs)
Calcium channel blockers (CCBs)

Mechanism of action. The exact mechanism by which the thiazide diuretics lower blood pressure has not been determined (Table 12.8). The thiazides initially inhibit the reabsorption of sodium from the distal convoluted tubule and part of the ascending loop of Henle in the kidney. Water and chloride ions passively accompany the sodium, producing diuresis. Because more sodium is presented to the site of sodium-potassium exchange, there is also an increase in potassium excretion. If sodium intake is increased, the potassium loss is exacerbated.

The thiazides' effect on blood pressure may occur through the following process: Initially, they reduce the extracellular fluid volume through their natriuretic action. This volume reduction returns to normal with continued therapy, but a slight decrease in interstitial volume may remain. Other effects of the thiazides that may contribute to their antihypertensive effects include changes in sodium and calcium concentrations and a reduced sensitivity to (this means that drugs reduce the body's response to the SNS which contributes to elevated blood pressure) the SNS.

Adverse reactions. Common adverse reactions associated with thiazides include hypokalemia (secondary to sodium-potassium exchange) and hyperuricemia (inhibits uric acid secretion) (Table 12.9). Hyperglycemia, hyperlipidemia, hypercalcemia (promotion of calcium reabsorption), and anorexia are other side effects. Hyperuricemia is of special concern when the patient has a history of gout. In the patient with diabetes, hyperglycemia—or impaired glucose tolerance—must be managed with diet or insulin alterations. There is a small chance of cross-hypersensitivity (allergy) between the sulfonamide oral medicine (antimicrobial agents) and the thiazides because of the similarity in their structures. The most common oral adverse reaction is xerostomia.

> Nonsteroidal antiinflammatory drugs reduce the antihypertensive effect of hydrochlorothiazide.

The most important dental drug interaction with the thiazides is with the NSAIDs. NSAIDs can reduce the antihypertensive effect of the thiazide diuretics. This interaction takes a few days to develop, and therefore a few doses of an NSAID can safely be used for acute pain control. A longer duration of use should be undertaken only with blood pressure monitoring. Patients often have their own blood pressure monitoring systems at home. Patients are often taking thiazide diuretics for their blood pressure and NSAIDs for arthritis. With long-term use of both agents, their blood pressure medication is adjusted to account for the concurrent use of an NSAID.

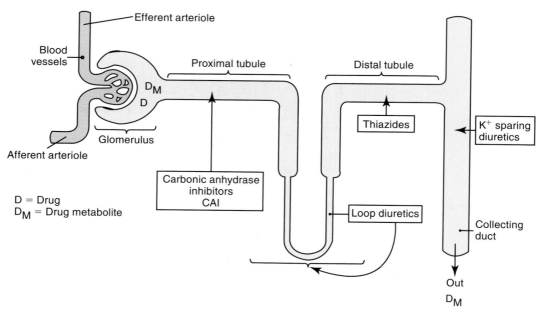

Fig. 12.6 Location of action of diuretics.

TABLE 12.8   Mechanisms of Action of the Antihypertensive Agents

Group	Subgroup, Example	Mechanism	Comments	
Diuretics	Thiazide, loop	Decrease PVR	Counteract Na retention from other agents	
Angiotensin-converting enzyme inhibitors		Reduce PVR; decrease aldosterone secretion	Reduces rate of bradykinin (vasodilator) inactivation	
Angiotensin receptor blockers	Losartan	Vasodilation; decrease aldosterone secretion		
Autonomic nervous system agents	β-Blockers	↓CO, ↓sympathetic outflow from central nervous system, reduces renin release	First-dose syncope; postural hypotension	
	α₁-Adrenergic blockers	Blocks α₁; decreases peripheral vascular resistance; relaxes arterial and venous smooth muscles		
Vasodilators	Hydralazine	Direct vasodilation, arteries, and arterioles	Headache, nausea, sweating, lupus-like syndrome	↓TPR, ↑HR and CO, use with β-blocker and diuretic
	Minoxidil	Arteriole dilation	Na/H₂O retention, reflex	
α₂-Adrenergic agonist, centrally acting	Clonidine	Reduces adrenergic outflow	Sedation, xerostomia	
	α-Methyldopa	Reduces adrenergic outflow		
Calcium channel blockers		Vasodilators; ↓TPR		

CO, Cardiac output; *H₂O,* water; *HR,* heart rate; *Na,* sodium; *PVR,* peripheral vascular resistance; *TPR,* total peripheral resistance; ↑, increase (in); ↓, decrease (in).

TABLE 12.9   Adverse Reactions of the Thiazides

Adverse Reaction
Hypokalemia (↓Potassium)
Hyperglycemia (↑Glucose)
Hyperlipidemia (↑Lipids)
Hyperuricemia (↑Uric acid, ↑calcium, ↓magnesium, ↑sodium)

Thiazides can cause hypokalemia and can therefore sensitize the myocardium which could lead to the development of arrhythmias. The potential for arrhythmias is exacerbated in patients taking digoxin, especially if digitalis toxicity is present. Epinephrine, as contained in local anesthetic mixtures, also has arrhythmogenic potential. Therefore in a dental situation in which a patient is taking thiazide diuretics and digitalis toxicity may be present, the epinephrine dose should be limited to the cardiac dose (see Chapter 9). The thiazide diuretics potentiate the action of the other antihypertensives, increasing the potential for hypotension. This drug interaction is used to therapeutic advantage so that lower doses of each drug are needed to control the patient's blood pressure.

Loop Diuretics

Loop diuretics can be considered the "strong cousins" of the thiazides. Furosemide (fur-OH-se-mide) (Lasix), the most commonly used loop diuretic, is the prototype drug. Furosemide acts on the ascending limb of the loop of Henle and has some effect on the distal tubule. Like thiazides, loop diuretics inhibit the reabsorption of sodium with a concurrent loss of fluids. Furosemide's side effects are similar to those of the thiazides and include hypokalemia and hyperuricemia. However, there is a higher risk of adverse reactions with furosemide because it is much more potent. Furosemide is used in management of hypertensive patients with HF. Loop diuretics can be used when rapid diuresis is required. As occurs with thiazides, NSAIDs can interfere with furosemide's antihypertensive action (see previous discussion on HCTZ).

Potassium-Sparing Diuretics

Potassium-sparing diuretics are "puny" diuretics with "potassium-catching" ability. Individual members of this group have different mechanisms of action, but all have weak diuretic action.

Spironolactone. Spironolactone (speer-on-oh-LAK-tone) (Aldactone) is chemically similar to aldosterone but competitively antagonizes its action (aldosterone antagonist). The result is sodium excretion through diuresis and loss of fluid volume. However, potassium ion is conserved because some of the potassium is reabsorbed at the expense of sodium in the sodium-potassium exchange system in the distal tubule.

Triamterene. Triamterene (trye-AM-ter-een) (Dyrenium), also a potassium-sparing diuretic, interferes with potassium-sodium exchange (active transport) in the distal and cortical collecting tubules and the collecting duct by inhibiting sodium-potassium-adenosine triphosphatase (Na^+-K^+-ATPase). The diuresis and potassium conservation that occurs resembles that of spironolactone.

The potassium-sparing diuretics act at different sites in the kidney from the thiazide diuretics. These two types of diuretics have the opposite effect on potassium loss. A combination product containing both is designed to reduce the amount of potassium loss and prevent hypokalemia. The combination of triamterene and HCTZ (Dyazide, Maxzide) is one of the most often used preparations.

Potassium Salts

K^+: potassium.

Although the potassium salts are not cardiac drugs, lack of potassium caused by the diuretics must be managed, often with potassium supplementation. Potassium is involved in many important physiologic processes, such as nerve impulses; contraction of smooth, cardiac, and skeletal muscles; and maintenance of normal renal function. It is indicated in the treatment of hypokalemia produced by diuretics. It is relatively contraindicated in patients with severe renal impairment or those receiving potassium-sparing diuretics (although there are a few exceptions to this statement). The most common adverse reaction of potassium occurs in the gastrointestinal tract and includes nausea and abdominal discomfort caused by gastrointestinal irritation. Patients taking potassium supplements should be questioned about their use of diuretics, and the possibility of cardiovascular disease should be explored when a drug history is taken. ACEIs should not be given to patients taking potassium supplements because hyperkalemia occurs with ACEIs. Examples of potassium supplements are K-Dur, K-Tab, Micro-K, K-Lyte, K-Lor, and Klor-Con (K, the element symbol for potassium, is used in their names).

Angiotensin-Converting Enzyme Inhibitors

Suffix: -pril.

ACEIs prevent the conversion of angiotensin I to angiotensin II. ACEI drugs are commonly used as antihypertensives. ACEIs are effective in treating hypertension and are well tolerated. They are less effective in black patients and other patients with low renin activity unless they are combined with a thiazide diuretic or CCB. These drugs have been found to prolong survival in patients with HF and low LVEF after a MI, to reduce mortality in patients with HF without low LVEF who are at high risk for adverse cardiovascular events, and to decrease proteinuria in patients with either diabetic or nondiabetic nephropathy. Examples include captopril (KAP-toe-pril) (Capoten), enalapril (e-NAL-a-pril) (Vasotec), and lisinopril (lyse-IN-oh-pril) (Prinivil, Zestril). The names of many ACEIs end in the suffix *-pril* (see Box 12.4).

Mechanism. A complex but important homeostatic mechanism involved in maintaining blood pressure is the renin-angiotensin-aldosterone system. This system adjusts the quantities of sodium and water retained (circulatory volume) and the peripheral resistance (blood vessels). When the kidney senses a decrease in blood pressure or flow, it releases renin, which catalyzes the conversion of angiotensinogen (inactive precursor) to angiotensin I. A second enzyme, ACE, converts angiotensin I to angiotensin II. This is the enzyme that is blocked by ACEIs (Fig. 12.7). Angiotensin II causes vasoconstriction (increasing peripheral vascular resistance) and stimulates the adrenal cortex to release aldosterone, facilitating water retention. When these events are blocked, the blood pressure is lowered. Cardiac output and heart rate are relatively unaffected. ACEIs retard the progression of diabetic nephropathy whether hypertension is present or not.

Adverse reactions. The two most common kinds of adverse reactions associated with the ACEIs are those related to the cardiovascular system and central nervous system (CNS) (Box 12.6).

Cardiovascular effects. Hypotension has produced dizziness, lightheadedness, and fainting. Tachycardia and chest pain have also been noted with use of ACEIs.

Central nervous system effects. CNS side effects include dizziness, insomnia, fatigue, and headache.

Gastrointestinal effects. Nausea, vomiting, and diarrhea can occur.

Respiratory effects. An increase in upper respiratory symptoms, including a dry, hacking cough, can occur. ACEIs can produce a dry cough in up to 10% of patients; this cough can occur within the first week of therapy and disappears after withdrawal of the drug. The cough begins as a tickle in the throat, leading to a dry, nonproductive, and persistent cough that may be worse at night or in the supine position. It occurs because blood levels of bradykinin, a potent stimulator of allergic reactions, including cough, rise when the ACEIs block ACE, the enzyme that normally destroys bradykinin.

Hyperkalemia. ACEIs can cause hyperkalemia, and potassium supplements and potassium-sparing diuretics should not be used with them.

Allergic-Like Reactions. Allergic-like reactions include the following:
- *Angioedema*: Swelling of the extremities, face, lips, mucous membranes, tongue, glottis, or larynx can occur, especially after the initial dose. If airway obstruction is severe, it can impair breathing or swallowing and could be fatal.
- Rash

Other effects. ACEIs should not be given to women who could be pregnant or could become pregnant because of the risk of teratogenicity. Rarely, pancreatitis, with symptoms of abdominal pain and abdominal distention, has occurred. Proteinuria is more common in patients who are taking higher doses or have renal impairment.

Oral adverse reactions. Dysgeusia, an altered sense of taste, is most commonly reported in patients taking captopril (6%). The loss of taste is usually reversible after a few months, even with continued drug treatment.

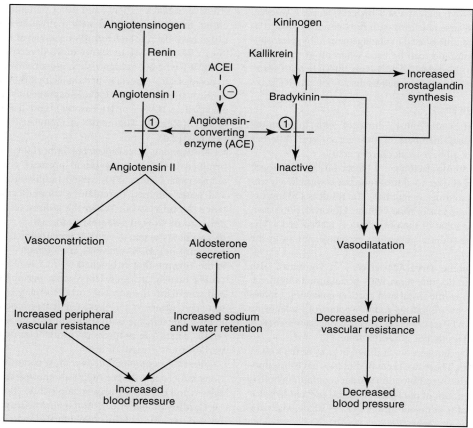

Fig. 12.7 Site of action of an angiotensin-converting enzyme inhibitor (ACEI).

BOX 12.6 Adverse Reactions of Angiotensin-Converting Enzyme Inhibitors

Hypotension
Allergic reactions
Neutropenia
Dry cough
Diabetic neuropathy

Autoimmune oral lesions, such as lichenoid or pemphigoid reactions, may have oral manifestations. This reaction may have a photosensitivity factor.

Dental drug interactions. The antihypertensive effectiveness of ACEIs is reduced by administration of the NSAIDs. A few doses of an NSAID are of little concern, but continuous dosing for several days might result in an increase in the patient's blood pressure. An ACEI may be used alone or in combination with a β-blocker, thiazide diuretic, or CCB. The ACEIs are commonly prescribed, and the dental team will treat many patients taking one or more of these agents.

Angiotensin Receptor Blockers

The ARBs act by attaching to the angiotensin II receptor and blocking the effect of angiotensin II. ARBs end with the suffix *-artan*. Losartan (loe-SAR-tan) (Cozaar) is the prototype. Losartan has a high affinity and selectivity for the type 1 angiotensin II receptor. It blocks the vasoconstrictor and aldosterone-secreting effects of angiotensin II. An increase in plasma renin level follows, thus causing vasodilation, decreased sodium and water retention, and reduction in blood pressure. ARBs are as effective as ACEIs in reducing blood pressure with equal

renoprotective and cardioprotective effects. Like ACEIs, ARBs are less effective in black patients and other patients with low renin activity unless combined with a diuretic or calcium channel blocker.

Adverse Reactions

Because ARBs work by blocking angiotensin II at its receptor, they are more specific than ACEIs and may be expected to cause fewer adverse reactions.

Central nervous system effects. CNS effects can include dizziness, fatigue, insomnia, and headache.

Upper respiratory infections. Upper respiratory infections occur more often in patients taking losartan. A dry cough and nasal congestion can also occur.

Gastrointestinal effects. Losartan can cause diarrhea.

Pain. Both muscle cramps and leg and back pain have been reported with losartan.

Angioedema. Rarely, angioedema can occur.

Teratogenicity. Fetal and neonatal morbidity and death can occur if losartan is administered to a pregnant woman.

Dental Drug Interactions

NSAIDs may antagonize the antihypertensive effect of losartan by inhibiting renal prostaglandin synthesis or by causing sodium and fluid retention.

Direct Renin Inhibitors

Aliskiren (Tekturna) is the first of a new class of drugs approved by the US Food and Drug Administration (FDA) for the treatment of hypertension. It is indicated for oral use either as monotherapy or in combination with other antihypertensive drugs. Aliskiren is a renin inhibitor that works by binding to renin, thereby reducing the levels of angiotensin I, angiotensin II, and aldosterone. Unlike ACEIs and ARBs, aliskiren does not appear to increase plasma renin activity. The most commonly reported adverse reactions include headache, dizziness, fatigue, cough, and upper respiratory tract infections. There have been reports of angioedema of the head and neck and hypotension with use of this agent.

Calcium Channel Blocking Agents

> Suffix: -dipine.

The common CCBs include the drugs verapamil (ver-AP-a-mil) (Isoptin, Calan), nifedipine (nye-FED-i-peen) (Procardia, Adalat), and diltiazem (dil-TYE-a-zem) (Cardizem). Many CCBs end in the suffix *-dipine* (see Box 12.4). These agents are used to treat hypertension and other cardiac conditions, such as arrhythmias and angina.

Mechanism

CCBs inhibit the movement of extracellular calcium ions into cells, including vascular smooth muscle and cardiac cells. The inhibition of calcium ion influx produces vasodilation, which causes coronary vasodilation and reverses vasospasms. By producing systemic vasodilation, the CCBs reduce the afterload on the heart (decrease the total peripheral resistance). These effects are useful in the treatment of both angina pectoris and hypertension.

Today, only long-acting CCBs are used. The short-acting calcium channel blockers were associated with a higher risk of MIs and fatalities when take at higher doses. This association may have been a result of the short-acting CCBs' ability to suddenly and powerfully lower blood pressure. The heart would overcompensate for this sudden drop by dramatically raising blood pressure. Long-acting CCBs have a gradual onset of action, which may allow time for the heart to adjust to the drop in blood pressure.

Pharmacologic Effects

Smooth muscle effects. Vascular smooth muscle is relaxed, and dilation of coronary and peripheral arteries and arterioles occurs, reducing preload. Other smooth muscle is relaxed but to a lesser extent. Orthostatic hypotension is uncommon. Some CCBs, such as nifedipine and its relatives, are more specific for this effect.

Cardiac muscle effects. The effect of the CCBs on the heart may reduce its rate, decrease myocardial contractility (negative inotropic effect), and slow AV nodal conduction. Less specific CCBs have some of both effects.

Adverse Reactions

Most side effects associated with the CCBs are merely extensions of their pharmacologic effects.

Central nervous system effects. CCBs can produce excessive hypotension, which can cause dizziness and lightheadedness. Dental patients taking them should be warned to rise from the dental chair slowly. Headache can occur in up to 10% to 20% of patients taking CCBs.

Gastrointestinal effects. Gastrointestinal side effects include nausea, vomiting, and constipation. Individual CCBs differ in the incidence of these various side effects.

Cardiovascular effects. Because CCBs have a depressant effect on the heart, they can cause bradycardia and edema. Flushing as a result of vasodilation should not be confused with an allergic or adverse reaction. Peripheral edema has been reported.

Other effects. Shortness of breath as a result of pulmonary edema has been reported. Nasal congestion and rhinitis may interfere with the administration of N_2O-O_2 for analgesia and anxiety relief.

Oral Manifestations

Gingival enlargement. The oral manifestations of the CCBs include xerostomia, dysgeusia, and gingival enlargement (formerly called *gingival hyperplasia*). Gingival enlargement has been reported most often with nifedipine, but diltiazem, verapamil, and other CCBs have been implicated.

Nifedipine's manufacturer originally reported the incidence of gingival enlargement as less than 0.5%. Manufacturers of both diltiazem and verapamil have mentioned gingival enlargement as an infrequently reported postmarketing event. Other studies have found the incidence for nifedipine to be 15% to 80%, depending on the criteria used. In one study, the incidence for diltiazem was determined to be 74%. These greatly varying rates of gingival enlargement may be the result of vastly differing criteria used in the studies (e.g., self-report by patients without prompting versus measuring gum changes in all patients). Studies with the highest rates evaluated the incidence of gingival enlargement versus a control group, prospectively.

The gingival enlargement can begin one to several months after the patient starts therapy with a CCB. Some investigators have found no relationship between the dose of the drug and the likelihood of a reaction, whereas others indicate that higher doses produce more severe reactions. Like gingival enlargement due to phenytoin, that due to nifedipine begins as nodular and firm tissue that bleeds easily on probing. The enlargement begins in the anterior labial dental papillae and can proceed eventually to include the lingual and palatal gingiva. The hyperplastic interdental papillae can eventually extend onto crown surfaces, interfering with the ability to chew.

Detailed oral hygiene instructions and more frequent recall appointments to reduce plaque load have been said to reduce this enlargement, but no well-controlled studies have confirmed this suggestion. The patient may be told to maintain scrupulous oral hygiene until more information is available.

On discontinuation of the CCB or switching to a drug outside the CCB group, the gingival enlargement usually reverts to normal tissue and does not reappear. This process may take weeks to months. If drug therapy cannot be discontinued because of the severity of the patient's cardiac condition, a gingivectomy or gingivoplasty may be required. Changing to another CCB does not appear to result in reversal of the enlargement.

Dental Drug Interactions

The CCBs are one of the few antihypertensive groups whose effect is not reduced by the NSAIDs. Both nausea and constipation, side effects of the CCBs, could be additive with the side effects produced by NSAIDs (e.g., ibuprofen) (nausea) and the opioids (e.g., codeine) (constipation).

β-Adrenergic Blocking Agents

β-Adrenergic blockers, one group of adrenergic blocking agents, are used to treat hypertension.

The adrenergic β-receptors are subtyped into β_1- and β_2-receptors (there also may be a β_3-receptor). They have been shown in clinical trials to decrease both the morbidity and mortality related to hypertension.

β_1-Receptor stimulation is associated with an increase in heart rate, cardiac contractility, and AV conduction. Stimulation of β_2-receptors produces vasodilation in skeletal muscles and bronchodilation in the pulmonary tissues. These receptors are initially described in Chapter 4, which discusses the autonomic nervous system drugs.

Many β-adrenergic blocking drugs are approved for use in the management of hypertension (see Box 12.4). Nonselective or nonspecific β-adrenergic receptor blocking drugs, such as propranolol (proe-PRAN-oh-lole), the prototype, block both β_1- and β_2-receptors. In usual doses, the selective, or specific, β-adrenergic receptor blocking drugs, such as metoprolol (me-toe-PROE-lole), block the β_1-receptors more than the β_2-receptors ($\beta_1 > \beta_2$). At larger doses, receptor selectivity disappears. Pindolol (PIN-doe-lole) and acebutolol (a-se-BYOO-toe-lole) have partial agonist activity and cause some β-stimulation while blocking catecholamine action. The selective β-blockers ($β_1 > β_2$) have some advantages in patients who may have preexisting bronchospastic disease, such as asthma, because they do not block the airway's bronchodilating action (not as likely to result in bronchoconstriction). They are less likely to cause a drug interaction with epinephrine.

β-Blockers lower blood pressure primarily by decreasing cardiac output. Other effects that may contribute to their antihypertensive effect include a lowering of plasma renin levels, reductions in plasma volume and venous return, a decrease in sympathetic outflow from the CNS, and a reduction in peripheral resistance. These drugs are often used as, either as single drugs or in combination with other antihypertensive drugs. They are usually recommended for treating hypertension in patients who also have HF, MI, or angina pectoris or suffer from migraine headaches. Large cardiovascular outcome trials have found that β-blockers are less effective than ACEIs, ARBs, and calcium channel blockers in preventing cardiovascular events such as stroke. They are also less effective in black patients.

> Suffix: -olol.

The side effects of the β-blocking agents include bradycardia, mental depression, and decreased sexual ability. The drug can cause symptoms of HF and CNS effects, such as confusion, hallucinations, dizziness, and fatigue, have been reported. Gastrointestinal tract effects include diarrhea, nausea, and vomiting. β-Blockers can produce xerostomia (very mild) or worsen a patient's lipid profile. Exacerbations of asthma, angina, and peripheral vascular disease have been seen.

Dental Drug Interactions

Nonselective β-blockers can have drug interactions with epinephrine. Patients pretreated with a nonspecific β-blocker, such as propranolol, and given epinephrine may have a twofold to fourfold increase in vasopressor response (blood pressure goes up more in patients pretreated with β-blockers than in untreated patients), resulting in hypertension. Via the vagus nerve, the increase in blood pressure triggers a reflex bradycardia.

The amount of caution required with this drug interaction depends on the patient's underlying cardiovascular disease, any potential increase in blood pressure, and the dose of the β-blocker the patient is taking. In patients with cardiovascular disease or higher blood pressure, the amount of epinephrine given to patients taking nonspecific β-blockers should be limited to the cardiac dose unless careful blood pressure monitoring accompanies the use of larger doses. Neither gingival retraction cord containing epinephrine nor 1:50,000 epinephrine should be used in patients with uncontrolled hypertension. Usual dental doses of epinephrine can be given to patients who are taking β-blockers provided that their blood pressure is under control. Box 12.4 separates the β-blockers into those without intrinsic sympathetic activity and those with intrinsic sympathetic intrinsic activity.

α- and β-Adrenergic Blocking Drug

Labetalol (la-BET-a-lole) (Trandate, Normodyne) is a β-adrenergic receptor blocking drug that also has α-receptor blocking activity. In addition to the typical β-blocking effects, labetalol also reduces peripheral resistance through its α-blocking action. Labetalol is used either alone or in combination with diuretics. Side effects and drug interactions are similar to those of the α- and β-adrenergic blockers.

α₁-Adrenergic Blocking Agents

The adrenergic blockers include the α-blockers and β-blockers, which were discussed earlier. Two α-receptor subtypes, $α_1$ and $α_2$, have been identified (see Box 12.4). Doxazosin (doks-AYE-zoe-sin) (Cardura) and terazosin (ter-AY-zoe-sin) (Hytrin) are examples of selective $α_1$-adrenergic blocking drugs.

Mechanism

The $α_1$-receptors, located on postsynaptic receptor tissues, produce vasoconstriction and increase peripheral resistance when stimulated. The $α_1$-blocking agents causes peripheral vasodilation in the arterioles and venules, which decreases peripheral vascular resistance. They have little effect on cardiac output or renal blood flow. They are more effective when combined with diuretics or β-blockers.

$α_1$-Adrenergic blockers result in a reduction in urethral resistance and pressure, bladder outlet resistance, and urinary symptoms. This effect accounts for their use in management of older men with enlarged prostate glands. Surgery can often be avoided in patients whose prostate enlargement is managed by drug therapy. If a man has both hypertension and benign prostatic hypertrophy (BPH), one can "kill two birds with one stone" by treating both disorders with an $α_1$-blocker.

Adverse Reactions

Orthostatic hypotension. Orthostatic hypotension can result in dizziness or syncope. A "first-dose orthostatic hypotensive reaction" sometimes occurs with the initial dose or with changes in the dose of doxazosin. Syncope is more likely to occur when the patient is volume depleted or sodium restricted. Both exercise and alcohol may exaggerate the effect.

Central nervous system effects. $α_1$-Adrenergic blockers can cause CNS depression, producing either drowsiness or excitation and headache. The patient should be told to use caution about doing anything that requires alertness until his or her response to the drug can be evaluated.

Cardiovascular effects. Tachycardia, arrhythmias, and palpitations can occur. Peripheral edema is another side effect related to the cardiovascular system.

Dental Drug Interactions

Nonsteroidal antiinflammatory drugs. NSAIDs, especially indomethacin, can reduce the antihypertensive effect of the $α_1$-blockers (Box 12.7). They produce this effect by inhibiting renal prostaglandin synthesis or causing sodium and fluid retention.

Epinephrine. The sympathomimetics can increase the antihypertensive effects of doxazosin. The $α_1$-blockers prevent the $α_1$-agonist effects (vasoconstriction) of epinephrine, leaving the $β_1$- and $β_2$-agonist effects (vasodilation) to predominate. The combined vasodilation can result in severe hypotension and reflex tachycardia.

Uses

In addition to the treatment of hypertension, both doxazosin and terazosin are indicated for the management of BPH. Difficulty in urination is reduced by taking these agents.

BOX 12.7 **Management of Dental Patients Taking α₁-Blocking Agents**

To avoid orthostatic hypotension dizziness, lightheadedness, or syncope: Raise patient from chair slowly.

To avoid drowsiness or nervousness: Use caution if other sedating drugs are necessary.

Nonsteroidal antiinflammatory drugs (NSAIDs) interfere with the antihypertensive effect of $α_1$-blockers.

Epinephrine (sympathomimetics) should not be used to treat hypotension.

Central α-Adrenergic Agonists

These other antihypertensive agents are used less than those previously described because they generally have more or less tolerated adverse reactions. Clonidine is used in some patients in whom the previously discussed antihypertensives are ineffective.

Clonidine

Clonidine (KLON-i-deen) (Catapres) is a CNS-mediated (centrally acting) antihypertensive drug. Clonidine reduces peripheral resistance through a CNS-mediated action on the α-receptor. Stimulation of pre-synaptic central α_2-adrenergic receptors results in decreased sympathetic outflow. Thus clonidine reduces heart rate, cardiac output, and total peripheral resistance. It is indicated for the management of essential hypertension and can be administered orally or with a transdermal patch (Catapres-TTS).

Adverse reactions. Adverse effects of clonidine include a high incidence of sedation and dizziness. Rapid elevation of blood pressure has occurred with its abrupt discontinuation. CNS depressants used in dental conscious-sedation techniques may contribute to postural hypotension when used in a patient taking clonidine.

Oral effects. The oral effects of clonidine include a high incidence of xerostomia (40%), parotid gland swelling, and pain. Another side effect is dysgeusia (unpleasant taste), the mechanism of which is unknown but may be related to xerostomia.

Methyldopa

The other centrally acting antihypertensive drug is methyldopa (meth-ill-DOE-pa) (Aldomet). Adverse effects and indications for use are similar to those for clonidine. The centrally acting antihypertensive drugs may be combined with diuretics in essential hypertension management.

Direct Vasodilators

Hydralazine (hye-DRAL-a-zeen) (Apresoline) exerts its antihypertensive effect by acting directly on the arterioles to reduce peripheral resistance (vasodilation). At the same time, a rise in heart rate and output occurs. Propranolol is often administered concurrently to reduce the reflex tachycardia and increase cardiac output. Hydralazine is commonly used in combination with the thiazides or other antihypertensive agents. Both diastolic and systolic blood pressures are reduced proportionately, and there is little orthostatic hypotension. The most commonly reported side effects associated with hydralazine are cardiac arrhythmias, angina, headache, and dizziness. A serious toxic reaction produces symptoms like those of systemic lupus erythematosus (lupus-like reaction).

Peripheral Adrenergic Neuron Antagonist

Originally used as a tranquilizer, reserpine (re-SER-peen) is currently used in low doses as an antihypertensive agent. Like guanethidine, reserpine depletes norepinephrine from the sympathetic nerve endings and can accumulate in the body. Adverse reactions include diarrhea, bad dreams, sedation, and even psychic depression leading to suicide. Reserpine increases the production of stomach acid and aggravates peptic ulcers. It can also cause galactorrhea, breast engorgement, and gynecomastia.

Management of the Dental Patient Taking Antihypertensive Agents

Although the antihypertensive drugs cause a variety of adverse reactions, many of them exert similar actions that can alter dental treatment (Box 12.8). Because the hypertension of patients taking antihypertensive medications may or may not be controlled, the blood pressure of each patient should be measured on each visit to the dental office. Not uncommonly, a patient whose blood pressure is "normal" on one visit might be hypotensive or hypertensive on a subsequent visit.

> **BOX 12.8 Management of the Dental Patient Taking Antihypertensives**
>
> Check for xerostomia and its management.
> If patient is taking a calcium channel blocker (CCB), check for gingival enlargement.
> Check blood pressure before each appointment.
> Avoid dental agents that add to side effects, such as opioids (sedation and constipation).
> If patient is taking a diuretic, check for symptoms of hypokalemia, which may exacerbate arrhythmias from epinephrine.
> If patient is taking an angiotensin-converting enzyme inhibitor (ACEI), check for symptoms of neutropenia.

Adverse Reactions

Xerostomia. Dry mouth is an adverse reaction associated with several of the antihypertensives. If the dental health care worker notices this effect, it is imperative to discuss with the patient the methods used to alleviate this discomfort.

Dysgeusia. With some antihypertensives, an altered sense of taste may occur, which may be related to xerostomia.

Gingival enlargement. CCBs have the ability to produce gingival enlargement. Meticulous oral hygiene and frequent recall appointments may minimize this effect.

Orthostatic hypotension. When a patient has been in a supine position and suddenly rises to an upright position, a sudden drop in blood pressure may occur. This side effect is called *orthostatic hypotension*. Patients taking antihypertensive agents who have been supine for some time should be slowly raised from that position. They should dangle their legs over the side of the chair or bed and wiggle them before rising to the standing position. The patient should be supported for a few steps to prevent syncope. Guanethidine causes this problem often; other agents produce variable amounts of orthostatic hypotension.

Constipation. Some antihypertensive agents (e.g., verapamil) can cause constipation, which could be additive with the constipation produced by the opioids. An increase in dietary fiber, a bulk laxative, or a stool softener may be considered if an opioid is prescribed for a patient receiving a constipation-producing antihypertensive medication.

Central nervous system sedation. Several antihypertensives (β-blockers, methyldopa) can produce sedation, which is additive to effects of other CNS depressants such as opioids or benzodiazepines.

ANTIHYPERLIPIDEMIC AGENTS

> LDL: bad cholesterol.
> HDL: good cholesterol.

Hyperlipidemia and hyperlipoproteinemia are elevations of plasma lipid concentrations above accepted normal values. These metabolic disorders include elevations in cholesterol and/or triglycerides and are associated with the development of arteriosclerosis, although the exact correlation is unknown. Many different types of hyperlipoproteinemias result in elevations of chylomicrons, very-low-density lipoproteins (VLDLs), low-density lipoproteins (LDLs), or combinations of these.

Foam cells in the actual blood vessel, which are more prevalent in uncontrolled diabetes, become filled with cholesterol esters. Accumulation of these esters leads to deposition of lipids in the arteries. Collagen and fibrin also accumulate, occluding the vessels. Atherosclerosis can lead to coronary artery disease, MI, and cerebral arterial disease. The endothelium over the plaques activates platelets,

150

leading to the formation of thrombi and clinical symptoms. Additional risk factors for development of complications include untreated hypertension, smoking, obesity, and alcohol use.

Cholesterol and other plasma lipids are transported in the blood in the form of protein complexes (lipoproteins) to make them more soluble in plasma. LDL-Cs are referred to as "bad cholesterol" because they deposit excess cholesterol in artery walls and are considered the most dangerous. High-density lipoproteins (HDL-Cs) are referred to as "good cholesterol" because they have the lowest cholesterol content and are considered beneficial (they carry cholesterol away from the blood vessels).

The newest guidelines from the ACC/AHA no longer recommend using specific cholesterol targets to determine treatment for patients with elevated cholesterol values. Fig. 12.8 reviews the newest recommendations. The focus is no longer on cholesterol numbers but on the patient's estimated 10-year atherosclerotic cardiovascular disease risk. HMG CoA (3-hydroxy-3-methylglutaryl coenzyme A) reductase inhibitors (statins) are the drugs of first choice for treating patients with atherosclerotic

cardiovascular disease, as recommended by the ACC/AHA. Lifestyle modifications, including adhering to a heart healthy diet, getting regular exercise, avoiding tobacco products, and maintaining a healthy weight, remain a critical component of lowering lipid levels and should be used in conjunction with cholesterol-lowering drugs (Table 12.10).

3-Hydroxy-3-Methylglutaryl Coenzyme A Reductase Inhibitors

Suffix: -statins.

The HMG CoA reductase inhibitors (statins) are the first choice of therapy for most patients with atherosclerotic heart disease and elevated cholesterol values and are further categorized as being of high or moderate intensity. They are often referred to as the "statins" because their generic names end in that suffix. Statins can also be used

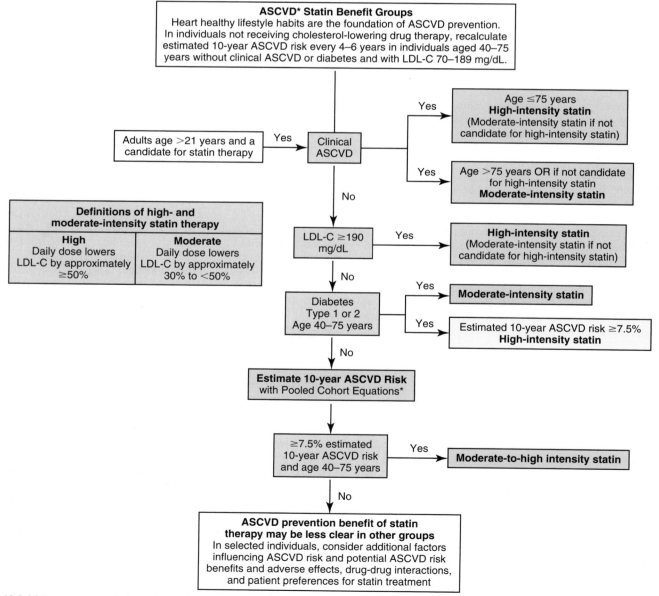

Fig. 12.8 Major recommendations for statin therapy for ASCVD prevention. Reprinted with permission Circulation. 2014;129:S1–S45 © 2014 American Heart Association, Inc.
*Atherosclerotic Coronary Vascular Disease.

TABLE 12.10   Effect of Antihyperlipidemic Agents on Serum Lipids

Type of Agent	EFFECT(S)				
	Chol	TGD	VLDL-C	LDL-C	HDL-C
HMG CoA Reductase Inhibitors ("Statins")					
Atorvastatin (Lipitor)	–	–	–	–	+
Fluvastatin (Lescol)	–	–	–	–	+
Lovastatin (Mevacor)	–	–	–	–	+
Pitavastatin (Livalo)					+
Pravastatin (Pravachol)	–	–	–	–	+
Rosuvastatin (Crestor)					+
Simvastatin (Zocor)	–	–	–	–	+
Bile Acid Sequestrants					
Cholestyramine (Questran, Prevalite)	–	±	±	–	+ (slight)
Colestipol (Colestid)	–	±	±	–	+ (slight)
Colesevelam (Welchol)					
Cholesterol Absorption Inhibitor					
Ezetimibe (Zetia)	–	–	–	–	+ (slight)
Statin Combination Products					
Ezetimibe/simvastatin (Vytorin)	–	–	–	–	+
Ezetimibe/atorvastatin (Liptruzel)	–	–	–	–	+
Niacin ER/Lovastatin (Advicor)	–	–	–	–	+
Niacin ER/simvastatin (Vytorin)	–	–	–	–	+
Niacin					
Niacin immediate-release over-the-counter	–	–	–	–	+
Niacin extended-release (Niaspan)	–	–	–	–	+
Niacin sustained-release (Slo-Niacin)	–	–	–	–	+
Fibrates					
Fenofibrate (Lipidil-DSC, TriCor)	–	–	–	–	+
Gemfibrozil (Lopid)	–	–	–	–	+
Fenofibric acid (Trilipix)				–	+
PCSK9 Inhibitors					
Alirocumab (Praluent)				–	
Evolocumab (Repatha)				–	
Fish Oil Capsules					
Iicosapentyl ethyl (Vascepa)	–	+	–	–	–
Omega-3 fatty acid (Lovaza)	–	+	–	–	–

Chol, Cholesterol; *HDL-C*, high-density lipoprotein cholesterol; *HMG CoA*, 3-hydroxy-3-methylglutaryl coenzyme A; *LDL-C*, low-density lipoprotein cholesterol; *TGD*, triglycerides; *VLDL-C*, very-low-density lipoprotein cholesterol; +, increases levels; –, decreases levels; ±, no change.

in combination with fenofibrate, niacin, colesevelam, or omega-3-fatty acids to lower triglycerides and increase HDLs in addition to lowering LDLs. The side effect profile of the statins is more desirable than that any of the other drugs used to treat hyperlipidemias. However, their use is contraindicated in women who are pregnant or nursing. They are assigned to FDA Pregnancy Category X.

Lovastatin (LOE-va-sta-tin) (Mevacor) was the first agent in this group. The statins lower cholesterol levels by inhibiting HMG CoA reductase, the rate-limiting enzyme in cholesterol synthesis. They may work because they are structural analogs of HMG CoA reductase and thereby inhibit that enzyme. Another possible mechanism of the HMG CoA reductase inhibitors may relate to the increase in the number of LDL receptors that occurs.

Adverse Effects

Adverse effects of HMG CoA reductase inhibitors include gastrointestinal complaints such as stomachache, constipation, diarrhea, and gas. Other side effects are myositis, rash, impotence, hepatotoxicity, blurred vision, and lens (in the eye) opacities. Myositis results in complaints of muscle pain. Liver function tests should be performed because of the statins' small potential for hepatotoxicity. These agents can increase the anticoagulant effect of warfarin.

Inhibitors of Intestinal Absorption of Cholesterol

Ezetimibe (Zetia) is approved to treat elevated cholesterol values and low HDL-cholesterol (HDL-C) values. This drug works by inhibiting the intestinal absorption of cholesterol. It can be used alone or in combination with an HMG CoA reductase inhibitor. It currently comes in combination with simvastatin (Vytorin) or atorvastatin (Liptruzet) to treat cholesterol via two different mechanisms of action. Ezetimibe decreases total cholesterol and LDL-C levels and increases HDL-C levels. These fixed-dose combinations lower LDL-C levels more than a statin alone. Side effects include fatigue, abdominal pain, and diarrhea.

Niacin

Niacin (NYE-a-sin) (nicotinic acid) is a B vitamin. In larger doses, niacin has a therapeutic effect. It lowers cholesterol levels by inhibiting the secretion of VLDL-Cs without accumulation of triglycerides in the liver. This reduces LDL synthesis. At these larger doses, niacin commonly produces cutaneous flushing (especially of the face and neck) and a sensation of warmth after each dose. The prostaglandin-mediated flushing is blocked by pretreatment with 81 to 325 mg of aspirin taken one-half hour before niacin is taken or by use of one tablet of ibuprofen daily. This side effect can also be minimized by initiation of therapy with a low dose of niacin with a slow increase over a period of weeks or by niacin ingestion after meals. Increasing the dose of niacin enough to produce a decrease in lipid levels without intolerable adverse effects is challenging. Hyperuricemia can occur and can be treated with allopurinol. Allergic reactions, cholestasis, and hepatotoxicity have been reported.

Dental Implications of Niacin

Hypotension may occur as a result of the vasodilation due to the niacin's effect on blood vessels, especially in patients taking antihypertensives. Such patients should be told to rise from the dental chair slowly to prevent orthostatic hypotension.

Cholestyramine

The bile acid-binding resins—cholestyramine (koe-less-TIR-a-meen) (Questran), colestipol (koe-LES-ti-pole) (Colestid), and colesevelam (Welchol)—lower cholesterol concentrations in the following manner. Cholesterol is a precursor required for the synthesis of the new bile acids. When the resins bind with the bile acids, they produce an insoluble product that is lost through the gastrointestinal tract. The bile acids must be replaced, and formation of new ones uses up cholesterol, thereby reducing cholesterol levels. Adverse reactions relate to the gastrointestinal tract and include constipation and bloating, but serious side effects are infrequent. These drugs are poorly tolerated because of their effects on the gastrointestinal tract and poor taste. Patients often stop using them for these reasons.

Fibric Acid Derivatives

The fibric acid derivatives, gemfibrozil, fenofibrate, and fenofibric acid, are used to treat hyperlipidemias, especially when triglycerides are elevated. These agents work by increasing lipolysis of triglycerides, decreasing lipolysis in adipose tissue, and inhibiting secretion of VLDL-Cs from the liver. They cause fewer gastrointestinal complaints than the bile acid-binding drugs but can promote gallstone formation (cholelithiasis). An altered sense of taste and hyperglycemia have been reported. Hematologic and liver function should be monitored routinely in patients taking fibric acid derivatives. Gemfibrozil and fenofibric acid should not be given with statins because of the increased risk for muscle cramping, myopathy, and rhabdomyolysis. Fenofibrate can be used in combination with statins.

PROPROTEIN CONVERTASE SUBTILISIN/KEXIN TYPE 9 INHIBITORS

Proprotein convertase subtilisin/kexin type 9 (PCSK9) is a protein in the liver that binds to LDL cholesterol receptors. PSCK9 binds to the LDL receptor and degrades it once the LDL particulates are taken from extracellular fluids into cells. As a result, there are fewer LDL receptors to go to the cell surface and pick up more LDL particulates that are then taken to the liver for metabolism. PCSK9 inhibitors are the newest in a class of drugs that have been shown to decrease LDL cholesterol by as much as 60%. These drugs are monoclonal antibodies that bind to and inactivate the PSCK9 protein thereby increasing the amount of LDL cholesterol that is metabolized in the liver.

Two PCSK9 Inhibitors have been approved for use in the United States are alirocumab (Praluent) and evolocumab (Repatha). These drugs are administered subcutaneously via self-administration with a pen device once or twice a month. They can be used in conjunction with HMG CoA reductase inhibitors. These drugs appear to be well tolerated. The most common side effect is injection site reactions. Other side effects reported include signs and symptoms of the common cold and the flu, itching, and allergic reaction.

Fish Oils

Long-chain omega-3 polyunsaturated fatty acids are present in cold water fish, including salmon, and are commercially available in capsules to treat elevated cholesterol values. They can decrease fasting triglyceride concentrations by 20% to 50% by reducing hepatic triglyceride production and increasing triglyceride clearance. Long-term use of fish oils may also raise HDL levels. Fish oil supplements are generally well tolerated. Adverse effects include belching, unpleasant fishy aftertaste, and worsening of glycemic control in diabetic patients.

Dental Implications of Elevated Cholesterol Levels

> Measure blood pressure and heart rate at each appointment.

Patients who take antihyperlipidemic agents are at a higher risk for developing hypertension and coronary artery disease. They also have increased risk for MI and cardiac arrest; dental health care workers should be prepared to handle such emergencies. The patient's blood pressure and heart rate should be measured before each appointment and recorded in the dental chart. If an emergency occurs, it is important to know the preemergency blood pressure and heart rate so that they can be compared with the current measurements. Because gastrointestinal and liver abnormalities are side effects associated with many of these drugs, the patient's ability to tolerate (in terms of side effects) to the agents taken should be determined before dental drugs are prescribed or suggested. The small possibility of liver abnormalities requires laboratory testing for abnormal liver function.

DRUGS THAT AFFECT BLOOD COAGULATION

Anticoagulants

Anticoagulants are drugs that in some way interfere with coagulation. The first anticoagulant was discovered when cows that ingested spoiled sweet clover silage became hemorrhagic. The toxic agent in the clover was found to be dicumarol, and warfarin is a close relative. Warfarin has been used as a rodenticide. When the rats eat the warfarin, they begin to bleed and eventually die. Therapeutically, anticoagulants are administered in an attempt to prevent clotting. Examples of indications for warfarin are after an MI, for thrombophlebitis, or to prevent a stroke. Warfarin is the most important oral anticoagulant and is the one used almost exclusively in therapy.

Hemostasis

Hemostasis is a normal mechanism in the body that is designed to prevent the loss of blood after injury to a blood vessel. The leaking vessel is plugged by a complicated process of clot formation. In the presence of a vascular injury, the entire clotting mechanism is initiated. Thromboplastin, factors V, VII, and X, and calcium ions form prothrombin, thrombin, and, finally, fibrinogen and fibrin. The fibrin, along with vascular spasms, platelets, and red blood cells, quickly forms the clot.

If the blood vessel's interior remains smooth, circulating blood does not clot. However, if internal injury to the vessel occurs and a roughened surface develops, intravascular clotting takes place. This process involves an intrinsic prothrombin activator that includes a platelet factor, factor V, factors VIII through XII, and calcium ions. The prothrombin activator, which was formerly called *thromboplastin,* converts prothrombin to thrombin. Thrombin then converts fibrinogen to fibrin, and clot formation occurs.

Many of the factors required in the clotting process are synthesized in the liver. Prothrombin (II) and factors VII, IX, and X require vitamin K for synthesis. Because warfarin antagonizes vitamin K, it interferes with the synthesis of four clotting factors, for an anticoagulant effect.

In certain diseases, intravascular clots can form. These clots, or thrombi, may break off, forming emboli that lodge in the smaller vessels of major organs, such as the heart, brain, and lungs, producing severe and even fatal thromboembolic disease. Anticoagulant therapy attempts to reduce intravascular clotting and prevent life-threatening situations. Each person's anticoagulant therapy must be adjusted to suit his or her needs. If the dose of the anticoagulant is too large, hemorrhage may occur. If the dose is too small, the danger of embolism remains.

Parenteral Anticoagulants

Heparin

Heparin (HEP-a-rin) is one of the most commonly used anticoagulant agents in hospitalized patients. Because it must be given by injection and cannot be used orally, its outpatient use is essentially nonexistent. Newer heparins, termed *low-molecular-weight heparins,* are being used, but until an oral dose form is developed, their use will be limited. Because its effect begins quickly, heparin is the first anticoagulant given to hospitalized patients with excessive clotting. Patients who might receive heparin are those with MI, stroke (embolism), or thrombophlebitis. When the heparin is started (as soon as possible), warfarin is also begun. Because warfarin's effect has a latent period, the heparin can provide immediate anticoagulant effect while warfarin's effect is building up. The effect of an overdose of heparin is antagonized by protamine sulfate, which immediately reverses its anticoagulant effects.

Low-Molecular-Weight Heparin

Low-molecular weight heparin (LMWH) inhibits factor Xa more than it inhibits thrombin as compared to unfractionated heparin which inhibits thrombin more than factor Xa. It has a longer half-life that permits fewer doses each day and a greater bioavailability that leads to a more predictable anticoagulant response. It is used to prevent or treat venous thromboembolism. Two examples of LMWHs are enoxaparin (Lovenox), dalteparin (Eisai), and they are administered subcutaneously. Enoxaparin is available in an autoinjector dose form which allows for patient self-administration. As with heparin, side effects include bleeding and bruising, especially at the site of injection.

Oral Anticoagulants

Warfarin

Warfarin (WAR-far-in) (Coumadin) is an oral anticoagulant (interferes with coagulation). It blocks γ-carboxylation of glutamate residues in the synthesis of factors VII, IX, and X; prothrombin (II); and endogenous anticoagulant protein C. Instead of the factors, incomplete and inactive molecules are formed that do not function properly. Warfarin also prevents the metabolism of the inactive vitamin K epoxide back to its active form.

Warfarin's pharmacologic effect is delayed when therapy begins and persists when therapy ends. This latent period in the onset of action of warfarin occurs for the following two reasons:

- The blood level of the warfarin accumulates over time until it plateaus or reaches steady state. The maximum effect for one dose occurs after five half-lives (1 half-live is 42 hours): 5×42 hours = 210 hours (or 9 days).
- Endogenous clotting factors II, VII, IX, and X have half-lives that are 60, 6, 24, and 40 hours, respectively. They must be depleted before the anticoagulant effect is maximized.

During reduction of the dose or discontinuation of warfarin therapy, there is a delay in the change in effect because the drug must be metabolized to be inactivated and the clotting factors must be synthesized again.

Monitoring. Warfarin's effect is monitored by means of the international normalized ratio (INR) (Fig. 12.9). The INR is a function of the prothrombin time (PT) of the patient, the control PT, and the international sensitivity index (ISI). The ISI is a function of the potency of the specific (human or rabbit) thromboplastin used in the particular laboratory. The advantage of the INR over the PT ratio is that INR values from any laboratory in the world can be compared, whereas the PT ratio varies among laboratories.

The therapeutic target INR (number at which the provider is trying to keep the patient's INR) for most indications, such as thrombophlebitis and AF, is between 2 and 3. For patients with a prosthetic heart valve, the target INR is between 2.5 and 3.5. The INR can range from 1 (INR without drug effect) to 4, although with overdose it can reach higher levels.

Because warfarin is orally effective and less expensive than heparin, it is used for the long-term treatment of thromboembolic diseases such as thrombophlebitis and MI.

Adverse reactions. The most common adverse effects associated with the warfarin are various forms of bleeding, including hemorrhage. Because of its narrow therapeutic index and because of numerous drug interactions, serious reactions can easily occur. One should look for petechial hemorrhages in the oral cavity. Ecchymoses can occur, even without concomitant trauma. With mild trauma, these effects may be seen in the oral cavity. Studies comparing the effects of lower and higher doses of warfarin in clot prevention found no advantage in use of higher doses but did find an increase in adverse reactions. Dosing of warfarin is now titrated to a lower INR than in the past.

Aspirin. The most serious drug interaction of warfarin is with aspirin (Table 12.11). Patients taking warfarin should not be given aspirin or aspirin-containing products ("cold preparations") because bleeding episodes or fatal hemorrhages can result. Aspirin interacts with warfarin in several ways. First, aspirin causes hypoprothrombinemia and alters platelet adhesiveness (see Chapter 5). These effects in themselves reduce clotting ability. Aspirin can also irritate the gastrointestinal tract, which might bleed more in a patient taking warfarin.

$$INR = \left[\frac{PT_{patient}}{PT_{control}} \right]^{ISI}$$

Fig. 12.9 The formula for the international normalized ratio *(INR)*. *ISI,* International sensitivity index; *PT,* prothrombin time.

TABLE 12.11   Drug Interactions Between Nonsteroidal Antiinflammatory Drugs and Warfarin

Severity	NSAID Examples
Major	Aspirin
Moderate	Indomethacin
	Meclofenamate
	Piroxicam
	Sulindac
Minor	Diclofenac
	Fenoprofen
	Ibuprofen
	Naproxen
	Acetaminophen (small)
None	Nonacetylated salicylates

NSAID, Nonsteroidal antiinflammatory drug.

TABLE 12.12   Drug Interactions Between Warfarin and Antiinfectives

Most	Metronidazole
	Erythromycin
	Ketoconazole (-azole antifungals)
	Cephalosporins
Some	Tetracycline
	Doxycycline
	Penicillin, ampicillin, amoxicillin, dicloxacillin
	Quinolones
Least	Clindamycin

BOX 12.9   Management of the Dental Patient Taking Warfarin (Coumadin)

Avoid aspirin and aspirin-containing compounds; acetaminophen and opioids can be used.

Oral hygiene with subgingival calculus removal can produce bleeding (oozing); use local pressure.

Determine underlying disease of patient.

Patient may have atrial fibrillation.

Patient should be free of infection before scaling/root planing is performed.

Some suggest prophylactic antibiotics after surgery.

Check with patient to ensure healing.

Another factor in the aspirin-warfarin interaction is related to protein binding of drugs. Warfarin is more than 99% bound to plasma proteins and about 1% free drug. The bound drug is merely a reservoir for the drug. Only the free drug (<1%) exerts the pharmacologic effect, decreased clotting. Because warfarin and aspirin compete for the same plasma protein-binding site, aspirin displaces the bound warfarin, thereby increasing the proportion of free (unbound) warfarin and hence potentiating its activity. Even a small increase in free warfarin can lead to a large increase in effect, leading to dire consequences, including hemorrhage. If an NSAID is to be used in a patient taking warfarin, ibuprofen or naproxen should be prescribed. These agents have only a minor interaction with warfarin, and a few doses can be given to the patient with an INR within the therapeutic target.

Acetaminophen. Acetaminophen and its effect on warfarin were prospectively analyzed. Hylek and colleagues (1998) studied patients taking warfarin in an attempt to identify factors that were associated with an INR above 6 (therapeutic INR = 2 to 3.5). A statistically significant association was found between acetaminophen use and the abnormal INR elevation. With higher doses of acetaminophen (9 g/week), there was a 10-fold increase in the likelihood of an abnormal INR. Whether there is a causal relationship between acetaminophen use and warfarin, toxicity has not been proven. Managing patients taking warfarin who need analgesics may require more frequent monitoring of the INR, especially with intermittent use of such agents.

Antibiotics. Antibiotics can also potentiate the effect of warfarin. Antibiotics reduce the bacterial flora in the gastrointestinal tract that normally synthesize vitamin K. This results in a decrease in the amount of vitamin K absorbed. Because warfarin also inhibits vitamin K-dependent factors, there is an added anticoagulant effect. If an antibiotic is to be used with warfarin, clindamycin has no effect; doxycycline, tetracycline, and amoxicillin have small effect; and erythromycin and metronidazole have the greatest effect in altering warfarin's anticoagulant action (Table 12.12). If the antibiotic is used for prophylaxis before a dental procedure (one dose), the interaction would not have a chance to develop.

Other agents. Induction of the microsomal enzymes increases warfarin's metabolism and reduces its effect. Phenobarbital induces the liver microsomal enzymes that would normally destroy the anticoagulant. Alcohol's effect on warfarin depends on the pattern of alcohol use. With chronic alcohol ingestion, the metabolism of warfarin is stimulated. Acute alcohol intoxication inhibits the metabolism of warfarin. Other agents that inhibit the metabolism of warfarin include cimetidine, disulfiram, and metronidazole.

Management of the dental patient taking warfarin. Box 12.9 summarizes the management of dental patients taking warfarin.

Most dental procedures require no change in dose of warfarin.

Bleeding. Historically, it was recommended that a patient taking warfarin reduce the dose or stop warfarin temporarily just prior to a dental procedure because of the increased risk for prolonged bleeding. However, according to current recommendations, based on data from a systemic review and meta-analysis of the literature, it is not necessary to reduce or discontinue therapy prior to dental therapy. Patients are at higher risk for clots, which could lead to a thromboembolism, a possibility that outweighs the consequences of prolonged bleeding, which can be controlled by local measures.

Analgesics. Aspirin and aspirin-containing products are absolutely contraindicated in patients taking warfarin unless the patient is taking one aspirin tablet daily for its anticoagulant effect. In this case, monitoring of warfarin effect is performed while the patient is taking aspirin. Acetaminophen or any opioid alone or together may be substituted if analgesia is desired. A few doses of ibuprofen or naproxen may be safely used if there is no other contraindication to their use.

Factor Xa Inhibitors

Rivaroxaban (Xarelto), apixaban (Eliquis) and edoxaban (Savaysa) are factor Xa inhibitors that prevent coagulation by selectively blocking the active site of factor Xa and do not require a cofactor (antithrombin III) for activity. Activation of factor X to factor Xa plays a central role in the coagulation cascade. All three drugs are indicated to reduce the risk of stroke and systemic embolism in patients with nonvalvular AF. Rivaroxaban and edoxaban are also indicated for the treatment of deep vein thrombosis (DVT) and pulmonary embolism (PE) and for the reduction in the risk of recurrence of DVT and PE. Rivaroxaban is also indicated for the prophylaxis of DVT that may lead to PE in patients undergoing hip or knee joint replacement. A systematic review of the literature has demonstrated that the treatment benefits with these drugs in comparison with warfarin are small and vary according to the control achieved by warfarin therapy. Patients already taking warfarin with excellent INR values may have little to gain by switching to a newer agent. The most common side effect associated with these drugs is an increased risk for bleeding, and they have the potential to cause serious, potentially fatal bleeding. As a result, the patient may be at an increased risk for bleeding during a dental appointment. In May of 2018, the Food and Drug Administration approved the use of the first Xa factor inhibitor antidote for the drugs rivaroxaban (Xarelto) and apixaban (Eliquis) when anticoagulation reversal is needed in life-threating or uncontrolled bleeding. An antidote still does not exist for edoxaban (Savaysa). Unlike warfarin, monitoring is not required. Aspirin and NSAIDs increase the patient's risk for bleeding if taken with the factor XA inhibitors (Box 12.10).

Direct Thrombin Inhibitor

Dabigatran (Pradaxa) is a direct thrombin inhibitor that is indicated for the prevention of stroke and systemic embolism in patients with nonvalvular AF. Thrombin enables the conversion of fibrinogen to fibrin during the coagulation cascade that results in the formation of the clot or thrombus. This drug directly prevents the clot from forming. The most common side effects are gastrointestinal effects and an increased risk for bleeding. Bleeding can be serious. As a result the patient is at increased risk for prolonged bleeding during a dental appointment. As with the factor XA inhibitors, a systematic review of the literature has demonstrated that the treatment benefits with this drug in comparison with warfarin is small. Patients already taking warfarin with excellent INR values may have little to gain by switching to a newer agent. Idarucizumab (Praxibind) is the only FDA-approved treatment to reverse the blood thinning effects of dabigatran in emergency situations. Aspirin and NSAIDs increase the patient's risk for bleeding if taken with this drug (see Box 12.10).

THIENOPYRIDINES

Clopidogrel

The drug clopidogrel (Plavix) is an inhibitor of adenosine diphosphate (ADP)-induced platelet aggregation that causes prolonged bleeding time. Clopidogrel is indicated for patients with recent history of MI or stroke, established peripheral arterial disease, or acute coronary artery syndrome. Its major side effects include thrombotic thrombocytopenic purpura (TTP) and increased bleeding. TTP can occur within as little as 2 weeks of the beginning of therapy. TTP is characterized by **thrombocytopenia** seen on peripheral smear, neurologic findings, renal dysfunction, and fever. It does not alter PT or INR values.

Clopidogrel can be taken with or without food. Patients taking this drug should be carefully managed in the dental office because of the risk for increased bleeding. The patient who has experienced excessive bleeding in the past should discontinue clopidogrel 5 days prior

to dental work or surgery. The patient's physician should be consulted before the patient discontinues clopidogrel therapy. NSAIDs should be avoided because of the risk for gastrointestinal bleeding. Aspirin use should also be avoided. Patients may be taking a combination of clopidogrel and aspirin to treat acute coronary syndrome. This should only be done under a doctor's supervision. NSAID use should especially be avoided in these patients.

Ticlopidine

The drug ticlopidine (tye-KLOE-pi-deen) is an irreversible inhibitor of ADP-induced platelet aggregation that causes prolonged bleeding time. Ticlopidine is indicated to decrease that chances of thrombotic stroke in patients with previous stroke. It is used in patients who are intolerant of aspirin. Its major side effect, neutropenia, is monitored by appropriate blood tests. An increase in infections could signal neutropenia. It does not alter the PT or INR values.

Ticlopidine is taken with food because it can cause diarrhea, nausea, and vomiting. Patients taking ticlopidine have increased bleeding after trauma or surgery. It takes 10 to 14 days to eliminate the bleeding effect. Bleeding can lead to ecchymoses, epistaxis, and perioperative bleeding. For emergency surgery, injectable methylprednisolone can reverse the prolonged bleeding to normal in a few hours. NSAIDs should be avoided because gastrointestinal bleeding can result from the combination. Patients taking this drug should be carefully managed in the dental office, but no laboratory tests are used to monitor ticlopidine.

Prasugrel

The drug prasugrel (Effient) in conjunction with aspirin is used for the prevention of a MI and stent thrombosis in persons with acute coronary syndrome undergoing percutaneous coronary intervention. It is contraindicated in persons with a history of stroke or transient ischemic attack. The risk for bleeding is greater in older persons.

Ticagrelor

Ticagrelor (Brilinta) is a platelet aggregation inhibitor and is used in conjunction with aspirin for the prevention of MI and stroke in persons with acute coronary syndrome. The most common side effects include shortness of breath and bleeding.

Streptokinase and Alteplase

Enzymes called *clot busters,* such as streptokinase (strep-toe-KYE-nase) (Streptase, Kabikinase) and the recombinant tissue-type plasminogen activator alteplase (AL-ti-plase) (tPA, Activase), are sometimes used in the therapy of DVT, arterial thrombosis, PE, and acute coronary artery thrombosis associated with MI. These may appropriately be termed *thrombolytic drugs* because they promote the conversion of plasminogen to plasmin, the natural clot-resolving enzyme. They are usually administered by direct vessel perfusion to the clot site. Considerable technical skill and immediate treatment of the thrombus, within 3 hours of the onset of symptoms, are required for satisfactory results. Because streptokinase is a foreign protein, allergic reactions can occur. Hemorrhage may result from the use of any of these drugs, which are contraindicated in patients at risk for hemorrhage.

Dipyridamole

The drug dipyridamole (dye-peer-ID-a-mole) (Persantine) is used to prolong the life of platelets in patients with prosthetic heart valves as adjunct to warfarin therapy. The artificial valves cause premature death of the platelets because of their mechanical effect (trauma) on the blood cells passing through the valves. Dipyridamole does not offer

---

BOX 12.10 Concerns in a Patient Taking Factor Xa or a Direct Thrombin Inhibitor

Anticoagulant effects, which can last up to 24 hours, cannot be reversed.

No antidote is available.

Status is not monitored with periodic measurements of international normalized ratio, possibly leading to lower treatment adherence rates.

Risk of bleeding is increased.

Patient should avoid aspirin and nonsteroidal antiinflammatory drugs (NSAIDs).

any additional anticlotting benefit over the use of aspirin and/or warfarin. It does not affect bleeding related to dental treatment.

Pentoxifylline

Pentoxifylline (pen-tox-IF-i-lin) (Trental) is a dimethylxanthine that improves blood flow via its hemorheologic effects, which include lowering blood viscosity and improving the flexibility of red blood cells. It is indicated for intermittent claudication due to chronic occlusive artery disease of the limbs. Side effects associated with pentoxifylline include cardiovascular and gastric symptoms. Dry mouth, bad taste, excessive salivation, and swollen neck glands have infrequently been reported. Pentoxifylline does not alter blood clotting.

DRUGS THAT INCREASE BLOOD CLOTTING

Hemostatic Agents (Fibrinolytic Inhibitors)

ε-Aminocaproic acid (EACA) and its analog, tranexamic acid (Cyklokapron), are similar to the amino acid lysine, and they inhibit plasminogen activation (synthetic inhibitor of fibrinolysis).

EACA and tranexamic acid are used intravenously, orally, or topically. Adverse effects include intravascular thrombosis, hypotension, and abdominal discomfort. Some literature recommends the use of topical tranexamic acid before dental procedures in patients taking warfarin who are at risk of bleeding. It is indicated in the treatment of hemorrhage after dental surgery.

■ DENTAL HYGIENE CONSIDERATIONS

- Measure the patient's blood pressure and pulse at every visit.
- Make sure that the patient is experiencing a minimal amount of stress, and maintain adequate pain control during each visit. Stress and pain can elevate blood pressure.
- Conduct a thorough medication/health history to avoid drug interactions.
- Evaluate the patient for adverse effects that may affect oral health care.
- If a local anesthetic with a vasoconstrictor is required, make sure that the patient can receive it. If the patient can, make sure the patient is given the lowest dose possible.
- Be careful when raising patients to the supine position. Raise the chair slowly.
- Review Boxes 12.2, 12.3, 12.7, 12.8, and 12.9 and Table 12.2.
- Although elevated cholesterol values do not affect oral health care, they often go hand in hand with high blood pressure. Always check the blood pressure and heart rate of patients with elevated cholesterol values.

- Antiarrhythmic medicines can cause arrhythmias. Always check the blood pressure and heart rate of patients with elevated cholesterol values.
- Patients with HF may have breathing difficulties when in the supine position. Work with the patient to find the most comfortable chair position. A semisupine position may be necessary.
- Some medicines may have GI adverse effects. NSAIDs should be avoided. Recommend acetaminophen for pain instead.
- Make sure that patients with angina have brought their NTG with them. Have them place the NTG on the tray where it is easily accessed.
- Lower-dose aspirin does not normally cause excess bleeding but in a patient taking it, blood clotting may take a little longer than normal.
- Patients taking anticoagulants are at an increased for bleeding during dental appointments. It may take longer for their blood to clot and the bleeding to stop. Apply pressure if necessary.

■ ACADEMIC SKILLS ASSESSMENT

1. What is angina and what are some of its causes?
2. What is the mechanism of action of NTG in treating angina and what are its adverse reactions?
3. Describe the role of nitrates in the treatment of angina.
4. Describe the interaction between nitrates and drugs used to treat erectile dysfunction.
5. What is hypertension and what is its prevalence in the United States?
6. Explain the pharmacologic effects of ACEIs in the treatment of hypertension.
7. Describe the current algorithm for treating hypertension. State the individual drug classes for treating compelling indications in patients with hypertension.
8. State the individual drug classes for treating hypertension, including pharmacologic effects, adverse effects, and any dental concerns.

9. What is the role of aspirin in anticoagulation therapy? List the other classes of anticoagulant drugs and describe mechanism of action, adverse effects, and dental concerns.
10. What is the relationship between elevated cholesterol values and heart disease?
11. Compare and contrast the classes of medication used to treat elevated cholesterol levels, including adverse effects and dental concerns.
12. Compare and contrast the classes of medication used to treat arrhythmias.
13. Compare and contrast the classes of medications used to treat HF, along with adverse effects and dental concerns.
14. Discuss the concern regarding the lack of INR monitoring with the factor XA and direct thrombin inhibitors. Are there any dental concerns in patients taking these drugs?

■ CLINICAL CASE STUDY

Nina Papadopoulos is 56 years old and has been coming to your practice for close to 15 years. Until recently, she would take only acetaminophen for an occasional headache. Mrs. Papadopoulos went to the doctor last week for her annual check-up. She had not been "feeling herself" for the last several months. Upon examination, Mrs. Papadopoulos learned that she has hypertension and elevated cholesterol values. Life has not been the same since. Mrs. Papadopoulos started having some chest pain, which was attributed to anxiety regarding her diagnosis. Now, in addition to acetaminophen, Mrs. Papadopoulos is taking lisinopril and chlorthalidone to treat hypertension and atorvastatin to treat cholesterol levels.

1. What is lisinopril and what is its role in the treatment of hypertension?
2. Are there any dental concerns associated with lisinopril?
3. What are the dental concerns associated with antihypertensive therapy? Counsel the patient about them.
4. What are the lifestyle modifications associated with treating hypertension?
5. What is chlorthalidone and what is its role in treating hypertension?

6. Why is atorvastatin used to treat elevated cholesterol values?
7. Discuss the new approach to treating elevated cholesterol values.
8. What are the dental concerns associated with elevated cholesterol values?
9. Should Mrs. Papadopoulos be doing anything else to lower her cholesterol levels besides taking medication?
10. Is acetaminophen contraindicated in a person taking medicines used to treat hypertension or elevated cholesterol?

REFERENCES

Hylek EM, Heiman H, Skates SJ, et al. Acetaminophen and other risk factors for excessive warfarin anticoagulation. *JAMA*. 1998;279:657–662.

Stone NJ, Robinson J, Lichtenstein AH, et al. 2013. ACC/AHA guideline on the treatment of blood cholesterol to reduce atherosclerotic cardiovascular risk in adults. *Circulation*. 2014;129:S1–S45, published online before publication on November 12, 2013.

13

Drugs for the Treatment of Gastrointestinal Disorders

http://evolve.elsevier.com/Haveles/pharmacology

LEARNING OBJECTIVES

1. Summarize the most common types of gastrointestinal diseases and their impact on oral health care.
2. Name and describe the types of drugs used to treat gastrointestinal diseases, their uses, adverse reactions, drug interactions, and any implications to dentistry, including
   - Discuss the role of H_2-receptor blockers in the treatment of peptic ulcer disease and gastroesophageal reflux disease.
   - Discuss the role of proton pump inhibitors and antibiotics in the treatment of peptic ulcer disease and gastroesophageal reflux disease.
   - Describe the role of antacids in the treatment of peptic ulcer disease and gastroesophageal reflux disease.

3. Discuss several miscellaneous gastrointestinal drugs that can be used and their possible side effects.
4. List the different types of laxatives and know the advantages and disadvantages of each.
5. List the medications used to treat diarrhea.
6. Define the term antiemetic and give examples of drugs used to treat vomiting and nausea.
7. Discuss the medications used to manage chronic inflammatory bowel disease (IBD).

GASTROINTESTINAL DRUGS

Many drugs, both over-the-counter (OTC) and prescription, are used for gastrointestinal diseases (Fig. 13.1). Some are used to treat specific gastrointestinal diseases, and others to provide symptomatic relief.

Gastrointestinal Diseases

Ulcers and gastroesophageal reflux disease (GERD) are common gastrointestinal tract diseases. With the discovery of the etiology of ulcers, the incidence of ulcers in the population has decreased substantially. Nonspecific complaints for GERD include burping, cramps, flatulence, fullness, and congestion in the stomach. The gastrointestinal tract is highly susceptible to emotional changes because it is innervated by the vagus nerve associated with the autonomic nervous system.

Gastroesophageal Reflux Disease

Gastroesophageal reflux disease: heartburn.

GERD, or "heartburn," is the most prevalent gastrointestinal disease in the US population. In this condition, the stomach contents, including the acid, reflux, or flow backward through the cardiac sphincter, up into the esophagus. Because the esophagus is not designed to endure the stomach's acid, irritation, inflammation, and erosion can occur. The pain from the inflamed esophagus may be severe and located in the middle of the chest, causing it to be interpreted as a heart attack and trigger an emergency room visit. The main problem is inadequate function of the lower esophageal sphincter, allowing backflow to occur. The symptoms of GERD are exacerbated by eating large meals (blowing up a balloon [stomach] increases the backpressure) and by assuming the supine position (gravity is no longer helping).

Close to 3 million Americans suffer from Barrett esophagus. This disorder occurs when the cells of the lower esophagus become damaged as a result of repeated exposure to stomach acid. This causes a change in the color and composition of esophageal cells. Barrett esophagus is most often diagnosed in patients with long-term GERD; however, only a small percentage of patients with GERD go on to develop Barrett esophagus. A diagnosis of Barrett esophagus is of concern because a small number of patients who have it can go on to have esophageal cancer. Barrett esophagus is normally diagnosed through endoscopy. Patients who present to a dental practice without a diagnosis of GERD or Barrett esophagus but with symptoms of taste changes and enamel erosion should be referred to their primary care physicians for further evaluation.

Lifestyle changes that can reduce symptoms include avoiding eating for 4 hours before bedtime, eating smaller meals more often, and raising the head of the bed with bricks or using several pillows. Some patients with either disorder that is not treated may have such severe symptoms that they cannot sleep lying down and must sit in a chair.

GERD is treated in two ways: one is to decrease the acid in the stomach and the other is to constrict the cardiac sphincter (the muscle between the stomach and the esophagus). If the sphincter is tighter, it is less likely that the contents will flow back into the esophagus. The histamine$_2$ (H_2) blocking agents and the proton pump inhibitors (PPIs) reduce or eliminate the stomach's acid. The gastrointestinal stimulants act by increasing the tone of the cardiac sphincter. Sometimes both of these approaches are required to make the patient asymptomatic. Antacids are used for acute relief of symptoms.

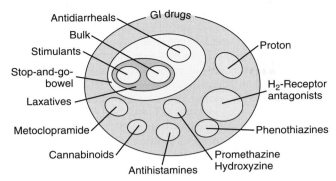

Fig. 13.1 Gastrointestinal (*GI*) drug groups.

Ulcers

Ulcers may occur in the stomach or small intestine. In the past, it was thought that ulcers were caused by "too much acid." However, in the last decade, it has been determined that most ulcers are related in some way to the presence of the organism *Helicobacter pylori*. Many ulcers can now be cured by using a combination of one or more antibiotics and an H_2-blocker or a PPI to reduce the acid in the stomach. Some ulcers, especially in the elderly, are secondary to the long-term use of nonsteroidal antiinflammatory drugs (NSAIDs). NSAID-induced ulcers occur because NSAIDs inhibit synthesis of prostaglandins (PGs), which are cytoprotective to the stomach.

Dental Implications

Box 13.1 summarizes the treatment of dental patients with **peptic ulcer disease (PUD)** and GERD.

DRUGS USED TO TREAT GASTROINTESTINAL DISEASES

Histamine₂-Blocking Agents

Histamine₂ receptor antagonists block and inhibit basal and nocturnal gastric acid secretion by competitive inhibition of the action of histamine at the H_2-receptors of the parietal cells. They also inhibit gastric acid secretion stimulated by other agents such as food and caffeine. All the members of this group, which are now available OTC, are listed in Table 13.1. Cimetidine (sye-MET-i-deen) (Tagamet) is discussed as the

---

BOX 13.1　Management of Dental Patients With Peptic Ulcer Disease or Gastroesophageal Reflux Disease

- Avoid the use of aspirin or NSAIDs because they can exacerbate an existing ulcer and further aggravate GERD.
- Patients with GERD may not be able to be in the supine position in the dental chair because of acid reflux.
- The dental hygienist should work with such patients to determine the best position for them.
- Some drugs may cause xerostomia. Patients should be encouraged to maintain good oral hygiene and drink plenty of water.
- Tart sugarless gum or candy can help with dry mouth.
- Patients should avoid caffeinated and alcohol-containing beverages or mouth rinses because they can exacerbate dry mouth.
- Patients presenting with taste changes and loss of tooth enamel should be referred to their primary care physicians for further evaluation.

GERD, Gastroesophageal reflux disease; *NSAIDs,* nonsteroidal antiinflammatory drugs.

---

prototype. However, it has largely been replaced by famotidine, ranitidine, and nizatidine because of their more tolerable side-effect profiles.

Uses

This group is indicated for the treatment of ulcers and the management of the symptoms of ulcers and GERD. H_2-blockers should be administered with meals and at bedtime. For maintenance, if only one dose is needed daily, the bedtime dose is most effective. If taken twice daily, agents are taken in the morning and at bedtime.

Because smoking increases acid production and reduces the effect of the H_2-blockers, smoking cessation assistance should be offered to dental patients who smoke.

Adverse Reactions

The side effects of cimetidine include central nervous system (CNS) effects such as slurred speech, delusions, confusion, and headache.

TABLE 13.1　Drugs Used to Treat Peptic Ulcer Disease and Gastroesophageal Reflux Disease

Drug Group	Available as a Prescription Drug?	Available as a Nonprescription Drug?
H₂-Receptor Blockers		
Cimetidine (Tagamet, Tagamet HB 200)	Yes	Yes
Famotidine (Pepcid/Pepcid AC)	Yes	Yes
Famotidine/calcium carbonate/ magnesium hydroxide (Pepcid Complete)	No	Yes
Nizatidine (Axid, Axid AR)	Yes	Yes
Ranitidine (Zantac, Zantac 75, Zantac 150)	Yes	Yes
Proton Pump Inhibitors		
Omeprazole (Prilosec, Prilosec OTC)	Yes	Yes
Omeprazole/sodium bicarbonate (Zegrid, Zegrid OTC)	Yes	Yes
Lansoprazole (Prevacid, Prevacid OTC)	Yes	Yes
Esomeprazole (Nexium)	Yes	Yes
Pantoprazole (Protonix)	Yes	No
Rabeprazole (AcipHex)	Yes	No
Dopamine Antagonists		
Metoclopramide (Reglan)	Yes	No
Antacids		
Sodium bicarbonate	No	Yes
Magnesium hydroxide	No	Yes
Aluminum hydroxide	No	Yes
Calcium carbonate	No	Yes
Prostaglandins		
Misoprostol (Cytotec)	Yes	No
Antiflatulents		
Simethicone (Mylicon, Gas-X)	No	Yes

Because cimetidine binds with the androgen receptors, it has antiandrogenic effects such as gynecomastia, reduction in sperm count, and sexual dysfunction (e.g., impotence). Unlike cimetidine, neither ranitidine nor famotidine has been found to possess antiandrogenic activity. Famotidine has been associated with dry mouth and taste alterations. Cimetidine's hematologic effects include granulocytopenia, thrombocytopenia, and neutropenia. Reversible hepatitis and abnormal liver function values have been reported with all of the H_2-blockers.

Cimetidine inhibits liver microsomal enzymes responsible for the hepatic metabolism of some drugs (cytochrome P-450 oxidase system), resulting in a delay in elimination and an increase in serum levels of some drugs, possibly producing toxicity. Ranitidine inhibits the P-450 enzymes much less than does cimetidine, and the other H_2-blockers have no effect on the P-450 enzymes. A few examples of drugs that are metabolized by the P-450 pathway are warfarin, metronidazole, lidocaine, phenytoin, theophylline, diazepam, and carbamazepine.

Dental Drug Interactions

The metabolism of the following drugs occasionally used in dentistry may be reduced by the administration of cimetidine:

Ketoconazole and itraconazole: Toxic levels of these antifungal agents may be produced if they are used continuously for the management of chronic fungal infections. H_2-receptor antagonists may increase gastrointestinal pH. Concurrent administration with H_2-receptor antagonists may result in a marked reduction in absorption of itraconazole or ketoconazole. Patients taking itraconazole or ketoconazole should take an H_2-receptor antagonist at a different time of the day.

Alcohol: The blood alcohol levels of persons who have ingested alcoholic beverages may be higher if they have been taking cimetidine.

Benzodiazepines: The metabolism of the benzodiazepines, such as diazepam and midazolam, may be slower. The recovery from use of these drugs might also be slower.

The other H_2-blockers are unlikely to have important dental drug interactions.

Proton Pump Inhibitors

PPIs are potent inhibitors of gastric acid secretion that are effective (in combination with the antibiotics) in healing duodenal ulcers and in monotherapy for the acute treatment and maintenance therapy of GERD. The mechanism of action involves the inhibition of the hydrogen/potassium adenosine triphosphatase (H +/K + -ATPase) enzyme system at the surface of the gastric parietal cell. Currently available PPIs are listed in Table 13.1. PPIs heal ulcers more rapidly than H_2-receptor blockers and other drugs. Tolerance does not occur with PPIs because the increased gastric-mediated histamine release cannot overcome proton pump blockade.

Adverse Reactions

Some of the most frequent side effects associated with PPIs include headache, diarrhea, abdominal pain, nausea, and dizziness. Although it is unknown whether a relationship exists between omeprazole and mucosal atrophy of the tongue and dry mouth, these side effects have been reported. Long-term use of PPIs, particularly at high doses, has been associated with an increased risk of osteoporotic fractures. Long-term use of PPIs has also been associated with hypomagnesemia. PPIs may also be associated with a greater risk of *Clostridium difficile*-associated diarrhea and community-acquired pneumonia. Gastroduodenal tumors have been reported in patients taking long-term omeprazole to treat Zollinger Ellison syndrome, although the tumors may be related to the syndrome itself. Their long-term use has also been associated with an increased risk for chronic kidney disease.

Mixed Anti-infective Therapy for Ulcer Treatment

Ulcers are closely related to the organism *H. pylori*. To treat ulcers, a combination of two antiinfective agents (tetracycline, metronidazole, clarithromycin, or amoxicillin), an H_2-blocker or a PPI, and bismuth subsalicylate (Pepto-Bismol) may be used. Common multidrug regimens are listed in Table 13.2. Newer combinations often use one antibiotic and a PPI, such as clarithromycin and esomeprazole. These agents are used for 2 weeks and result in a cure in many patients.

TABLE 13.2   Common Multidrug Regimens for *Helicobacter pylori*

Drug	Daily Dose	Duration	Comments
Triple Therapy			No longer preferred. Consider if no prior macrolide exposure and clarithromycin resistance < 15%
Clarithromycin +	500 mg bid	14 days	
amoxicillin	1 gm bid	14 days	
or			
Metronidazole +	500 mg tid	14 days	
a PPI	standard PPI dose	14 days	
Bismuth Quadruple Therapy			Preferred first-line therapy. Good for prior macrolide exposure or true penicillin allergy.
Bismuth subsalicylate (Pepto-Bismol) +	262 or 525 mg qid	10–14 days	
Metronidazole +	250 mg qid or 500 mg tid or qid	10–14 days	
Tetracycline +	500 mg tid or qid	10–14 days	
PPI	Standard dose	10–14 days	
Concomitant Quadruple Therapy			Preferred first-line, more convenient dosing
Clarithromycin +	500 mg bid	10–14 days	
Amoxicillin +	1 gm bid	10–14 days	
Metronidazole +	500 mg bid	10–14 days	
PPI	Standard dose	10–14 days	

bid, Twice a day; *PPI,* proton pump inhibitor; *qid,* four times a day; *tid,* three times a day.

TABLE 13.3 Drugs Used to Treat Other Gastrointestinal Disorders

Drug Group	Subgroup	Examples
Antidiarrheals	Opioid-like agents	Loperamide (Imodium)
		Diphenoxylate (in Lomotil)
	Adsorbents	Kaolin and pectin (Kaopectate)
Antiemetics	Phenothiazines	Prochlorperazine (Compazine)
	Antihistamines	Meclizine (Bonine)
		Dimenhydrinate (Dramamine)
		Trimethobenzamide (Tigan)
	Cannabinoids	Dronabinol (Marinol)
		Nabilone (Cesamet)
Agents used in the treatment of inflammatory bowel disease	Nonaspirin salicylates	Sulfasalazine (Azulfidine)
		Mesalamine (Rowasa, Pentasa, Asacol)
		Olsalazine (Dipentum)
	Adrenocorticosteroids	Prednisone
	Immune modifiers	Cyclosporine
		Azathioprine (Imural)
		Mercaptopurine (6-MP, Purinethol)
	Antibiotics	Metronidazole (Flagyl)

Antacids

Antacids are used to treat a variety of gastric conditions, by both self-medication and recommendation of the patient's prescriber. Acute gastritis and symptoms of ulcers are sometimes managed with antacids. Acute gastritis, the most common type of gastric distress, is termed *heartburn* or *upset stomach*. The symptoms include epigastric discomfort or a burning feeling. The symptoms of gastric ulcers can be managed with antacids.

Antacids are drugs that partially neutralize hydrochloric acid in the stomach. If the pH is raised to 3 or 4, the erosive effect of the acid is decreased and pepsin activity is reduced (Table 13.3).

Sodium bicarbonate rapidly neutralizes gastric acid. Its major disadvantage is that it can lead to alkalosis. It also contains sodium and so is contraindicated in patients with cardiovascular disorders who are to minimize sodium intake. For these reasons, it is not recommended, although it is still used by the lay public.

Calcium carbonate, aluminum and magnesium salts, and magnesium-aluminum hydroxide gels are the active ingredients in all other antacids. Calcium salts may cause acid rebound, constipation, or hypercalcemia. Aluminum salts can produce constipation. Magnesium salts produce osmotic diarrhea. Hypermagnesemia has been reported in patients with renal disease.

Drug interactions with the antacids include altering the absorption of other drugs from the gastrointestinal tract. Drugs whose absorption is inhibited include tetracyclines, digitalis, iron, chlorpromazine, and indomethacin. Conversely, levodopa's absorption is increased because stomach emptying time is shortened. Mixing aluminum and magnesium salts in a single preparation balances the effects on the bowel.

Miscellaneous Gastrointestinal Drugs

Misoprostol

Misoprostol (mye-soe-PROST-ole) (Cytotec), a synthetic prostaglandin $E2_\alpha$ ($PGE2\alpha$), is indicated in the management of NSAID-induced ulcers. Both H_2-blockers and PPIs reduce the symptoms of NSAID-induced

ulcers but do not prevent the ulcers. Misoprostol increases gastric mucus and inhibits gastric acid secretion. Its side effects include stomach distress and diarrhea (caused by PGs). The US Food and Drug Administration (FDA) has assigned misoprostol to pregnancy category X because it stimulates uterine contractions and will induce labor.

Sucralfate

Sucralfate (soo-KRAL-fate) (Carafate), a complex of aluminum hydroxide and sulfated sucrose (a polysaccharide with antipeptic activity), is used to treat duodenal ulcers. In the stomach, the aluminum ion splits off, leaving an anion that is essentially nonabsorbable. Sucralfate combines with proteins, forming a complex that binds preferentially with the ulcer site. It can be thought of as a "bandage" for ulcers. It inhibits the action of pepsin and absorbs the bile salts. Its acid-neutralizing capacity does not contribute to its antiulcer action. Constipation is the most common side effect reported (2.2%). Other side effects (<0.3%) include dry mouth, nausea, rash, and dizziness. Sucralfate must be taken on an empty stomach and can inhibit the absorption of tetracycline.

Metoclopramide

The drug metoclopramide (met-oh-KLOE-pra-mide) (Reglan) is a dopaminergic antagonist. Its dopamine-blocking action facilitates cholinergic effects within the gastrointestinal tract. Metoclopramide stimulates the motility of the upper gastrointestinal tract without stimulating secretions and also relaxes smooth muscle innervated by dopamine. It relaxes the pyloric sphincter and increases peristalsis in the duodenum, resulting in accelerated gastric emptying time. It also increases the tone of the lower esophageal sphincter. Its antiemetic property is the result of its antagonism of dopamine receptors both centrally and peripherally.

Metoclopramide is indicated for the relief of symptoms associated with diabetic gastroparesis (gastric stasis) and improves delayed gastric emptying time. Another indication is short-term therapy for gastroesophageal reflux with symptoms. The most common CNS side effects are restlessness, drowsiness, and fatigue, which occur in 10% to 25% of patients. Parkinson-like reactions can occur in up to 10% of patients. Gastrointestinal side effects include nausea and diarrhea. Additive CNS depression may occur when other CNS depressants are used concomitantly.

Simethicone

Simethicone (Mylicon, Gas-X) is an agent used to relieve flatulence (gas). It lowers the surface tension and breaks up gas pockets so they can be expelled.

Laxatives and Antidiarrheals

Laxatives

Self-medication with laxatives is a common practice among the lay public. Although a few indications for the use of laxatives exist, overuse of these agents is common and habituation can result. The myth that "regular" bowel habits are essential has led to this practice. Abuse of these substances occurs in bulimic patients. Short-term, occasional use of laxatives for constipation and their use before diagnostic procedures (barium enema) are legitimate indications. The types of laxatives are as follows (Table 13.4):

Bulk laxatives: Bulk laxatives are preferred because they are the safest and act most like the normal physiology of humans. They contain polysaccharides or cellulose derivatives that combine with intestinal fluids to form gels. The gels increase peristalsis and facilitate movement through the intestine. Patients who have constipation problems can increase their intake of fiber or use any bulk laxative daily without problems.

Lubricants: Mineral oil, a lubricant that was previously often used for constipation, is no longer recommended. It can be absorbed if

TABLE 13.4 Available Laxatives

Drug Group	Subgroup	Examples
Laxatives	Bulk	Psyllium seed husks (Metamucil)
		Carboxymethylcellulose
		Methylcellulose (Citrucel)
		Polycarbophil (FiberCon)
	Stool softeners, emollient	Docusate (dioctyl sodium sulfosuccinate, DSS, Colace)
	Stimulants	Magnesium hydroxide (milk of magnesia [MOM])
		Bisacodyl (Dulcolax)
		Cascara sagrada
		Senna
		Casanthranol
		Castor oil
	Hyperosmotic	Phenolphthalein
		Glycerin
		Lactulose
		Salts (magnesium citrate, hydroxide, oxide, or sulfate; sodium phosphate)

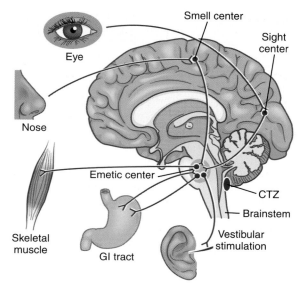

Fig. 13.2 The chemoreceptor trigger zone *(CTZ)* and other sites that activate the emetic center. *GI,* Gastrointestinal. (From McKenry L, Tessier E, Hogan MA. *Mosby's Pharmacology in Nursing.* 22nd ed. St. Louis: Mosby; 2006.)

used over a long period and can interfere with the absorption of the fat-soluble vitamins (A, D, E, and K).

Stimulants: Stimulant laxatives act by producing local irritation of the intestinal mucosa. Because of their potent effect, intestinal cramping can result. Bisacodyl, a member of this group, is often used before bowel surgery or radiologic examinations but should not be used for simple constipation.

Stool softeners (emollients): Dioctyl sodium sulfosuccinate, an anionic detergent, wets and softens the stool by accumulating water in the intestine. This and other such agents should be limited to short-term use, although they are nontoxic.

Osmotic (saline) laxatives: Magnesium sulfate or phosphate produces its laxative effect by osmotically holding water. It should be used with caution in patients who have renal impairment.

Mu receptor antagonists: Naloxegol (Movantik), naldemedine (Symproic), and methylnaltrexone (Relistor) are mu opioid receptor antagonists that are used to treat opioid-induced constipation in patients with chronic pain that is noncancerous. They block mu receptors in the gastrointestinal tract which decreases the constipating effects of opioids. The most common side effects are diarrhea, abdominal pain, and headache.

Chloride channel activator: Lubiprostone (Amitiza) works by enhancing the chloride-rich intestinal fluid secretions, thereby increasing intestinal fluid secretions which then increase intestinal motility, allowing for the passage of stool. It is used to treat chronic idiopathic constipation, opioid-induced constipation in chronic pain not related to cancer, and irritable bowel syndrome with constipation. The most common side effects include nausea, diarrhea, abdominal pain, and headache.

Antidiarrheals

Drugs used to treat diarrhea are either adsorbents or opioid-like in action. Antidiarrheals are used to minimize fluid and electrolyte imbalances. In certain poisonings or infections, antidiarrheals are contraindicated. The most common adsorbent combination used to treat diarrhea is kaolin and pectin (Kaopectate). The opioids, such as diphenoxylate with atropine (Lomotil) and loperamide (OTC Imodium), are the most effective antidiarrheal agents. They decrease peristalsis by acting directly on the smooth muscle of the gastrointestinal tract.

Antiemetics

Drugs used to induce vomiting and to prevent vomiting are used for certain gastrointestinal tract problems. Vomiting may occur for a variety of reasons, such as motion sickness, pregnancy, drugs, infections, and radiation therapy, and many sites within the body can activate the emetic center to cause vomiting (Fig. 13.2). Choice of the drug to treat vomiting depends, to some extent, on the cause of the vomiting.

Phenothiazines

Phenothiazines (e.g., prochlorperazine [Compazine]) are used to control severe nausea. Their side effects include sedation and extrapyramidal symptoms, including tardive dyskinesia (see Chapter 15). Promethazine (Phenergan), a phenothiazine with antihistaminic and anticholinergic properties, is used in dentistry to treat nausea and vomiting associated with surgery and anesthesia. It also has sedative and antisialagogue action. It is sometimes used concurrently with opioids to minimize the nausea they produce.

Anticholinergics

Anticholinergics can be used for the nausea and vomiting associated with motion sickness and labyrinthitis. Both dimenhydrinate (Dramamine) and meclizine (Bonine) possess antiemetic, antivertigo, and antimotion sickness action. Because they have antihistaminic action, sedation is a side effect. A scopolamine transdermal patch (Transderm Scōp) is placed behind the ear and releases medication over a 3-day period. It is used for motion sickness on ships and boats. It is contraindicated whenever anticholinergics are used (see Chapter 4). Dry mouth, blurred vision, sedation, and dizziness have been reported with use of the patch.

Antihistamines

The agent diphenhydramine (Benadryl), an antihistamine with antiemetic properties, commonly produces sedation. Hydroxyzine (Atarax) is used in dentistry as an antiemetic or antianxiety agent.

Trimethobenzamide

The drug trimethobenzamide (Tigan) has an antiemetic effect that is mediated through the chemoreceptor trigger zone. It produces sedation, agitation, headache, and dry mouth. It is available orally or as a suppository that contains 2% benzocaine (should be avoided in patients allergic to ester local anesthetics).

Metoclopramide

Metoclopramide (Reglan) can control the nausea and vomiting of cancer patients receiving chemotherapeutic agents. It acts both centrally (dopamine antagonist) and peripherally (stimulates release of acetylcholine). It is also indicated for the management of gastric motility disorders such as diabetic gastric stasis.

5-HT₃ Receptor Antagonists

Ondansetron (Zofran), dolasetron (Anzemet), granisetron (Kytril), and palonosetron (Aloxi) control the nausea and vomiting due to postoperative and cancer chemotherapeutic agents. These agents work by blocking 5-HT_3 receptors in the CNS and the chemoreceptor trigger zone. The most common adverse effects include constipation or diarrhea, headache, and dizziness. The 5-HT_3 receptor antagonists do not cause sedation.

Cannabinoids

The cannabinoids dronabinol (droe-NAB-i-nol) (Marinol) and nabilone (NAB-i-lone) (Cesamet) are psychoactive substances derived from *Cannabis sativa* L. (marijuana) and are controlled substances listed by the FDA as schedule III drugs. Their effects are similar to those of marijuana. These agents are indicated to treat the nausea, vomiting, and weight loss associated with cancer chemotherapy and to treat the anorexia associated with weight loss in patients who have acquired immunodeficiency syndrome (AIDS). Cannabinoids can be abused. Tolerance and both physical and psychologic dependence can occur with their use. Close supervision is required when these agents are administered. Side effects include drowsiness and dizziness. Perceptual difficulties, muddled thinking, and elevation of mood can also occur.

Agents Used to Manage Chronic Inflammatory Bowel Disease

> Inflammatory bowel disease: IBD.

Chronic **inflammatory bowel disease** (IBD) is divided into two subcategories: ulcerative **colitis** and Crohn disease (Fig. 13.3). Although ulcerative colitis is probably multifactorial, an autoimmune response is thought to be associated with it. Crohn disease extends through all layers of the intestinal wall, whereas ulcerative colitis involves only the mucosa. Crohn disease can involve the whole intestine, but the colon is most commonly affected. Ulcerative colitis involves the rectum and may involve the distal part of the colon but does not involve the small intestine. Smoking is protective against ulcerative colitis, and smoking cessation may exacerbate the disease. NSAIDs should be used with caution in patients with IBD.

Antiinflammatory drugs are usually the first line of therapy in the treatment of IBD. These drugs include sulfasalazine (Azulfidine), mesalamine (Apriso), balsalazide (Colazal), and olsalazine (Dipentum). They reduce the symptoms of IBD by decreasing inflammation. Side effects include nausea, vomiting, diarrhea, headache, and heartburn, which occur more frequently with sulfasalazine. Corticosteroids (see Chapter 16) are used for moderate to severe IBD that does not respond to other therapies.

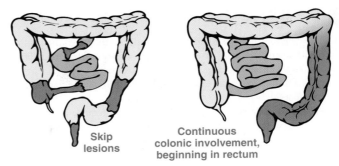

Fig. 13.3 Crohn disease *(left)* and ulcerative colitis *(right).* (From Kumar V, Abbas AK, Fausto N, Aster JC. *Robbins and Cotran Pathologic Basis of Disease.* 9th ed. St. Louis: Saunders; 2010.)

Immunosuppressant drugs, such as 6-mercaptopurine (Purinethol) and azathioprine (Imuran), work by blocking the immune reaction that contributes to inflammation. Side effects include nausea, vomiting, and diarrhea. Other drugs used to treat IBD, such as laxatives, colonic stimulants, and osmotic agents, are indicated for patients whose disease does not respond to fiber supplementation. Loperamide (Imodium) and atropine/diphenoxylate (Lomotil) are antidiarrheal agents that are also used to treat IBD in patients with diarrhea-predominant irritable bowel syndrome (IBS). Antispasmodics, such as hyoscyamine and dicyclomine, are best used on an as-needed basis for acute attacks of abdominal pain or before meals in patients with postprandial symptoms.

Infliximab (Remicade), adalimumab (Humira), certolizumab pegol (Cimzia), vedolizumab (Entyvio), and golimumab (Simponi) are the newest agents approved by the FDA to treat ulcerative colitis. They work by neutralizing tumor necrosis factor (TNF). Infliximab finds TNF in the bloodstream and removes it before it causes inflammation in the gastrointestinal tract. These drugs have been linked to an increased risk of infection, especially tuberculosis, and may also raise the risks for blood problems and hepatitis.

CELIAC DISEASE

Celiac disease is an autoimmune disorder that can occur in genetically predisposed people where the ingestion of gluten, a protein found in wheat, barley, and rye, damages the microvilli of the small intestine. It is estimated to affect 1 in 100 people worldwide. Almost 200,000 people are diagnosed each year and 3,000,000 Americans suffer from it. Celiac disease is hereditary and people with a first-degree relative with celiac disease have a 1:10 chance of developing it too. It is characterized by diarrhea, abdominal distension, malabsorption, pale, loose, greasy stool, and failure to thrive in young children. Many people have no symptoms. It is diagnosed by serology blood testing for certain antibodies and genetic testing for human leukocyte antigens. If the patient tests positive for celiac disease, then an endoscopy is necessary to determine the extent of tissue damage to the small intestine. The patient must be consuming gluten in order for these tests to be done. The only treatment for celiac disease is a gluten-free diet. In December of 2017, FDA issued a guidance titled, "Gluten in Drug Products and Associated Labeling Recommendations." The intent of this guidance is to encourage drug manufacturers to state whether or not their drug products are gluten-free. The starch often used in manufacturing prescription drugs could contain gluten. It should be noted that the vast majority of prescription and nonprescription drugs do not contain gluten.

DENTAL HYGIENE CONSIDERATIONS

- The dental hygienist should always conduct a thorough medication/health history to avoid drug interactions or prescribing medications that could exacerbate a gastrointestinal disorder.
- NSAIDs and aspirin can exacerbate PUD and GERD. Acetaminophen can be used instead.
- Patients with gastrointestinal disorders may require a semisupine position in the dental chair. The dental hygienist should work with such patients to determine what is best for them.

- Evaluate patients with GERD for tooth enamel erosion and an altered sense of taste. Refer these patients to their primary care physicians for follow-up.
- Review the information in Box 13.1.

ACADEMIC SKILLS ASSESSMENT

1. What are some of the risk factors for GERD?
2. Are there any dental concerns associated with GERD?
3. What is the role of antacids, H_2-receptor antagonists, and PPIs in the treatment of GERD?
4. What are the dental concerns associated with the medications used to treat GERD?
5. Compare and contrast the different antacids.
6. What is the role of sucralfate in the treatment of PUD?
7. What is the rationale for using antibiotics to treat PUD?
8. Are there any dental concerns associated with PUD?
9. What are some common adverse effects of antidiarrheals, antiemetics, and laxatives?
10. Are there dental concerns associated with antiemetics? If so, what are they?

CLINICAL CASE STUDY

Linda Thompson is a 45-year-old executive with a local advertising agency and is new to your practice. Upon completion of her medication health history, you learn that she is taking omeprazole 20 mg daily for constant heartburn. She is purchasing this agent at her local grocery store because this strength is available over the counter. She "doesn't have time" to see her physician. Her job is rather stressful, and she is continually working late to meet deadlines. As a result, Ms. Thompson drinks 10 cups of coffee a day, which is actually down from her normal 15 to 20 cups a day. Unfortunately, she frequents fast-food places for lunch and snacks. She tries to keep dinner with her family somewhat healthy. Ms. Thompson's other medications include ibuprofen for headaches, and she has started taking Pepcid AC (over the counter) to help with her heartburn. She takes at least 600 to 1200 mg of ibuprofen at least twice a week.

1. What is the prevalence of gastroesophageal reflux disease (GERD) in the United States and why is this of importance?
2. What is omeprazole and what is its role in treating GERD?
3. What are the adverse effects associated with GERD?
4. Are there any dental concerns associated with GERD? What should Ms. Thompson be told about them?
5. What effect can NSAIDs have on GERD?
6. Can NSAIDs cause PUD?
7. What should Ms. Thompson be told about her ibuprofen use in regard to GERD and peptic ulcer disease?
8. What is Pepcid AC, and what are some of its dental concerns?

14

Drugs for the Treatment of Seizure Disorders

http://evolve.elsevier.com/Haveles/pharmacology

LEARNING OBJECTIVES

1. Define epilepsy and briefly summarize the various types of seizures.
2. Discuss drug therapy of patients with epilepsy and describe the general adverse reactions to antiepileptic agents.
3. Summarize the pharmacologic effects, adverse reactions, and drug interactions of the main antiepileptics—valproate, lamotrigine, levetiracetam, oxcarbazepine, carbamazepine, and phenytoin.
4. Discuss ethosuximide and benzodiazepines (two miscellaneous antiepileptics) and describe the workings of each.
5. Provide several examples of new types of antiepileptics, including the mechanism of action, indications, and adverse reactions of each.
6. Outline the dental treatment of patients with epilepsy.

EPILEPSY

Epilepsy comprises a group of disorders that involve a chronic stereotyped recurrent attack of involuntary behavior or experience or changes in neurologic function caused by electrical activity in the brain that can be recorded via an electroencephalography (EEG). This activity can be localized or generalized. Each episode is termed a *seizure*. The seizure may be accompanied by motor activity, such as convulsions, or by other neurologic changes (e.g., sensory or emotional).

Because seizure disorders are estimated to affect approximately 1% of the population, the dental team is likely to encounter a patient with epilepsy. The antiepileptic agents are used long term, so potential adverse reactions that might alter dental treatment must be considered.

> Idiopathic (cause unknown).

There are many etiologies for epilepsy, including infection, trauma, toxicity to exogenous agents, genetic or birth influences, circulatory disturbances, metabolic or nutritional alterations, neoplasms, hereditary factors, fevers, and degenerative diseases. The majority of epileptic patients have *idiopathic* epilepsy; this term is used when the cause is unknown.

Epilepsy has been classified based on causes, symptoms, duration, precipitating factors, postictal state (postseizure), and aura. Currently, The International Classification of Epileptic Seizures divides seizures into two major groups and a miscellaneous group (Table 14.1). The two major groups are partial seizures and generalized seizures. Partial seizures are divided into simple and complex attacks. The most common generalized seizures are (1) tonic-clonic and (2) absence.

Generalized Seizures

Generalized seizures are divided into two large groups: (1) absence and (2) tonic-clonic types. Consciousness is lost in both types.

Little movement occurs in absence seizures, but in tonic-clonic seizures, major movement of large muscle groups occurs. Often, the patient may experience an aura (a brief period of heightened sensory activity) before the onset of the seizure. It may be characterized by numbness, nausea, or unusual sensitivity to light, odor, or sound.

Absence Seizures

> Absence seizure: brief loss of consciousness with little movement.

The symptoms of absence seizures include a brief (few seconds) loss of consciousness with characteristic EEG waves and little movement. Absence seizures usually begin during childhood and disappear in middle age. The patient is usually unaware that these seizures are occurring, and body tone is not lost. There is no aura or postictal state, and the patient quickly returns to normal activity. The drug of choice in the treatment of typical absence seizures is ethosuximide.

> Postictal state: altered state of consciousness after a seizure.

Management of absence seizures poses no problems for the dental team. The team's main concern when treating patients with absence seizures is the adverse reactions that can occur from long-term administration of the drugs used to treat the disease.

Tonic-Clonic Seizures

> Tonic-clonic seizure: longer periods of loss of consciousness and major activity of the large muscles of the body.

The generalized tonic-clonic seizures include longer periods of loss of consciousness and major motor activity of the large muscles of the body. As the seizure begins, the body becomes rigid and the patient falls to the floor. Urination, apnea, and a cry may be present. Tonic rigidity is followed by clonic jerking of the face, limbs, and body. The patient may bite the cheek or tongue. Finally, the patient becomes limp and comatose. Consciousness returns gradually, with postictal confusion, headache, and drowsiness. Some patients experience prodromal periods of varying durations, but a true aura does not occur. Because this

TABLE 14.1 International Classification of Epileptic Seizures

Generalized seizures	Tonic-clonic Myoclonic Akinetic Absence
Partial seizures	Simple Complex Secondarily generalized Temporal lobe
Miscellaneous	Status epilepticus Unilateral seizures Unclassified seizures

TABLE 14.2 Antiepileptic Drugs of Choice

	DRUGS	
Seizure Disorder	First Choice	Alternatives
Primary Generalized Seizures		
Tonic-clonic	Lamotrigine Levetiracetam Valproate*	Perampanel Topiramate Zonisamide
Absence	Ethosuximide Valproate	Clonazepam Lamotrigine Levetiracetam Zonisamide
Atypical absence, atonic, myoclonic	Lamotrigine Levetiracetam Valproate*	Clobazam Clonazepam Felbamate Rufinamide Topiramate Zonisamide
Status epilepticus	Diazepam (Valium) IV Phenytoin (Dilantin) IV Phenobarbital (Luminal) IV	
Partial Seizures		
Simple Complex Secondarily generalized	Carbamazepine Lamotrigine Levetiracetam Oxcarbazepine	Brivaracetam Clobazam Eslicarbazepine Gabapentin Lacosamide Perampanel Phenytoin Pregabalin Topiramate Valproate Zonisamide

*Not approved by US Food and Drug Administration (FDA) for this indication.
IV, Intravenous.

seizure type involves the violent movement of major muscle groups, it is more likely to result in serious injury to the patient. Valproate, lamotrigine, and levetiracetam are considered the drugs of choice for treating generalized tonic-clonic seizures (Table 14.2).

Status Epilepticus

> Tonic: stiffening of limbs.
> Clonic: limbs and face begin to jerk.

Status epilepticus seizures are continuous tonic-clonic seizures that last longer than five minutes or recur before the end of the postictal period of the previous seizure. This is an emergency situation, and rapid therapy is required, especially if the seizure activity has produced hypoxia. Parenteral benzodiazepines, such as diazepam (Valium), are the drugs of choice to control this seizure type (see Chapter 11).

Partial (Focal) Seizures

Partial seizures involve activation of only part of the brain, and the location of the activity determines the clinical manifestation. When consciousness is not impaired, the attack is called a *simple partial attack.* When consciousness is impaired, the attack is termed a *complex partial attack.* In contrast to absence seizures, which last a few seconds, complex partial seizures last several minutes. Some patients with complex partial seizures have an aura, and full consciousness is slow to return. For the partial seizures, lamotrigine, carbamazepine, levetiracetam, and oxcarbazepine are used (see Table 14.2).

DRUG THERAPY OF PATIENTS WITH EPILEPSY

> Dosing of antiepileptics is difficult.

Drug therapy of the patient with epilepsy has variable efficacy, from complete control of all seizures to reduction in the frequency of seizures. Antiepileptic agents may be used singly or in combination. The goal is to control seizures and minimize potential adverse reactions. Some newer antiepileptics are able to treat previously untreatable seizures, but more serious side effects can accompany them. General principles on the management of the dental patient taking any antiepileptic agents are listed in Box 14.1.

The antiepileptic drug used to treat a specific patient depends on the type of seizures the patient has. Because these agents are usually taken for life, their long-term toxicity becomes an important consideration in choosing a particular antiepileptic agent and determining the drug's dental implications.

BOX 14.1 Dental Management of Patients Taking Antiepileptic Agents

- Review emergency management of epileptic patients (remove hands and dental instruments from mouth, turn head to side).
- Take a thorough medical and drug history including medications and frequency of seizures.
- Additive central nervous system (CNS) depression—use additional CNS depressants cautiously.
- Additive gastrointestinal adverse reactions—use drugs that are gastric irritants cautiously (e.g., nonsteroidal antiinflammatory drugs [NSAIDs]).
- Drug interactions—induction of hepatic microsomal enzymes, metabolizes certain drugs more quickly (lowers blood level and effect).
- Dental drugs affected—propoxyphene, doxycycline.

General Adverse Reactions of Antiepileptic Agents

Central Nervous System Depression

Depressed central nervous system (CNS) function is a common side effect of the antiepileptic agents. Tolerance often develops to these sedative effects while the antiepileptic effect persists. Impairment of learning and cognitive abilities occurs in some patients. Behavior alterations reported include both hyperactivity and sedation. Another CNS side effect is exacerbation of a seizure type that is not being treated. This CNS depression is additive with other CNS depressants such as the opioids. If another CNS drug is given to the patient, the dose should be reduced.

Gastrointestinal Distress

Gastrointestinal distress, including anorexia, nausea, and vomiting, can occur with most antiepileptics. These effects can be minimized by taking the drugs with food. Agents with adverse reactions related to the gastrointestinal tract, for example, nonsteroidal antiinflammatory drugs (NSAIDs) or opioids, should be prescribed cautiously.

Drug Interactions

> Antiepileptic drug interactions.

Many drug interactions can occur with the antiepileptics. They may interact with themselves, with each other, or with other drugs. The mechanisms of drug interactions include altering absorption or renal excretion and inducing or inhibiting metabolism. The outcome may alter the levels of the inducing drug itself, another concomitant antiepileptic, or some other drug that is extensively metabolized by the liver microsomal enzymes.

The most important drug interaction of the antiepileptics involves stimulation of the hepatic microsomal enzymes. Inducing these enzymes results in a reduction in the blood level of the affected drugs (those metabolized by the liver enzymes). Fig. 2.11A shows the normal, unaffected enzyme situation. When the enzymes are stimulated (Fig. 2.11B), the level of the affected drug (D) is reduced because it is being metabolized more quickly, producing its metabolite (D_m).

Drug interactions with the older antiepileptics, such as phenytoin, carbamazepine, and valproate, are more significant than those with other drug groups because of these agents' narrow therapeutic indexes. If the level of an older antiepileptic drug is altered sufficiently by a drug interaction, either toxicity (level too high) or loss of seizure control (level too low) can result. Before any changes or additions are made to a patient's therapy, the possibility of drug interactions should be considered.

Idiosyncratic reactions. A wide range of idiosyncratic reactions occurs with the antiepileptics. Dermatologic side effects include rash, Stevens-Johnson syndrome, exfoliative dermatitis, and erythema multiforme. Drug-induced systemic lupus erythematosus and hematologic effects have also been reported with most of these agents.

Teratogenicity/growth. Reports have associated the antiepileptic agents with alteration in growth, profound effects being seen on fetal development and in children receiving antiepileptic medications during growth and development. The teratogenic potential of the antiepileptics has been documented. Several have been implicated in the production of fetal anomalies. However, antiseizure therapy may be necessary. In some instances the mother's seizures may be more damaging to fetal development than the drug itself. In this case, the risk-to-benefit benefit ratio must be considered.

Withdrawal. Abrupt withdrawal of any antiepileptic medication can precipitate seizures. Although many patients require medication for life, certain seizure types tend to disappear as patients grow older. In these patients, gradual withdrawal of their seizure medications under controlled conditions can be undertaken after an appropriate interval of drug use.

Valproate

> Valproate used: divalproex (Depakote).

A group of antiepileptic agents that are not structurally related to any other antiepileptics are the valproates, which include valproic (val-PRO-ik) acid, valproate (val-PRO-ate) sodium, and divalproex (dye-VAL-pro-ex) sodium. The term *valproate* is used here to refer to all of these agents. Divalproex sodium is a 1:1 ratio of valproic acid and valproate sodium. The mechanism of action of valproate may be its effect on sodium or potassium channels, a reduction in aspartate levels, or an increase in the inhibitory neurotransmitter γ-aminobutyric acid (GABA). Clinical trials have shown that it is effective and usually well tolerated in patients being treated for myoclonic and atonic seizures. It is often used first in treating patients with generalized tonic-clonic seizures on the basis of results presented in the medical literature, although this use is not approved by the US Food and Drug Administration (FDA).

Other uses. Valproate is FDA approved for migraine prophylaxis and bipolar disorder.

Adverse Reactions

Gastrointestinal effects. Indigestion, nausea, and vomiting are the most frequent adverse effects associated with valproate. They can be minimized by giving the drug with meals or increasing the dose very gradually. Divalproex sodium may have fewer adverse gastrointestinal effects than its components. Other gastrointestinal side effects are hypersalivation, anorexia, increased appetite, cramping, diarrhea, and constipation.

Central nervous system effects. Sedation and drowsiness have been reported with valproate. Rarely, ataxia, headache, and nystagmus have been noted. Some children exhibit hyperactivity, aggression, and other behavioral disturbances. Weight gain and an increase in appetite have been reported.

Hepatotoxicity. The idiosyncratic toxicity of valproate is hepatotoxicity. Dose-related changes in liver enzyme levels often occur in affected patients. Deaths due to hepatic failure have also been reported. Because valproic acid can produce serious hepatotoxicity, liver function tests should be performed. Signs of hepatotoxicity include nausea, vomiting, abdominal pain, loss of appetite, and diarrhea.

Bleeding

> Platelet aggregation inhibited.

Valproate inhibits the second phase of platelet aggregation; therefore, bleeding time may be prolonged. Thrombocytopenia, petechiae, bruising, and hematoma have been reported. Platelet counts, bleeding time measurements, and coagulation studies should be performed before surgical procedures.

Teratogenicity. Several reports suggest an association between the use of valproate in pregnant women and an increase in birth defects (particularly neural tube defects).

Drug Interactions

Other CNS depressants can have an additive CNS depressant effect when used with valproate. Valproate inhibits the metabolism of phenobarbital, producing excessive sedation. Valproate has also been associated with drug interactions with phenytoin, resulting in decreased action of valproate and increased phenytoin action. Because valproate can affect bleeding, other drugs that affect bleeding should be used cautiously. Box 14.2 summarizes the management of dental patients taking valproic acid.

BOX 14.2   Dental Management of Patients Taking Valproic Acid (Depakote)

- Additive bleeding is a risk: Use caution with drugs that can alter coagulation.
- Look for signs of hepatotoxicity.

Lamotrigine

Lamotrigine belongs to the class of sodium-channel-blocking antiepileptic drugs. Table 14.3 reviews the FDA-approved indications for lamotrigine therapy. A review of the literature has found that lamotrigine appears to be as effective as carbamazepine and better tolerated in elderly patients newly diagnosed with partial or generalized seizures. It is also preferred over ethosuximide in children with absence seizures because it is better tolerated.

Other uses. Lamotrigine is FDA approved for maintenance therapy of bipolar disorder. It can also improve depression in some patients with epilepsy.

Adverse Reactions

The adverse reactions associated with lamotrigine therapy are similar to with most other antiepileptic drugs. Dizziness, ataxia, somnolence, headache, diplopia, nausea, vomiting, rash, insomnia, and incoordination are the most commonly reported adverse effects. Stevens-Johnson syndrome, a life-threatening dermatologic reaction, is rare but usually occurs during the first 2 months of therapy. Lamotrigine is more tolerable than carbamazepine and topiramate because it has fewer adverse cognitive effects.

Drug Interactions

Lamotrigine does not induce or inhibit cytochrome P-450 enzymes. Carbamazepine can decrease lamotrigine levels, and valproate increases lamotrigine levels more than twofold.

Levetiracetam

The exact mechanism of action of levetiracetam is unknown. It is thought to inhibit presynaptic calcium channels, an effect that is believed to impede impulse conduction across synapses. Table 14.3 reviews the FDA-approved indications for levetiracetam. It is commonly used as monotherapy for partial-onset and generalized tonic-clonic seizures and may also be effective in children with Lennox-Gestaut syndrome and absence seizures.

Adverse Reactions

The most commonly reported adverse reactions include dizziness, somnolence, and weakness. Behavioral changes such as suicidal ideation, aggressive behavior, irritability, hostility, and psychosis have been reported, especially in patients with psychiatric disorders. Stevens-Johnson syndrome has also been reported. It appears to have a low incidence of adverse cognitive effects.

Drug Interactions

No clinically significant drug interactions have been reported with levetiracetam. It does not inhibit CYP-450 enzymes nor is it a substrate of this system.

Oxcarbazepine

Oxcarbazepine is chemically similar to carbamazepine but causes less induction of hepatic enzymes and does not induce its own metabolism. Table 14.3 reviews its FDA-approved indications. This agent is as effective as phenytoin, carbamazepine, and valproate for the treatment of partial seizures and may be better tolerated. Most of its clinical effect is attributed to its 10-monohydroxy metabolite, which has a half-life of 8 to 10 hours.

Adverse Effects

The most commonly reported adverse effects of oxcarbazepine are somnolence, dizziness, diplopia, ataxia, nausea, and vomiting. The extended-release dose form, taken with food, can increase both the peak concentration of the drug and the likelihood of adverse effects. Stevens-Johnson syndrome has occurred with its use. Cross-sensitivity with carbamazepine hypersensitivity occurs in 20% to 30% of patients.

Drug Interactions

Oxcarbazepine induces CYP-3A4/5 enzymes and inhibits CYP-2C19 enzymes. It can increase phenytoin levels by 40%. Its active metabolite is reduced in the presence of such drugs as phenobarbital and phenytoin.

Carbamazepine

Carbamazepine for trigeminal neuralgia.

Structurally related to the tricyclic antidepressants, carbamazepine (kar-ba-MAZ-e-peen) (Tegretol) is used to treat seizures. Table 14.2 lists the specific seizure disorders that it can treat. Carbamazepine is discussed in greater detail than the newer drugs because of its impact on oral health care.

Other uses. Carbamazepine is of special interest in dentistry because of its use in the treatment of trigeminal neuralgia (tic douloureux). It is also indicated in the treatment of bipolar depression.

Pharmacologic Effects

The mechanism of action involves blocking sodium channels, which then stops the propagation of nerve impulses. Other effects of carbamazepine include inhibition of high-frequency repetitive firing in neurons and presynaptic decrease in synaptic transmission.

Adverse Reactions

Carbamazepine can have many types of adverse reactions; some are serious, but most patients seem to tolerate the medication well. CNS depression and gastrointestinal tract problems are most common.

Central nervous system effects. Carbamazepine can produce dizziness, vertigo, drowsiness, fatigue, ataxia, confusion, headache, nystagmus, and visual (diplopia) and speech disturbances. Activation of a latent psychosis, abnormal involuntary movements, depression, and peripheral neuritis occur rarely.

Gastrointestinal effects. Gastrointestinal side effects include nausea, vomiting, and gastric distress. Abdominal pain, diarrhea, constipation, and anorexia have also been noted. Taking carbamazepine with food can reduce its chance of producing nausea and vomiting.

Hematologic effects. Fatal blood dyscrasias, including aplastic anemia and agranulocytosis, have been reported in relation to carbamazepine therapy. These effects usually occur within 4 months and have been reported in elderly patients taking carbamazepine for trigeminal neuralgia (may be caused by the higher doses used). Thrombocytopenia and leukopenia have also been reported. Because of the hematologic adverse effects, it is necessary to perform laboratory tests to monitor these patients. Patients should be made aware of the symptoms of blood dyscrasias and warned to stop the drug and report any of the symptoms immediately. The dental team should observe the oral cavity of any patient taking carbamazepine with these side effects in mind (look for petechiae and signs of infection).

TABLE 14.3 Antiepileptic Drugs

Drug	Mechanism	FDA-Approved Indications	Adverse Reactions
Brivaracetam (Briviact)	Displays a high and selective affinity for synaptic vesicle protein 2A (SV2A) in the brain, which may contribute to its antiepileptic effects	Monotherapy and adjunctive therapy of partial seizures in patients ≥16 years of age	Somnolence, dizziness, fatigue, nausea, vomiting
Eslicarbazepine (Aptiom)	Thought to involve the inhibition of voltage-gated sodium channels.	Monotherapy and adjunctive therapy of partial-onset seizures in adults	Dizziness, somnolence, nausea, headache, diplopia, tremor, hyponatremia, Stevens-Johnson syndrome
Felbamate (Felbatol)	Antagonist to glycine (stimulant neurotransmitter)	Adjunctive therapy or monotherapy for partial seizures with or without generalization	Bone marrow depression (agranulocytosis, aplastic anemia), severe hepatitis. Monitor liver function. Third-line drug. Available on a very limited basis
Fosphenytoin (Cerebyx)	Stabilizes neuronal membranes	Acute seizures, status epilepticus	Parenteral use
Gabapentin (Neurontin)	GABA (γ-aminobutyric acid) analog but does not interact with GABA receptor	Adjunctive treatment of partial seizures with and without secondary generalizations in adults and children ≥3 years of age	Somnolence, dizziness, ataxia, fatigue, nystagmus, blurred vision, confusion. Edema weight gain and movement disorders have been reported. Does not induce or inhibit hepatic microsomal enzymes
Lacosamide (Vimpat)	Selectively enhances slow inactivation of voltage-gated sodium channels	Monotherapy or adjunctive therapy for adults with partial onset seizures	Dizziness, headache, nausea, vomiting, fatigue, ataxia, diplopia, somnolence, tremor. Classified as a schedule V controlled substance because of reports of euphoria.
Lamotrigine (Lamictal)	Inactivates sodium channels	Adjunctive therapy for partial seizures, primary generalized tonic-clonic seizures, or generalized seizures of the Lennox-Gestaut syndrome in patients ≥2 years of age	Dizziness, headache, nausea, somnolence, diplopia, rash/hypersensitivity, Stevens-Johnson syndrome (rare)
Levetiracetam (Keppra)	Exact mechanism of action is unknown	Adjunctive therapy for partial seizures in adults and children ≥1 month of age, for primary generalized tonic-clonic seizures n adults and children ≥6 years of age, and for myoclonic seizures in adults and adolescents ≥12 years of age	Dizziness, somnolence, weakness, irritability, behavioral changes, hallucinations, psychosis. No clinically significant pharmacokinetic drug interactions. Low incidence of adverse cognitive effects. Stevens-Johnson syndrome has been reported
Oxcarbazepine (Trileptal)	Exact mechanism of action is unknown	Monotherapy and adjunctive therapy for partial seizures in adults and children ≥4 years of age and adjunctive therapy for partial seizures in children ≥2 years of age	Somnolence, dizziness, diplopia, ataxia, nausea, vomiting, Stevens-Johnson syndrome reported. Does not cause induction of its own metabolism. Less induction of hepatic enzymes
Perampanel (Fycompa)	Targets and antagonizes AMPA (α-Amino-3-hydroxy-5-methyl-4-isoxazolepropionic acid) glutamate receptors which then decreases seizure activity	Monotherapy and adjunctive treatment for partial-onset seizures in patients ≥12 years of age	Dizziness, drowsiness, weight gain, mood changes, ataxia, vertigo, nausea, fatigue, suicidal ideation, aggressive behavior. Controlled Substance III scheduled drug because of abuse and dependence
Phenobarbital	Prolongs or potentiates the effects of GABA	Alone or in combination for the treatment of generalized tonic-clonic and partial seizures	Sedation, excitement, and hyperactivity in children. Stomatitis, which may preclude serious skin reactions such as Stevens-Johnson syndrome
Pregabalin (Lyrica)	In vitro, pregabalin reduces the calcium-dependent release of several neurotransmitters	Adjunctive therapy for partial seizures in adults	Somnolence, dizziness, ataxia, weight gain, dry mouth, blurred vision, peripheral edema, abnormal thinking. Schedule V controlled substance because it caused euphoria in some clinical trials
Rufinamide (Banzel)	Thought to involve the stabilization of the sodium channel inactive state, effectively keeping the ion channels closed	Adjunctive therapy for Lennox-Gestaut syndrome in patients ≥4 years of age	Somnolence and vomiting, headache, dizziness, fatigue, nausea, diplopia, tremor
Tiagabine (Gabitril)	Inhibitor of GABA uptake	Adjunctive therapy for partial seizures in patients ≥12 years of age	Dizziness, nervousness, tremor, depression; rash idiosyncratic

Continued

TABLE 14.3   Antiepileptic Drugs—cont'd

Drug	Mechanism	FDA-Approved Indications	Adverse Reactions
Topiramate (Topamax)	Blocks sodium channels, potentiates GABA at different site from that of other drugs	Monotherapy or adjunctive therapy for partial/primary generalized tonic-clonic seizures in adults and children ≥2 years of age Adjunctive therapy for Lennox-Gastaut syndrome in children ≥2 years of age	No effect on metabolism, some drug interactions, reduced effectiveness of birth control pills
Vigabatrin (Sabril)	Believed to be the result of irreversible GABA inhibition	Monotherapy for infantile spasms and adjunctive therapy for complex partial seizures refractory to other AEDs in persons ≥10 years of age	Only available through a restricted distribution program due to concerns about retinal toxicity and permanent visual field loss.
Zonisamide (Zonegran)	In vitro trials suggest a blockade of sodium channels	Adjunctive therapy for partial seizures in adults	Somnolence, dizziness, confusion, anorexia, nausea, diarrhea, weight loss, Stevens-Johnson syndrome, agranulocytosis, psychosis

FDA, US Food and Drug Administration; *AED,* Antiepileptic Drug.

Dermatologic effects. Rashes, urticaria, photosensitivity reactions, and altered skin pigmentation can occur. Erythema multiforme, erythema nodosum, and aggravation of systemic lupus erythematosus have been reported. Alopecia can also occur.

> Alopecia: Male pattern baldness.

Oral effects. Dry mouth, glossitis, and stomatitis can sometimes be seen in patients taking carbamazepine. A child who is taking chewable carbamazepine, often four times daily, is exposed to sugar for an extended period (sticks to teeth). The pediatric dose form of carbamazepine contains 63% sugar in its chewable tablet. The parents should be questioned about the child's medication use and the oral hygiene methods being used.

Drug Interactions

Carbamazepine can decrease the effect of doxycycline, warfarin, theophylline, and oral contraceptives. Carbamazepine's effects may be increased by erythromycin, isoniazid, propoxyphene, and calcium channel blockers. The dental management of patients taking carbamazepine is presented in Box 14.3.

Phenytoin

Phenytoin is a hydantoin that works by blocking the sustained high-frequency repetitive firing of action potentials. Phenytoin is used to treat both generalized tonic-clonic and partial seizures with complex symptomatology. Although phenytoin has traditionally been considered a drug of choice for treating generalized tonic-clonic seizures, it is no longer considered a drug of choice because of its complicated pharmacokinetics, adverse effects, and many drug interactions. However, it is discussed in detail here, owing to its impact on oral health care. Because phenytoin is associated with gingival enlargement, the dental team plays an integral role in the management of patients who use or have used this agent.

Adverse Reactions

The adverse reactions associated with phenytoin are frequent, affect many body systems, and may be serious (rare). Because of phenytoin's narrow therapeutic index, adverse reactions associated with elevated blood values can occur. The chance for toxicity is also increased because phenytoin's metabolism is a saturable process. Phenytoin has a propensity for drug interactions because of its enzyme-stimulating property.

BOX 14.3   Dental Management of Patients Taking Carbamazepine (Tegretol)

- Check for dry mouth, glossitis, and stomatitis.
- Additive bleeding is a risk: Use caution with drugs that can alter coagulation.
- Look for symptoms of blood dyscrasias.
- Check for flu-like symptoms.
- Monitor white blood cell counts.
- Consider drug interactions—doxycycline (reduced doxycycline effect) and erythromycin (increased carbamazepine).
- Perform appropriate laboratory testing (if carbamazepine being prescribed by dentist for trigeminal neuralgia):
  - Hematologic tests
  - Ophthalmologic examination
  - Complete urinalysis
  - Liver function tests
- Emphasize oral hygiene; for a child using chewable carbamazepine tablets, the large amount of sugar could predispose to a higher caries rate.

Gastrointestinal effects. Gastrointestinal adverse reactions to phenytoin are not uncommon. Taking the medication with food can reduce them. Other drugs with the potential for adverse gastrointestinal tract effects, such as NSAIDs or opioids, should be used carefully.

Central nervous system effects. The CNS effects of phenytoin include mental confusion, nystagmus, ataxia, slurred speech, blurred vision, diplopia, amblyopia, dizziness, and insomnia. Because these effects are dose related, they can often be controlled by a reduction in dose.

> Amblyopia: Impaired vision in an eye that otherwise appears normal—lazy eye.

Dermatologic effects. Skin reactions to phenytoin range from rash to (rarely) exfoliative dermatitis, lupus erythematosus, and Stevens-Johnson syndrome. Some patients experience irreversible hypertrichosis or hirsutism (excessive hairiness) on the trunk and face. This is one reason that alternative drugs are often selected, especially in a girl or young woman.

Vitamin deficiency. Deficiency produced by phenytoin may involve vitamin D and folate. Osteomalacia may result from phenytoin's interference with vitamin D metabolism. The first symptoms of folate deficiency may be oral mucosal changes such as ulcerations and glossitis. Treatment involves administering folic acid.

Teratogenicity/growth. Fetal hydantoin syndrome is the term given to the congenital abnormality associated with maternal ingestion of phenytoin (Fig. 14.1). It consists of craniofacial anomalies, microcephaly, nail/digit hypoplasia, limb defects, growth deficiency, and mental retardation. Thickening of facial structures and coarsening of facial features have been noted.

Gingival enlargement

> Gingival enlargement.

Another adverse reaction to phenytoin, gingival enlargement (previously referred to as *gingival hyperplasia*), occurs in approximately 50% of all long-term patients. The name change is the result of a greater understanding of the nature of the enlargement. In approximately 30% of affected patients, gingival enlargement is severe enough to require surgical intervention.

Symptoms. The clinical symptoms that occur with gingival enlargement may appear as little as a few weeks or as much as a few years after initial drug therapy. It often begins as a painless enlargement of the gingival margin. The gingiva is pink and does not bleed easily unless other factors are present. With time, the interproximal papillae become involved and finally coalesce to cover even the occlusal surfaces of the teeth. The hyperplasia is more commonly located in the anterior rather than the posterior surfaces, and the buccal rather than the lingual surfaces. The affected areas of the mouth, in descending order of severity, are the maxillary anterior facial, mandibular anterior facial, maxillary posterior facial, and mandibular posterior facial areas. In the affected patient, both normal and abnormal tissue may be found. Edentulous areas are rarely involved. As the tissue begins to enlarge, it becomes more fibrotic or dense. Patients may experience tooth movement, which may result in the loss of teeth.

The better the patient's oral hygiene, the less likely the lesions are to occur or the less severe they will be if they do occur. Younger patients are more likely to experience this adverse reaction. Controversy exists about the contribution of dose and duration of therapy to the risk for the development of gingival enlargement.

Etiology. The cause of phenytoin gingival enlargement is unknown. Many causes have been investigated, including alteration in the function of the adrenal gland, hypersensitivity or allergic reaction, immunologic reaction, and vitamin C or folate deficiency. Because it is known that phenytoin may be found in the saliva, some investigators suggest a local etiology.

Management. The management of phenytoin-induced gingival enlargement requires consultation between dental personnel and the patient's physician. Some possible alternatives are as follows:

Choose another antiepileptic drug. Choosing another effective antiepileptic drug is one method of handling the gingival enlargement caused by phenytoin.

Discontinue phenytoin. Patients who have stopped taking phenytoin experience a decrease in gingival enlargement over a 1-year period. Surgical intervention should wait until at least 18 months after cessation of therapy because some patients experience additional reduction in the enlargement even after 1 year.

Improve oral hygiene. Meticulous oral hygiene may delay the onset or decrease the rate of formation of enlargement. Avoiding irritating restorations may also reduce enlargement. Even with ideal oral hygiene, enlargement is not always totally preventable, and once formed it is not easily reversed.

Consider gingivectomy. When gingival enlargement interferes with plaque control, esthetics, or mastication and when oral hygiene has not been successful in controlling enlargement, surgical elimination

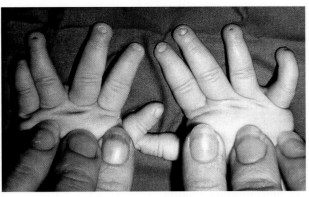

Fig. 14.1 Infant with fetal hydantoin syndrome. Hypoplasia of nails and distal phalanges. (From Graham JM, Jr. *Smith's Recognizable Patterns of Human Deformation.* 3rd ed. St. Louis: Saunders; 2008.)

BOX 14.4   Dental Management of Patients Taking Phenytoin (Dilantin)

- If patient has nausea, avoid drugs that are gastric irritants.
- Monitor for gingival enlargement.
- Provide extensive oral hygiene instruction.
- Schedule more frequent oral prophylaxis.

---

is indicated. It is not a permanent solution because if the patient continues taking phenytoin, enlargement quickly returns in most cases and can progress to the presurgical level in a short period.

Consider other drugs. Although many types of drugs, such as diuretics, corticosteroids, mouthwashes, vitamin C, folic acid, and antihistamines, have been tried for the treatment of this condition, none has been shown to be effective in controlled trials.

Box 14.4 summarizes the management of dental patients taking phenytoin.

Ethosuximide

The drug of choice for the treatment of absence seizures is ethosuximide (eth-oh-SUX-i-mide) (Zarontin) (see Table 14.2). Its mechanism of action may involve inhibiting the T-type calcium channels. It is ineffective in partial seizures with complex symptoms and in tonic-clonic seizures. In the treatment of mixed seizures, agents effective against tonic-clonic seizures must be used in addition to ethosuximide.

Gastrointestinal adverse effects include anorexia, gastric upset, cramps, pain, diarrhea, and nausea and vomiting. CNS adverse effects include drowsiness, hyperactivity, headache, and hiccups. Ethosuximide has been associated with blood dyscrasias, a positive direct Coombs' test result, systemic lupus erythematosus, Stevens-Johnson syndrome, and hirsutism. Oral effects reported with ethosuximide include gingival enlargement and swelling of the tongue.

Benzodiazepines

Benzodiazepines, such as clonazepam (kloe-NA-ze-pam) (Klonopin) and clobazam (Onfi) are used orally as antiepileptic adjuvants. Diazepam (Valium), lorazepam (Ativan), and midazolam (Versed) are used parenterally to treat recurrent tonic-clonic seizures or status epilepticus.

Clonazepam is used as an adjunct to treat absence seizures not responsive to ethosuximide. Drowsiness and ataxia occur often.

Behavioral disturbances and adverse neurologic effects can occur. Other side effects reported relate to the gastrointestinal tract and to the dermatologic and hematologic systems. Oral manifestations include increased salivation, coated tongue, dry mouth, and sore gums. This agent is also used as an adjunct in the treatment of certain mental illnesses.

Clobazam is used as an adjunctive treatment for seizures associated with Lennox-Gastaut syndrome in patients 2 years or older. The most common adverse effects are somnolence, pyrexia, lethargy, drooling, and constipation. Like other benzodiazepines, clobazam can cause anterograde amnesia, ataxia, and withdrawal symptoms. It is classified as a schedule IV controlled substance.

Other Antiepileptic Agents

There are many other drugs available to treat the many different types of epilepsy. Phenobarbital and the newer antiepileptics are reviewed in Table 14.3.

DENTAL TREATMENT OF THE PATIENT WITH EPILEPSY

The dental team should not treat a patient who has a history of seizure disorders without reviewing the management of patients with epilepsy, including the procedures for handling a patient experiencing tonic-clonic seizures. Preventive measures include a detailed seizure history, treatment planning to avoid excessive stress and missed medications, and education of the entire dental office staff. The management of the patient experiencing tonic-clonic seizures should include moving the patient to the floor if possible, tilting the patient's head to one side to prevent aspiration, and removing objects from the patient's mouth before the seizure to prevent fracture of teeth. The use of tongue blades is not recommended because the blades may split, causing additional trauma in the oral cavity.

NONSEIZURE USES OF ANTIEPILEPTICS

Neurologic Pain

Several antiepileptics are used to manage chronic pain syndromes. An example is carbamazepine, which is used to treat trigeminal neuralgia and atypical facial pain. Phenytoin has also been used to treat neurologic pain. Valproic acid has been used for migraine headache prophylaxis. Gabapentin is FDA approved for the treatment of neuropathic pain. Pregabalin is also FDA approved for the treatment of neuropathic pain and fibromyalgia. Topiramate is FDA approved for migraine prophylaxis.

Psychiatric Use

> Antiepileptics for bipolar disorder.

Carbamazepine, valproic acid, clonazepam, and gabapentin have been used in the treatment of certain mental disorders (see Chapter 15). They are sometimes called *mood stabilizers* in this context. They can be used to "level out," or stabilize, the mood in a patient with bipolar disorder. Thus, a patient taking an antiepileptic drug may or may not have a seizure disorder.

▮ DENTAL HYGIENE CONSIDERATIONS

- Conduct a thorough health history to determine the type, duration, and frequency of seizures.
- Determine when the client had his or her last seizure.
- Conduct a detailed medication history to avoid drug interactions and adverse effects.
- Determine whether the patient is experiencing any adverse effects of antiseizure medications.

- Find out how often the patient takes his or her medication and whether it was taken on the day of the appointment.
- Several antiseizure medications can affect oral health care. Always examine the patient for gingival enlargement or overgrowth.
- Have the patient describe his or her seizure symptoms and how the seizure resolves itself.
- Review the information in Boxes 14.2 to 14.4.

▮ ACADEMIC SKILLS ASSESSMENT

1. What is gingival hyperplasia and how can it be treated?
2. Discuss methods to minimize gingival enlargement.
3. What is the mechanism of action of phenytoin and what are its clinical uses?
4. What is hirsutism? Why would this be a concern among girls and young women?
5. What are some of the gastrointestinal adverse reactions associated with phenytoin?
6. What should a patient be told about the concomitant use of an NSAID and phenytoin?
7. What are the dental concerns associated with the CNS adverse reactions of phenytoin?
8. What is carbamazepine and what is its role in treating seizure disorders?
9. What are the major classes of adverse reactions associated with carbamazepine therapy?
10. Can any of the CNS adverse reactions affect oral health care?
11. Why should a parent be concerned about the pediatric dose form of carbamazepine?
12. What would you tell a parent about the pediatric dose form of carbamazepine?
13. What are the dental concerns associated with carbamazepine and what should a parent be told about them?
14. Discuss the role of valproate in the treatment of generalized tonic-clonic seizures. Include adverse effects and any impact on oral health care.
15. What is the role of the newer antiepileptic drugs, lamotrigine, levetiracetam, and oxcarbazepine, in the treatment of seizure disorders? What makes them more appealing than older drugs?

CLINICAL CASE STUDY

Sam Jones is 17 years old and has been coming to your practice for nearly 12 years. His medication/health history is significant for generalized tonic-clonic seizures. He was receiving carbamazepine when he was much younger but was switched to phenytoin because of a high incidence of dental caries. Last year, his physician switched him to levetiracetam because he could not tolerate phenytoin. He is in today for his scheduled maintenance oral examination.

1. What is carbamazepine and what is its role in treating seizure disorders?
2. What may have been causing the increased incidence of caries in Sam?
3. What should a patient and parents or caregivers be told about the pediatric dose form of carbamazepine?
4. What are the adverse effects associated with phenytoin therapy?
5. Discuss the adverse effects that may have led to Sam's inability to tolerate phenytoin.
6. What is levetiracetam and what is its role in treating generalized tonic-clinic seizures?
7. Are there any dental concerns associated with levetiracetam?

15

Drugs for the Treatment of Central Nervous System Disorders

(e) http://evolve.elsevier.com/Haveles/pharmacology

LEARNING OBJECTIVES

1. Name and describe the three categories of functional disorders discussed in this chapter.
2. Outline some basic precautions that the dental health care professional should keep in mind when treating patients with psychiatric disorders.
3. Discuss antipsychotic agents and their mechanism of action as well as the following:
   - Identify first-generation antipsychotics their adverse reactions, drug interactions, uses, and dental implications.
   - Identify second-generation antipsychotics, their adverse effects, drug interactions, uses, and dental implications.

4. Discuss antidepressant agents, including:
   - Describe the mechanism of action and adverse reactions of selective serotonin reuptake inhibitors.
   - Describe the mechanism of action and adverse effects of serotonin norepinephrine reuptake inhibitors.
   - Describe the mechanism of action, adverse reactions, and drug interactions of the tricyclic antidepressants.
5. Name several other types of antidepressants and their possible adverse reactions and dental implications.
6. List several drugs used to treat bipolar disorder.

Many drugs have the ability to affect mental activity. Some are used in the treatment of psychiatric disorders. The dental health care worker is most likely to encounter the use of these agents in dental patients for whom they have been prescribed by psychiatrists or other physicians. Because these agents are so widely prescribed and can alter a patient's dental treatment, the dental health care worker must understand their pharmacologic effects, adverse reactions, and dental implications.

Agents used in the treatment of the major psychiatric disorders are discussed in this chapter. Those used to treat anxiety are discussed in Chapter 11. The antiepileptic drugs used as "mood stabilizers" are discussed in Chapter 14. Because the psychotherapeutic drugs are classified by therapeutic use, a brief discussion of the common psychiatric illnesses follows.

PSYCHIATRIC DISORDERS

There are many psychiatric disorders. Psychiatric disorders can be categorized as psychoses, affective disorders, or anxiety disorders (Fig. 15.1).

Schizophrenia: Split or loss of reality.

The psychoses are discussed first. Schizophrenia, the most common type of psychosis, is an extensive disturbance of the patient's personality function with a loss of perception of reality. Schizophrenia is derived from the word meaning "splitting," and in context it refers to the patient's splitting from reality (not into multiple personalities). The patient's ability to function in society is impaired because of altered thinking. The impaired thinking of patients with schizophrenia may be so detached from reality and their delusions or paranoia

(e.g., someone is out to get me) so severe that their illness could lead to committing serious crimes, including assassination attempts or murders. Patients may suffer from hallucinations, delusions, or agitation. The positive symptoms of psychosis include agitation and auditory hallucinations. Other patients may be introspective and uninvolved. The negative effects of psychosis include flat affect and apathy (Box 15.1).

The etiology of schizophrenia is not specifically known, but a familial pattern is often seen. The biochemical actions of the brain and even brain anatomy have been demonstrated to be different in some patients with schizophrenia from those in normal individuals.

Affective disorders include endogenous and exogenous depression and bipolar disorder or mania with or without depression.

Major depressive disorder, or depression, is the result of biologic, psychological, and social factors. Biologic factors consist of low levels of the neurotransmitters serotonin, norepinephrine (NE), and dopamine, or a combination of the three in the brain. Psychological and social factors are related to specific external life events. Whether there are actually two types of depression separated by circumstances of occurrence is questionable. Theories for several different types of depression based on the biochemical situation in the brain have been developed, but no one has been able to demonstrate the types. Patients who exhibit alternating periods of depression and excitation (mania, elation) have bipolar (*bi*, two) depression, also known as manic-depressive disorder.

Anxiety disorders are less severe than psychoses but can also be helped by drug therapy. Examples are anxiety, panic disorder, phobias, and obsessive-compulsive disorder. Psychophysiologic (somatic) disorders are those that have an emotional origin but manifest as physiologic symptoms. Personality disorders include sexual deviation, alcoholism, and drug dependence. Anxiety disorders are now

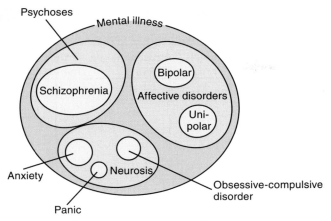

Fig. 15.1 Classification of common mental illnesses.

BOX 15.1   Symptoms of Psychoses

Positive
Hallucinations, auditory
Delusions
Unwanted thoughts
Disorganized behavior
Agitation
Distorted speech, communication

Negative
Flat affect
Unemotional lack of emotion
Apathetic, passivity
Abstract thinking difficult
Spontaneity and goals lacking
Thought and speech impaired
Lack of pleasure
Social withdrawal

---

managed with antidepressants because of the concerns of abuse/dependence with benzodiazepines. Situational anxiety-related problems can be treated with benzodiazepines. Divisions of these different mental disorders have been and are continually changing to reflect either a greater knowledge or a political or "fad" perspective (What is "normal" anyway?).

This presentation is an oversimplification of the classifications of psychiatric disorders. The drug groups discussed in this chapter are antipsychotic agents, used to treat psychoses; antidepressant agents, used to treat affective disorders; and lithium, used to treat bipolar disorder. The benzodiazepines, used to treat anxiety and panic disorders, are discussed in Chapter 11.

Before the antipsychotic drugs were introduced into the management of psychiatric disorders, many physical methods were used to treat patients. Only electroconvulsive therapy (ECT, shock therapy) is still used in the treatment of depression. With the use of neuromuscular blocking agents, ECT therapy has become much safer. ECT produces the fastest results of any treatment for depression. It is reserved for patients whose disease is refractive to antidepressant therapy. Some memory loss occurs during the treatment (several sessions).

Use caution in verbal interaction with patient.

When treating patients with mental disorders, the dental hygienist should observe the following general precautions:

Communication: Patients with various mental disorders may perceive comments or movement from dental health care workers as threatening. Even normal office discussions may be perceived differently from how they are intended. For example, small talk with a peer may be interpreted as a conspiracy by the patient. What you say around and to the patient should be carefully monitored. (I once asked a patient, "How are you?" and the patient replied in a loud and angry voice, "Why are you asking me that question?")

Compliance: Patients undergoing drug therapy for the treatment of psychoses often do not take their medication as prescribed. A thorough health history including the patient's medication and its dosage should be obtained.

Suicide: Depressed patients may attempt suicide. When patients are severely depressed, they have no motivation and usually do not act on any irrational thoughts of suicide. After the start of antidepressant therapy, partial improvement gives them the motivation to attempt suicide before the full antidepressant effects have developed. Children and teens appear to be at a higher risk for suicide with antidepressant therapy, especially with the newer class of drugs.

ANTIPSYCHOTIC AGENTS

Antipsychotic drugs are used for the treatment of schizophrenia, schizoaffective disorder, delusional disorder, and other types of psychosis. The first-generation antipsychotic drugs are more likely to treat the positive symptoms (agitation, hallucinations, delusions) than the negative symptoms (apathy, social withdrawal, blunted affect) of schizophrenia. Some symptoms may improve rapidly with antipsychotic therapy, but chronic schizophrenia may take weeks to months to respond. Most patients require maintenance therapy with antipsychotics, which can help reduce the rate of relapse. Patients can be treated with either first- or second-generation antipsychotics. The second-generation antipsychotics are now used more commonly than the first-generation agents even though clinical trials have not demonstrated a clear advantage in efficacy, except for clozapine and possibly olanzapine. However, the second-generation antipsychotic drugs are better tolerated. Table 15.1 lists available antipsychotic drugs, their adult usual daily dose ranges for maintenance therapy, and their adverse effect profiles.

Mechanism of Action

There are several differences between the first-generation and second-generation antipsychotic agents. The first-generation antipsychotic agents were primarily dopamine antagonists (Fig. 15.2). The second-generation agents have action at more than one receptor, for example, the dopamine, serotonin (5-HT), and NE receptors, improving their efficacy. The side effects of the second-generation antipsychotics are less than those of the first-generation antipsychotics. Like the first-generation antipsychotics, the second-generation agents are effective against the positive effects associated with psychoses. However, unlike the first-generation antipsychotics, the second-generation antipsychotic agents are effective against the negative effects.

Pharmacologic Effects
First-Generation Antipsychotics
The pharmacologic effects of the first-generation antipsychotic agents are as follows.

Antipsychotic effect. All antipsychotics have antipsychotic effects, such as slowing of the psychomotor activity in an agitated patient and calming of emotion with suppression of hallucinations and delusions. These agents are active against the positive effects of psychosis but have

TABLE 15.1   Antipsychotic Agents

| Drug Name Generic (Trade) | Daily Dose (mg)* | Sedation | Severity of Side Effects | | |
			Extrapyramidal Effects	Anticholinergic Effects	Orthostatic Hypotension
First-Generation Antipsychotics					
High Potency					
Fluphenazine (Prolixin)	10 qd	1	3	1	1
Haloperidol (Haldol)	5 bid	1	3	1	1
Medium Potency					
Loxapine (Loxitane)	60–100 in 2–4 divided doses	1	2	1	1
Perphenazine (Trilafon)	24 mg in divided doses				
Thiothixene (Navane)	10 bid	1	3	1	2
Low Potency					
Chlorpromazine (Thorazine)	200 bid	3	2	3	3
Thioridazine (Mellaril)	100–200 bid	3	1	3	3
Second-Generation Antipsychotics					
Aripiprazole (Abilify) Orally disintegrating (generic)	10–30 qd 10–15 mg qd	1	2	1	2
Asenapine (Saphris)	5–10 bid	1	2	1	1
Brexpiprazole (Rexulti)	2–4 mg qd	1	2	1	3
Cariprazine (Vraylar)	1.5–6 mg qd	3	3	3	1
Clozapine (Clozaril)[†]	300–900 divided bid or tid	4	1	4	4
Iloperidone (Fanapt)	6–12 bid	1	0–1	2	2
Lurasidone (Latuda)	40–160 qd	2	2	1	1
Olanzapine (Zyprexa) Orally disintegrating (Zyprexa Zydis)	10–20 qd	2	2	3	2
Paliperidone (Invega)	6–12 qd	1	2	1	2
Quetiapine (Seroquel) Extended release (Seroquel XR)	150–750 in 2 or 3 divided doses 400–800 qd	3	2	0	2
Risperidone (Risperdal) Orally disintegrating (Risperdal M-TAB)	4–6 qd	1	2	1	2
Ziprasidone (Geodon)	20–80 bid	2	2	1	2

*Usual oral dose for outpatient treatment in mg/day.
[†]Agranulocytosis; weekly white blood cell (WBC) counts needed.
0, Nonexistent; *1*, very low; *2*, low; *3*, moderate; *4*, high; *qd*, once daily; *bid*, twice a day; *qid*, four times a day; *tid*, three times a day.

little effect on the negative effects. Second-generation antipsychotics differ in that they appear to be effective against both the positive and negative symptoms of schizophrenia.

Antiemetic effect. The antiemetic effect of first-generation antipsychotics is a result of depression of the chemoreceptor trigger zone, an area in the brain that causes nausea and vomiting. These agents are useful in the symptomatic treatment of certain types of nausea and vomiting. Historically, prochlorperazine (Compazine) has been used for this effect.

Adverse reactions. Table 15.1 lists the side effects of the first-generation antipsychotic agents, and Fig. 15.3 demonstrates the relative side effects of several first-generation antipsychotic agents. Management of patients taking these agents involves minimizing the troubling side effects in each patient. Though first-generation antipsychotics are used less commonly than second-generation antipsychotics, the former's adverse effects are discussed in greater detail because they can negatively affect oral health care.

Sedation. First-generation antipsychotics differ in the degree of sedation and drowsiness they produce. The degree of sedation is one factor that determines which antipsychotic agent is prescribed. Tolerance develops to the sedative effect but not to the antipsychotic effect.

Akinesia: Loss of voluntary movement.
Akathisia: Inability to sit still.
Tardive dyskinesia: Abnormal, involuntary movements.

Extrapyramidal effects. The most common type of adverse reactions associated with these agents results from stimulation of the extrapyramidal system. All first-generation antipsychotics have this effect, although the incidence of the reaction varies. The following types of extrapyramidal effects can occur:
- Acute dystonia, consisting of muscle spasms of the face, tongue, neck, and back

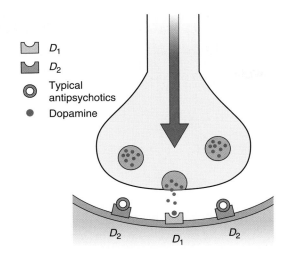

Fig. 15.2 Conventional antipsychotics act to block postsynaptic dopamine (D) receptors. Conventional antipsychotics have a greater affinity for D_2 receptors than for D_1 receptors. (From McKenry L, Tessier E, Hogan MA. *Mosby's Pharmacology in Nursing.* 22nd ed. St. Louis: Mosby; 2006.)

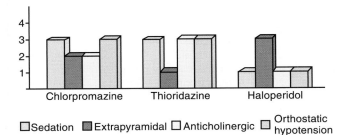

Fig. 15.3 Comparison of the severities of adverse reactions of selected antipsychotics.

- **Parkinsonism,** with symptoms of resting tremor, rigidity, and akinesia
- **Akathisia,** or increased compulsive motor activity
- **Tardive dyskinesia,** involuntary, repetitive body movements involving the tongue, lips, face, and jaw

Its onset is gradual and the movements are coordinated and rhythmic. This effect is exacerbated by drug withdrawal. The involuntary movements, especially those involving the face, jaw, and tongue, can make home care difficult if not impossible. Performing oral prophylaxis is difficult because of the strength of the oral facial and tongue muscles.

The dental hygienist should discuss the patient's side effects with his or her physician if oral prophylaxis cannot be performed. A dosage or drug change may be instituted by the patient's psychiatrist. With the availability of the second-generation agents, extrapyramidal side effects can be greatly minimized.

The extrapyramidal side effects of first-generation antipsychotics can cause severe intermittent pain in the region of the temporomandibular joint (TMJ). This pain is produced by a spasm of the muscles of mastication. In an acute attack, it becomes difficult or impossible to open or close the jaw. Should muscle spasm be present, force should not be exerted to open the patient's mouth for dental treatment because dislocations of the mandible can occur.

Treatment of an acute spasm of the mandible must be undertaken after consultation with the patient's prescribing physician. Alternatives include decreasing the antipsychotic dose, adding an anticholinergic medication to counteract the spasm, or changing the patient's antipsychotic medication to one with fewer extrapyramidal effects. The anticholinergics used to treat the extrapyramidal side effects of the antipsychotics include benztropine (Cogentin) and trihexyphenidyl (Artane).

Orthostatic hypotension. Because these agents depress the central sympathetic outflow and block the peripheral adrenergic receptors (α-sympathetic blockers), they can cause orthostatic hypotension, which is additive with the effect of other CNS depressants. When a patient rises rapidly from the supine position, a compensatory tachycardia can accompany the orthostatic hypotension.

Other cardiovascular effects. These agents have also been reported to cause tachycardia.

Seizures. Because first-generation antipsychotics lower the seizure threshold, seizures may be more easily precipitated in a patient taking such an agent, especially one with a previous history of epilepsy.

Anticholinergic effects

Xerostomia with older antipsychotics.

The anticholinergic effects of first-generation antipsychotics produce blurred vision, xerostomia, and constipation. This is especially significant because the anticholinergic effects of other medications the patient may be taking are additive. The anticholinergics, such as benztropine, which are used to treat the extrapyramidal symptoms, are additive, too. The dental hygienist should be aware of the presence of xerostomia and should question patients regarding their method of managing it.

Second-Generation Antipsychotics

Second-generation antipsychotics have a relatively low incidence of extrapyramidal effects and are less likely to cause tardive dyskinesia and neuroleptic malignant syndrome than first-generation agents. Clozapine, olanzapine, and quetiapine do, however, cause a significant amount of weight gain. Table 15.2 reviews some of the adverse effects of the second-generation antipsychotics.

Agranulocytosis. Clozapine causes agranulocytosis or granulocytopenia in about 1% of patients taking it. As a result, patients require weekly blood cell count monitoring. Because it produces potentially life-threatening agranulocytosis, clozapine should be tried only after several trials of other agents have failed. Frequent white blood cell counts with differential are required during therapy. With the release of newer atypical antipsychotic agents, use of this agent has decreased.

Metabolic effects. The second-generation antipsychotics have been associated with a higher risk of hyperglycemia, diabetes, and metabolic syndrome. All second-generation antipsychotics are required by the US Food and Drug Administration (FDA) to carry a product label warning regarding hyperglycemia and diabetes. It is important to monitor patient plasma glucose and cholesterol levels. Patients should be encouraged to maintain a healthy diet and lifestyle.

Tachycardia. Ziprasidone significantly prolongs the QT/QTc interval on electrocardiograms (ECGs). Periodic ECGs should be performed in patients taking this drug.

Drug Interactions
Central Nervous System Depressants

First-generation antipsychotics interact in an additive or even potentiating fashion with all CNS depressants, including benzodiazepines, alcohol, general anesthetics, and opioid analgesics. Persons taking a combination of these drugs can experience increased sedation, confusion, dizziness, and impaired cognitive abilities. Sedation and respiratory depression can occur with the use of both first-generation antipsychotics and any central nervous system depressant drug.

TABLE 15.2 Selected Adverse Effects of Second-Generation Antipsychotics

Drug	Diabetes	Weight Gain	QTc Prolongation	Prolactin Elevation
Aripiprazole	0–1	1	0–1	0–1
Asenapine	1	2	1	2
Brexpiprazole	1	2	0	0–1
Cariprazine	0–1	1	0	0
Clozapine	4	4	1	0–1
Iloperidone	2	2	2	0–1
Lurasidone	0–1	0–1	0–1	0–1
Olanzapine	4	4	1	1
Paliperidone	2	3	1	3
Quetiapine	2	3	1	0–1
Risperidone	2	3	1	3
Ziprasidone	0–1	0–1	2	1

QTc, Corrected QT interval; *0,* nonexistent; *1,* very low; *2,* low; *3,* moderate; *4,* high.

Epinephrine

Epinephrine, used as a vasoconstrictor in local anesthetic solutions, can be safely used in patients taking first-generation antipsychotics. However, because the first-generation antipsychotics are α-adrenergic blockers, epinephrine should not be used to treat vasomotor collapse (acute drop in blood pressure) because it could cause a further decrease in blood pressure. This occurs because of the predominant β-agonist (vasodilating) activity of epinephrine in the presence of the conventional antipsychotics (α-blockers). However, the use of epinephrine-containing local anesthetics in patients taking antipsychotics is acceptable in dentistry.

Anticholinergic Agents

To control excessive extrapyramidal stimulation, first-generation antipsychotic therapy is often combined with anticholinergic drugs such as benztropine (Cogentin). This combination is bound to exacerbate antimuscarinic peripheral effects, such as xerostomia, urinary retention, constipation, blurred vision, and inhibition of sweating.

Uses
For Antipsychotic Effects

Antipsychotics are the drugs of choice for treatment of schizophrenia.

For Antiemetic Effects

Because first-generation antipsychotics prevent or inhibit vomiting, they are useful in the treatment of some types of nausea and vomiting. Prochlorperazine (proe-klor-PAIR-a-zeen) (Compazine) has traditionally been used.

Bipolar Disorder

Second-generation antipsychotics are used to treat and rapidly control symptoms of acute mania. Reports in the medical literature show that they may be effective in preventing recurrent episodes of mania and depression.

Depression

The use of second-generation antipsychotics with antidepressants may be helpful when the response to an antidepressant is not adequate. Quetiapine and oral aripiprazole are FDA-approved for the adjunctive treatment of major depressive disorder.

Other Uses

Intractable hiccups and certain drug withdrawals have been successfully treated with first-generation antipsychotics.

BOX 15.2 Management of the Dental Patient Taking Antipsychotic Agents

- Use caution with patient interactions (patient may misinterpret verbal or nonverbal actions).
- Check for xerostomia and its management.
- Emphasize oral hygiene instruction.
- Extrapyramidal dyskinesia may make oral hygiene more difficult.
- Check the temporomandibular joint for extrapyramidal side effects (mouth may be difficult to open; do not force).
- Sedation from antipsychotics is additive with sedative effects of other agents.
- Epinephrine can be safely used in a dental local anesthetic.
- Encourage patient to rise slowly from the dental chair to minimize orthostatic hypotension.
- Disease may make following an oral care program difficult for the patient (depends on disease severity).

Dental Implications

The dental management of patients taking antipsychotics is summarized in Box 15.2.

Sedation

Sedation, an adverse reaction to the first-generation antipsychotics, is additive with that of other sedating agents.

Anticholinergic Effects

The atropine-like effects of first-generation antipsychotics are additive with those of other agents; this combination can lead to toxic reactions, including tachycardia, urinary retention, blurred vision, constipation, and xerostomia. The dental hygienist should be aware that patients may use sugar-containing candy to counteract xerostomia. Use of sugarless products or artificial saliva (Orex, Xero-Lube, Moi-Stir) should be recommended. Patients should be encouraged to stay away from caffeine-containing beverages because they can exacerbate dry mouth. They should also avoid alcohol-containing mouth rinses because alcohol can also exacerbate dry mouth.

Orthostatic Hypotension

Orthostatic hypotension effect can be minimized by raising the dental chair slowly and assisting the patient's first few steps.

Epinephrine

> Epinephrine can be used with antipsychotics.

Epinephrine should be avoided in the management of an acute hypotensive crisis in a patient taking an antipsychotic. It may be safely used in local anesthetic solutions for dental patients.

Temporomandibular Joint Pain

As a result of the first-generation antipsychotics' extrapyramidal effects, the muscles of mastication may be in spasm.

Tardive Dyskinesia

Tardive dyskinesia is irreversible and should be reported to the patient's physician.

ANTIDEPRESSANT AGENTS

Antidepressant agents are used not only to manage depression but also for a variety of other uses, such as chronic pain adjuvant therapy and migraine headache prophylaxis. One should question the patient to determine the indication for which an antidepressant is being prescribed. The dental hygienist should not assume that the patient is being treated for depression. Until the late 1950s, there was no widely accepted pharmacologic treatment for depression. Forms of mild depression were treated with psychotherapy, and severe depression was treated with ECT. Several classes of antidepressants are currently available, including selective serotonin reuptake inhibitors (SSRIs), serotonin-norepinephrine reuptake inhibitors (SNRIs), tricyclic antidepressants (TCAs), monoamine oxidase inhibitors (MAOIs), bupropion, mirtazapine, nefazodone,

and vilazodone. Improvement can be seen in as little as 2 weeks, but it may take 4 to 8 weeks to achieve substantial benefit.

ECT is still used in the treatment of severely suicidal patients and in cases of depression resistant to antidepressants. In the case of suicidal thoughts, ECT works faster than any antidepressant drug.

The antidepressants may block NE and/or serotonin (5-HT) reuptake (Table 15.3 and Figs. 15.4 and 15.5), produce sedation, and have anticholinergic side effects. One theory of their mechanism of action involves blocking reuptake of NE and/or 5-HT. Another involves downregulation of the β-adrenergic receptors.

Selective Serotonin Reuptake Inhibitors

SSRIs are recommended as first-line therapy for the treatment of major depression. They are generally well tolerated, safe, and effective. There is no convincing data showing that one SSRI is better than another. The SSRIs have specific action on inhibiting the reuptake of 5-HT. Fluoxetine (floo-OX-uh-teen) (Prozac) was the first member of this group, and others have followed. Sertraline (SER-tral-leen) (Zoloft), paroxetine (pa-ROKS-e-teen) (Paxil), citalopram (Celexa), and escitalopram (Lexapro) are other members of this group. Their antidepressant action is equivalent to that of TCAs. Their advantage lies in their adverse reaction profile, which differs from that of TCAs (see Table 15.3).

Adverse Reactions

Central nervous system effects. The SSRIs tend to produce CNS stimulation (activation) rather than CNS depression. Headache, dizziness, tremor, agitation, sweating, and insomnia are side effects associated with stimulation. Weight loss or weight stabilization occurs more often than the weight gain that occurs with TCAs. Somnolence and fatigue have also been reported.

TABLE 15.3 Commonly Used Antidepressants

Drug Name Generic (Trade)	Usual Adult Dose (mg)*	Side Effects					Blocks Reuptake	
		Anticholinergic Effect	Sedation	Orthostatic Hypotension	Weight Gain	Nausea, Diarrhea	NE	SERT
Selective Serotonin Reuptake Inhibitors (SSRIs)								
Citalopram (Celexa)	40 qd	0	0	0	3	0	0	5
Escitalopram (Lexapro)	10–20 qd	0	0	0	0	0	0	5
Fluoxetine (Prozac)	20 qd	0–1	0–1	0–1	0	3	0–1	5
Sertraline (Zoloft)	50–100 qd	0	0–1	0	0	3	0–1	5
Paroxetine (Paxil)	20 qd	0	0–1	0	1	3	0–1	5
Serotonin-Norepinephrine Reuptake Inhibitors								
Desvenlafaxine (Pristiq)	50 qd	1	0	1	0	3	3	3
Venlafaxine (Effexor)†	75 tid	1	0	1	0	3	3	3
Venlafaxine, extended-release (Effexor XR)	75–225 qd	1	0	1	0	3	3	3
Duloxetine (Cymbalta)	60 qd or 30 bid	0–1	0–1	0–1	0–1	3	0–1	5
Levomilnacipran (Fetzima)	40–120 qd	3	0	0	0	2	3	3
Tricyclic—Tertiary Amines								
Amitriptyline (Elavil)	100–300 qd	4	4	2	4	0	2	4
Desipramine (Norpramin, Pertofrane)	100–300 qd	1	1	1	1	0	3	2
Imipramine (Tofranil)	100–300 qd	2	2	3	4	1	2	4
Nortriptyline (Pamelor, Aventyl)	50–150 qd	2	2	1	1	0	2	3

Continued

TABLE 15.3   Commonly Used Antidepressants—cont'd

Drug Name Generic (Trade)	Usual Adult Dose (mg)*	Side Effects					Blocks Reuptake	
		Anticholinergic Effect	Sedation	Orthostatic Hypotension	Weight Gain	Nausea, Diarrhea	NE	SERT
Other Antidepressants								
Bupropion (Wellbutrin), generic	100 tid	2	2	1	0	1	0–1	0–1
Bupropion, sustained-release 12-hr	150 bid	2	2	1	0	1	0–1	0–1
Wellbutrin SR	150 bid							
Aplenzin	348 qd							
extended-release (24-hour) -generic								
Forfivo XL 450 qd	300 qd	2	2	1	0	1	0–1	0–1
Nefazodone (Serzone)‡	200 bid	1	2	1	0	1	0–1	3
Trazodone (Desyrel)	300 divided bid	1	4	2	2	1	0	3
Mirtazapine (Remeron)‡	30–45	2	3	2	0	3	3	3
Vilazodone (Viibryd)	40	0–1	0–1	0–1	0–1	0–1	0–1	5
Vortioxetine (Trintellix)	10–20 qd	1	0–1	0	0	3	0–1	5
Monoamine Oxidase Inhibitors								
Isocarboxazid (Marplan)	30–40 per day, divided	1	2	2	1	0	NA	NA
Phenelzine (Nardil)	30 bid	1	2	2	1	0	NA	NA
Tranylcypromine (Parnate)	20–30 bid	1	1	2	1	0	NA	NA

*Usual adult daily dose (mg).
†In divided doses.
‡Antagonizes α₂-adrenergic receptors.
0, Nonexistent; *1,* very low; *2,* low; *3,* moderate; *4,* high; *bid,* twice a day; *NA,* not applicable; *NE,* norepinephrine; *qd,* once daily; *SERT,* serotonin reuptake inhibitors; *tid,* three times a day.

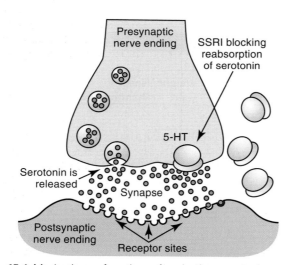

Fig. 15.4 Mechanism of action of selective serotonin reuptake inhibitors. *5-HT,* Serotonin; *SSRI,* selective serotonin reuptake inhibitor.

Gastrointestinal effects. Nausea and diarrhea occur in about 15% to 30% of patients taking SSRIs. Anorexia, dyspepsia, and constipation have been reported.

Oral effects. Oral side effects include xerostomia (10%–15%), taste changes, aphthous stomatitis, glossitis, and, rarely, increased salivation, salivary gland enlargement, and tongue discoloration or edema. The SSRIs differ less in incidence of the side effects.

Other effects. The SSRIs often cause sexual dysfunction. The incidence varies but may be more than 75% with some agents. Excessive sweating is another common side effect. Palpitations have been reported. Citalopram can cause significant QT interval prolongation, and escitalopram may also prolong the QT interval.

SSRIs have different effects on the CYP-450 isoenzymes and can interact with many other drugs.

Serotonin-Norepinephrine Reuptake Inhibitors

The SNRIs are also considered first-line therapy for the treatment of depression. It is not clear, however, whether they offer any advantage over SSRIs. These drugs work by inhibiting the reuptake of both serotonin and NE. Examples are venlafaxine (Effexor), desvenlafaxine (Pristiq), duloxetine (Cymbalta), and levomilnacipran (Fetzima) (see Table 15.3). They appear to be more selective for serotonin than NE. Their adverse effects are similar to those of the SSRIs but can include sweating, tachycardia, elevated blood pressure, and urinary retention. The abrupt discontinuation of these drugs can lead to withdrawal characterized by symptoms of anxiety, which may be attributed to their short half-lives. Dosages of these drugs should be slowly tapered off to reduce the risk of withdrawal.

Tricyclic Antidepressants

The TCAs are sometimes referred to as the first-generation antidepressants because they were developed and marketed before the other agents. However, they are no longer first-line therapy and are reserved for patients with moderate to severe treatment-resistant depression. Table 15.3 lists the antidepressants with their usual adult outpatient daily doses in milligrams. All TCAs are similar in their antidepressant effectiveness, differing only in side-effect profile. These drugs work by blocking the reuptake of both serotonin and NE to varying degrees.

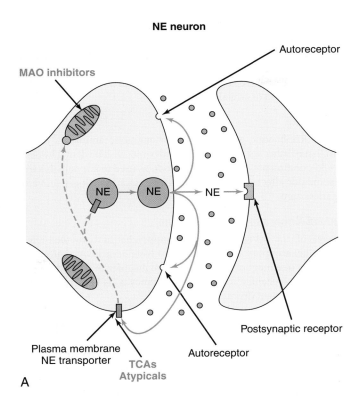

NE neuron

MAO inhibitors

Autoreceptor

Plasma membrane NE transporter

TCAs Atypicals

Postsynaptic receptor

Autoreceptor

A

5-HT neuron

MAO inhibitors

Autoreceptor

Plasma membrane 5-HT transporter

TCAs SSRIs Atypicals

Postsynaptic receptor

Autoreceptor

B

Fig. 15.5 Noradrenergic *(top)* and serotonergic *(bottom)* synapses and sites at which antidepressants may exert their actions. Tricyclic antidepressants *(TCAs)*, selective serotonin reuptake inhibitors *(SSRIs)*, and some atypical antidepressants *(Atypicals)* inhibit the reuptake transporter for norepinephrine *(NE)* and/or serotonin *(5-HT)*. Monoamine oxidase *(MAO)*, which is targeted by MAO inhibitors, is localized at the outer mitochondrial membrane. (From Minneman KP, Wecker L. *Brody's Human Pharmacology: Molecular to Clinical.* 4th ed. Philadelphia: Mosby; 2005.)

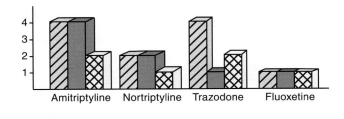

☒ Sedation   ■ Anticholinergic   ☒ Orthostatic hypotension

Fig. 15.6 Relative severities of side effects of some antidepressants.

Adverse Reactions

Some of the widely diverse adverse reactions associated with the TCAs resemble those of the antipsychotic agents (Fig. 15.6; see Table 15.3). Their adverse effects are discussed in more detail than the other antidepressants because they can negatively affect oral health care.

Central nervous system effects. Almost all of the TCAs induce some degree of sedation.

Anticholinergic effects. These agents possess distinct anticholinergic effects resulting in xerostomia, blurred vision, constipation, and urinary retention. Some tolerance can develop with continued use.

Cardiac effects. TCAs can cause tachycardia and orthostatic hypotension. The most serious peripheral side effect associated with the TCAs is cardiac toxicity. They can cause cardiac conduction delays which can lead to arrhythmias. TCAs are more dangerous in an overdose situation than SSRIs because of their cardiac effects.

Drug Interactions

TCAs potentiate (1) the behavioral actions of the amphetamines and other CNS stimulants and (2) the pressor effect of injected sympathomimetics, such as epinephrine. These agents also interact with MAOIs, resulting in severe toxic reactions. Additive anticholinergic effects are seen if TCAs are administered with other agents that have anticholinergic action.

Monoamine Oxidase Inhibitors

> MAOIs: many drug interactions.

MAOIs are a large variety of drugs that have the ability to inhibit monoamine oxidase. MAOIs have many adverse effects, and an overdose can lead to a severe toxic reaction. Adverse effects include sleep disturbances, orthostatic hypotension, sexual dysfunction, and weight gain. MAOIs interact with many drugs, such as amphetamines, and with foods, such as cheeses, wines, and fish, precipitating a hypertensive crisis and even death. Patients taking MAOIs are given detailed food prohibitions because of the chance of drug-food interactions. Because of the potential for life-threatening situations, MAOIs are used as drugs of last choice. A patient taking an MAOI should not be given any drug unless the prescriber has first consulted a reference source on drug interactions.

Other Antidepressants
Bupropion

Bupropion (byoo-PROE-pee-on) (Wellbutrin [and Wellbutrin SR]) is a dopamine-NE reuptake inhibitor that has been on the market and then off the market; in 1993 it was back on the market with increased warnings regarding the possibility of developing seizures at higher doses. About 0.4% of patients treated with bupropion have experienced seizures. This incidence may be 4 times greater than with the TCAs and as much as 10 times greater with TCAs at higher doses. Because of its seizure potential, bupropion is reserved for patients whose depression is not responsive to other agents. Gastrointestinal effects, such as constipation, nausea, and vomiting, occur in about 20% of patients. Neurologic effects, such as dry mouth (28%), headache (25%), excessive sweating, and tremors, have been reported. Agitation (32%) and dizziness (22%) also occur. Divided doses, slow titration of doses, and careful patient selection can minimize seizure risk.

Trazodone

Trazodone (TRAZ-oh-done) (Desyrel) is a serotonin modulator antidepressant unrelated chemically to TCAs. It appears to have antidepressant effects equivalent to those of TCAs. Its advantages are that it has fewer anticholinergic effects (e.g., xerostomia) and that it is less cardiotoxic even at higher doses. Its disadvantages are that it is highly sedative and that it has been associated with painful priapism requiring surgical intervention and leaving some patients permanently impotent.

Nefazodone, Mirtazapine, Vilazodone, and Vortioxetine

Nefazodone (nef-AY-zoe-done) (Serzone), vilazodone (Viibryd), mirtazapine (Remeron), and vortioxetine (Trintellix) are examples of newer antidepressants. They are indicated for the treatment of depression. Nefazodone, like trazodone, is a 5-HT modulator, and vilazodone and vortioxetine are serotonin reuptake inhibitors. Mirtazapine is an NE-5-HT modulator. The incidence of xerostomia is greater than 10% and sexual dysfunction often occurs with nefazodone. Nefazodone raises the serum levels of alprazolam, triazolam, and digoxin. Nefazodone carries a black box warning regarding its potential to cause life-threatening hepatic failure. Mirtazapine causes somnolence, weight gain, constipation, and dry mouth. Vilazodone and vortioxetine have an adverse effect profile similar to that of the SSRIs. There is little evidence available to support vilazodone's claim of a lower incidence of weight gain or sexual dysfunction.

Suicide and Antidepressants

All antidepressants carry a black box warning about suicidal ideation and behavior (suicidality). According to the results of an FDA analysis of placebo-controlled antidepressant trials, there is an increased risk of suicidality in children, adolescents, and young adults ($\leq$24 years of age), information about which is included in the package inserts. All depressed children, adolescents, and adults should be monitored for suicidal ideation and behavior regardless of antidepressant or nontherapy.

Dental Implications

The management of dental patients taking antidepressants is summarized in Box 15.3.

Sympathomimetic Amines

Vasoconstricting drugs (sympathomimetic amines) in the local anesthetic solution must be administered with caution to patients taking TCAs, which may potentiate the vasopressor (increased blood pressure) response to epinephrine. In the usual cardiac dose (0.04 mg), the sympathomimetic amines present in a local anesthetic solution can be safely administered to patients without preexisting arrhythmias. Caution should be used if epinephrine is necessary in a patient taking either citalopram or escitalopram.

Xerostomia

The anticholinergic effect of sympathomimetic amines is additive with that of other agents that produce dry mouth. The dental hygienist should question patients about the products used to alleviate this troublesome side effect and suggest alternatives such as artificial saliva and sugarless gum.

Second-Generation Antipsychotics

Several of the second-generation antipsychotics (extended-release quetiapine, aripiprazole, brexpiprazole) have been FDA-approved for adjunctive treatment of major depressive disorder. A fixed-dose combination of olanzapine and fluoxetine (Symbyax) is FDA-approved for treatment-resistant depression.

DRUGS FOR TREATMENT OF BIPOLAR DISORDER

Lithium is generally the drug of choice for maintenance treatment of bipolar disorder. Bipolar disorder is characterized by elevated moods and periods of depression. The elevated mood is known as hypomania or mania as mood elevation increases. Other agents commonly used today include a variety of antiepileptics, such as carbamazepine, valproate, and lamotrigine, and the second-generation antipsychotics.

Lithium

Lithium (LITH-ee-um) (Eskalith, Lithobid) is used in the treatment of bipolar disorder, which is characterized by cyclic recurrence of mania alternating with depression. The side effects, which can be minimized by monitoring serum lithium levels, include polyuria, fine hand tremor, thirst, and, in more severe cases, slurred speech, ataxia, nausea, vomiting, and diarrhea. Patients undergoing lithium therapy should be observed for signs of overdose toxicity, which may be exhibited as CNS symptoms, including muscle rigidity, hyperactive deep reflexes, excessive tremor, and muscle fasciculations. Because lithium is handled in the body like sodium, changes in sodium levels can affect lithium levels. Salt intake and sweating can also change lithium levels. Some nonsteroidal antiinflammatory drugs (NSAIDs) can decrease lithium clearance, leading to an increase in lithium levels (Box 15.4).

Antiepileptic Drugs

In the treatment of bipolar depression (mania), several antiepileptic agents have been used. The manic phase has been treated

---

BOX 15.3   Management of the Dental Patient Taking Antidepressant Agents

- Use caution in patient interactions.
- An antidepressant is used for other than depression; ask patient why he or she is taking it.
- Check for xerostomia and its management.
- Epinephrine may increase the vasopressor response (blood pressure response). Limit dose of epinephrine to 0.04 mg if blood pressure is a concern.
- Limit total amount of any potentially lethal drugs prescribed if patient is depressed.
- Increase motivation for good oral hygiene (usually improves with treatment of depression).

BOX 15.4   Management of the Dental Patient Taking Lithium

- Monitor toxicity related to lithium levels; sweating and salt intake can alter levels.
- Tremors may interfere with oral hygiene.
- Drowsiness is additive with effects of other central nervous system depressants.
- Xerostomia or excessive salivation reported.
- Naproxen (and other nonsteroidal antiinflammatory drugs) can cause lithium toxicity.

with antiepileptics such as carbamazepine, lamotrigine, valproate, and gabapentin. Valproate, lamotrigine, and carbamazepine are approved by the FDA for treatment of bipolar disorder. Valproate is used more often than lithium because of its more tolerable side-effect profile.

Second-Generation Antipsychotics

All of the atypical antipsychotics have been approved for the long-term treatment of bipolar disorder as well as for acute treatment of bipolar disorder. Olanzapine and aripiprazole are approved for relapse prevention of bipolar disorder.

DENTAL HYGIENE CONSIDERATIONS

- Some patients are still reluctant to state that they have a mental health illness.
- Ask questions pertaining to mental health in a nonthreatening manner.
- Remind the patient that all information is confidential and that the intent of gathering information is to ensure that the patient receives the necessary oral health care.
- Determine which medications the patient is taking. Many medications used to treat psychiatric disorders can affect oral health care.

Such medications also have many potential drug interactions with medications prescribed in a dental practice.
- Check the patient's blood pressure and pulse at each office visit, because many of the medications used to treat psychiatric disorders can cause orthostatic hypotension or tachycardia.
- Review Boxes 15.2 to 15.4.

ACADEMIC SKILLS ASSESSMENT

1. State the major pharmacologic effects of first- and second-generation antipsychotics.
2. State the adverse reactions attributable to the first- and second-generation antipsychotics.
3. How does risperidone differ from haloperidol?
4. What are the dental concerns associated with both first- and second-generation antipsychotics? How would you discuss them with the patient?
5. Explain the drug interactions between epinephrine and the first-generation antipsychotics and epinephrine and the TCAs. Identify the clinically significant interactions.
6. What differentiates one group of antidepressants from another?
7. Describe the advantages of the second-generation antipsychotics.
8. List three adverse reactions associated with the TCAs.
9. State the advantages and disadvantages of the SSRIs over the TCAs.
10. Describe two advantages of the SSRI and SNRI antidepressants over the TCAs.
11. Name the agent used to treat bipolar affective disorders and describe its effect on saliva.
12. Describe the effect of the NSAIDs on lithium.
13. Discuss the roles of valproate, carbamazepine, and the second-generation antipsychotics in the treatment of bipolar disorder.
14. What are MAOIs and what are their adverse reactions?

CLINICAL CASE STUDY

Suzanne Fernandez is 44 years old and has been coming to your practice for close to 2 years. She has no medical problems and takes only over-the-counter analgesics and cough and cold products. Mrs. Fernandez has noticed that lately she has not been feeling herself. She feels "blue" and nothing seems to make her happy. Mrs. Fernandez tells you that she went to her physician last week, who started Mrs. Fernandez on fluoxetine. Mrs. Fernandez will be having a cavity filled today, and the dentist plans to use a local anesthetic with a vasoconstrictor.

1. What is Mrs. Fernandez's diagnosis?
2. What are some of the signs and symptoms of depression, and who does it affect?
3. How does fluoxetine work?
4. Are there any drug interactions which you need to be aware of?
5. Does fluoxetine have any dental adverse reactions or concerns?
6. What should Mrs. Fernandez be told about potential drug interactions or dental adverse reactions?

16

Adrenocorticosteroids

LEARNING OBJECTIVES

1. Define adrenocorticosteroids and describe how the body releases them.
2. Summarize the classification, administration, mechanism of action, and pharmacologic effects of adrenocorticosteroids.
3. Describe the various adverse reactions and uses of adrenocorticosteroids, including their application to dentistry.
4. List several examples of corticosteroid products and describe the ways in which they are differentiated.
5. List several dental implications to the use of steroids.

The term *adrenocorticosteroids* (a-dree-noe-KOR-ti-KO-ster-oids) (adrenal corticosteroids, adrenocorticoids, corticosteroids, or steroids) refers to a group of agents secreted by the adrenal cortex. The dental team should be aware of the effects, adverse reactions, and dental implications of these agents for at least the following reasons:

Use in dentistry: These compounds are used topically or systemically for the treatment of oral lesions associated with inflammatory diseases.

Long-term therapy: The adrenocorticosteroids, or *steroids* as they are commonly called, are prescribed for many patients with chronic systemic diseases such as asthma and arthritis. If taken long term in high enough doses, these agents can cause a variety of adverse reactions that may influence the patient's dental treatment.

MECHANISM OF RELEASE

> Negative feedback mechanism.

The adrenocorticosteroids are naturally occurring compounds secreted by the adrenal cortex. Their release is triggered by a series of events (Fig. 16.1). First, a stimulus such as stress (1) causes the hypothalamus (2) to release corticotropin-releasing hormone (CRH) (3), which acts on the pituitary gland (4). Under the influence of CRH, the pituitary gland secretes adrenocorticotropic hormone (ACTH) (5), which stimulates the adrenal cortex (6) to release hydrocortisone (7). Hydrocortisone then acts on both the pituitary (8) and the hypothalamus (9) to inhibit the release of CRH and ACTH, respectively. This mechanism is called negative feedback. Exogenous steroids act in the same way as hydrocortisone (10); that is, they inhibit the release of CRH and ACTH. With long-term administration of steroids, ACTH release is suppressed and the adrenal gland atrophies. If the administration of the exogenous steroid is then abruptly stopped, a relative steroid deficiency results. This can cause severe problems, including adrenal crisis.

CLASSIFICATION

> Glucocorticoids.
> Mineralocorticoids.

The adrenocorticosteroids can be divided into two major groups: the glucocorticoids, which affect intermediate carbohydrate metabolism, and the mineralocorticoids, which affect the water and electrolyte composition of the body. The major glucocorticoid present in the body is cortisol (hydrocortisone). Without stress, the normal adult secretes about 20 mg of hydrocortisone daily. A 10-fold increase can occur with stress. Maximal secretion occurs between 4 a.m. and 8 a.m. in people with a normal schedule. The chemical structures of the synthetic agents and the naturally occurring adrenocorticosteroids, such as hydrocortisone, are similar. Many chemical modifications have been made in an attempt to produce synthetic glucocorticoids with fewer adverse reactions and more specific activity.

Although the term *adrenocorticosteroids* refers to those steroids secreted by the adrenal cortex and includes both the glucocorticoids and the mineralocorticoids, this chapter discusses primarily the action of glucocorticoids because of their more common use.

DEFINITIONS

The following terms are used in this chapter:

Addison disease: Disease/condition produced by a deficiency of adrenocorticosteroids.

Adrenocorticosteroids/corticosteroids/steroids: Steroidal components released from the adrenal cortex, including glucocorticoids and mineralocorticoids.

Adrenocorticotropic hormone (ACTH): Agent secreted by the pituitary that causes the release of hormones from the adrenal cortex.

Cushing syndrome: Disease/condition produced by an excess of adrenocorticosteroids.

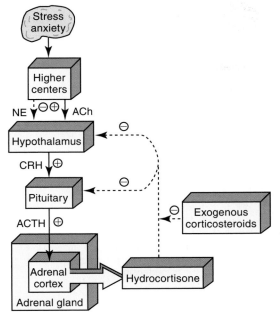

Fig. 16.1 The body's release of adrenocorticoids. *ACh,* Acetylcholine pathways; *ACTH,* adrenocorticotropic hormone; *CRH,* corticotropin-releasing hormone; *NE,* norepinephrine pathways; +, stimulates release; –, inhibits release.

Glucocorticoids: Adrenocorticosteroids that primarily affect carbohydrate metabolism.
Mineralocorticoids: Adrenocorticosteroids that affect the body's sodium and water balance (fluid levels).

ROUTES OF ADMINISTRATION

Glucocorticoids are available in a wide variety of dose forms. They are routinely used topically, orally, intramuscularly, and intravenously. Systemic effects are commonly obtained when the drug is administered orally or parenterally, but topical administration may rarely cause systemic effects. If a large quantity of a steroid is applied topically, especially if the skin is denuded or an occlusive dressing such as plastic wrap is applied, systemic effects can occur. Table 16.1 shows the relative potencies of selected topical corticosteroid products.

MECHANISM OF ACTION

> Effect has lag time.

The mechanism of action of the steroids involves binding to a specific receptor and forming a steroid-receptor complex. The complex then translocates into the nucleus and alters gene expression (turns genes on or off), resulting in the regulation of many cellular processes. Because of the mechanism, a lag time exists in the action of the steroids, and the relationship between their effects and blood levels is poor. Other effects of glucocorticoids are mediated by catecholamines producing vasodilation or bronchodilation.

> Many effects.

The antiinflammatory action of glucocorticoids results from their profound effects on the number, distribution, and function of peripheral leukocytes and from their inhibition of phospholipase A. The use of steroids results in an increase in the concentration of neutrophils and a decrease in the lymphocytes (T and B cells), monocytes, eosinophils, and basophils. Steroids induce the synthesis of a protein that inhibits phospholipase A, decreasing the production of both prostaglandins and leukotrienes from arachidonic acid.

These agents, responsible for the delayed phase of acute inflammation, act synergistically. Steroids also inhibit interleukin-2, migration inhibition factor, and macrophage inhibition factor.

PHARMACOLOGIC EFFECTS

The pharmacologic effects and the adverse reactions of corticosteroids are closely related (Fig. 16.2). The effects for which they are used include their antiinflammatory action and suppression of allergic reactions. They also suppress the immune response. Corticosteroids are palliative rather than curative. The glucocorticoid effects and the mineralocorticoid effects are listed in Box 16.1. Many of these effects produce adverse reactions and are discussed in the following section.

ADVERSE REACTIONS

The adverse reactions of corticosteroids are proportional to the dose, frequency and time of administration, and duration of treatment. With prolonged therapy and sufficiently high doses, the following side effects occur.

TABLE 16.1 Relative Potency of Selected Topical Corticosteroid Products

Potency	Drug Generic (Trade)	Dose Form	Strength (%)
Super high	Clobetasol propionate (Temovate)	Cream, ointment	0.05
High	Fluocinolone acetonide (Lidex)	Cream	0.2
Medium	Triamcinolone acetonide (Aristocort, Flutex, Kenalog)	Ointment	0.1
	Betamethasone valerate (Valisone)	Cream	0.1
Low	Fluocinolone acetonide (Synalar)	Cream, ointment	0.025
	Triamcinolone acetonide (Aristocort)	Cream, ointment, lotion	0.025
		Cream, ointment, lotion	0.1
		Cream, ointment	0.5
	Hydrocortisone (Cortaid, Anusol, Hytone, Dermacort, Penecort, Cetacort)	Lotion	0.25
		Cream, ointment, lotion, aerosol	0.5
		Solution	0.5
		Aerosol	1
		Cream, ointment, lotion	2.5

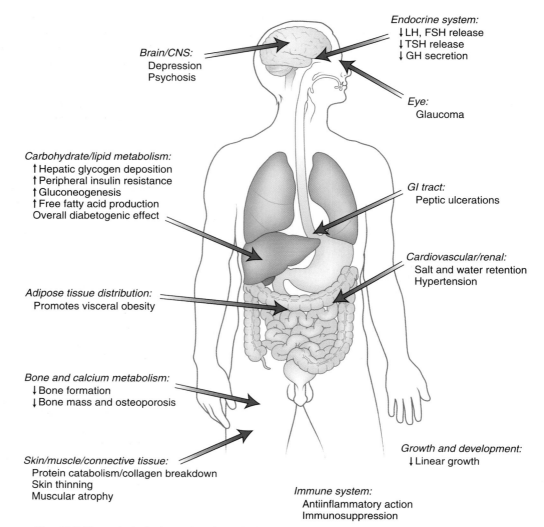

Fig. 16.2 The principal sites of action of glucocorticoids in humans highlighting some of the consequences of glucocorticoid excess. ↑, Increase (in); ↓, decrease in; *CNS*, central nervous system; *FSH*, follicle-stimulating hormone; *GH*, growth hormone; *GI*, gastrointestinal; *LH*, luteinizing hormone; *TSH*, thyroid-stimulating hormone. (From Melmed S, Polonsky KS, Kronenberg HM. *Williams' Textbook of Endocrinology.* 12th ed. Philadelphia: Saunders; 2012.)

Metabolic Changes

Moon face (round), buffalo hump (fat deposited on back of the neck), truncal obesity, weight gain, and muscle wasting give patients the Cushing syndrome appearance (Fig. 16.3). Hyperglycemia (diabetes-like) may be aggravated or initiated, especially in prediabetic patients. More antidiabetic medication may be required.

Infections

Corticosteroids decrease resistance to infection. Because of their anti-inflammatory action, they may also mask its symptoms. Patients taking long-term glucocorticoid therapy are given isoniazid, an antituberculosis agent, to prevent tuberculosis.

Central Nervous System Effects

Changes in behavior and personality, including euphoria (with increasing dose), agitation, psychoses, and depression (with decreasing dose), can occur.

Peptic Ulcer

Because corticosteroids stimulate an increase in production of stomach acid and pepsin, they may exacerbate peptic ulcers. Healing is impaired, and the ulcer may perforate.

Impaired Wound Healing and Osteoporosis

The catabolic effects of steroids that result from impaired synthesis of collagen can interfere with wound healing. This same process can cause osteoporosis or delay growth in children. If the osteoporosis affects alveolar bone, tooth loss may occur. Thinning bones can also result in fractures without trauma in patients on long-term steroid therapy. Muscle wasting, bruising, and abdominal striae are other symptoms associated with catabolism.

Ophthalmic Effects

Because corticosteroids can increase intraocular pressure, they may exacerbate glaucoma. Cataracts are also associated with steroids.

BOX 16.1 Glucocorticoid and Mineralocorticoid Effects

Glucocorticoid Effects
Broad
Decrease carbohydrate metabolism
Antiinflammatory
Antiallergenic
Increases enzyme action
Negatively affects membrane function
Increases nucleic acid synthesis

Specific
Catabolism
Increased gluconeogenesis
Decreased glucose use
Inhibition of protein synthesis
Increased protein catabolism
Decreased growth
Decreased bone density
Decreased resistance to infection

Mineralocorticoid Effects
Increased sodium retention
Increased potassium loss
Edema and hypertension

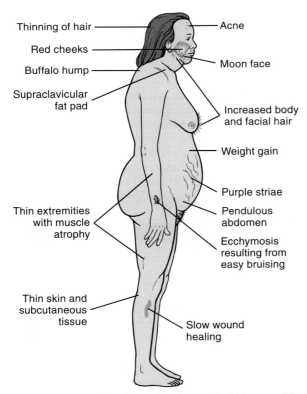

Fig. 16.3 Body image alterations with glucocorticoid therapy. (Modified from Lewis SM, Heitkemper MM, Dirksen SR. *Medical-Surgical Nursing: Assessment and Management of Clinical Problems.* 7th ed. St. Louis: Mosby; 2007.)

Electrolyte and Fluid Balance
Glucocorticoids that possess some mineralocorticoid action can cause sodium and water retention. Hypertension or congestive heart failure may be worsened. Hypokalemia may also result.

Adrenal Crisis
With prolonged use, adrenal suppression can occur. If a stressful situation arises, the adrenal gland cannot respond adequately. Symptoms of adrenal crisis include weakness, syncope, cardiovascular collapse, and death.

Dental Effects
Oral tissue changes may occur in patients taking corticosteroids. Their mucosal surfaces heal more slowly, are more likely to have infection, and are more friable. In the patient using an oral steroid inhaler for asthma, oral candidiasis may result. This may be prevented by rinsing the mouth after inhaler use.

USES

Medical Uses
There are many conditions for which corticosteroids may be administered (Box 16.2). Patients with these conditions should be questioned about past use of systemic steroids.

Replacement
Patients with hypofunction of the adrenal cortex (Addison disease) need replacement of glucocorticoid and mineralocorticoid activity. Usually, hydrocortisone is used to restore glucocorticoid activity, and desoxycorticosterone to restore mineralocorticoid activity. The patient with a hyperfunctioning adrenal cortex (Cushing syndrome) may undergo surgical removal of a majority of the gland. In this case, replacement therapy is needed.

BOX 16.2 Conditions for Which Corticosteroids May Be Used

Corticosteroid Deficiency
Addison disease (deficiency of steroids)

Autoimmune Diseases
Arthritis, rheumatoid
Collagen diseases
Pemphigus vulgaris
Psoriasis
Systemic lupus erythematosus
Scleroderma

Gastrointestinal Disease
Crohn disease
Ulcerative colitis
Inflammatory bowel disease (IBD)

Others
Hematologic conditions
Hypercalcemia
Organ transplants
With chemotherapy (antiemetic)
Asthma

Emergencies

Corticosteroids are used in emergency situations for the treatment of shock or adrenal crisis, as discussed in Chapter 21.

Inflammation/Allergy

The most extensive use of the corticosteroids in both medicine and dentistry is in the treatment of a wide variety of inflammatory and allergic conditions. These agents are not curative but merely ameliorate symptoms through their antiinflammatory activity. Some conditions that have been treated with corticosteroids are rheumatoid arthritis, rheumatic fever, systemic lupus erythematosus, scleroderma, inflammation of the joints and soft tissues, acute bronchial asthma, severe and acute allergic reactions, and severe allergic dermatoses. Prednisone (PRED-ni-sone) is the most common corticosteroid used orally.

> Topical steroids.

Topical corticosteroids are used for a variety of skin conditions, which involve various dermatoses or "irritations." The steroids can be divided into several classes depending on their relative maximum potencies*: the least efficacious to the most efficacious and in between. An example of the weakest is hydrocortisone (hye-droe-KOR-ti-sone), an example of a medium-potency agent is triamcinolone (trye-am-SIN-oh-lone) acetonide, and an example of the most potent is augmented betamethasone (bay-ta-METH-a-sone) dipropionate.

Dental Uses

Because of the adrenocorticosteroids' antiinflammatory action, they are administered topically, intra-articularly, or orally in several dental situations. The use of steroids in dentistry has had mixed success, and double-blind controlled studies are needed to determine unequivocally their proper place in the therapeutic armamentarium.

Oral Lesions

Systemically administered steroids are often effective in the treatment of oral lesions associated with noninfectious inflammatory diseases, including erythema multiforme, lichen planus, pemphigus, desquamative gingivitis, and benign mucous membrane pemphigoid. It is imperative that an infectious etiology for an oral lesion, such as herpes, be ruled out.

Aphthous Stomatitis

The evidence for the benefit of adrenocorticosteroids in the treatment of aphthous stomatitis seems clear. Triamcinolone acetonide (Kenalog in Orabase) has been advocated. Orabase is a mineral oil gel base that sticks to the oral mucosa, forming a plastic-like surface. Other topical steroids, such as fluocinonide and fluocinolone (floo-oh-SIN-oh-lone), can be used topically.

Temporomandibular Joint

Arthritis (inflammation) of the temporomandibular joint (TMJ) also responds to the systemic administration of steroids. If only this joint is affected, an intra-articular injection can often decrease the pain and improve joint movement.

Uses in Oral Surgery

> Weigh pros and cons.

The adrenocorticosteroids have been used in oral surgery to reduce postoperative edema, trismus, and pain. Although the decrease in edema with steroid use can be easily documented, the magnitude of the benefit must be weighed against the potential risk of infection and decreased healing. The safety and effectiveness of these agents have not been proved in double-blind controlled studies.

Pulp Procedures

The adrenocorticosteroids have been used in pulp capping, in pulpotomy procedures, and for the control of hypersensitive cervical dentin. Their use in these situations is currently empirical or experimental.

CORTICOSTEROID PRODUCTS

Selected synthetic corticosteroids are arranged in Table 16.2 according to their duration of action: short, intermediate, and long. The relative antiinflammatory and salt-retaining activities and equivalent oral doses are given, with hydrocortisone arbitrarily assigned the value of 1 for each activity. The other agents are then given values in relation to those of hydrocortisone. For example, prednisone, which is given an antiinflammatory activity of 4, has four times as much antiinflammatory action as hydrocortisone. Therefore only one-fourth as much prednisone is required to have the same effect as that produced by hydrocortisone. The mineralocorticoid, or salt-retaining, properties of the glucocorticoids are also compared with those of hydrocortisone. For example, triamcinolone does not increase salt retention, whereas hydrocortisone does.

Table 16.2 lists the equivalent oral doses in milligrams based on 20 mg of hydrocortisone, the amount normally secreted daily by an adult without stress. One can see that 0.75 mg of dexamethasone or 5 mg of prednisone is approximately equivalent to 20 mg of hydrocortisone.

TABLE 16.2 Selected Oral Corticosteroids

Group	Drug Name	ACTIVITY* Antiinflammatory	ACTIVITY* Salt Retention	Equivalent Oral Dose (mg)
Short acting	Hydrocortisone	1	1	20
	Prednisone	4	0.3–0.5	5
	Methylprednisolone	5	0.3–0.5	4
Intermediate acting	Triamcinolone	5	0	4
	Prednisolone	4	0	5
Long acting	Dexamethasone	30	0	0.8
	Betamethasone	25	0	0.8

*See text for explanation of numbers, deleted trade names because all of those drugs are available as the generic and generic products are used, very rarely is a trade name product dispensed.

*Using the strict definition of potency and efficacy, the term *potency* as used to refer to topical steroids is really efficacy.

DENTAL IMPLICATIONS

Box 16.3 summarizes the management of dental patients taking steroids. The patient's risk for requiring additional steroid dosing prior to a dental procedure is based on the patient's risk category (Fig. 16.4). Patients with primary adrenal insufficiency are more likely to be at higher risk than those with secondary adrenal insufficiency (see Box 16.2). Because steroids suppress immune reaction, with long-term administration of steroids, infections are more likely to occur and healing is delayed. These factors are important in the dental patient, especially if a surgical procedure is to be performed. Because the symptoms of infection may be masked, the wound site should be carefully examined.

Adverse Reactions

Gastrointestinal Effects

Adrenocorticosteroids stimulate acid secretion; patients taking these agents should be given other ulcerogenic medications, such as the salicylates or the nonsteroidal antiinflammatory agents, with caution.

Blood Pressure Changes

The blood pressure of patients taking corticosteroids should be measured because these agents can exacerbate hypertension. The more mineralocorticoid action an agent has, the more likely the agent is to raise blood pressure.

Glaucoma

Other agents that can induce or exacerbate glaucoma, such as the anticholinergics, should be used with caution in patients taking adrenocorticosteroids.

BOX 16.3 Management of Dental Patient Who Is Taking or Has Taken Corticosteroids

Most dental patients taking steroids who are having normal dental treatment DO NOT need additional corticosteroids. Supplemental steroids may be required if a patient has severe dental fears or for major surgical procedures.

Precautions to Avoid Stress
- Obtain good anesthesia.
- Check blood pressure.
- Provide postoperative analgesics (as needed).

No Supplementation Needed, Depending on Risk Category*
- Steroid therapy stopped >1 year ago
- Dose <20 mg/day hydrocortisone (HC) or 5 mg/day prednisone
- Dose >40 mg/day HC or 10 mg/day prednisone
- Duration of therapy <1 month
- Every-other-day therapy
- Topical use—rash, asthma inhaler, nose spray

Supplementation May Be Needed Depending on Risk Category*
- Dose 20–40 mg HC or 5–10 mg prednisone/day
- Duration of therapy >1 month
- Topical use (see above) in very large doses or over entire body

Supplemental Steroid Doses
- For patients at minor risk*:
- 25 mg HC or 5 mg prednisone on day of surgery
- For patients at moderate risk*:
- 50–75 mg HC on day of surgery and for at least one postoperative day
- For patients at major risk*:
- 100–150 mg HC on day of surgery and for at least one postoperative day

*See Fig. 16.4.

Behavioral Changes

A patient's bizarre behavior may be explained by the presence of, or withdrawal from, adrenocorticosteroids. Psychosis, euphoria, or depression might be seen.

Osteoporosis

Dental radiographs may demonstrate osteoporosis in patients taking long-term adrenocorticosteroids. More than 50% bone loss is required for osteoporosis to be detected radiographically. These patients are more likely to suffer fractures either with or without trauma.

Infection

Because of the antiinflammatory activity of the adrenocorticosteroids, they may mask the symptoms of an infection. They decrease a patient's ability to fight infection by suppressing migration of polymorphonuclear leukocytes, thus reducing lymph system action.

Delayed Wound Healing

Because the adrenocorticosteroids cause delayed wound healing, special precautions should be taken when surgical procedures are performed in the oral cavity. Friability of the tissue also requires special care during closure of wounds, and extra sutures may be required.

Adrenal Crisis

> Only with severe stress.

The body releases corticosteroids and epinephrine from the adrenal gland when a person experiences stress. Under normal conditions, when the body sends a message (ACTH) to the adrenal gland, it is stimulated and secretes hydrocortisone. Because the adrenal gland of a normal person is regularly stimulated when the person experiences stress, the adrenal gland stays ready for a message to put out hydrocortisone. The body does not differentiate between the hydrocortisone (endogenous) it secretes and the hydrocortisone or prednisone (exogenous) received by any route. When a patient is taking long-term prednisone, the steroid provides negative feedback to the hypothalamus (reduces release of CRH) and the pituitary (reduces release of ACTH).

With prolonged administration of steroids, suppression of the hypothalamic-pituitary-adrenal axis occurs. With suppression, the body does not quickly respond to stress with release of hydrocortisone. Suppression is proportional to the potency of the agent, the dose of the agent, and the duration of administration. The longer the duration, the higher the dose, and the greater the potency of the steroid, the quicker the suppression occurs. Once suppression occurs, it can take weeks or months for the adrenal gland to respond normally. Without the proper response to stress, adrenal crisis is possible. The crisis occurs because of a relative lack of corticosteroids during stress, such as a dental appointment for a patient with dental phobia. It may be necessary to administer adrenal steroids before a stressful dental procedure to prevent crisis. A consultation with the patient's physician is helpful. Generally, low doses and very high (mega) doses do not present problems; problems may occur, however, with mid-range doses.

Periodontal Disease

Steroids have actions that can contribute to periodontal disease. First, they interfere with the body's response to infection (inflammatory mediators are inhibited). Second, steroids can cause osteoporosis, which may reduce the bony support for the teeth.

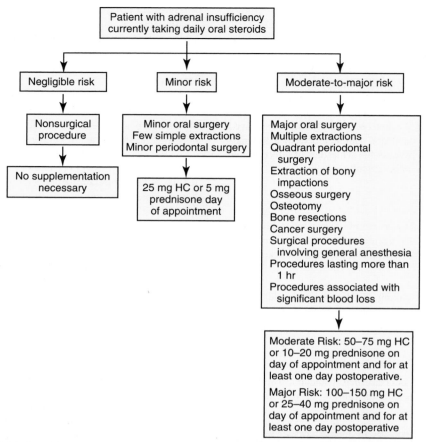

Fig. 16.4 Steroid supplementation decision tree for patients with adrenal insufficiency. *HC,* Hydrocortisone. (From Sharuga CR. Corticosteroid supplementation: is it still relevant? *Dimens Dent Hyg.* 2008;6:16–17.)

Steroid Supplementation

> 5–10 mg prednisone/day.

Several researchers have found that adrenal crisis is a rare event in dentistry, especially for patients with secondary adrenal insufficiency—which is due to steroid use for certain medical conditions (see Box 16.2). More often than not, patients with secondary adrenal insufficiency do not require steroid supplementation for most routine dental procedures, including nonsurgical periodontal therapy. Patients with Addison disease (primary adrenal insufficiency) may need steroid supplementation, depending on the risk associated with the procedure (see Fig. 16.4). Minor surgical procedures under a local anesthetic may not require steroid supplementation. The local anesthetic provides pain control, which reduces the amount of cortisol that the body needs during a stressful situation.

There are many ways of using supplemental steroids in patients who use steroids long term and are to undergo a stressful dental procedure. Fig. 16.4 illustrates a method of determining whether or not supplementation is necessary. If the patient is considered to be at minor risk, the dose of hydrocortisone is 25 mg or prednisone 5 mg on the day of the procedure. If the patient is considered to be at moderate to major

risk, the dose is hydrocortisone 50–150 or prednisone 10–40 mg on the day of the procedure and for at least one postoperative day.

Another method of determining whether a patient requires supplementation is to consider both the dose and duration of the patient's corticosteroid use. With both low doses (<20 mg hydrocortisone or 5 mg prednisone) and very high doses (immunosuppressive; >40–60 mg/day hydrocortisone or 10–15 mg/day prednisone), no additional steroid supplementation is needed. With some intermediate doses of steroids (estimated to be between 20 and 40 mg/day hydrocortisone or 5 and 10 mg/day prednisone), additional steroids may be indicated if the procedure is likely to cause severe stress.

Regardless of the method chosen, the patient's physician should always be consulted if there is any doubt as to whether or not the steroid dose needs to be supplemented.

Topical Use

Steroids are used in dentistry to manage certain oral conditions, such as aphthous stomatitis, related to inflammatory or immune mechanisms. Both topical and systemic steroids are used in these instances. The relative potencies of selected topical glucocorticoids are listed in Table 16.1.

DENTAL HYGIENE CONSIDERATIONS

- Obtain a detailed medication history in order to avoid drug interactions and adverse reactions.
- Obtain a detailed health history because corticosteroids can interfere with or exacerbate several medical illnesses.
- Corticosteroids can elevate blood pressure, so it is important that the dental hygienist check the patient's blood pressure and pulse at each visit.
- Encourage the patient to avoid the use of nonsteroidal antiinflammatory drugs (NSAIDs) and aspirin, which can cause gastrointestinal (GI) upset and ulcers. Corticosteroids also increase the risk for GI upset and ulcer.
- Corticosteroids can cause behavioral changes that could interfere with the patient's ability to sit through an appointment. The appointment may need to be rescheduled if the patient can not cooperate.
- Corticosteroids can mask the symptoms of infection and delay wound healing. Antibiotics may be necessary for patients using corticosteroids on a long-term basis.
- Check for symptoms of osteoporosis of the jaw and bone because corticosteroids can increase the risk of osteoporosis.
- Review the information in Box 16.3.

ACADEMIC SKILLS ASSESSMENT

1. Compare and contrast the activity of the glucocorticoids and mineralocorticoids.
2. List the routes of administration for the steroids used in dentistry.
3. What are the dental concerns associated with steroids?
4. Are there any drug interactions to be aware of?
5. Describe the three major uses of the steroids in medicine.
6. Explain how to evaluate a patient undergoing corticosteroid therapy and how to determine whether the patient's physician should be consulted. State what problems could arise from dental treatment and how these adverse effects could be monitored.
7. Define the terms *Cushing syndrome* and *Addison disease*.
8. Both hypofunctioning and hyperfunctioning of the adrenal cortex require steroid replacement therapy. What are the dental concerns regarding this therapy?

CLINICAL CASE STUDY

Ted Hamilton is a 45-year-old man with a history of myasthenia gravis. He takes oral steroids to treat the myasthenia gravis. Mr. Hamilton is otherwise healthy and takes occasional over-the-counter analgesics and cough and cold preparations. He is at your practice today for a maintenance oral examination.

1. Should steroid-dependent patients receive prophylaxis with antibiotics prior to a dental procedure? Why or why not?
2. Mr. Hamilton needs to have a root canal and new crown. Should he receive an antibiotic after this procedure? Why or why not?
3. What are the adverse reactions associated with steroids?
4. What are the dental concerns associated with steroids?
5. Are there any drug interactions that Mr. Hamilton should be aware of?
6. What should the dental hygienist tell Mr. Hamilton about the dental concerns associated with steroids?

REFERENCE

Sharuga CR. Corticosteroid supplementation: is it still relevant? *Dimens Dent Hyg.* 2008;6:16–17.

17

Drugs for the Treatment of Respiratory Disorders and Allergic Rhinitis

http://evolve.elsevier.com/Haveles/pharmacology

LEARNING OBJECTIVES

1. Summarize the two groups of respiratory diseases.
2. Name and describe the mechanisms of action of several types of drugs used to treat respiratory diseases.
3. Discuss the types of drugs used to treat respiratory infections, including the implications to dentistry.
4. Define allergic rhinitis and describe the dental implications, pharmacologic effects, adverse reactions, and toxicity of antihistamines.
5. Describe the dental implications, pharmacologic effects, and adverse reactions of the intranasal corticosteroids.

6. Discuss montelukast, cromolyn sodium, and ipratropium bromide and describe their role in treating allergic rhinitis. Also describe the adverse reactions of ipratropium bromide.
7. Describe the use of decongestants, including:
   - Discuss the pharmacologic effects, adverse reactions, and uses in treating allergies.
   - Discuss the use of intranasal decongestants as an alternative to oral decongestants.

Diseases of the respiratory tract are common, so dental hygienists are sure to encounter patients taking drugs for these diseases (Fig. 17.1). Because the medications given to treat these diseases can affect dental treatment, the dental hygienist should be aware of the effects of these drugs on the patient and how these drugs can alter the dental treatment plan.

Diseases that are treated with respiratory drugs include asthma, chronic obstructive pulmonary disease (COPD), and upper respiratory tract infections (Fig. 17.2). Respiratory drugs come from a wide range of drug groups, from adrenergic drugs for bronchodilation to corticosteroids for reducing inflammation. Drugs that increase expectoration and reduce coughs are also included in this discussion. Many drugs used to treat respiratory problems are administered topically via the lungs by the use of a metered-dose inhaler (MDI).

RESPIRATORY DISEASES

Noninfectious respiratory diseases are divided into two groups: (1) asthma and (2) COPD (see Fig. 17.2). COPD is further divided into chronic bronchitis and emphysema. Other respiratory problems are related to respiratory infections, principally viral or bacterial.

Asthma

> Asthma: Reversible airway obstruction with inflammation.

One common respiratory disease is asthma. It is characterized by reversible airway obstruction and is associated with reduction in expiratory airflow. A few hours later, inflammation occurs, resulting in an increase in secretions in the lungs and swelling in the bronchioles. Asthma is classified as being either intermittent or persistent. Persistent asthma is further categorized as mild, moderate, or severe. Patients with intermittent asthma experience symptoms less than two

times a month and the symptoms do not interfere with normal activity. Persistent asthma occurs anywhere from more than twice a week to all day long. Persistent asthma can cause minor limitation of normal activities, and severe persistent asthma can severely limit the patient's normal activities. When asthma is treated, both components of the disease must be addressed. The *National Asthma Education and Prevention Program Expert Panel Report 3*, published in October 2007, presents the latest recommendations of the National Heart Lung and Blood Institute regarding asthma therapy. Table 17.1 reviews the stepwise approach for managing asthma in children older than 12 years and adults.

Asthma may be precipitated by allergens, pollution, exercise, stress, or upper respiratory infection (allergic reaction to viruses), certain medications (nonsteroidal antiinflammatory drugs). The patient with status asthmaticus has persistent life-threatening bronchospasm despite drug therapy. Environmental pollution may also play an important role in the increase in asthma. The dental hygienist should manage dental patients with asthma so as to induce minimal stress. Patients should bring their fast-acting β_2-agonist inhalers to be used prophylactically or in the management of an acute asthmatic attack in the dental office. Signs of asthma include shortness of breath and wheezing. By observing and asking the patient about asthma control before the dental appointment, the dental hygienist can prevent an acute attack. β_2-adrenergic agonists, xanthines, cromolyn, corticosteroids, leukotriene (LT) altering agents, and antimuscarinics are used to treat this disease (Fig. 17.3).

Chronic Obstructive Pulmonary Disease

> Chronic obstructive pulmonary disease: Irreversible airway obstruction.

COPD is characterized by irreversible airway obstruction which occurs with either chronic bronchitis or emphysema. Smoking is associated with almost all cases of COPD. Chronic bronchitis is a result

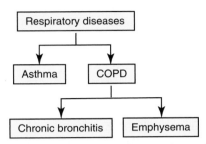

Respiratory drugs

β₂-Agonists
Corticosteroids
Leukotriene modifiers
Mast cell inhibitors
Anticholinergic drugs
Methylxanthines

Fig. 17.1 Respiratory drug groups.

Respiratory diseases
→ Asthma
→ COPD
→ Chronic bronchitis
→ Emphysema

Fig. 17.2 Respiratory diseases. *COPD,* Chronic obstructive pulmonary disease.

TABLE 17.1 Treatment of Asthma

Step	Asthma Severity	Preferred Therapy	Alternatives
1	Intermittent	SABA, as needed	
2	Mild persistent	Low-dose ICS	LM
3	Moderate persistent	Low-dose ICS + LABA or medium-dose ICS	Low-dose ICS + LM
4	Severe persistent	Medium-dose ICS + LABA	Medium-dose ICS + LM
5	Severe persistent	High-dose ICS + LABA	Consider omalizumab for patients with allergies
6	Severe persistent	High-dose ICS + LABA + oral corticosteroids	Consider omalizumab for patients with allergies

ICS, Inhaled corticosteroid; *LM,* leukotriene modifier; *LABA,* long-acting β₂-agonist; *SABA,* short-acting β₂-agonist.

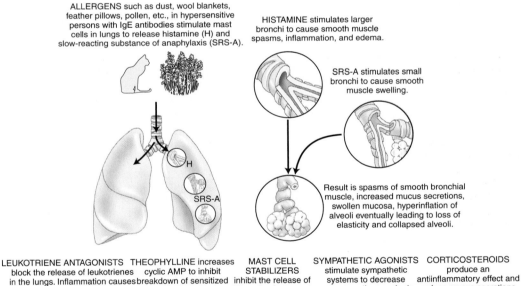

ALLERGENS such as dust, wool blankets, feather pillows, pollen, etc., in hypersensitive persons with IgE antibodies stimulate mast cells in lungs to release histamine (H) and slow-reacting substance of anaphylaxis (SRS-A).

HISTAMINE stimulates larger bronchi to cause smooth muscle spasms, inflammation, and edema.

SRS-A stimulates small bronchi to cause smooth muscle swelling.

Result is spasms of smooth bronchial muscle, increased mucus secretions, swollen mucosa, hyperinflation of alveoli eventually leading to loss of elasticity and collapsed alveoli.

LEUKOTRIENE ANTAGONISTS block the release of leukotrienes in the lungs. Inflammation causes an increase in leukotrienes, substances that constitute the slow-reacting substance of anaphylaxis (SRS-A).

THEOPHYLLINE increases cyclic AMP to inhibit breakdown of sensitized mast cells that stimulate the release of histamine, serotonin, and SRS-A.

MAST CELL STABILIZERS inhibit the release of histamine from mast cells to reduce allergic effects.

SYMPATHETIC AGONISTS stimulate sympathetic systems to decrease mucus secretions and relax bronchial muscle spasms.

CORTICOSTEROIDS produce an antiinflammatory effect and reduce mucus secretions and tissue histamine.

Fig. 17.3 Overview of the effects of various antiasthmatic medications. *IgE,* Immunoglobulin E. (From McKenry L, Tessier E, Hogan MA. *Mosby's Pharmacology in Nursing.* 22nd ed. St. Louis: Mosby; 2006.)

of chronic inflammation of the airways and excessive sputum production. Emphysema is characterized by alveolar destruction with air space enlargement and airway collapse. Tables 17.2 and 17.3 review the recommended treatment regimens for COPD. The antimuscarinics are the first-line agents, but β₂-adrenergic agonists are also used to produce bronchodilation in patients with this disease. In many instances patients receive a combination MDI containing an antimuscarinic drug and a β₂-agonist. COPD is associated with an increase in the incidence of bronchospasm and with fixed airway obstruction. Patients with upper respiratory tract infections also often take β₂-

adrenergic agonists for bronchoconstriction, antihistamines to reduce secretions, expectorants to thin sputum, and antitussives to control coughing. Each drug group is discussed separately in the section on respiratory infections.

In the normal person, the drive for ventilation (breathing) is stimulated by an elevation in the partial pressure of carbon dioxide (Paco₂). The partial pressure of oxygen (Pao₂) can vary widely without stimulating ventilation in the normal patient. Patients with COPD, because their ventilation is compromised, experience a gradual rise in Paco₂ over time. Because this mechanism becomes resistant

TABLE 17.2   US Food and Drug Administration-Approved Drugs Used to Manage Asthma

Group	Example(s)	Mechanism of Action	Adverse Reactions	Dental Drug Implications
β_2-Adrenergic Agonists (Inhaler)				
Short acting*	Albuterol (ProAir HFA, Proventil HFA, Ventolin HFA, ProAir RespiClick)* Metaproterenol (Alupent, generic) Levalbuterol (Xopenex HFA)	Stimulates β_2-receptors (bronchodilation)	Nervousness, dry mouth, throat irritation, fast or irregular heartbeat	Increased risk for dry mouth (rinse mouth to prevent) Can increase heart rate
Long acting	Salmeterol (Serevent Diskus)† Formoterol (Foradil Aerolizer)†	Stimulates β_2-receptors (bronchodilation)	Nervousness, dry mouth, throat irritation, fast or irregular heartbeat	Increased risk for dry mouth (rinse mouth to prevent) Can increase heart rate
Corticosteroids				
Inhaled	Beclomethasone (QVAR) Budesonide (Pulmicort Flexhaler) Ciclesonide (Alvesco) Flunisolide (Aerospan HFA) Fluticasone propionate (Flovent HFA, Flovent Diskus) Fluticasone furoate (Arnuity Ellipta) Mometasone furoate (Asmanex HFA, Asmanex Twisthaler)	Reduces inflammation, inhibits release of inflammatory substances	Cough, dysphonia (hoarseness)	Oral candidiasis (rinse mouth to prevent), unpleasant taste, xerostomia
Oral	Prednisone (Deltasone, Meticorten)	Reduces or prevents inflammatory processes	Hyperglycemia, osteoporosis, fluid retention	Suppresses adrenal gland Healing slower Infection more likely, symptoms masked
Inhaled Corticosteroids/Long-Acting β_2-Agonists				
Corticosteroid/β_2-agonist	Fluticasone/salmeterol (Advair HFA, Advair Diskus, AirDuo RespiClick) Budesonide/formoterol (Symbicort HFA) Fluticasone furoate (Breo Ellipta) Mometasone/formoterol (Dulera)	The steroids reduce airway inflammation and the β_2-agonists cause bronchodilation	Nervousness, dry mouth, throat irritation, fast or irregular heartbeat, cough, dysphonia (hoarseness)	Increased risk for dry mouth (rinse mouth to prevent) Can increase heart rate Oral candidiasis (rinse mouth to prevent), unpleasant taste
Leukotriene Modifiers				
LT pathway antagonist	Zafirlukast (Accolate) [PO] Montelukast (Singulair) [PO]	Blocks the action of cysteinyl leukotrienes (LT receptor antagonist)	Nausea, CNS depression, increase in LFTs, myalgia, headache	Erythromycin lowers zafirlukast levels (40%); inhibitor of cytochrome P-450 3A/4 Aspirin raises zafirlukast levels (45%) [PO 20 bid]
LT pathway synthesis inhibitor (LPI)	Zileuton (Zyflo) [PO] Zileuton, extended release (Zyflo CR)	Inhibits 5-lipoxygenase that catalyzes production of LT (LTD_4 and LTE_4)	Headache, dyspepsia, nausea, abdominal pain, asthenia	
Mast Cell Degranulation Inhibitors				
Mast cell stabilizers	Cromolyn (Intal, (NasalCrom) [IH] Nedocromil (Tilade) [IH—see benefit in 2 weeks]	Mast cell stabilizer (degranulation inhibitor); affects cells of inflammation	Nausea, headache, cough, epistaxis	Taste perversion (bad, unpleasant), burning mouth/throat; sputum increased; swollen parotid glands; dry throat
Methylxanthines				
Methylxanthines	Theophylline‡ (Theo-Dur, Slo-Bid) [PO]	Direct smooth muscle relaxant	Gastric reflux, headache, tachycardia, insomnia, nausea, trembling, nervousness	Erythromycin may increase theophylline levels

(Continued)

TABLE 17.2 US Food and Drug Administration-Approved Drugs Used to Manage Asthma—cont'd

Group	Example(s)	Mechanism of Action	Adverse Reactions	Dental Drug Implications
Anti-IgE Antibody				
Anti-IgE antibodies	Omalizumab (Xolair)	Keeps IgE from binding to mast cells and basophils, thereby preventing an inflammatory response	Injection site pain and bruising	
Anti-Interleukin-5 Antibodies				
	Mepolizumab (Nucala) Reslizumab (Cinqair)	Inhibit interleukin-5 signaling which reduces the production and survival of eosinophils	Mepolizumab: headache, injection site reactions, back pain, fatigue Hypersensitivity reactions Reslizumab: oropharyngeal pain, anaphylaxis, hypersensitivity reactions	

*Use for an acute attack.
†Do not use in an emergency, delayed onset (>1 hour), prolonged effect (12 hours).
‡Relative of caffeine found in coffee and cola beverages.
bid, Twice a day; *BP*, blood pressure; *CNS*, central nervous system; *IH*, inhalation; *IgE*, immunoglobulin E; *LFTs*, liver function tests; *LT*, leukotriene; *PO*, by mouth.

TABLE 17.3 Treatment of Chronic Obstructive Pulmonary Disease

Patient Group	Criteria	Initial	Persistent or Severe Symptoms	Further Exacerbations
Group A	Occasional dyspnea or few symptoms; ≤1 exacerbations that did not lead to hospitalizations	Inhaled ipratropium as needed *or* SABA as needed *or* LAMA *or* LABA		
Group B	Moderate to severe dyspnea; ≤1 exacerbations that did not lead to hospitalizations	LAMA *or* LABA	LAMA + LABA	
Group C	Occasional dyspnea or few symptoms; ≥1 exacerbations leading to hospital admission or ≥2 exacerbations	LAMA (preferred) *or* LABA		LAMA + LABA (preferred) *or* LABA + ICS
Group D	Moderate to severe dyspnea or symptoms; ≥1 exacerbations leading to hospital admission or ≥2 exacerbations	LABA + LAMA		ICS + LABA + LAMA *or* ICS + LABA *or* ICS + LABA + LAMA + PDE₄ inhibitor *or* ICS + LABA + LAMA + azithromycin

ICS, Inhaled corticosteroid; *LABA*, long-acting β₂-agonist; *LAMA*, long-acting antimuscarinic agent; *PDE₄*, phosphodiesterase-4; *SABA*, short-acting β₂-agonist.

to changes in Paco₂, a new stimulus emerges, the partial pressure of Pao₂. The patient's ventilation is then driven by a decrease in Pao₂. If a patient with COPD is given oxygen and the Pao₂ rises, the stimulant to breathing is removed, and apnea may be induced. For patients with severe COPD, it is suggested that the rate of oxygen administration be limited to less than 3 L/min. Other literature recommends that in the patient with severe COPD, oxygen by nasal cannula be used during a dental appointment, especially if pain or stress is expected (increased oxygen demand).

DRUGS USED TO TREAT RESPIRATORY DISEASES

Metered-Dose Inhalers

Inhalers: quick onset, low toxicity.

The MDI, developed in the 1950s, provides a useful method to administer certain medications to the respiratory tree (Fig. 17.4). It is the preferred route of delivery for most asthma drugs. Its advantages include the following:

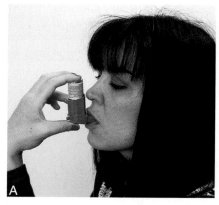

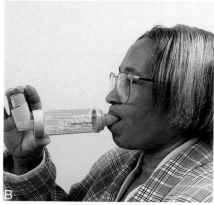

Fig. 17.4 (A) Metered-dose inhaler (MDI) for treatment of respiratory conditions. (B) MDI with spacer. (From Potter PA, Perry AG, Stockert P, Hall A. *Fundamentals of Nursing.* 8th ed. St. Louis: Mosby; 2013.)

- It delivers the medication directly into the bronchioles, thereby keeping the total dose low and side effects minimal.
- The bronchodilator effect is greater than that of a comparable oral dose.
- The inhaled dose can be accurately measured.
- The onset of action is rapid and predictable (versus unpredictable response with orally administered agents).
- The MDI is compact, portable, and sterile, making it ideal for the ambulatory patient.

Disadvantages of MDIs are that they are difficult to use properly (particularly for children) and they can be abused, with a resultant decrease in response. Additional patient education is required to get the most from this dose form. Often, a "spacer" is placed between the MDI and the mouth to increase the amount of drug delivered to the lungs (see Fig. 17.4B). Medications currently available in MDIs include β-agonists, both specific and nonspecific; corticosteroids; cromolyn; and antimuscarinic drugs.

Chlorofluorocarbons (CFCs), which have ozone-depleting properties, have been phased out as propellants in MDIs. Nonchlorinated hydrofluoroalkane propellants, which do not deplete the ozone layer, have replaced CFCs.

Sympathomimetic Agents

Sympathomimetic or adrenergic agonists produce bronchodilation by stimulating the β-receptors in the lungs. Chapter 4 discusses the presence of β-receptors in the heart (β_1) (tachycardia) and lungs (β_2) (bronchodilation). With the development of selective β_2-agonists, bronchodilation with fewer cardiac side effects can be achieved. The selective β_2-agonists, used orally, by inhalation, and parenterally, are currently one of the mainstays of respiratory therapy.

Short-Acting β_2-Agonists

> Albuterol: β_2 agonist.

Asthma. The short-acting β_2-agonists have specificity for the respiratory tree. Side effects include nervousness, tachycardia, and insomnia. Short-acting β_2-agonists, such as albuterol, may be administered by inhalation (metered dose or nebulization with an air compressor) or orally (tablet or liquid). Table 17.2 lists some short- and long-acting β_2-agonists and their routes of administration. The first line of treatment for intermittent asthma is a short-acting β_2-agonist (see Table 17.1). The short-acting β_2-agonists are the drugs of choice for the emergency treatment of an acute attack of asthma. Studies have found that the overuse of these agents results in airway hyperresponsiveness and a decrease in the lung's response to them. Therefore these agents should be used primarily for the treatment of acute problems, not for the management of normal breathing function. One major mistake that many asthmatic patients make is to rely on the albuterol inhaler and omit using the steroid inhaler. They do so because the albuterol gives an immediate response.

Chronic obstructive pulmonary disease. Short-acting β_2-agonists can be used for acute relief in patients with intermittent symptoms of COPD (see Table 17.3). These patients typically present with mild airflow obstruction and their symptoms are usually due to exertion. These drugs can improve forced expiratory volume in one second and can relieve symptoms. In patients with COPD, β_2-agonists are sometimes combined with antimuscarinic drugs (Table 17.4).

Long-Acting β_2-Agonists

Asthma. Long-acting β_2-agonist inhalers (see Tables 17.1 and 17.2) are used in conjunction with low-dose inhaled corticosteroids to treat patients with persistent asthma that is not well-controlled by low-dose inhaled corticosteroids alone. Long-acting β_2-agonists improve lung function, decrease symptoms, and reduce exacerbations of asthma and rescue uses of short-acting β_2-agonists. They are not recommended as monotherapy for asthma. Long-acting β_2-agonists carry a black box warning from the US Food and Drug Administration (FDA) about a higher risk of asthma-related deaths; this warning is the result of the report of a high number of asthma-related deaths with salmeterol therapy during a clinical trial. Long-acting β_2-agonists are best administered in a fixed-dose combination in the same inhaler with an inhaled corticosteroid (see Table 17.2). Long-acting β_2-agonists are combined with corticosteroid inhalers so that two different drugs, at lower doses, can be used to treat persistent asthma, thereby improving adherence to therapy.

Chronic obstructive pulmonary disease. Patients with COPD who have moderate to severe airflow obstruction and chronic symptoms can benefit from maintenance treatment with long-acting β_2-agonists (see Table 17.3). These drugs improve lung function and quality of life and lower exacerbation rates in patients with the disease (see Table 17.4). With the exception of indacaterol (once-daily dosing), the long-acting β_2-agonists are administered twice a day.

Corticosteroids

> Steroid inhaler: for inflammation.

Asthma

Inhaled corticosteroids are the most effective long-term treatment option for control of symptoms in all patients with mild, moderate, or severe persistent asthma (see Table 17.1). Randomized, controlled clinical trials have demonstrated that inhaled corticosteroids are more effective than LT modifiers, long-acting β_2-agonists, cromolyn, and

TABLE 17.4 Some Drugs Approved by US Food and Drug Administration for Treatment of Chronic Obstructive Pulmonary Disease

Drug	Delivery Device(s)
Inhaled Short-Acting Antimuscarinic	
Ipratropium (Atrovent HFA)	HFA MDI, nebulizer
Inhaled Short-Acting β_2-Agonist/Short-Acting Antimuscarinic Combinations	
Albuterol/Ipratropium (Combivent, Combivent Respimat, DuoNeb)	Chlorofluorocarbon MDI, MDI, nebulizer
Inhaled Long-Acting β_2-Agonists	
Indacaterol (Arcapta Neohaler)	DPI
Salmeterol (Serevent Diskus)	DPI
Formoterol (Foradil Aerolizer, Perforomist)	DPI, nebulizer
Arformoterol (Brovana)	Nebulizer
Olodaterol (Striverdi Respimat)	ISI
Inhaled Long-Acting Antimuscarinic Agents	
Tiotropium (Spiriva HandiHaler)	DPI
Aclidinium (Tudorza)	DPI
Glycopyrrolate (Seebri Neohaler)	DPI
Inhaled Corticosteroid/Long-Acting β_2-Agonist Combinations	
Fluticasone propionate/salmeterol (Advair Diskus, Advair HFA, AirDuo RespiClick)	DPI
Fluticasone furoate/vilanterol (Breo Ellipta)	DPI
Budesonide/formoterol (Symbicort)	MDI
Phosphodiesterase-4 Inhibitor	
Roflumilast (Daliresp)	Oral tablets

CFC, Chlorofluorocarbon; *DPI,* dry powder inhaler; *HFA,* hydrofluoroalkaline; *MDI,* metered-dose inhaler; *ISI,* inhalation spray inhaler.

theophylline in improving pulmonary function, preventing symptoms and exacerbations, reducing the need for emergency room visits, and decreasing the number of asthma-related deaths. Most patients experience a positive response at relatively low doses. The optimal dose may decrease or increase over time but it should always be tailored to the lowest possible dose. Dose depends on the inhaled corticosteroid and the inhaler device. Common inhalers contain beclomethasone (be kloe-METH-a-sone) (Qvar) and fluticasone (Flovent) (see Table 17.2). Patients taking these corticosteroids have a significant improvement in pulmonary function, with a decrease in wheezing, tightness, and cough. The orally inhaled corticosteroids are especially useful in reducing inflammation and therefore the secretions and swelling that occur within the lungs after an asthma attack occurs. Although the steroids produce no immediate benefit in an acute asthmatic attack, they hasten recovery and decrease morbidity in these patients. They also reduce airway hyperreactivity.

The side effects of steroids vary, depending on route of administration, frequency of intake, duration of intake, total dose, and the preexisting diseases a patient may have.

Long-term oral corticosteroid therapy, such as with prednisone, may be necessary in some severely asthmatic patients and even in patients with moderate asthma, especially during respiratory infections. Prolonged systemic use of such agents, however, can result in adrenal suppression, poor wound healing, and immunosuppression. Supplemental steroids may need to be considered if adrenal suppression has occurred (see Chapter 16).

Candidiasis of the oral cavity can result from the long-term use of an inhalation corticosteroid. When the dental health professional performs an oral examination of any patient using steroid inhalers, any symptoms of candidiasis should be noted and treated. Patients using oral corticosteroid inhalers should be advised to rinse the mouth and gargle with water after using the inhaler to minimize the chance of candidiasis.

Chronic Obstructive Pulmonary Disease

Inhaled corticosteroid monotherapy is not approved for COPD. Inhaled corticosteroids in combination with long-acting β_2-agonists or in addition to a long-acting β_2-agonist can be used to treat COPD (see Tables 17.3 and 17.4).

Leukotriene Modifiers

LTs are synthesized by the enzyme 5-lipoxygenase from arachidonic acid, which also produces prostaglandins (PGs). The LTs are produced by cells of inflammation and produce bronchoconstriction, increased mucus secretion, mucosal edema, and greater bronchial hyperreactivity. The LT pathway inhibitors block the effects of the release of LTs. These agents are used to manage patients with asthma that is not controlled by β_2-agonists and corticosteroid inhalers.

Zileuton (Zyflo) is a 5-lipoxygenase inhibitor that works by preventing the synthesis of the LTs. Zafirlukast (Accolate) and montelukast (Singulair) are LT-receptor antagonists (LTRAs). They are not as effective as the corticosteroid inhalers. Both are effective when taken orally. Some patients have better responses than others, but who will have a better response cannot be predicted.

The adverse reactions of these agents include irritation of the stomach mucosa, headache, and alteration of liver function test values. Zafirlukast has a drug interaction with erythromycin and aspirin, and increases the effect of warfarin. Caution should be exercised when giving this agent to patients taking drugs metabolized by cytochrome P-450 isoenzyme 2C9 (tolbutamide, phenytoin, and carbamazepine) or 3A/4 (dihydropyridines, cyclosporin, astemizole, and cisapride). Erythromycin lowers the level of zafirlukast by about 40%. Aspirin raises zafirlukast levels by about 50%. Zafirlukast has recently been found to raise the level of theophylline in the blood. This finding may be explained by the fact that zafirlukast is an inhibitor of cytochrome P-450 3A/4 and a substrate for cytochrome P-450 2C9. Both zafirlukast and zileuton have been reported to cause life-threatening hepatic injury. Alanine aminotransferase levels need to be monitored, and patients should discontinue the drug immediately if abdominal pain, nausea, jaundice, itching, or lethargy occurs. Also, there have been reports of mood changes in patients taking montelukast.

Cromolyn

> Inhibits mast cell degranulation.

An agent that is effective only for the prophylaxis of asthma and not for treatment of an acute attack is cromolyn (KROE-moe-lin) (Intal, Nasalcrom). It has no intrinsic bronchodilator, antihistaminic, or anti-inflammatory action. Cromolyn prevents the antigen-induced release of histamine, LTs, and other substances by sensitized mast cells. It appears to do so by preventing the influx of calcium provoked by immunoglobulin E (IgE) antibody-antigen interaction on the mast cell. This effect accounts for the group name that these drugs have been given: mast cell degranulation inhibitors. Cromolyn is the least toxic of all asthma medications. It is currently available in a metered-dose form like the other inhalation agents. Nedocromil (Tilade) is similar in action to cromolyn.

The advantage of cromolyn is its safety. It may be used prophylactically by patients with chronic asthma or taken before exercise-induced asthma.

Methylxanthines

The xanthines and methylxanthines consist of theophylline (thee-OFF-i-leen) (Theo-Dur, Slo-Bid), caffeine, and theobromine. Theophylline, used as a bronchodilator, can be combined with ethylenediamine to produce aminophylline (am-in-OFF-i-leen), which is more soluble. Theophylline is used to treat persistent asthma and the bronchospasm associated with chronic bronchitis and emphysema. Bronchodilation is the major therapeutic effect desired.

Side effects associated with the methylxanthines include central nervous system (CNS) stimulation, cardiac stimulation, increased gastric secretion, and diuresis. Patients often complain of nervousness and insomnia. Erythromycin can increase the serum levels of theophylline, leading to toxicity.

Intravenous aminophylline and rapidly absorbed oral liquid preparations are used to manage acute asthmatic attacks and status asthmaticus. To manage persistent asthma, sustained-release preparations in tablet or capsule form are used. Blood drug levels may be measured in patients undergoing long-term theophylline therapy to determine whether the dose they are taking is appropriate. Current literature suggests that the use of theophylline should be limited to patients whose asthma or COPD is not controlled with other agents. When the chance of theophylline toxicity is weighed against the potential therapeutic benefit, theophylline is often omitted from an asthmatic patient's therapeutic regimen.

Antimuscarinic

> Ipratropium: first choice for chronic obstructive pulmonary disease.

Inhaled antimuscarinic drugs appear to inhibit vagally mediated reflexes by antagonizing the action of acetylcholine, thereby causing bronchodilation. Ipratropium (i-pra-TROE-pee-um) bromide (Atrovent) is a short-acting antimuscarinic available for oral inhalation for people with COPD. Tiotropium bromide (Spiriva) is an inhaled long-acting antimuscarinic drug used to treat COPD. Side effects, including dry mouth and bad taste, are minimized with administration by inhalation. Both drugs have a cross-hyperreactivity with peanut and soybean allergies. Ipratropium bromide's bronchodilating effect is additive with that of the β-agonists. It is available as in combination with albuterol sulfate (Combivent) and is used in the patient with COPD who is using a regular aerosol inhalation bronchodilator and continues to have evidence of bronchospasm. Neither ipratropium bromide nor tiotropium bromide is approved by the FDA for treatment of asthma.

Anti-Immunoglobulin E Antibodies

Omalizumab (Xolair) is the first in a new class of medications introduced to treat asthma due to allergens. It is a recombinant humanized monoclonal antibody that prevents IgE from binding to mast cells and basophils, thereby preventing the release of inflammatory mediators after allergen exposure (see Table 17.2). This drug is FDA-approved for adjunctive use in patients at least 12 years of age who have well-documented specific allergies and moderate-to-severe persistent asthma that is not well-controlled with an inhaled corticosteroid with or without a long-acting β2-agonist. Omalizumab is administered as a subcutaneous injection every 2 to 4 weeks. It is expensive. Adverse effects include injection-site pain and bruising. Anaphylaxis can occur within 2 hours of injection but sometimes 4 days later. It is advised that patients be kept under observation for 2 hours after the first three injections and for 30 minutes after subsequent injections. Patients are educated about the signs and symptoms of anaphylaxis and when to self-administer injectable epinephrine.

Interleukin-5 Antibody Antagonists

Mepolizumab (Nucala) and reslizumab (Cinqair) are the first in a new class of drugs approved by the FDA to treat severe asthma in patients with elevated eosinophil levels. Interleukin-5 is the major cytokine that is responsible for growth, differentiation, recruitment, activation, and survival of eosinophils that are thought to play a role in the allergy process. These drugs inhibit the signaling of interleukin-5 which blocks the production of eosinophils and results in decreased inflammation and a reduction in asthma symptoms. However, their mechanism of action in controlling asthma symptoms has not been established. Nucala is indicated for those over the age of 12 and Cinqair is indicated for persons over 18 as add-on maintenance therapy for severe asthma with an eosinophilic type. Nucala is administered subcutaneously every 4 weeks. Side effects include injection-site reactions, headache, fatigue, and back pain. Hypersensitivity reactions have also been reported. Cinqair is administered intravenously every 4 weeks in a health care setting by a health professional because of the risk of anaphylaxis. The most common adverse reaction is oropharyngeal pain. There have been reports of hypersensitivity reactions.

Agents Used to Manage Upper Respiratory Infections

Nasal Decongestants

Nasal decongestants are α-adrenergic agonists that act by constricting the blood vessels of the nasal mucous membranes. Some examples of these include pseudoephedrine (soo-doe-e-FED-rin) (Sudafed, Sucrets, in Actifed) and phenylephrine (fen-ill-EF-rin) (Neo-Synephrine, Sinex, Allerest). Many nasal decongestants are available over-the-counter (OTC) for both local and systemic use (see also Table 4.5). Long-term topical use of decongestants may result in rebound swelling and congestion. Therefore decongestant nose sprays should not be used for more than a few days. Unwanted side effects of adrenergic stimulation may occur. Phenylephrine (Neo-Synephrine) is used topically as a nasal spray, and phenylpropanolamine is used systemically as a decongestant (α-agonist action). Pseudoephedrine, both an α-adrenergic agonist and a β-adrenergic agonist, is used systemically as a nasal decongestant.

Expectorants and Mucolytics

Expectorants are drugs that promote the removal of exudate or mucus from the respiratory passages. Liquefying expectorants are drugs that promote the ejection of mucus by decreasing its viscosity. Mucolytics destroy or dissolve mucus.

Some expectorants act through their ability to cause reflex stimulation of the vagus nerve, which increases bronchial secretions. Guaifenesin (gwye-FEN-e-sin), the most popular expectorant, is contained in a variety of OTC products mixed with other active ingredients. Robitussin is available as guaifenesin alone (Robitussin plain) and mixed with an antitussive agent (Robitussin DM).

Mucolytics are enzymes that are able to digest mucus, decreasing its viscosity. Acetylcysteine (Mucomyst) is a mucolytic used to loosen secretions in pulmonary diseases, including cystic fibrosis. It is also used orally as an antidote for acetaminophen toxicity.

Antitussives

Antitussives may be opioids or related agents used for the symptomatic relief of nonproductive cough. Opioids are the most effective, but because of their addicting properties, other agents are often used. Codeine-containing cough preparations are commonly used, but their histamine-releasing properties may precipitate bronchospasm.

Dextromethorphan (dex-troe-meth-OR-fan) (the DM in cough medicines such as Robitussin DM), an opioid-like compound, suppresses the cough reflex through its direct effect on the cough center. It does not cause the release of histamine. It may potentiate the effects of CNS depressants. It is available both alone and in combination with other ingredients. By impairing coughing, dextromethorphan may not allow the secretions to be cleared from the lungs.

DENTAL IMPLICATIONS OF THE RESPIRATORY DRUGS

About 10% of the population has some type of pulmonary disease, so patients taking medications for asthma, emphysema, or chronic bronchitis are often encountered in dental practice. A patient with severe COPD can have pulmonary hypertension, increasing the risk for cardiac arrhythmias. Stress should be minimized and adrenal supplementation instituted for patients taking long-term oral steroids and the dental procedures are likely to produce severe stress. Patients prone to development of respiratory failure, if given oxygen (either alone or with nitrous oxide) or CNS depressants, may manifest acute respiratory failure. Aspirin should be avoided in patients with asthma, and erythromycin may alter the metabolism of theophylline (Box 17.1). Emergency equipment and medications should be available when these patients are undergoing dental treatment (see Table 21.1 and Box 21.3).

ALLERGIC RHINITIS

Allergic rhinitis is an inflammation of the nasal airways that occurs when an allergen is inhaled in an individual with a sensitized immune system. The allergen triggers the response of the antibody IgE, which binds to mast cells and basophils containing histamine. The release of histamine causes itchy, watery eyes and runny nose. Symptoms vary in severity among those affected by allergies. Allergic rhinitis can be seasonal or perennial. Seasonal allergic rhinitis is usually caused by

BOX 17.1 Management of the Dental Patient With Asthma

- Avoid aspirin, nonsteroidal antiinflammatory drugs (NSAIDs) because of the risk of these drugs precipitating an asthma attack.
- Sulfiting agents in local anesthetic agents with a vasoconstrictor could increase the risk for bronchoconstriction.
- Avoid erythromycin with theophylline, which could lead to toxicity.
- Review emergency treatment of asthma with staff.
- Have patient's albuterol inhaler available for use.
- Watch for oral candidiasis with use of an inhaled steroid; have patient rinse mouth to prevent.
- Patients on long-term oral (PO) steroid therapy may need supplemental steroids for severe stress.
- Patient management: reduce stress.
- Use nitrous oxide (N_2O) with caution if needed for sedation.

pollen from trees, grass, and flowers and lasts several weeks to months. Perennial allergic rhinitis is a result of sensitivity to different allergens, such as house dust and animal dander, and lasts throughout the year. Fig. 17.5 illustrates the inflammatory process.

The most effective method of treating allergic rhinitis is to eliminate the source of allergen. If this is not possible, medication is necessary.

Antihistamines (H_1-receptor antagonists). The common term *antihistamine* refers to agents that are H_1 antihistamines or H_1-blockers. They are widely used drugs, and dental hygienists should be familiar with them for the following reasons:

- Many patients have seasonal allergies or allergic rhinitis (e.g., hay fever) that make dental treatment difficult. The dentist may prescribe, or the patient may self-medicate with, antihistamines before a dental procedure to reduce the symptoms of hay fever and make it easier for the patient to breathe.
- A mild allergic reaction to a drug may be treated with antihistamines in the dental office. If the allergic reaction is severe, epinephrine is the drug of choice.
- Patients taking antihistamines may experience side effects, such as xerostomia, but the second-generation antihistamines have less anticholinergic effect.

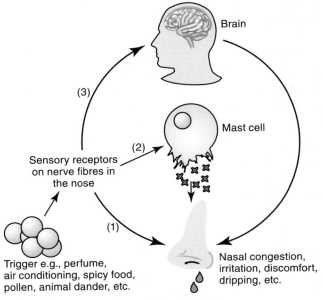

Fig. 17.5 Inflammatory process of allergic rhinitis.

- Antihistamines, especially first-generation, interact with many other drug groups and their CNS effects are additive with those of other CNS depressants.

Pharmacologic Effects

The first-generation H_1 antihistamines, also called H_1-blockers, have several pharmacologic effects, including antihistaminic, anticholinergic, antiserotonergic, and sedative effects. Second-generation H_1 antihistamines penetrate poorly into the CNS and so are less likely to cause sedation. Because they have a chemical structure similar to that of histamine, they can bind with the H_1-receptor and prevent or block the action of histamine (if it is released). Table 17.5 reviews the both the first- and second-generation H_1 antihistamines.

Fig. 17.6 compares the relative sedative, antihistaminic, and anticholinergic effects of five common antihistamines: brompheniramine (brome-fen-EER-a meen) (Dimetane), chlorpheniramine (klor-fen-EER-a-meen) (Chlor-Trimeton), diphenhydramine (dye-fen-HYE-dra-meen) (Benadryl), fexofenadine (feks-oh-FEN-a-deen) (Allegra), and loratadine (lor-A-ti-deen) (Claritin).

The pharmacologic effects of antihistamines can be divided into those caused by blocking of histamine at the H_1-receptor and those independent of this effect.

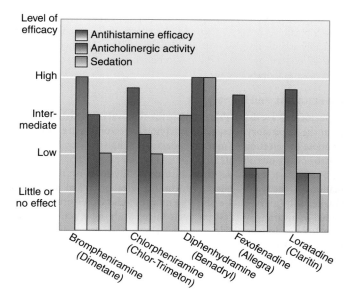

Fig. 17.6 Comparison of efficacy and adverse effects of selected antihistamines. (From Lilley LL, Harrington S, Snyder JS. *Pharmacology and the Nursing Process.* 5th ed. St. Louis: Mosby; 2007.)

TABLE 17.5   Selected Oral Drugs for Allergic Rhinitis

Drug Name	Antihistamine Activity	Single Adult Dose	Dosing Interval (hr)	Sedative Effects	Anticholinergic Activity
Some First-Generation Antihistamines					
Diphenhydramine (Benadryl)*	+/++	25–50 mg	6–8	+++	+++
Clemastine (Tavist)	+/++	1 mg	12	++	+++
Chlorpheniramine* (Chlor-Trimeton)	++	4 mg	4–6	+	++
Second-Generation Antihistamines					
Acrivastine (Semprex)*	++/+++	8 mg	4–6	±	±
Acrivastine/pseudoephedrine (Semprex D)*	++/+++	8 mg/60 mg	4–6	±	±
Cetirizine (Zyrtec)*	++/+++	5–10 mg	24	++	±
Cetirizine/pseudoephedrine (Zyrtec D)*	++/+++	5 mg/120 mg ER tab	12	++	±
Desloratadine (Clarinex)*	++/+++	5	24	±	±
Desloratadine/pseudoephedrine:	++/+++			±	±
Clarinex-D 12 hour*		2.5 mg/120 mg ER tab	12		
Clarinex-D 24 hour*		5 mg/24 mg ER tab	24		
Fexofenadine (Allegra)*	++/+++	60 mg	12	±	±
		180 mg	24		
Fexofenadine/pseudoephedrine:	++/+++			±	±
Allegra D 12 hour*		60 mg/120 mg ER tab	12		
Allegra D 24 hour*		180 mg/240 mg ER tab	24		
Levocetirizine (Xyzal)*	++/+++	5 mg	24	±	±
Loratadine (Claritin)*	++/+++	10 mg	24	±	±
Loratadine/pseudoephedrine (all are ER tablets):	++/+++			±	±
Alavert-D 12 hour*		5 mg/120 mg	12		
Claritin-D 12 hour*		5 mg/120 mg	12		
Claritin D-24 hour*		10 mg/240 mg	24		
Leukotriene Modifier					
Montelukast (Singulair)	++	10 mg	24	−	−

ER tab, Extended-release tablet.

++++, Very high; +++, high; ++, moderate; +, low; ±, may have some effect; −, no effect.

*Available over the counter.

H₁-Receptor Blocking Effects

Counteracts histamine's effects.

Antihistamines, which are H₁-antagonists, competitively block or antagonize histamine's effect at the following sites:

Capillaries permeability: When the capillary permeability produced by histamine is blocked, less tissue edema occurs from the transport of the serum into the intracellular spaces.

Vascular smooth muscle (vessels): The antihistamines block the dilation of the vascular smooth muscle that histamine produces.

Nonvascular (bronchial) smooth muscle: Because other autacoids (physiologically active substance produced by and acting within the body [i.e.; bradykinin]) are also released in an anaphylactic reaction, antihistamines are not effective in counteracting all the bronchoconstriction present during that reaction.

Cutaneous nerve endings: Antihistamines can suppress the itching and pain associated with histamine-mediated release of inflammatory chemical mediators (cytokines, LT, PGs) at the cutaneous nerve endings.

Other Effects (Unrelated to H₁-Blocking Effects)

CNS effects: The antihistamines produce varying degrees of CNS depression.

Anticholinergic effects: Antihistamines block acetylcholine receptors to varying degrees and produce an anticholinergic effect (cholinergic blockade) that is weaker than but similar to that of atropine.

Adverse Reactions

Like the pharmacologic effects of the antihistamines, the adverse reactions vary among the different agents. Fig. 17.6 shows how adverse reactions and pharmacologic effects vary among antihistamines.

Central Nervous System Depression

Sedation is the most common side effect associated with the first-generation antihistamines, and it may be accompanied by dizziness, tinnitus, incoordination, blurred vision, and fatigue. Patients who are given first-generation antihistamines should be warned against operating a motor vehicle or signing important documents. Sedation with first-generation antihistamines is additive with that caused by other CNS depressant drugs.

As with all drugs that depress the CNS, stimulation or excitation can occur in a few cases. Symptoms include restlessness, excitation, and, in severe cases, convulsions. CNS stimulation is more common in children, elderly patients, and those who use a larger dose than prescribed. The nonsedating H₁-blockers, such as loratadine (Claritin), produce less sedation because they do not penetrate the brain as easily.

Anticholinergic Effects

Anticholinergic: xerostomia.

The first-generation H₁ antihistamines can cause anticholinergic effects such as xerostomia. The importance to the dental hygienist is that anticholinergic effects lead to xerostomia and xerostomia leads to numerous dental problems. Xerostomia can cause an increased caries rate in patients taking antihistamines on a long-term basis. In patients taking antihistamines long term, the mouth should be observed for symptoms of xerostomia and counseling about techniques to manage it should be presented.

The nonsedating antihistamines have much less anticholinergic effect and are less likely to cause xerostomia. Loratadine (Claritin) is a heavily advertised nonsedating antihistamine.

Toxicity

Antihistamine poisoning has become more common in recent years because of the easy accessibility of the agents in OTC preparations promoted as sleep aids. Excitation predominates in small children, and sedation can occur in adults. Death usually results from coma with cardiovascular and respiratory collapse. The treatment is directed at specific symptoms.

Adverse Reactions of Intranasal Dose Form

Intranasal antihistamines can cause nasal discomfort, epistaxis, and headache, and there have been reports of somnolence. Nasal mucosal irritation has been reported with the long-term use of intranasal antihistamines. Patients have reported a "bad taste" with intranasal azelastine.

Intranasal corticosteroids. Intranasal corticosteroids are very effective for the treatment of moderate to severe allergic rhinitis and are considered first-line therapy (Table 17.6). These drugs work by decreasing inflammation in the airways. They are used to control the symptoms rhinorrhea, itching, sneezing, and nasal congestion. Intranasal corticosteroids are effective when given once daily. Onset of action is about 12 hours although full relief may take up to 7 days. The intranasal spray can also decrease ocular symptoms in patients with seasonal rhinitis.

Adverse effects. Intranasal corticosteroids can cause mild dryness, irritation, burning, or bleeding of the nasal mucosa, sore throat, epistaxis, and headache. Ulceration and mucosal atrophy have been reported. Growth suppression in children has not been reported with the newer intranasal corticosteroids (ciclesonide, fluticasone, propionate, mometasone). There were reports in the literature that beclomethasone might slightly slow the growth rate in children.

Leukotriene modifiers.

Leukotrienes have a role in allergy and inflammation.

During an allergic reaction, cysteinyl LT is released in the nasal mucosa, causing nasal congestion. The LTRA montelukast (Singulair) is approved for the treatment of seasonal and perennial allergic rhinitis. It provides relief for sneezing, itching, discharge, and congestion but is

TABLE 17.6	Selected Nasal Sprays for Allergic Rhinitis
H₁ Antihistamines	Azelastine (Astelin 0.1%, Astepro 0.1%, 0.15%) Olopatadine (Patanase)
Corticosteroids	Beclomethasone dipropionate (Beconase, QNasl) Budesonide (Rhinocort Aqua)* Ciclesonide (Omnaris, Zetonna) Flunisolide (Nasalide) Fluticasone furoate (Veramyst) Fluticasone propionate (Flonase)* Mometasone furoate (Nasonex) Triamcinolone acetonide (Nasacort AQ)*
H₁ Antihistamine/ corticosteroid	Azelastine/fluticasone propionate (Dymista)
Mast cell stabilizer	Cromolyn sodium (Nasalcrom)*
Anticholinergic	Ipratropium bromide (Atrovent)

*Available without a prescription.

less effective than H_1 antihistamines and intranasal corticosteroids. It is usually used as adjunct therapy with H_1 antihistamines and intranasal corticosteroids.

Montelukast is generally well tolerated. However, there are post-marketing reports of psychiatric symptoms (thoughts of suicide) and sleep disturbances.

Mast cell stabilizers. Cromolyn sodium inhibits mast cell degranulation and mediator release when given before allergen exposure. When taken before the onset of triggers, it prevents allergic rhinitis symptoms. It is well tolerated with few adverse effects. It must be used four times a day and is less effective than intranasal corticosteroids.

Intranasal anticholinergic drugs. Ipratropium bromide, a quaternary amine drug, blocks acetylcholine receptors, thereby decreasing rhinorrhea in persons with allergic rhinitis. It is poorly absorbed systemically and does not readily cross the blood-brain barrier. This agent can cause dry nose and mouth, epistaxis, and pharyngeal irritation. If inadvertently placed in the eye, ipratropium bromide can raise intraocular pressure. It should be used with caution in patients with glaucoma.

Decongestants

Oral decongestants. The oral decongestants, pseudoephedrine and phenylephrine, are α-adrenergic agonists that cause a vasoconstriction of the nasal mucosa. They are thought to primarily stimulate α_1-adrenergic receptors on the venous sinusoids. These agents are used to treat the congestion associated with allergic rhinitis, not sneezing or mucosal discharge. They are often used with H_1 antihistamines. Phenylephrine, though less effective than pseudoephedrine, is now in many OTC oral decongestant products because of the legal restrictions placed on the sale of pseudoephedrine.

Adverse effects. The most common adverse effects associated with oral decongestants include insomnia, excitability, headache, nervousness, anorexia, palpitations, and tachycardia. Other adverse effects are arrhythmias, hypertension, nausea, vomiting, and urinary retention. These agents should be used with caution in patients with cardiovascular disease, hypertension, diabetes, hyperthyroidism, closed-angle glaucoma, and bladder neck obstruction.

Intranasal decongestants. Because they are less likely to have systemic adverse effects, intranasal decongestants are an alternative to oral decongestants. However, they can cause stinging, burning, sneezing, and dry throat or nose. They should be used for no more than 3 to 5 consecutive days in order to avoid rebound congestion. Rebound congestion is treated by discontinuing the intranasal decongestant and then having the patient use an intranasal corticosteroid or possibly undergoing a short course of oral steroids to help control symptoms.

DENTAL HYGIENE CONSIDERATIONS

- Always conduct a thorough medication/health history in order to avoid causing drug interactions and prescribing medications that could exacerbate a respiratory illness.
- Patients with emphysema or chronic obstructive pulmonary disease (COPD) should not receive nitrous oxide because of their diminished oxygen capacity.
- Nonsteroidal antiinflammatory drugs (NSAIDs) can exacerbate an asthma attack and should be avoided. Acetaminophen can be used instead.
- Oral steroid inhalers can cause candidiasis, and patients using them should be examined for symptoms at each visit.
- Oral steroid inhalers, oral β_2-agonist inhalers, and oral antimuscarinic inhalers can cause dry mouth.
- Instruct patients on the importance of good oral health care after using their inhalers.
- Patients with respiratory disorders may require a semi-supine position. Work with patients to determine what is best for them.
- Review the information in Box 17.1.

- Obtain a detailed medication history to avoid drug interactions.
- First-generation and, to a lesser extent, second-generation antihistamines can cause sedation.
- The combination of sedating antihistamines with opioid analgesics or antianxiety drugs can increase the patient's risk for sedation.
- Instruct the patient to avoid driving or any other task that requires thought or concentration if a sedating antihistamine is necessary.
- First-generation antihistamines can cause significant xerostomia.
- Ipratropium bromide can cause xerostomia.
- Instruct the patient to drink plenty of water and to chew tart, sugarless gum or candy in order to avoid or minimize xerostomia.
- Remind the patient that caffeinated beverages and alcohol can exacerbate xerostomia.
- Remind the patient that even though fruit juices may help with xerostomia, they raise the risk for caries.
- Check blood pressure and heart rate of any patient taking oral decongestants either alone or in combination with an antihistamine.

ACADEMIC SKILLS ASSESSMENT

1. Discuss different methods of minimizing an asthma attack in the dental office.
2. What is the role of steroids in the treatment of asthma?
3. Why are oral, inhaled steroids the preferred dose form in the treatment of asthma?
4. What is the role of β_2-adrenergic agonists in the treatment of asthma?
5. What are the dental concerns associated with β_2-adrenergic agonists? What would the dental practitioner tell a patient about them?
6. What are first-generation antihistamines and how do they work?
7. What are the pharmacologic effects of first-generation antihistamines?
8. What are the adverse reactions associated with first-generation antihistamines? Can they lead to toxicity?

9. What would the dental practitioner tell a patient about adverse reactions, with a special emphasis on those with dental implications?
10. What drug interactions associated with first-generation antihistamines are of dental concern?
11. What are the adverse reactions of second-generation antihistamines?
12. What are the advantages of second-generation antihistamines over first-generation antihistamines?
13. How do intranasal corticosteroids work, and how do they differ from antihistamines?
14. What is the role of ipratropium bromide in the treatment of allergic rhinitis?
15. What is the role of cromolyn sodium in the treatment of allergic rhinitis?
16. Why are oral decongestants combined with antihistamines in the treatment of allergic rhinitis?

CLINICAL CASE STUDY

Lance Saville is a 65-year-old male with COPD who has been coming to your practice for 19 years. His medication/health history is significant for COPD (emphysema). He is being treated with tiotropium (Spiriva) and an albuterol inhaler as needed. He is in the office today to have a cavity filled. The dentist will use a local anesthetic with a vasoconstrictor.

1. What is tiotropium and what is its role in the treatment of COPD?
2. What are the adverse effects associated with tiotropium?
3. What are the dental considerations associated with tiotropium?
4. What are the potential drug interactions between albuterol and the vasoconstrictor?
5. Can nitrous oxide be used in this patient? Why or why not?

CLINICAL CASE STUDY

John Esposito is 55 years old and has a history of seasonal allergies that are getting worse by Mr. Esposito's account. He saw his general physician last month because none of the non-prescription drugs he had used were working. Also, his oral decongestant was making him dizzy and was causing his heart rate to rise. The doctor then started Mr. Esposito on cetirizine and the intranasal corticosteroid fluticasone (Flonase) to treat his symptoms. Mr. Esposito is finally feeling relief from his symptoms today. He is also happy to knew that both of these medicines are now available without a prescription.

1. What is the mechanism of action of second-generation antihistamines?
2. Are there any adverse effects associated with cetirizine that would affect this patient's oral health care?
3. What is fluticasone and how does it work?
4. What are the adverse effects associated with fluticasone?
5. Are there any oral adverse effects associated fluticasone?
6. What other classes of drugs can be used if these drugs are not effective?
7. Do any of the other classes of drugs affect oral health, and if so, how?

18

Drugs for the Treatment of Diabetes Mellitus

http://evolve.elsevier.com/Haveles/pharmacology

LEARNING OBJECTIVES

1. Describe the importance of the hormones released by the endocrine glands in maintaining homeostasis, including
   - Discuss the two primary hormones secreted by the pancreas and their role in relation to diabetes mellitus.
   - Define diabetes mellitus and describe the two types of this disease, its complications, and issues involving dentistry, cautions, and contraindications in the treatment of patients with diabetes.

2. Describe the systemic complications of diabetes and the evaluation of the dental patient with diabetes.
3. Discuss the goals of therapy and describe the types of drugs used to treat diabetes.
4. Discuss four new drugs being used to treat diabetes and summarize their mechanism of action and possible adverse effects.
5. Discuss the treatment of hypoglycemia.

Hormones are secreted by endocrine glands and transported by the blood to target organs, where they are biologically activated. The endocrine gland discussed in this chapter is the pancreas (Fig. 18.1). The hormones released by the endocrine glands help maintain homeostasis by regulating body functions and are controlled themselves by feedback systems. In most of these systems, the hormone released has a negative feedback effect on the secretion of the hormone stimulating substance. Patients with diabetes mellitus (DM) being treated in the dental office may be taking medication to help lower their plasma glucose levels.

PANCREATIC HORMONES

Two primary hormones secreted by the islets of Langerhans of the pancreas are insulin and glucagon. Insulin promotes fuel storage (pack the bags: glucose out of blood), whereas glucagon promotes fuel mobilization (empty the bags: glucose into blood) in the body. Other hormones secreted by the pancreas are islet amyloid polypeptide (IAPP; amylin) and pancreatic peptide. Their functions have not yet been elucidated.

DIABETES MELLITUS

Diabetes mellitus is a group of metabolic disorders characterized by persistent hyperglycemia. DM is currently classified as types I and II (Table 18.1).

Over 30 million people in the United States have diabetes, of which 23.1 million have an actual diagnosis of diabetes while the remaining 7.2 million remain undiagnosed. The vast majority of these people, 90% to 95%, are diagnosed with type 2 diabetes. Both environmental and genetic factors are believed to contribute to the pathogenesis of type 2 diabetes. It is thought that the hyperglycemia leads to the many complications of diabetes.

Fasting blood sugar (FBS) > 126 mg/dL.

Symptoms and complications usually result from inadequate or poorly timed secretion of insulin from the pancreas and/or insulin resistance of the pancreatic islet cells (β cells). (Fig. 18.2 outlines the body's physiologic response to changes in plasma glucose levels.) The criterion for the diagnosis of DM is (1) two consecutive fasting plasma glucose levels or the more commonly used term of fasting blood sugars (FBSs) higher than 126 mg/dL or (2) a hemoglobin A_{1c} value of 6.5% or higher or (3) a 2-hour plasma glucose level of 200 mg/dL or higher during an oral glucose tolerance test or (4) a randomly measured plasma glucose level of 200 mg/dL or higher in a patient with the classic symptoms of hyperglycemia or hyperglycemic crisis.

Diabetes is primarily characterized by hyperglycemia and glycosuria. Other characteristics include hyperlipemia, azoturia, ketonemia, and, when the deficiency is severe, ketoacidosis. Patients usually experience general weakness, weight loss, polyphagia, polydipsia, and polyuria. Patients with type 2 diabetes often experience weight gain.

Types of Diabetes
Type 1
Type 1 diabetes usually develops in persons younger than 30 years and results from an autoimmune destruction of the pancreatic β cells. The type 1 autoimmune response may be triggered by an infection, a slow virus, environmental insults, or some as yet unknown factor. It is associated with a complete lack of insulin secretion, increased glucagon secretion, rapid onset of disease, ketosis, and severe symptoms. Type 1 diabetes must be treated with injections of insulin because the pancreas does not produce any insulin. Without insulin, type 1 DM is fatal.

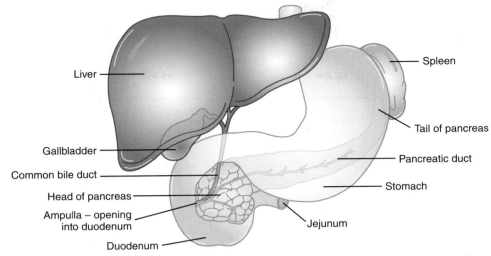

Fig. 18.1 The pancreas. (From Applegate E. *The Anatomy and Physiology Learning System.* 4th ed. St. Louis: Saunders; 2011.)

TABLE 18.1	Diabetes Types 1 and 2	
Property	**Type 1**	**Type 2**
Age of onset	<30 years	>40 years
Onset of symptoms	Acute	Gradual
Incidence of cases	10%	90%
Etiology	Autoimmune reaction	Insulin resistance, excess hepatic glucose production, diminished insulin secretion
Genetic influence	Just a little	Quite a bit
Receptors	Normal	Defective
Plasma insulin	No	Normal or elevated then over time reduced
Ketoacidosis	Yes	No

Type 2

Type 2 diabetes usually develops in persons older than 40 years. However, more and more cases of type 2 diabetes are being reported in persons younger than 20 years. This development is being attributed to a much more sedentary lifestyle and lack of exercise in the US population. Fast food has replaced traditional home-cooked food, and video games and television have replaced physical activity; as a result, obesity is dramatically on the rise. Obesity is a major risk factor for development of type 2 diabetes. This disease is associated with the ability of the pancreas to secrete enough insulin to prevent ketoacidosis but not enough to normalize the plasma glucose level. The insulin secreted does not reduce the glucose levels in the serum to normal levels, for a variety of possible reasons (Box 18.1).

Insulin resistance develops because of prolonged hyperglycemia and resulting hyperinsulinemia. Type 2 diabetes involves a slower onset of disease, less severe symptoms, and lack of ketoacidosis. Tissue insensitivity to insulin, a deficiency of the pancreas's response to glucose, and obesity lead to impaired insulin action. In the presence of hyperglycemia, the resistance of the tissues to insulin and the impaired β cells' response are exaggerated. Normal serum glucose levels improve these parameters toward normal.

Type 2 diabetes is treated first with diet and exercise, then with orally acting agents, and, if these modalities fail, with insulin.

Therefore, patients with type 2 diabetes may be taking insulin either with or without oral agents. Because of the etiology of the hyperglycemia in patients with type 2 diabetes, moderate improvement of diet and/or an increase in exercise can produce a large improvement in the glucose levels. Exercise increases the sensitivity of the cells to insulin. Unfortunately, these behavior modifications are difficult to carry out on a routine basis for almost all patients.

Dental Implications of Diabetes

Uncontrolled diabetes causes a pronounced susceptibility to dental caries. This mainly occurs through decreased salivary flow (xerostomia) related to fluid loss. The loss is secondary to an increase in urination that occurs because of poor use of carbohydrates and the glucose that is excreted via the kidneys (water follows glucose). The complications of xerostomia are a result of the lack of its normal functions: lubricating, cleansing, regulating pH, destroying microorganisms and their products, and maintaining the integrity of the oral structures.

A dry, cracking oral mucosa with the presence of mucositis, ulcers, infections, and an inflamed painful tongue may result. Any change in the glucose level in saliva probably contributes little to the higher caries rate.

Xerostomia

Patients with DM are at a higher risk for xerostomia, especially as they age. A decrease in salivary flow can lead to mouth ulcers, inflammation of the tongue or mucosal tissues, and tooth deterioration. Diabetes causes blood vessels to thicken, thereby slowing down blood flow to the teeth and gums. As a result, teeth and gums become less healthy and less resistant to oral bacteria in dental plaque.

Periodontal Disease

Patients with uncontrolled or undiagnosed diabetes are more prone to periodontal disease. However, the periodontal status of the patient with well-controlled diabetes has been somewhat more controversial. Despite the fact that some investigators have reported a lack of correlation between diabetes and an increase in the rate of periodontal disease, many other studies have come to the opposite conclusion. (It may be that if diabetes control is good, there is hardly any effect on periodontal status, whereas if diabetes control is poor, there is a greater effect.)

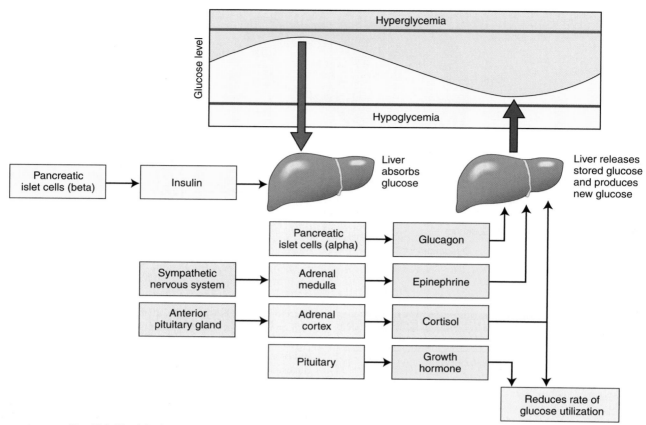

Fig. 18.2 Physiologic response to changes in blood glucose levels. (From McKenry L, Tessier E, Hogan MA. *Mosby's Pharmacology in Nursing.* 22nd ed. St. Louis: Mosby, 2006.)

BOX 18.1   Possible Causes of Type 2 Diabetes

- β cells in the pancreas have a reduced or delayed response to glucose.
- Secretion of insulin is delayed so that blood glucose values are elevated.
- Because cells in the body have insulin resistance (are not as sensitive to insulin as normal cells), more than the usual amount of insulin is required to produce a response. This is known as reduced insulin sensitivity; ultimately, insulin receptors do not respond to insulin at all.
- "Pooped out" pancreas (P³) (a euphemism). Because of the delay in insulin secretion and insulin resistance, the insulin released from the pancreas does not effectively lower the blood glucose level. The pancreas is working "overtime" secreting a lot of insulin but without producing the desired results (decrease in blood sugar). Eventually, the pancreas cannot continue to supply this increased production to keep up with the need for insulin. Either a relative (as a result of resistance) or absolute lack of insulin occurs.
- Adipose tissue secretes a group of hormones called *adipokines* that may impair glucose tolerance.

Periodontal findings include inflammatory and degenerative changes ranging from mild gingivitis to painful periodontitis with a widened periodontal ligament, multiple abscesses, putrescent exudates from periodontal pockets, and increased tooth mobility caused by destruction of supporting alveolar bone. Although it may be more severe, periodontal disease in diabetic patients appears to be similar to that found in nondiabetic patients. The diabetic state probably serves as a predisposing factor that can accelerate the periodontal destruction originated by microbial agents. The proposed etiology for the periodontal changes seen in the patient with diabetes includes microangiopathy of the tissues, thickening of capillary basement membranes, changes in glucose tolerance factor (more glucose), altered polymorphonuclear leukocyte function, and enhanced collagenase activity.

Issues in Dental Care

Dental appointments for diabetic patients should not interfere with meals and should involve minimal stress. In the patient with controlled diabetes, oral surgical procedures should be performed 1.5 to 2 hours after the patient has eaten normal breakfast and taken regular antidiabetic medication. Following surgery, the patient should receive an adequate caloric intake to prevent hypoglycemia. With general anesthesia, patients are often instructed to have nothing by mouth (NPO), should take half of their usual dose of insulin, and receive intravenous 5% glucose in distilled water (D_5W).

Patients with diabetes have fragile blood vessels, delayed wound healing, and a tendency to development of infections; therefore surgical therapy in such patients should be approached with caution. Scaling and soft tissue curettage usually are tolerated well. The bulk of the literature suggests that prophylactic use of antibiotics should be avoided, although many practitioners routinely use antibiotics. If infection is present or if infection ensues, it should be aggressively treated. Measures to reduce the possibility of infection should be used (sterilize instruments, rinse mouth before procedures). The oral complications of diabetes are summarized in Table 18.2.

TABLE 18.2   Oral Complications of Diabetes Mellitus

Complication	Comment(s)	Treatment
Xerostomia	Increase in caries Problem with tasting Problem swallowing Wetting food difficult Problem with mastication Mucositis, ulcers, desquamation Painful tongue	Saliva lubricates, cleanses, regulates acidity; has electrolytes, glycoproteins, antimicrobial enzymes
Slightly elevated blood glucose	In parotid saliva	Not clinically significant
Caries rate	Some say less Some say more	Result of diabetic diet Glucose in saliva
Microvascular disease—small blood vessel disease	Less blood flow to oral cavity	Infection more difficult to treat (antibiotic cannot reach site)
Altered immunity/white blood cell abnormality	Less ability to fight microorganisms	Get infections more easily Periapical abscesses Periodontal abscesses
Increased acidity	Oral infection reduces diabetes control; more insulin needed Oral infection after surgery	Infection treated, better insulin control (need less)
Neuropathy	From diabetes	Numbness, burning, tingling, pain in nerves
Infections	Candidiasis Mucormycosis	Fungal infections more likely
Symptoms	Burning mouth syndrome	Unknown cause
Delayed, impaired healing	With oral trauma	Collagen poorly formed

All complications worsen with hyperglycemia, either acute or chronic. An acute fasting glucose (mg/dL) measurement with a glucose monitor is reflective of glucose at that moment, and long-term glucose levels measured by HgA_{1c} concentration are reflective of glucose control over the previous 2 to 3 months. Oral complications of hyperglycemia are xerostomia, infection, poor healing, increased caries, candidiasis, gingivitis, periodontal diseases, periapical abscess, and burning mouth syndrome.

Cautions and Contraindications

Drugs that may decrease insulin release or increase insulin requirements, such as epinephrine, glucocorticoids, and opioid analgesics, should be used with caution in patients with diabetes. Caution should also be exercised with use of general anesthetics because of the possibility of acidosis. If diabetes is in good control, these drugs can be used.

Systemic Complications of Diabetes

The systemic complications of diabetes include actions affecting almost all the body tissues and organs.

Cardiovascular Complications

The incidence of cardiovascular problems is higher in patients with diabetes. Macroangiopathy, microangiopathy, and hyperlipidemia are common. Atherosclerosis is also more common in these patients.

Retinopathy

Because microvascular disease affects the blood supply to the retina, the functioning of the retina is impaired. In fact, diabetes is the major cause of blindness in adults.

Neuropathy

Neuropathy is another complication of diabetes. It leads to reduction in, and sometimes absence of, feeling, especially in the lower extremities. A variety of sensations, including pain and burning, have been reported. The complaints of pain and discomfort of the tongue and other oral structures are related to diabetic neuropathy. Drugs used to manage this problem include amitriptyline, carbamazepine, phenytoin, and capsaicin (made from hot peppers). The neurologic problems of diabetes can produce atony of the gastrointestinal (GI) tract (diabetic gastroparesis). Metoclopramide is used to manage this complication.

Infections

Gangrene can occur in the peripheral extremities, especially the feet and legs. It stems from the deficiencies of diabetes: depressed immunity, less effective white blood cells, microvascular changes (less blood), and neuropathy (cannot feel the problem).

Healing

Slower healing must be taken into account so that precautions are taken during surgery. Related to this problem is the likelihood of infection, which exacerbates the healing problem.

Evaluation of the Dental Patient With Diabetes

Asking a patient "How well is your diabetes controlled?" does not often produce usable information. In actuality, the answer patients give to this question does not relate to the actual control of the patient's diabetes. Some questions for the patient that might provide useful information are "What numbers have you been getting for your blood sugar or glucose? What was your number this morning? When did you last test your blood glucose? What were the results?" No matter what the number is, one should not be judgmental.

Both the oral and systemic complications of diabetes are exacerbated by poor glucose control. There are two laboratory measurements useful to evaluate a patient's glucose control: plasma glucose and glycosylated hemoglobin levels (Table 18.3). Plasma glucose is a measure of the patient's glucose control at the time that the blood is sampled. It does not reflect the patient's overall glucose control. The second measurement is

TABLE 18.3 Test Results for Normal Patient and Patient With Diabetes

Result	Normal	Goal	Action Required
Fasting plasma glucose (mg/dL)	<110	80–120	140
Glycosylated hemoglobin (HbA$_{1c}$) (%)	<6	<7	>8

of glycosylated hemoglobin (HbA$_{1c}$). Because this value reflects glucose control over a 2- to 3-month period, it more accurately measures the patient's overall serum glucose control. Of course, a relationship exists between all the blood glucose levels and the glycosylated hemoglobin value.

Goals of Therapy

The primary goal of treating diabetes is to maintain hemoglobin A$_{1c}$ levels as close to normal as possible. An abundance of conclusive evidence from long-term, randomized clinical trials has proved that keeping hemoglobin A$_{1c}$ levels as close as possible to the normal range decreases the incidence and progression of the microvascular complications of type 2 diabetes. For every percentage point drop in hemoglobin A$_{1c}$, the risk of microvascular complications decreases by 40%. Early intervention also appears to contribute to a reduction in macrovascular complications. Intensive therapy with multiple insulin formulations for patients with diabetes demonstrated similar results. The American Diabetes Association Standards of Medical Care in Diabetes recommends a hemoglobin A$_{1c}$ level below 7% to reduce the incidence and progression of microvascular and macrovascular complications in patients with both type 1 and type 2 diabetes.

DRUGS USED TO MANAGE DIABETES

Insulins

Insulin (IN-su-lin) is usually administered by subcutaneous injection because its large molecular size prevents it from being absorbed from the GI tract. Insulin is the only treatment for type 1 diabetes and is often used in patients with type 2 diabetes. The major differences among the currently used types of insulin are onset and duration of action. The older preparations were prepared from beef or pork pancreases, but human insulin is now used exclusively. Human insulin is produced by two different processes: through recombinant deoxyribonucleic acid (rDNA) synthesis and by modifying porcine (pig) insulin. Both compounds are identical to the human insulin secreted by people. Recombinant DNA synthesis produces human insulin by gene splicing carried out by *Escherichia coli*. The processing of pork insulin involves transpeptidation of the pork insulin until it is the same as human insulin. Pig insulin has only two amino acids that are different from those in human insulin.

Table 18.4 lists insulin preparations, their peak effects, and their durations of action. The most common insulins used in clinical practice are human regular and neutral protein Hagedorn (NPH) (isophane insulin suspension) insulin. Lispro is made by exchanging two amino acids in the structure of human insulin. This change results in insulin with a faster onset of action. Lispro insulin is commonly used to obtain tighter control of blood glucose.

The most common adverse reaction associated with any insulin product is hypoglycemia. Besides hypoglycemia, inhaled insulin can cause shortness of breath, dry mouth, and cough.

The dental hygienist should be most concerned about a hypoglycemic reaction (Box 18.2) in the dental patient with diabetes who takes insulin. This reaction can be caused by an unintentional insulin overdose (insulin shock), failure to eat, or increased exercise or stress. Symptoms that can be explained by a greater release of epinephrine from the adrenals include sweating, weakness, nausea, and tachycardia. Symptoms caused by glucose deprivation of the brain include headache, blurred vision, mental confusion, incoherent speech, and, eventually, coma, convulsions, and death.

Another side effect associated with insulin is an allergic reaction, usually caused by noninsulin contaminants. Lipodystrophy at the injection site causes atrophy of the subcutaneous fatty tissue. The incidence of these reactions has decreased because the newer insulin preparations are purer and because patient education about changing the injection site has improved.

TABLE 18.4 Selected Insulin Preparations

Type	Preparation	Onset	Peak	Duration
Rapid-acting	Insulin aspart (NovoLog) Insulin lispro (Humalog) Insulin glulisine (Apidra)	10–30 min	30–3 hr	3–5 hr
	Insulin inhalation powder (Afrezz)	10–30 min	12–15 min	About 3 hr
Short-acting	Insulin regular (Novolin R, Humulin R)	30–60 min	2.5–5 hr	4–12 hr
Intermediate-acting	Insulin NPH (Humulin N, Novolin N)	1–2 hr	4–8 hr	16–24 + hr
Long-acting	Insulin detemir (Levemir) Insulin glargine (Lantus, Toujeo, Basaglar) Insulin degludec (Tresiba)	1 hr 1–2 hr	No peak No peak	20 hr 24 hr
Combination insulin	Novolin 70/30, Humulin 70/30 (insulin NPH 70% and regular insulin 30%)	30–60 min	2–12 hr	18–24 hr
	Novolog Mix 70/30 (Insulin aspart protamine suspension 70% and insulin aspart injection 30%)	10–20 min	1–4 hr	18–24 hr
	Humalog Mix 75/25 (insulin lispro protamine suspension 75% and insulin lispro injection 25%)	10–30 min	1–6.5 hr	14–24 hr
Long-acting insulin/GLP-1 Receptor Agonist	Insulin degludec/liraglutide (Xultophy)	1–9 hr	No peak	Based upon individual components
	Insulin glarine/lixisenatide (Soliqua)	1–4 hr	No peak	Based upon individual components

GLP-1, Glucagon-like peptide-1; *NPH,* neutral protein Hagedorn.

BOX 18.2 Management of the Dental Patient Taking Insulin or Oral Hypoglycemics

- Hypoglycemia—Question patient regarding last meal ingested.
- Infection more likely—Monitor closely and give antibiotics if needed (treat aggressively).
- Healing prolonged—Monitor patient after any surgical procedure.
- Drug interactions—Large doses of salicylates may produce hypoglycemia.
- Give patient an appointment in morning, after he or she has eaten breakfast and injected insulin or taken an oral hypoglycemic agent.
- Provide a quick glucose source for hypoglycemia (cake icing, orange juice).
- Check for oral complications related to diabetes.
- Ask patient what the results of his or her blood glucose monitoring have been (if checked).

BOX 18.3 Examples of Oral Antidiabetic Combination Therapies

Pioglitazone & metformin (Actoplus Met)
Glyburide & metformin (Glucovance)
Glipizide & metformin (Metaglip)
Sitagliptin & metformin (Janumet)
Linagliptin & metformin (Jentadueto)
Empagliflozin & metformin (Synjardy)
Saxagliptin & metformin (Kombiglyze)
Repaglinide & metformin (Prandimet)
Pioglitazone & glimepiride (Duetact)
Rosaglitazone & metformin (Avandamet)
Alogliptin & metformin (KAZANO)
Alogliptin & pioglitazone (OSENI)
Canagliflozin & metformin (Invokarnet)
Dapagliflozin & metformin (Xigduo)
Empagliflozin & linagliptin (Glyxambi)
Insulin degludec & liraglutide (Xultophy 100/3.6)
Insulin glargine & lixisenatide (Soliqua 100/33)

Oral Antidiabetic Agents

There are currently 10 groups of oral agents used to treat diabetes, referred to as *oral antidiabetics*. They are used only to treat type 2 diabetes. Each group works by a different mechanism and has a different adverse reaction profile. The oldest group of oral antidiabetic agents, the sulfonylureas, are also known as *oral hypoglycemic agents*. The other nine groups are more precisely referred to as the *antihyperglycemic agents* because they lower an elevated blood glucose value but do not produce hypoglycemia by themselves. Many of these groups can be used in combination with each other. Box 18.3 lists available combination products.

Fig. 18.3 summarizes the mechanisms of action of the various types of antidiabetic agents.

Sulfonylureas

For many years, the sulfonylureas were the only orally active agents used to manage diabetes. There are two major groups, first-generation and second-generation sulfonylureas. Their actions are similar, but the second-generation agents are more potent than the first-generation agents so their doses are smaller. Second-generation sulfonylureas

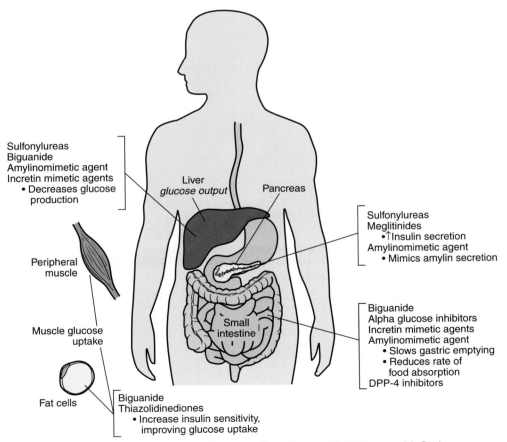

Fig. 18.3 Mechanisms of action of antidiabetic agents. (From Clayton BD, Willihnganz M. *Basic Pharmacology for Nurses*. 16th ed. St. Louis: Mosby, 2013.)

have replaced first-generation sulfonylureas because they are less toxic and easier to dose than first-generation sulfonylureas. Glyburide, one of the most commonly used oral sulfonylureas, is discussed as the prototype.

The mechanism of action of the sulfonylureas (Fig. 18.4) includes stimulation of the release of insulin from the β cells of the pancreas, reduction of glucose from the liver, reduction in serum glucagon levels, and increase in the sensitivity of the target tissues to insulin (probably secondary to reduced hyperglycemia).

Sulfonylureas are indicated for the treatment of patients with type 2 diabetes who cannot be treated with diet and exercise alone. Adverse reactions of the sulfonylureas include blood dyscrasias, GI disturbances, cutaneous reactions, and liver damage. Aspirin can interact with the sulfonylureas, producing a decrease in serum glucose levels. This is not clinically significant unless the diabetes is especially brittle. Table 18.5 lists the first- and second-generation sulfonylureas, their average daily doses, and their durations of action.

Biguanides

Metformin (met-FOR-min) (Glucophage) is a member of the biguanide group (Table 18.6). It lowers blood glucose but, used alone, does not produce hypoglycemia. Metformin increases hepatic and peripheral insulin sensitivity, resulting in decreased hepatic glucose production (by reducing gluconeogenesis). It also increases peripheral skeletal muscle uptake of glucose.

Metformin may be used alone, in combination with a sulfonylurea, or with insulin for management of type 2 diabetes.

Adverse reactions to metformin are primarily related to the GI tract (30%) and include anorexia, dyspepsia, flatulence, nausea, and vomiting. This agent can cause headache and interfere with vitamin B_{12} absorption. It accumulates in renal and hepatic impairment. Lactic acidosis, its most serious side effect, is rare. Factors predisposing to lactic acidosis include alcoholism, binge drinking, and renal or hepatic dysfunction. Metformin is contraindicated in patients with these conditions or patients who are fasting, because metformin predisposes a patient to lactic acidosis. Oral manifestations include a metallic taste. The dose ranges from 1500 to 2550 mg divided into two or three daily doses.

Meglitinides

Repaglinide (Prandin) and nateglinide (Starlix), although structurally different from the sulfonylureas, bind to adenosine triphosphate (ATP)-sensitive potassium channels on β cells and increase insulin release. These drugs stimulate the release of insulin from the pancreas. Insulin release is glucose-dependent and requires functioning β cells. These drugs are rapidly absorbed from the GI tract, resulting in peak plasma levels of insulin within 30 to 60 minutes and return to baseline before the next meal. They must be taken with meals. If a meal is missed, the drug should not be taken. Blood glucose control with these drugs is comparable to that with sulfonylureas. Repaglinide may be a

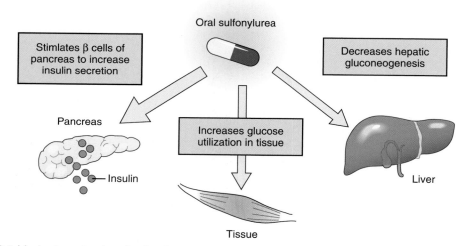

Fig. 18.4 Mechanism of action of sulfonylureas. (From McKenry L, Tessier E, Hogan MA. *Mosby's Pharmacology in Nursing.* 22nd ed. St. Louis: Mosby, 2006.)

TABLE 18.5   Antidiabetic Agents: Sulfonylureas

Drug	Total Daily Dose; How Divided (mg)	Onset (hr)	Peak (hr)	Duration (hr)
First Generation				
Chlorpropamide (Diabinese)	250–750 qd	1	2–4	24–72
Second Generation				
Glimepiride (Amaryl)	1–4 qd (max: 8 mg qd)	0.5–1.5	2–3	12–24
Glipizide (Glucotrol)	5–20 qd or bid (max: 40 mg qd)	1–1.5	1–3	10–24
Glipizide (Glucotrol-XL)	5–20 qd	—	6–12	24
Glyburide, nonmicronized (DiaBeta, Micronase)	2.5–20 qd or bid (max: 20 mg qd)	2–4	3.4–4.5	12–24
Glyburide, micronized (Glynase PresTab)	1.5–12 qd or bid (max: 12 mg qd)	1	2.3–3.5	24

bid, Twice a day; *qd,* daily.

TABLE 18.6 Oral Antidiabetic Agents

Drug	Dose	Mechanism	Adverse Reactions	Oral/DDI	Comments
Biguanides					
Metformin (Glucophage) Extended release (Glucophage XR, Glumetza)	1500–2550 mg in divided doses 500–2000 qd, usually with the evening meal	Decreases hepatic production of glucose, ↑ peripheral and hepatic insulin sensitivity and peripheral glucose uptake	Diarrhea, nausea, vomiting, lactic acidosis (serious)	Metallic taste Dl-EtOH acute/chronic, elevates lactate concentration, especially without food	Alone or in combination with a sulfonylurea
Fortamet	500–2500 qd, usually with the evening meal				
Meglitinides					
Nateglinide (Starlix)	60–120 mg tid before meals	Bind to ATP-sensitive potassium channels on β cells; ↑ insulin release	Hypoglycemia, weight gain	Clarithromycin, rifampin	Combined with metformin or a thiazolidinedione
Repaglinide (Prandin)	1–4 mg PO tid before meals	Bind to ATP-sensitive potassium channels on β cells; ↑ insulin release	Hypoglycemia, weight gain	Clarithromycin, rifampin	Same as above
Thiazolidinediones					
Pioglitazone (Actos)	15–45 mg qd	Improve the action of insulin in muscle and fat tissue	Weight gain, fluid retention, reports of hepatotoxicity	None reported	Alone or in combination with metformin, a sulfonylurea, or insulin
Rosiglitazone (Avandia)	4–8 mg qd or divided	Same as above	Same as above	None reported	Same as above
DPP-4 Inhibitors					
Alogliptin (Nesina)	25 mg PO qd	Inhibits DPP-4 enzyme responsible for the inactivation and degradation of the incretin hormones thereby lowering serum glucose concentration	Pancreatitis		
Linagliptin (Tradjenta)	5 mg PO qd	Inhibits DPP-4 enzyme responsible for the inactivation and degradation of the incretin hormones thereby lowering serum glucose concentration			
Saxagliptin (Onglyza)	2.5–5 mg PO qd	Inhibits DPP-4 enzyme responsible for the inactivation and degradation of the incretin hormones thereby lowering serum glucose concentrations			
Sitagliptin (Januvia)	100 mg PO qd	Inhibits DPP-4 enzyme responsible for the inactivation and degradation of the incretin hormones thereby lowering serum glucose concentration	Weight gain	None	
Alpha-glucosidase Inhibitors					
Acarbose (Precose)	25–100 mg tid with first bite of meal (max: 300 mg qd)	Delays digestion (breakdown) of ingested carbohydrate, so delays glucose absorption,* producing a smaller rise in BG	GI: abdominal pain, flatulence (77%), diarrhea, pain	None reported	Alone or in combination with a sulfonylurea
Miglitol (Glyset)	50–100 mg tid	Same as above	GI: flatulence (42%), diarrhea, abdominal pain, no hypoglycemia alone	No dental drug interactions	Same as above

continued

TABLE 18.6   Oral Antidiabetic Agents—Cont'd

Drug	Dose	Mechanism	Adverse Reactions	Oral/DDI	Comments
GLP-1 Receptor Agonist					
Albiglutide (Tanzeum)	30 or 50 mg SC once per week	Helps to stimulate insulin secretion in the presence of glucose, lowers serum glucagon levels, increases satiety	Nausea, vomiting, diarrhea, risk of hypoglycemia when used with a sulfonylurea	Avoid the use of anticholinergic drugs because of delayed gastric emptying. Semaglutide—Can cause retinopathy, complications can occur in persons that already have retinopathy	Approved for use as an alternative to starting insulin in patients with type II diabetes who have not achieved adequate control with metformin, a sulfonylurea, or both
Dulaglutide (Trulicity)	0.75 or 1.5 mg SC once per week				
Exenatide (Byetta)	5–10 μg SC bid before breakfast and dinner				
Exenatide, extended release (Bydureon BCise)	2 mg SC once per week				
Liraglutide	1.2 or 1.8 mg SC once per day				
Victoza	0.6 to 1.8 mg SC once per day				
Saxenda	0.6 to 3 mg SC once per day				
Lixisenatide (Adlyxin)	20 mcg SC once per day				
Semaglutide (Ozempic)	0.25 mg SC once weekly for 4 weeks, then increase to 0.5 mg SC once weekly, can be increased to 1 mg SC once weekly if needed after 4 weeks at 0.5 mg				
SGLT-2 Inhibitor					
Canagliflozin Invokana	100–300 mg before the first meal of the day	Reduces renal reabsorption of glucose and increases urinary glucose excretion	Female genital mycotic infections, urinary tract infection, increased urination, can increase the risk for hypoglycemia with insulin or insulin secretagogues, hypotension	None reported	Adjunct to diet and exercise to improve glycemic control in adults with type 2 diabetes mellitus
Dapagliflozin (Farxiga)	5–10 mg qd				
Empagliflozin (Jardiance)	10–25 mg qd				
Ertugliflozin (Steglatro)	5–15 mg qd				
Amylinomimetic Agent					
Pramlintide (Symlin)	60–120 μg SC tid before main meals	Modulation of gastric emptying, prevention of postprandial rise in plasma glucagon levels, increased satiety	Nausea, vomiting, diarrhea, risk of hypoglycemia when used with a sulfonylurea or insulin	Same as above	Type 1 diabetes: Adjunct therapy for patients who cannot achieve adequate glycemic control with mealtime insulin therapy. Type 1 diabetes: Adjunct therapy for patients who cannot achieve adequate glycemic control with mealtime insulin therapy with or without concurrent sulfonylurea and/or metformin therapy
Bile Acid Sequestrant					
Colesevelam (Welchol)	3.75 gm qd or divided bid	Bile-acid sequestrant used to lower LDL cholesterol. Reduces HbA$_{1C}$ when given with metformin, sulfonylureas, or insulin.	Constipation, nausea, dyspepsia	Interferes with the absorption of other oral drugs	Adjunct to diet and exercise in patients with type I diabetes

BG, Blood glucose; bid, twice a day; DDI, dental drug interactions; EtOH, alcohol; GI, gastrointestinal; LDL, low density lipoprotein; PO, by mouth; qd, every day; tid, three times a day.
*Does not produce hypoglycemia alone; reduces the insulinotropic and weight-increasing effects of sulfonylureas.

useful alternative to a sulfonylurea in patients with renal impairment or in patients who eat sporadically. Both drugs are approved by the US Food and Drug Administration (FDA) for combined use with metformin or a thiazolidinedione (see Table 18.6).

Hypoglycemia appears to occur less often with repaglinide and nateglinide than with sulfonylureas.

Thiazolidinediones

> Reduces insulin resistance.

Pioglitazone (Actos) and rosiglitazone (Avandia) are the only two thiazolidinediones available in the United States (see Table 18.6). These drugs increase the insulin sensitivity of adipose tissue, skeletal muscle, and the liver. They can take up to 6 to 14 weeks to achieve maximum effect. Both are FDA approved as monotherapy or in combination with metformin, a sulfonylurea, or insulin. Rosiglitazone is also approved as a third drug with both metformin and a sulfonylurea. Thiazolidinediones have an additive blood glucose-lowering effect when used in combination with metformin, sulfonylureas, or insulin.

Hepatotoxicity has rarely been reported with rosiglitazone and pioglitazone. The FDA recommends checking serum alanine aminotransferase (ALT) levels before starting therapy and periodically thereafter. These drugs should not be used in patients with underlying liver disease or with ALT levels greater than 2.5 times the upper limit of normal. Other common adverse effects are weight gain and fluid retention.

Dipeptidyl-Peptidase-4 Inhibitors

Sitagliptin (Januvia) is an oral dipeptidyl-peptidase-4 (DPP-4) inhibitor that has been approved for use in the treatment of type 2 diabetes as monotherapy or in combination with metformin, a sulfonylurea, or a thiazolidinedione, but not with insulin. It inhibits the DPP-4 enzyme that is responsible for the inactivation and degradation of the incretin hormones glucagon-like peptide-1 (GLP-1) and glucose-dependent insulinotropic polypeptide. These GI hormones potentiate insulin synthesis and release by pancreatic β cells and decrease glucagon production by pancreatic α cells, thereby lowering serum glucose concentration. Modest weight gain may occur with this drug. DPP-4 has a neutral or positive effect on cholesterol levels. The incidence of hypoglycemia increases when DDP-4 is used in combination with a sulfonylurea. Table 18.6 reviews all DPP-4 inhibitors.

α-Glucosidase Inhibitors

Acarbose (Precose) is an α-glucosidase inhibitor (see Table 18.6). Simply, it slows the breakdown of ingested carbohydrates so that postprandial hyperglycemia is reduced. It is a competitive, reversible inhibitor of GI tract enzymes: intestinal α-glucosidase and pancreatic α-amylase. The intestinal glucosidases hydrolyze saccharides to glucose or other monosaccharides that can be absorbed. The pancreatic amylase hydrolyzes complex starches to oligosaccharides in the intestine. Through inhibition of these enzymes, glucose availability and therefore absorption are delayed and postprandial hyperglycemia is lowered.

Acarbose can be used alone or with other agents, including insulin, sulfonylureas, and biguanides. Its major adverse effect is flatulence (77%), which is produced by bacteria acting on the undigested carbohydrates and producing gas. Other GI tract adverse reactions include diarrhea, abdominal pain, and distention. These effects are often tolerated if the dose of the drug is increased slowly and after the drug has been used for some time. Anemia and elevated transaminase values have been reported.

Glucagon-Like Peptide-1 Receptor Agonists

Exenatide (Byetta) is the first in a new class of drugs called *incretin mimetics* that has an amino acid sequence similar to human GLP-1 and in the presence of glucose acts to stimulate insulin secretion. Exenatide (Byetta) is indicated as an alternative to starting insulin in patients with type 2 diabetes in whom adequate control has not been achieved with metformin, a sulfonylurea, or both. This group of drugs lowers hemoglobin A1C levels by 1% to 1.5% and lowers weight by about 3 to 6 pounds. Studies have shown that these drugs also reduce cardiovascular risk. This drug is available as a subcutaneous injection. Liraglutide (Victoza) is a newer drug in this category. It is also available as a subcutaneous injection. It is indicated as adjunct therapy to diet and exercise in patients with type 2 diabetes (see Table 18.6). Table 18.6 reviews all the GLP-1 agonists.

The most commonly reported adverse effects for both drugs are nausea, vomiting, and diarrhea. There is the risk of acute pancreatitis in patients taking exenatide. There is also a risk for mild-to-moderate hypoglycemia with either drug when used in combination with a sulfonylurea. The dose of the sulfonylurea may have to be lowered if either of these drugs is started.

Sodium Glucose Transporter-2 Inhibitors

Canagliflozin (Invokana) is the first sodium-glucose cotransporter-2 (SGLT-2) inhibitor used to treat type 2 diabetes (see Table 18.6). This drug lowers plasma glucose levels by blocking the reabsorption of glucose in the kidneys, thereby causing excess glucose to be eliminated in the urine. This group of drugs lowers hemoglobin A1C levels by 0.7% and leads to about a 5-pound weight loss. Studies have shown that these drugs also reduce cardiovascular risk. They are indicated as adjunct treatment to diet and exercise in patients with type 2 diabetes. Canagliflozin use is contraindicated in patients with renal disease.

Adverse effects include genital yeast infections, urinary tract infections, increased urination, nausea, and constipation. Because of its effect on the kidneys, the drug should not be used in patients with severe renal impairment or end-stage renal disease or who are undergoing renal dialysis. Table 18.6 reviews all the SGLT-2 inhibitors.

Pramlintide

Pramlintide (Symlin) is an amylinomimetic agent that is responsible for modulation of gastric emptying, prevention of the postprandial rise in plasma glucagon, and satiety, which leads to decreased caloric intake and potential weight loss.

It is approved for type 1 diabetes as an adjunct treatment in patients who use mealtime insulin therapy and in whom desired glucose control has not been achieved despite optimal insulin therapy. It is also indicated for type 2 diabetes as an adjunct treatment in patients who use mealtime insulin therapy and in whom desired glucose control has not been achieved despite optimal insulin therapy with or without a concurrent sulfonylurea agent and/or metformin. Like exenatide, pramlintide is available as a subcutaneous injection and should be given immediately before major meals. The most commonly reported adverse effects are nausea, vomiting, and headache.

Bile Acid Sequestrants

Colesevelam (Welchol) is a bile-acid sequestrant that is used to lower low-density lipoprotein (LDL) cholesterol (see Table 18.6). Its mechanism of action in treating type 2 diabetes is unclear. It has been approved by the FDA as an adjunct to diet and exercise for the treatment of type 2 diabetes. Colesevelam can cause constipation, nausea, and dyspepsia, and can raise serum triglyceride concentrations. It also can interfere with the absorption of other oral drugs.

TREATMENT OF HYPOGLYCEMIA

One can prevent hypoglycemia by remembering that "An ounce of prevention is worth a pound of cure." It is easy to question patients about their insulin use and dietary intake. The treatment of hypoglycemia depends on whether a patient retains the swallowing reflex. In the early stages, when the patient is awake, the treatment consists of giving any of the following: fruit juice, cake icing, glucose gel, soluble carbohydrates. If the patient is unconscious and lacks a swallowing reflex, treatment consists of intravenous dextrose (50%). Intravenous glucose fluids and glucagon can be given. Because changes in behavior and in vital signs occur with hypoglycemia, dental teams should be able to use an oral product to manage their hypoglycemic patients. One of these items should be readily available in the dental office for emergencies.

Clinically, it is often difficult to distinguish an insulin reaction hypoglycemia (low glucose) from hyperglycemia (high glucose). It is useful to give a patient sugar for two reasons. First, the small amount of sugar used to treat hypoglycemia will do little additional harm if hyperglycemia is present. Second, the dental office is not equipped to treat hyperglycemia. Insulin should not be administered in a dental office emergency; the patient should be taken immediately to a hospital emergency room.

Glucagon

Glucagon is a polypeptide hormone produced by the β cells of the pancreas. Glucagon's role is as an antagonist to insulin. Higher levels of glucagon are present in the blood of patients with diabetes, even when normal blood glucose levels are maintained. Glucagon may be used parenterally for the emergency treatment of hypoglycemia, but glucose is usually preferred.

DENTAL HYGIENE CONSIDERATIONS

- Patients with diabetes are at an increased risk for caries and other oral disorders. Encourage such patients to maintain excellent home oral health care.
- Review the information in Box 18.2 and Table 18.2.

- Patients with diabetes are at an increased risk for infection and delayed wound healing. Antibiotics may be necessary.
- Hypoglycemia can occur if the patient has taken his or her medicine but has not eaten. Be prepared to treat hypoglycemia if it should occur.

ACADEMIC SKILLS ASSESMENT

1. What is diabetes and what are its signs and symptoms?
2. Compare and contrast type 1 and type 2 diabetes.
3. What are some of the dental concerns associated with diabetes, and how would the dental practitioner counsel a pediatric patient and their parent or caregiver with diabetes?
4. When during the day should a diabetic patient's dental appointment be scheduled, and why?
5. Describe the commonly used types of insulin and state their most common usage pattern.
6. What are the adverse reactions associated with insulin?
7. Name four oral hypoglycemic agents (from different groups) and state two side effects of this group of drugs.

CLINICAL CASE STUDY

Carter Edwards is a 10-year-old boy who has been coming to your practice for close to 6 years. He tries his best to brush his teeth at least twice a day (just like you told him). However, he is an active child and brushing his teeth is not always on his agenda. He does floss at least three times a week and he is quite proud of this. About 4 years ago, however, Carter was diagnosed with diabetes. Carter is fortunate in that his physician is working with him and his parents to maintain good control of his blood glucose levels without restricting his diet too much. Carter receives a combination of insulin that is administered as Novolin 70/30 (NPH/regular insulin). He is here today for his scheduled oral maintenance examination. He did remember to eat before coming in for his appointment, and he has brought some juice with him.

1. What is diabetes and what are its signs and symptoms?
2. Compare and contrast type 1 and type 2 diabetes.
3. What are some of the dental concerns associated with diabetes, and how would the dental hygienist counsel Carter and his parents about them?
4. When should Carter's dental appointment be scheduled and why?
5. What is the rationale for Carter bringing juice to his dental appointment?
6. Compare and contrast the different types of insulin.
7. What are the adverse reactions associated with insulin?
8. Should Carter be treated with an antibiotic after his dental procedure? Why or why not?

BIBLIOGRAPHY

ADVANCE Collaborative Group, et al. Intensive blood glucose control and vascular outcomes in patients with type 2 diabetes. N Engl J Med. 2008;358:2560.

American Diabetes Association. Diagnosis and classification of diabetes mellitus. Diabetes Care. 2010;33(Suppl 1):S62–S69.

American Diabetes Association. Standards of medical care for patients with diabetes mellitus. Diabetes Care. 2003;26(Suppl 1):S33–S54.

Drugs for type 2 diabetes: treatment guidelines. Med Lett Drugs Ther. 2008;50:47–54.

Eurich DT, Majumdar SR, McAlister FA, Tsuyuki RT, Johnson JA. Improved clinical outcomes associated with metformin in patients with diabetes and heart failure. Diabetes Care. 2005;28:2345.

In brief: a new indication for colesevelam (Welchol). Med Lett Drugs Ther. 2008;50:33.

Nathan DM, Buse JB, Davidson MB, et al. Management of hyperglycemia in type 2 diabetes: a consensus algorithm for the initiation and adjustment of therapy: a consensus statement from the American Diabetes Association and the European Association for the Study of Diabetes. Diabetologia. 2006;49:1711.

Diabetes Control and Complications Trial Research Group. The effect of intensive treatment of diabetes on the development and progression of long-term complications in insulin-dependent diabetes mellitus. N Engl J Med. 1993;329:977–986.

Drugs for the Treatment of Other Endocrine Disorders

http://evolve.elsevier.com/Haveles/pharmacology

LEARNING OBJECTIVES

1. Discuss pituitary hormones, the functions of the anterior and posterior pituitary glands and describe the negative feedback mechanism that takes place in endocrine glands.
2. Provide an overview of the thyroid hormones, conditions known as hypothyroidism and hyperthyroidism, and antithyroid drugs.
3. Summarize the major female and male sex hormones and describe several types of hormonal contraceptives.
4. Discuss other agents that affect sex hormone systems.

Hormones are secreted by endocrine glands and transported by the blood to target organs, where they are biologically active. Endocrine glands include the pituitary, thyroid, parathyroids, pancreas, adrenals, gonads, and placenta (Fig. 19.1). They help maintain homeostasis by regulating body functions and are controlled themselves by feedback systems. In most of these systems, the hormone released has a negative feedback effect on the secretion of the hormone-stimulating substance. Patients being treated in the dental office may be taking these hormones to treat various diseases.

Drugs that affect the endocrine system include the hormones secreted by the endocrine glands, synthetic hormone agonists and antagonists, and substances that influence the synthesis and secretion of hormones. The most important clinical application of these drugs is their use in replacement therapy, such as in the treatment of diabetes mellitus (DM) (insulin) (see Chapter 18) and hypothyroidism (levothyroxine). Additional applications include diagnostic procedures, contraception, and the treatment of glandular hyperfunction, cancer, and other systemic disorders.

PITUITARY HORMONES

> Pituitary: master gland.

The pituitary gland (hypophysis) is a small endocrine organ located at the base of the brain. It has been called the *master gland* because of its regulatory effect on other endocrine glands and organs of the body. It secretes peptide hormones that regulate the thyroid, adrenal, and sex glands; the kidney and uterus; and growth.

In addition to their regulatory effect, the pituitary hormones have a trophic effect that is necessary for the maintenance of many systems. For example, without the gonadotropins, the entire reproductive system fails; without growth hormone and thyrotropin, normal growth and development are impossible.

The secretion of pituitary hormones is influenced by peripheral endocrine glands via hormonal feedback mechanisms and by neurohumoral substances from the hypothalamus. When the hypothalamus releases specific hormone-releasing substances, the specific pituitary hormone is released.

Pituitary deficiency (hypopituitarism) can produce a loss of secondary sex characteristics, decreased metabolism, dwarfism, diabetes insipidus, hypothyroidism, Addison disease, loss of pigmentation, thinning and softening of the skin, decreased libido, and retarded dental development. Hypersecretion of pituitary hormones can produce sexual precocity, goiter, Cushing disease, acromegaly, and giantism. There are two parts to the pituitary gland: the anterior lobe (adenohypophysis) and the posterior lobe (neurohypophysis).

Anterior Pituitary

> Anterior pituitary: gland that stimulates hormones.

The anterior lobe of the pituitary gland secretes growth hormone, or somatotropin; luteinizing hormone (LH); follicle-stimulating hormone (FSH); thyroid-stimulating hormone (TSH), or thyrotropin; adrenocorticotropic hormone (ACTH), or corticotropin; and prolactin (Fig. 19.2). β-Lipotropin, secreted by the pituitary, is a precursor to β-endorphin (see Chapter 6).

Genetic engineering has been able to produce human growth hormone since 1987. Human growth hormone is used medically to treat children who lack it and illicitly by body builders and weight lifters to develop muscles. (Some say that in athletic events at which the contestant's urine is tested, e.g., the Olympics, growth hormone cannot be detected as easily as the androgenic steroids.)

Pharmaceutical gonadotropin-releasing hormone (GnRH) is a synthetic analog. One example, leuprolide, stimulates the pituitary function and is used to treat infertility. GnRH agonists are used to treat prostate cancer and endometriosis. The secretions from the anterior pituitary that stimulate other glands are used to test the function of the stimulated glands.

FSH-like products, which stimulate follicle growth, and LH-like products, which induce ovulation, are used in the treatment of infertility. Although LH itself is not available, human chorionic gonadotropin (hCG), which is almost identical in structure, can be used as an

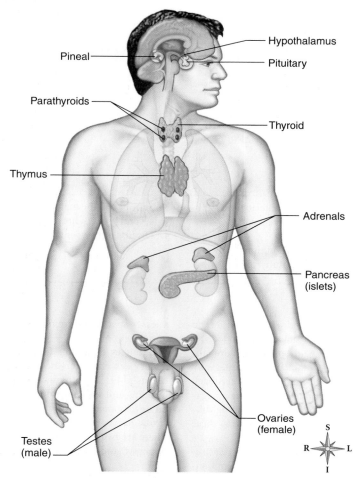

Fig. 19.1 Locations of the major endocrine glands. (From Patton KT, Thibodeau GA. *Anatomy and Physiology.* 8th ed. St. Louis: Mosby; 2013.)

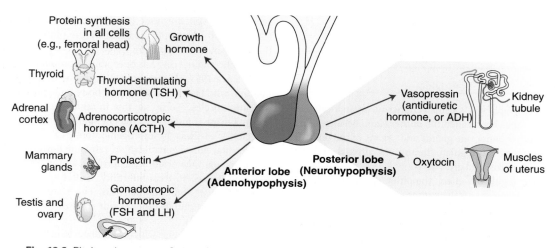

Fig. 19.2 Pituitary hormones. Some of the major organs of the anterior and posterior lobes and their principal target organs. *FSH,* Follicle-stimulating hormone; *LH,* luteinizing hormone. (From Lilley LL, Collins SR, Snyder JS. *Pharmacology and the Nursing Process.* 7th ed. St. Louis: Mosby; 2014.)

LH substitute for deficiency. Human menopausal gonadotropin (hMG) contains FSH and LH and is commercially available as menotropin (Pergonal). This preparation is used in infertility to stimulate development of ovarian follicles. When follicular maturation has occurred, the hMG is discontinued and hCG is given to induce ovulation.

Bromocriptine

Bromocriptine (broe-moe-KRIP-teen) (Parlodel), an ergot derivative, inhibits pituitary function. Although not a hormone, it is a dopamine agonist that suppresses prolactin levels. Bromocriptine is used to treat prolactin-secreting adenomas (**hyperprolactinemia**), acromegaly, and Parkinson disease.

Posterior Pituitary

> Posterior: vasopressin and oxytocin.

The posterior pituitary gland secretes two hormones: vasopressin (antidiuretic hormone [ADH]) and **oxytocin**. Vasopressin (vay-soe-PRES-in) (Pitressin) has vasopressor and ADH activity and is used for treatment of transient diabetes insipidus. Synthetic analogs of vasopressin (desmopressin [DDAVP, Stimate] and lypressin [Diapid]) are used for long-term treatment of pituitary diabetes insipidus and to treat certain clotting disorders (hemophilia A and **von Willebrand disease**). Available as nasal solutions, these two analogs have the same action as vasopressin but are longer acting.

Oxytocin (oks-i-TOE-sin) (Pitocin, Syntocinon), administered either by injection or intranasally, is used to induce labor, control postpartum hemorrhage, and induce postpartum lactation.

THYROID HORMONES

The thyroid gland secretes two iodine-containing thyroid hormones: **triiodothyronine** (T_3) and **tetraiodothyronine** (T_4, thyroxine). Calcitonin, another hormone secreted by the thyroid, regulates calcium metabolism. Thyroid hormones act on virtually every tissue and organ system of the body and are important for energy metabolism, growth, and development. Vulnerability to stress, altered drug response, and altered orofacial development are all possible manifestations of thyroid dysfunction. The head and neck examination performed by dental practitioners can identify some thyroid abnormalities. Swallowing can accentuate the thyroid to allow palpitation. The consistency of the gland varies with the abnormality.

Thyroid hormones are synthesized from iodine and tyrosine and stored as a complex protein until TSH stimulates their release. The actions of the thyroid hormones include those on growth and development, calorigenic effects, and metabolic effects. In frogs, thyroid hormone can transform a tadpole into a frog.

Iodine

> Iodine deficiency: goiter.

Normal function of the thyroid gland requires an adequate intake of **iodine** (approximately 50–125 mg/day). Without it, normal amounts of thyroid hormones cannot be made, TSH is secreted in excess, and the thyroid hypertrophies. This thyroid hypertrophy is called *simple goiter* or *nontoxic goiter*. Because iodine is not abundant in most foods, simple goiter is prevalent in some areas of the world. Marine life is the only common food that is naturally rich in iodine. Use of iodized salt (contains potassium iodide [KI]) has decreased the incidence of simple goiter in many countries. Iodine is currently used in

conjunction with an antithyroid drug in hyperthyroid patients being prepared for surgery.

Iodide in high concentrations suppresses the thyroid in a still poorly understood manner. It may produce gingival pain, excessive salivation, and sialadenitis as side effects.

Hypothyroidism

> ↓ Thyroid function in a child: cretinism.

In the small child, hypofunction of the thyroid is referred to as **cretinism**. In the adult, this condition is called **myxedema** or *simple hypothyroidism*. The main characteristics are mental and physical retardation. Such patients are usually drowsy, weak, and listless and exhibit an expressionless, puffy face with edematous tongue and lips. Oral findings in children usually include delayed tooth eruption, malocclusion, and increased tendency to development of periodontal disease. The teeth are usually poorly shaped and carious. The gingiva is either inflamed or pale and enlarged. The cretinous child is often uncooperative and difficult to motivate for plaque control. Diagnostic radiographs and routine dental prophylaxis in these patients may require special assistance.

Hypothyroid patients have difficulties withstanding stress and tend to be abnormally sensitive to all central nervous system (CNS) depressants, including the opioids and sedatives. If opioid analgesics are used, their doses should be reduced. Hypothyroid pregnant women tend to produce offspring with large teeth.

Thyroid hypofunction is rationally and effectively treated by oral administration of exogenous thyroid hormones. The most common thyroid hormone used for replacement therapy is levothyroxine (lee-voe-thye-ROX-een). Box 19.1 lists preparations used for thyroid **hormone replacement therapy**.

Hyperthyroidism

> ↑ Thyroid function: Graves, Plummer, or Hashimoto disease.

Diffuse toxic goiter (**Graves disease**) and toxic nodular goiter (Plummer disease) are the two forms of thyroid hyperfunction. Diffuse toxic goiter is characterized by a diffusely enlarged, highly vascular thyroid gland. It is common in young adults and is considered a disorder of the immune response. Toxic nodular goiter is characterized by nodules within the gland that spontaneously secrete excessive amounts of hormone while the rest of the glandular tissue is atrophied. It occurs primarily in older patients and usually arises from long-standing nontoxic goiter.

Hashimoto disease, a chronic inflammation of the thyroid associated with an autoimmune response, causes hypothyroidism. **Antithyroglobulin** antibody can be detected. It occurs in middle-aged women, often concomitantly with other autoimmune diseases.

BOX 19.1   Thyroid and Antithyroid Agents

Thyroid Replacements
Levothyroxine sodium ($L–T_4$) (Synthroid)
Liothyronine sodium ($L–T_3$) (Cytomel)
Liotrix ($T_3 + T_4$) (Euthroid, Thyrolar)
Thyroid (desiccated thyroid, Armour thyroid)

Antithyroid drugs
Propylthiouracil (PTU)
Methimazole (Tapazole)

Excessive levels of circulating thyroid hormone produce thyrotoxicosis. The adverse effects include excessive production of heat, increases in sympathetic activity, neuromuscular activity, and sensitivity to pain, ophthalmopathy, exophthalmos (protruding eyes), and anxiety. Oral manifestations are accelerated tooth eruption, marked loss of the alveolar process, diffuse demineralization of the jawbone, and rapidly progressing periodontal destruction.

The cardiovascular system is especially hyperactive because of a direct inotropic effect, increased peripheral oxygen consumption, and greater sensitivity to catecholamines. Epinephrine is relatively contraindicated in patients with hyperthyroidism. The potentiating effects of excess thyroid hormone and epinephrine on each other could result in cardiovascular problems such as angina, arrhythmias, and hypertension. β-Blockers, such as propranolol, are used to counteract the tachycardia.

In addition to their greater sensitivity to pain, hyperthyroid persons have an increased tolerance to CNS depressants. They may require higher than usual doses of sedatives, analgesics, and local anesthetics.

No treatment should be begun to any patient with a visible goiter, exophthalmos, or a history of taking antithyroid drugs until approval is obtained from the patient's physician. Medical management of the condition is important before any elective surgery is performed. A surgical procedure or an acute oral infection could precipitate a hyperthyroid crisis known as thyroid storm. Hydrocortisone should be administered intravenously, and cold towels should be placed on the patient. The use of epinephrine should be avoided in poorly treated or untreated thyrotoxic patients. The cardiac dose of epinephrine can be used carefully. Even in patients with controlled hyperthyroid disease who are considered to be euthyroid, stress should be kept at a minimum, preoperative sedation should be considered, and the dental team should be alert for signs of hypothyroidism or hyperthyroidism.

Treatment of hyperthyroidism usually includes one of the options highlighted in Box 19.2. The two most common treatments are radioactive iodine (^{131}I) and thyroidectomy. ^{131}I is usually the drug of choice for patients older than 21 years. It is taken internally and sequestered by the gland; localized destruction of thyroid tissue results. Side effects of radioactive iodine include a metallic-like taste that can last for several weeks and nausea which usually subsides within a few days. Radioactive iodine can also cause swollen salivary glands which can last for several weeks. It is a result of iodine being absorbed into the salivary gland. This can be treated by sucking on a tart candy (i.e., lemon drop) a day after treatment. This stimulates saliva flow. Thyroidectomy is the surgical approach to hyperthyroidism. Both radioactive iodine and thyroidectomy usually result in hypothyroidism because a dose that produces an inadequate effect would require repeating the procedure. If a patient has been adequately treated for hyperthyroidism with either radioactive iodine or thyroidectomy and is taking supplemental thyroid (as needed [prn]), then that patient may be treated like a euthyroid patient.

Antithyroid Agents

Antithyroid drugs, such as propylthiouracil (PTU) and methimazole (Tapazole), are used in patients who cannot tolerate surgery or treatment with radioactive iodine (iodine-131 [^{131}I]). These drugs interfere directly with the synthesis of thyroid hormones by inhibiting the iodination of tyrosine moieties and the coupling of the iodotyrosines. Adverse reactions associated with PTU include fever, skin rash, and leukopenia. The most serious adverse reaction is agranulocytosis, which can lead to poor wound healing, oral ulcers or necrotic lesions, and oral infections. Paresthesia of facial areas and loss of taste are also seen. Not only are antithyroid drugs used over prolonged periods to bring a hyperactive thyroid to the euthyroid state, they are also given before thyroidectomy to reduce the possibility of thyroid storm, a life-threatening acute form of thyrotoxicosis.

Propranolol, a β-blocker, is often given concomitantly with antithyroid agents to prevent tachycardia and tremors.

FEMALE SEX HORMONES

There are both male and female sex hormones, and most sex hormones occur in both sexes but in different proportions.

The two major female sex hormones are the estrogens (ES-troejenz) and progestins (proe-JES-tins) (e.g., progesterone [proe-JES-terone]). Products containing these hormones are listed in Table 19.1. Female sex hormones are secreted primarily by the ovaries but also

BOX 19.2   Hyperthyroidism Treatment Options

Drugs
Iodide
Antithyroid drugs
Radioactive iodine (iodine-131 [^{131}I])

Surgery
Partial thyroidectomy

TABLE 19.1   Selected Female Hormone Dose Forms and Doses

Hormones	Equivalent Dose
Estrogens	
Conjugated estrogens (Premarin)	0.3–1.25 mg/day
Esterified estrogens (Menest)	0.3–1.25 mg/day
Estradiol transdermal system (Estraderm)	0.05 mg or 0.1 mg patch applied twice weekly
Estradiol (Estrace)	0.5–2 mg/day (cyclic pattern)
Estropipate (Ogen)	0.75 mg/day
Progestins	
Medroxyprogesterone (Provera)	5 or 10 mg for 5–10 days for amenorrhea
Norethindrone (Micronor)	0.35 mg/day
Parenteral Progestins	
Medroxyprogesterone (Depo-Provera):intramuscular	150 mg q 3 months
Oral Estrogen-Progestin Combinations	
Estradiol/norgestimate (Prefest)	1 mg estradiol/day × 3 days, followed by 0.09 mg norgestimate—1 mg estradiol/day × 3 days, repeated
Estradiol/norethindrone acetate (Activella)	1 tablet (1 mg estradiol/0.5 mg norethindrone acetate) daily
Ethinyl estradiol/norethindrone acetate (Femhrt)	1 tablet (2.5 μg ethinyl estradiol/0.5 mg norethindrone acetate) daily
Conjugated Estrogen/Medroxyprogesterone	
Premphase	0.625 mg/day estrogen days 1–14, then 0.625 mg/day estrogen/5 mg medroxyprogesterone for days 15–28
Prempro	0.3 estrogen/1.5 mg medroxyprogesterone per day for 28 days in one tablet

by the testes and placenta. They are largely responsible for producing the female sex characteristics, developing the reproductive system, and preparing the reproductive system for conception.

Estrogen and progesterone levels vary daily. These changes depend on the pituitary gonadotropic hormones FSH and LH. The interrelationship among these hormones during the female sexual cycle is as follows: On day 1 of an average 28-day cycle, when the menstrual flow begins, the secretions of FSH and LH begin to increase. Their release is caused by a reduction in the blood levels of estrogen and progesterone, which normally inhibit it. In response to increased FSH, an ovarian egg matures, and the follicle in which it is contained grows and begins to produce and secrete estrogen. For reasons not entirely understood, on approximately day 12, the rate of secretion of FSH and LH increases markedly, to cause a rapid swelling of the follicle that culminates in ovulation on day 14.

Following ovulation, LH causes the secretory cells of the follicle to develop into a corpus luteum that secretes large quantities of estrogen and progesterone. This causes a feedback decrease in the secretion of both FSH and LH. On approximately day 26, the corpus luteum completely degenerates. The resultant reduction in estrogen and progesterone leads to menstruation and increased release of FSH and LH. The FSH initiates growth of new follicles to begin a new cycle. Fig. 19.3 illustrates the steps in the typical female menstrual cycle.

Estrogens

In addition to their role in the female sexual cycle, estrogens are largely responsible for the changes that take place at puberty in girls. They promote the growth and development of the vagina, uterus, fallopian tubes, breasts, and axillary and pubic hair. Estrogens increase both the deposition of fat in subcutaneous tissues and the retention of salt and water. They also cause increased osteoblastic activity and early fusion of the epiphyses.

The most potent endogenous estrogen is 17β-estradiol. The liver readily oxidizes it to estrone, which in turn can be hydrated to estriol. Because synthetic estrogens can be administered orally, they are used for therapy and contraception. Table 19.2 lists some estrogens and progestins used for birth control.

In addition to their presence in oral contraceptives, estrogens are used to treat menstrual disturbances (dysmenorrhea, dysfunctional uterine bleeding), osteoporosis, atrophic vaginitis, nondevelopment of the ovaries, hirsutism, cancer, and symptoms of menopause (particularly vasomotor instability [hot flashes and night sweats]). Estradiol transdermal system (Estraderm) is applied to the skin twice a week to treat the vasomotor symptoms of menopause.

The most common side effects of estrogen therapy are nausea and vomiting. With continued treatment, tolerance develops and these symptoms usually disappear. Other side effects are uterine bleeding, vaginal discharge, edema, thrombophlebitis, weight gain, and hypertension. Estrogen therapy may also promote endometrial carcinoma in postmenopausal women. This risk may be canceled out by administration of a progestin (e.g., medroxyprogesterone [Provera]) for the last 10 days of the cycle. Studies have found a slight increase in the risk for breast cancer in women using estrogen therapy as part of oral contraceptives or hormone replacement therapy. This risk returns to normal within 5 years of discontinuing hormone replacement therapy and 10 years after stopping oral contraceptives.

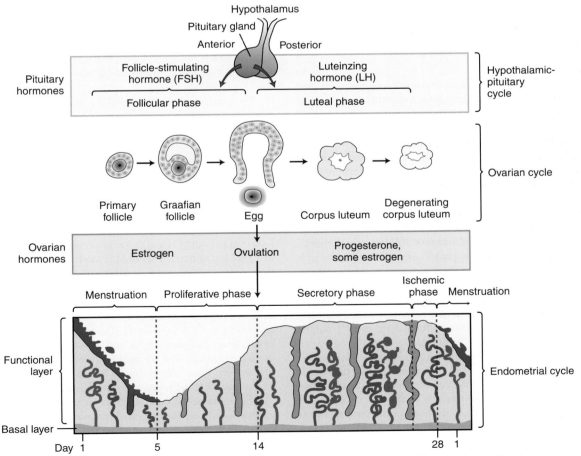

Fig. 19.3 The menstrual cycle. (From McKenry L, Tessier E, Hogan MA. *Mosby's Pharmacology in Nursing.* 22nd ed. St. Louis: Mosby; 2006.)

TABLE 19.2 Selected Hormonal Contraceptive Drugs

Trade Name(s)	Estrogen	Progestin
Norinyl 1/50, Necon 1/50	Mestranol	Norethindrone
Desogen, Ortho-Cept	Ethinyl estradiol	Desogestrel
Kelnor; Zovia 1/35, 1/50	Ethinyl estradiol	Ethynodiol
Levora, Nordette, Triphasil	Ethinyl estradiol	Levonorgestrel
Brevicon; Minasterin 24 Fe; Modicon; Ovcon-35, Ovcon-50; Tri-Norinyl; Norinyl 1 + 35; Ortho-Novum 1/35	Ethinyl estradiol	Norethindrone
Ortho-Cyclen, Ortho Tri-Cyclen	Ethinyl estradiol	Norgestimate
Lo/Ovral, Ogestrel	Ethinyl estradiol	Norgestrel
Newer Oral Contraceptives		
Seasonale (0.03 mg/0.15 mg)	Ethinyl estradiol	Levonorgestrel
Yaz, Ocella	Ethinyl estradiol	Drospirenone
NuvaRing (contraceptive vaginal ring)	Ethinyl estradiol	Etonogestrel

Effect on Oral Tissues

Estrogens influence the gingival tissues. For example, changes in sex hormone levels during the life of the female are related to the development of gingivitis at puberty (puberty gingivitis), during pregnancy (pregnancy gingivitis), and after menopause (chronic desquamative gingivitis). Conscientious plaque control helps minimize these conditions. The increase in gingival inflammation may occur even with a decrease in the amount of plaque. This may be a result of higher levels of prostaglandin E (PGE), estradiol, and progesterone in the saliva.

Other side effects of estrogens are discussed in the section on oral contraceptives.

Progestins

The corpus luteum is the primary source of progesterone during the normal female sexual cycle. Progesterone promotes secretory changes in the endometrium and prepares the uterus for implantation of the fertilized ovum. If implantation does not occur by the end of the menstrual cycle, progesterone secretion declines, and the onset of menstruation occurs. If implantation takes place, the developing trophoblast secretes chorionic gonadotropin, which sustains the corpus luteum, thus maintaining progesterone and estrogen levels and preventing menstruation. Other effects of progesterone include suppression of uterine contractility, proliferation of the acini of the mammary gland, and alteration of transplantation immunity to prevent immunologic rejection of the fetus.

Medroxyprogesterone (me-DROKS-ee-proe-JESS-ter-one) (Provera), a progestin, is used orally by postmenopausal women in conjunction with estrogens. It prevents the increase in the risk of uterine cancer that can occur with unopposed estrogen. Women who have had a hysterectomy do not need to take medroxyprogesterone with estrogens.

Progestins alone are used in a variety of dose forms. Parenteral medroxyprogesterone (Depo-Provera) is administered every 3 months as a contraceptive. Progestin-only "minipills," such as Micronor, (see Table 19.1) are used orally for contraception in patients in whom estrogens are contraindicated. They must be taken each day of the month and are slightly less effective than the combination oral contraceptive products. These agents are very infrequently used.

A progestational agent can be administered in the form of an intrauterine device (IUD) impregnated with a progestational agent (Progestasert) These implants can cause prolonged, spotty, and irregular menstrual bleeding or amenorrhea; however, many women find them convenient and problem free.

The primary use of the progestins is as one of the ingredients in almost all oral contraception combinations. The second most common use is in combination with estrogen for postmenopausal women. Other uses of the progestational agents include the treatment of endometriosis, dysmenorrhea, dysfunctional uterine bleeding, and premenstrual tension.

Hormonal Contraceptives

Oral contraceptives, the most common dose forms of hormonal contraceptives, consist of estrogens and progestins in various combinations. They are the most common birth control pills and are more than 99% effective (if patient compliance is perfect). Preparations that contain a progestin alone (the "minipill") are slightly less effective and produce less regular menstrual cycles but do not have most of the side effects of the estrogen contained in the combination preparation.

The compounds most commonly found in oral contraceptives are the estrogens, ethinyl estradiol and mestranol, and the progestins, norgestrel, norethindrone, and norethynodrel. The combination-type of oral contraceptive is taken for 21 days of each month. With a 28-day pack, the five or seven pills in the fourth week contain no active ingredient but remind the patient to take a pill every day. After the third week, the menstrual cycle occurs. At least three different formulations exist: the fixed combination, the biphasic (two different strengths of tablets), and the triphasic (three different types of tablets with varying amounts of the estrogenic and progestogenic component). The biphasic and triphasic agents are said to mimic the "natural" hormones more closely. No documented advantage has been demonstrated for any of the three combinations.

Seasonale (ethinyl estradiol/levonorgestrel) is the newest in combination oral contraceptive. Seasonale is different in that it is an extended-cycle oral contraceptive. Women take Seasonale for 3 months. Seasonale is taken once daily until the last tablet in the extended-cycle tablet dispenser is taken. The active tablets ($n = 84$) are pink, and the inactive tablets ($n = 7$) are white. The new dispenser is started the very next day. As a result, women bleed only once every 3 months (four menstrual periods a year).

The contraceptive vaginal ring is a new dose form that introduces hormonal contraception into the body. NuvaRing is the only combination dose form in this group. It contains ethinyl estradiol and etonogestrel. The patient inserts the ring for 3 weeks, during which the ring continuously releases low doses of ethinyl estradiol and etonogestrel. The ring is removed at the start of the fourth week, and the patient then experiences bleeding (her period). She inserts a new ring on day 29 of her cycle, after being ring-free for a week. Patients must insert the new ring on the same day each month.

Hormonal contraceptives interfere with fertility by inhibiting the release of FSH and LH and therefore preventing ovulation. Early follicular FSH and midcycle FSH and LH increases are not seen. In addition, these contraceptive agents interfere with impregnation by altering the endometrium and the secretions of the cervix.

The side effects associated with hormonal contraceptives include increased tendency to clot (produces thrombophlebitis and thromboembolism) and carcinogenicity. The minor side effects, nausea, dizziness, headache, weight gain, and breast discomfort, resemble those of early pregnancy and are mainly attributable to the estrogen in the preparation. These effects usually last only several weeks. Other side effects include blood pressure elevation and liver damage.

The hormones in contraceptives increase gingival fluid, stimulate gingivitis, and have been reported in some studies to be associated with gingival inflammation similar to but not as prominent as that seen in pregnancy. Other studies have not shown any significant differences between the plaque scores, gingival scores, or loss of attachment in users and nonusers of oral contraceptives. This discrepancy may be based partly on differences in dose among studies. In addition, this effect may not be evident in all users but may be of clinical significance only in women who are highly susceptible to oral soft tissue disorders. In any case, the dentist and dental hygienist should be aware that hormonal contraceptives do have the potential to cause or aggravate gingival inflammation.

Hormonal contraceptives are also associated with a significant increase in the frequency of dry socket after extractions. This risk can be minimized by performing extractions during days 23 through 28 of the patient's tablet cycle. For patients taking Seasonale, extractions should be limited to the end of the extended-cycle tablet dispenser, when the patient is taking the white tablets. Contraindications to the use of oral contraceptives include thromboembolic disorders, significant dysfunction of the liver, known or suspected carcinoma of the breast or other estrogen-dependent neoplasm, and undiagnosed genital bleeding.

The side effects of oral contraceptives are many and can impact on oral health care. Box 19.3 discusses the management of dental patients taking oral contraceptives.

In light of the increased use of antibiotics in periodontal therapy, the importance of the antibiotic-hormonal contraceptive interaction must be mentioned (Table 19.3). Certain antibiotics have been said to reduce the effectiveness of hormonal contraceptives. They are thought to do so indirectly by suppressing the intestinal flora and thus diminishing the availability of hydrolytic enzymes to regenerate the parent steroid molecule. Consequently, plasma concentrations of the steroid are said to be abnormally low, and the steroid is cleared more rapidly from the body than under normal circumstances. Some writers recommend that the patient use an additional method of contraception

until the end of her cycle. Other suggestions include the substitution of topical for systemic antibiotics, if possible, and the use of hormonal contraceptives with higher levels of the estrogen component. The latter suggestion should be acted on only by the patient's physician. Although all antibiotics have been implicated in this drug interaction, the incidence is indeed rare. If the patient is in the last week (week 3) or the placebo week (week 4) of her cycle, the chance of hormonal contraceptive therapy failure is even slimmer. In our litigation-conscious society, there should be documentation in the dental chart that the patient was informed about the rare chance of a drug interaction between oral contraceptives and antibiotics (see Table 19.3).

MALE SEX HORMONES

Androgens

The main androgen, testosterone, has both androgenic and anabolic effects. Because there is overlap between androgens and anabolic steroids, separating them is difficult. Table 19.4 lists the male hormones and their antagonists and the female hormone antagonists. Androgens are responsible for the development of secondary male sex characteristics. Their anabolic action results in an increase in tissue protein and nitrogen retention in the body. Other actions of the androgens include greater osteoblastic activity, epiphyseal closure (cannot grow any taller), and a rise in sebaceous gland activity (increased acne).

BOX 19.3 Management of the Dental Patient Taking Oral Contraceptives

Estrogen-Related
Increased incidence of postextraction dry socket
Chloasma or melasma; use caution with dental light
Increased susceptibility to *Candida* organisms; check oral cavity; check after antibiotic therapy
Decreased glucose tolerance; check blood glucose level if needed
Increased thromboembolic disease; for long appointments, give a break
Antibiotics said to reduce effectiveness of oral contraceptives; take precautions
These agents can increase blood pressure; check blood pressure
Gingivitis and periodontitis; check; more frequent recall appointments are needed if found
Patient may be taking calcium supplementation for bones; she should avoid the concomitant use of calcium supplements with tetracycline or doxycycline

Progestin-Related
Melasma or chloasma; use caution with dental light
Thrombophlebitis; check for symptoms; refer patient to physician if symptoms worsen

TABLE 19.3 Dental Drug Interactions With Oral Contraceptives

Drug	Interaction
Penicillin	Decreased effectiveness of OC
Tetracyclines	Decreased effectiveness of OC
Acetaminophen	Increased hepatotoxicity of acetaminophen
Benzodiazepines	Increased clearance of benzodiazepines

OC, Oral contraceptives.

TABLE 19.4 Examples of Male Hormones, Agonists, and Antagonists, and Female Hormone Antagonists

Drug Group	Examples	Indications
Male Reproductive System		
Androgens	Testosterone Methyltestosterone	Deficiency of testosterone, estrogen-dependent malignancy
Anabolic agents	Methandrostenolone (Dianabol) Nandrolone Stanozolol	Body builders use illicitly
Antiandrogens	Flutamide (Eulexin)	Advanced or metastatic prostate carcinoma in males
	Nilutamide (Nilandron) Bicalutamide (Casodex)	
	Finasteride (Propecia, Proscar)	Inhibits 5-α-reductase; baldness, benign prostatic hypertrophy
Female Reproductive System		
Gonadotropin-releasing hormone	Gonadorelin (Factrel)	Stimulates release of FSH and LH; used to test hypothalamus and pituitary gland function
Nonpituitary chorionic gonadotropin	Gonadotropin, chorionic (A.P.L., Pregnyl)	Infertility
Menotropins	Menotropins (Pergonal)	Infertility; like FSH and LH
Antiestrogens	Danazol (Danocrine) Tamoxifen (Nolvadex)	Endometriosis Early and advanced hormone receptor–positive breast cancer

Continued

TABLE 19.4   Examples of Male Hormones, Agonists, and Antagonists, and Female Hormone Antagonists — cont'd

Drug Group	Examples	Indications
	Fulvestrant (Faslodex)	Advanced breast cancer
	Toremifene (Fareston)	Advanced breast cancer
	Raloxifene (Evista)	Prevents breast cancer in selected high-risk populations of women
	Bazedoxifene/estrogen (DuaVee)	Treatment of menopause symptoms and postmenopausal osteoporosis
	Clomiphene (Clomid, Serophene)	Infertility; increases FSH and LH
	Nafarelin (Synarel)	Endometriosis; gonadotropin-releasing hormone agonist; stimulates LH and FSH
Aromatase inhibitors	Anastrozole (Arimidex)	Advanced breast cancer
	Exemestane (Aromasin)	Advanced breast cancer
	Letrozole (Femara)	Advanced breast cancer

FSH, Follicle-stimulating hormone; *LH,* luteinizing hormone.

Androgenic steroids are used medically in the treatment of breast cancer or for replacement therapy (Box 19.4). Puberty gingivitis can occur in relation to hormonal changes. Treatment includes subgingival debridement and oral hygiene instructions.

Androgens are used illicitly by body builders, weight lifters, and other athletes for gains in muscle mass. Many athletic events now test participants' urine for the presence of anabolic steroids. Because of their abuse, androgenic steroids are classified by the US government as Schedule III controlled substances (same category as Tylenol #3). The

BOX 19.4   Androgenic Anabolic Steroids

Androgenic/Anabolic Steroids and Their Indications

- Testosterone deficiency: androgen replacement therapy in the treatment of delayed male puberty, postpartum breast pain and engorgement, inoperable breast cancer, male hypogonadism
- Methyltestosterone (Metandren, Android) Therapy: hypogonadism, delayed puberty, impotence, and climacteric symptoms
- Use in women: palliative treatment of metastatic breast cancer; postpartum breast pain and/or engorgement
- Used with estrogen in postmenopausal women
- Nandrolone (Androlone, Deca-Durabolin): metastatic breast cancer, anemia of renal insufficiency
- Oxymetholone (Anadrol): anemias caused by antineoplastics
- Danazol (Danocrine): endometriosis, hereditary angioedema
- Stanozolol (Winstrol): hereditary angioedema
- Fluoxymesterone (Halotestin)
- Methandrostenolone (Dianabol)

Antiandrogens and Their Indications

- Bicalutamide (Casodex), nilutamide (Nilandron): in combination therapy with luteinizing hormone–releasing hormone (LH-RH) agonist analogs for prostatic carcinoma
- Finasteride (Proscar): benign prostatic hyperplasia (BPH), prostatic cancer; alopecia

side effects of androgenic steroids include nausea, cholestatic jaundice, hepatocellular neoplasms, increased serum cholesterol, habituation, and depression and excitation. In females, virilization (acne, hirsutism, deepening voice, clitoral enlargement, male-like baldness) occurs. Considering the potential for side effects, the illicit use of these agents is difficult to understand.

OTHER AGENTS THAT AFFECT SEX HORMONE SYSTEMS

Other agents that affect sex hormones may either act like the hormones or inhibit the action of the naturally occurring sex hormones (Tables 19.4 and 19.5). Hormones from the opposite sex are often used to manage prostate, breast, and uterine cancers because the cancers are often stimulated by the patients' own sex hormones. For example, prostate cancer is often stimulated by testosterone, so men with prostate cancer are given estrogens to inhibit the cancer's growth.

Clomiphene

Clomiphene (KLOE-mi-feen) (Clomid, Serophene) has the ability to induce ovulation in some anovulatory women. Clomiphene lowers the number of estrogenic receptors (antiestrogen) by binding to them. The hypothalamus and pituitary then falsely interpret the situation as low estrogen levels and increase their secretion of LH, FSH, and gonadotropins. Because clomiphene is a partial estrogen agonist, it acts as a competitive inhibitor of endogenous estrogen. Ovarian stimulation then results. Its side effects include hot flashes, eye problems, headaches, and constipation. Other side effects result from the symptoms of ovulation. Clomiphene is used to treat infertility in women and has been used experimentally for men also. The chance of multiple pregnancies increases about six times with clomiphene treatment. Female dental patients being treated with clomiphene should be considered to be pregnant unless known not to be.

Leuprolide

Leuprolide (loo-PROE-lide) (Lupron) is a GnRH analog used intramuscularly in the management of endometriosis and to treat infertility. It suppresses production of male and female steroids as a result of a decreased level of LH and FSH.

Tamoxifen

Tamoxifen (ta-MOKS-i-fen) (Nolvadex) is a competitive inhibitor of estradiol at the receptor. It is indicated in the treatment of

TABLE 19.5   Other Agents That Affect Sex Hormone Systems

Drug	Action	Indication
Clomiphene (Clomid, Serophene)	Estrogen antagonist and agonist	Infertility
Leuprolide injections (Lupron, ELIGARD)	Initially, increases LH and FSH; continuous administration results in reduced LH and FSH	Infertility
Tamoxifen (Nolvadex)	Estrogen agonist-antagonist Antiestrogen	Breast cancer
Toremifene (Fareston)	Estrogen agonist-antagonist	Breast cancer
Danazol (Danocrine)	Estrogen antagonist Antiestrogen	Endometriosis

FSH, Follicle-stimulating hormone; *LH,* luteinizing hormone.

early and advanced estrogen receptor-positive breast cancer in both premenopausal and postmenopausal women. It is also approved by the US Food and Drug Administration (FDA) for the prevention of breast cancer in women at high risk for the disease.

Danazol

Danazol (DA-na-zole) (Danocrine) possesses weak progestational and androgenic action. It suppresses ovarian function and prevents the LH and FSH midcycle surge. Its side effects include weight gain, unwanted hair growth all over the body, a decrease in breast size, acne, lowered voice, headache, and hot flashes. It is used to treat endometriosis and fibrocystic breast disease in women.

Aromatase Inhibitors

Aromatase inhibitors are the newest in a group of drugs to help treat breast cancer. These drugs reduce almost the entire amount of estrogen made in the bodies of postmenopausal women. One of the advantages of aromatase inhibitors is that because they cut off the estrogen supply, they tend to have fewer side effects than tamoxifen, especially stroke, blood clots, and uterine cancer. However, women taking aromatase inhibitors are at a higher risk for osteoporosis because they have less estrogen to protect bone density. These agents are indicated for the treatment of advanced breast cancer in postmenopausal women. Anastrozole is also FDA-approved for women with early-stage disease right after surgery and in premenopausal and postmenopausal

women with metastasis. Exemestane is FDA-approved for women with early-stage disease who have already received 2 to 3 years of tamoxifen therapy, and letrozole is FDA-approved in women with hormonally responsive tumors right after surgical treatment of the tumors and in women with early-stage disease who have completed 5 years of tamoxifen therapy.

Selective Estrogen Receptor Modulators

Selective estrogen receptor modulators (SERMs) are a class of drugs that act on the estrogen receptor. Raloxifene and bazedoxifine are the two SERM FDA-approved for us in the United States. Bazedoxifine comes in combination with conjugated estrogen. What makes this group of drugs different is that it has different effects on different tissues. These drugs are competitive partial agonists on the estrogen receptor resulting in either estrogenic or antiestrogenic effects depending on the specific tissue in question as well as the amount of the intrinsic activity of the drug. Raloxifene is used for the treatment of postmenopausal osteoporosis and the prevention of breast cancer in high-risk populations. Bazedoxifine/conjugated estrogen is used to treat menopause symptoms and postmenopausal osteoporosis. The more common side effects of raloxifene include hot flashes, headache, dizziness, increased sweating, nausea, and vomiting. The more common side effects of bazedoxifine include muscle spasms, diarrhea, dyspepsia, upper abdominal pain, oropharyngeal pain, dizziness, and neck pain.

■ DENTAL HYGIENE CONSIDERATIONS

- Regardless of the disease state being treated, the dental hygienist should obtain a detailed medication/health history from the patient.
- Patients who are hyperthyroid may require higher doses of local anesthetics or CNS depressant medications until they are considered euthyroid.
- Epinephrine use should be avoided in patients who are hyperthyroid.
- Patients who are hypothyroid may require lower doses of CNS depressant drugs. These patients should be counseled about the increased risk for sedation and the need to avoid driving or any activity that requires thought or concentration.
- The dental hygienist should review the importance of good home oral hygiene with all patients taking oral contraceptives because of the potential for gingivitis and gingival inflammation.

- Extractions should be performed on days 23 to 28 of a woman's oral contraceptive cycle to avoid dry socket.
- Always check the patient's blood pressure because oral contraceptives and hormone replacement therapy can elevate blood pressure.
- Have patients take a break and stretch their legs if the dental procedure is longer than 30 minutes. Oral contraceptives and hormone replacement therapy can cause thrombophlebitis.
- Review the information in Box 19.3 for all patients taking oral contraceptives.
- Patients taking anabolic steroids and male sex hormones can experience mood changes. Appointments may need to be rescheduled if patients become aggressive or psychotic.
- Anabolic steroids and male sex hormones can also elevate blood pressure, so always check the patient's blood pressure at each visit.

■ ACADEMIC SKILLS ASSESSMENT

1. What are the functions of the hypothalamus and the pituitary gland?
2. How are hormones released into the body, and what mechanism inhibits their release?
3. How do oral contraceptives work, and what are their clinical uses?
4. What are some of the adverse reactions associated with oral contraceptives?

5. What are the dental concerns associated with oral contraceptives?
6. Describe the dental effects of hypothyroidism and hyperthyroidism.
7. What is the difference between hypoglycemic agents and antihyperglycemic agents?
8. What are the legal and illegal uses of male sex hormones. Are there any dental concerns associated with them?

■ CLINICAL CASE STUDY

Melissa Williams, a 16-year-old girl, has been coming to your practice for 12 years. She has always been a healthy child with no medication history with the exception of ibuprofen or acetaminophen. According to her mom, she has been experiencing symptoms of anxiety, which was first attributed to "teenage hormones." This started happening right after her last appointment 6 months ago. Today, Mrs. Williams tells you that Melissa had a sports physical 3 weeks

ago with their family physician. It was during this appointment that the Williamses learned that Melissa's symptoms were more than "teenage hormones." Melissa presented with a resting heart rate of 100, symptoms of anxiety, and an inability to concentrate. The doctor immediately sent Melissa for thyroid hormone measurements. Melissa was then diagnosed with hyperthyroidism. Today, you note a cavity that needs to be filled.

1. What is hyperthyroidism, and what are its signs and symptoms?
2. What are some of the dental concerns associated with hyperthyroidism, and how would the dental hygienist counsel Melissa and her parents about them?
3. What are the drug interactions associated with hyperthyroidism?
4. What dose of an opioid analgesic be used in a patient just starting antithyroid therapy?

5. Can epinephrine be used in a patient newly diagnosed with hyperthyroidism? Why or why not?
6. What drugs are used to treat hyperthyroidism?
7. Do these drugs have any dental concerns?

Antineoplastic Drugs

LEARNING OBJECTIVES

1. Discuss antineoplastic agents and summarize their use, mechanisms of action, and classification.
2. Describe several adverse drug effects associated with antineoplastic agents.

3. Discuss the dental implications of patients planning to take or actively taking antineoplastic drugs.

Antineoplastic agents were designed to treat malignancies. A relatively new use of these agents is in the management of diseases with an inflammatory component such as psoriasis, rheumatoid arthritis, and systemic lupus erythematosus. Depending on their use, these agents are prescribed by oncologists, rheumatologists, or oral pathologists (for oral conditions related to systemic autoimmune diseases). For patients taking these agents to treat malignancies, the dental hygienist should be aware of the relationship between the timing of the treatments and the effects on the bone marrow. The dental hygienist should be familiar with the side effects of these agents, especially their oral manifestations.

Current research is elucidating many different mechanisms involved in the etiology of cancer, including genetics, viruses, deleted or damaged tumor-suppressor genes, specific oncogenes, and changes in both ribonucleic acid (RNA) and deoxyribonucleic acid (DNA) that affect the growth of cells. Many animal carcinogens have been identified, but proving carcinogenic potential in humans is much more difficult.

> Environmental carcinogens.

Many human carcinogens are environmental carcinogens, for example, polychlorinated biphenyls (PCBs) from transformers. Other known carcinogens are tobacco smoke, aflatoxins (produced by moldy peanuts), sunlight (increase in malignant melanoma and squamous cell carcinoma), radiation, chemicals, dioxin, and benzene. Most authorities believe that the herpes viruses and papillomaviruses have a potential for producing cancerous changes. Patients with a history of certain diseases, such as hepatitis, have a higher incidence of liver cancer than patients without such history.

Normal cells have a mechanism to turn off cell growth with certain signals. In cancer, however, a change in the cells occurs so that they continue to grow. With a lack of control (switch does not turn off), the abnormal neoplastic cells continue to grow. The cell-surface antigens appear similar to the normal fetal types, so the body does not mount an immune response. The tumor stem cells have chromosomal abnormalities, repetitions, and select subclones. With repeated cycles, the cells can migrate or metastasize to distant sites, thereby spreading the cancer. For example, cancer that begins in the breast may spread to the bone or liver.

USE OF ANTINEOPLASTIC AGENTS

Antineoplastic agents, sometimes called *cancer chemotherapeutic agents,* are used clinically to interfere with the neoplastic cells. The antineoplastic agents interfere with some function of the malignant cells. They suppress the growth of the cells and attempt to destroy and prevent the spread of malignant cells. (Fig. 20.1 illustrates the way in which cancer cells respond to chemotherapy.) These agents are used either alone or in combination with irradiation or surgery, depending on the type of malignancy being treated. Each type of malignancy may be sensitive to each of the three modalities: drugs, irradiation, or surgery.

> Drugs effective for some cancers.

For treatment of certain malignancies, for example, the leukemias, choriocarcinoma, multiple myeloma, and Burkitt lymphoma, drugs are considered the primary choice. Often, combinations of several antineoplastic agents, used in conjunction with surgery and/or irradiation, may affect a cure that each procedure alone could not. Certain cancers are relatively insensitive to antineoplastic agents. These cancers are treated with either irradiation and/or surgery. Box 20.1 lists malignancies and their likelihood of sensitivity to cancer chemotherapy agents.

The current philosophy for the use of the antineoplastic agents involves treating the initial stages of disease very aggressively. This approach promises more chance of controlling and curing the disease but also involves many severe side effects, including some that affect the oral cavity. The treatment of some cancers involves the removal of cells from the bone marrow before administration of the chemotherapy or irradiation. In the past, the dose administered would have been fatal. However, after treatment is complete, the cells taken from the bone marrow are returned to the patient's body, and they begin making the blood elements that are made in bone marrow. Gene therapy is being used, and many advances are continuing to be made. New research is attempting to use the body's immune system to fight the cancer cells.

MECHANISMS OF ACTION

The efficacy of antineoplastic agents is based primarily on their ability to interfere with the metabolism or reproductive cycle of the tumor

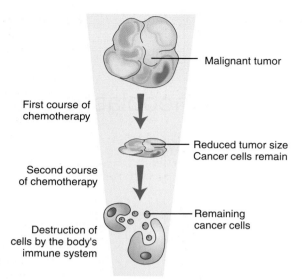

Fig. 20.1 Cancer cell response to chemotherapy. (From McKenry L, Tessier E, Hogan MA. *Mosby's Pharmacology for Nursing.* 22nd ed. St. Louis: Mosby, 2006.)

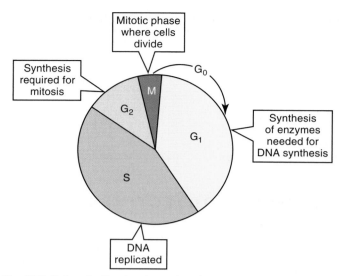

Fig. 20.2 Cell cycle. See text for explanation.

Cells in a resting stage that are not in a process of cell division are described as being in the G_0 stage. Cells enter the cycle from the G_0 stage. In some tumors, a large proportion of the cells may be at the G_0 level. These cells are difficult to reach and destroy.

> May be cell cycle–specific or cell cycle–nonspecific.

Most of the antineoplastic agents are labeled as being either cell cycle–specific (Table 20.1 and Fig. 20.3), indicating that they are effective only at specific phases of cellular growth, or cell cycle–nonspecific, indicating that they are effective at all levels of the cycle (effective both in the resting and the proliferating cells). For example, the alkylating agents interfere with the malignant cells during all phases of the reproductive cycle and the resting stage (G_0) and therefore are classified as cycle independent.

A major problem with treating neoplastic cells is that the cell growth is exponential. Before diagnosis is made, a large cell load must be present. If 10^{12} cells are present and 99.9% of the cells are killed, 10^9 cells would remain; if 99.9% of those cells were killed, 10^6 cells would still be present. Mixing several chemotherapeutic agents can increase the chance of killing more cells because they work by different mechanisms and have different adverse reactions.

Resistance to chemotherapy occurs by either of the following methods:

De novo resistance: The neoplasm was always resistant to the chemotherapeutic agents.

Acquired resistance: Resistance occurs through the natural selection of mutations.

BOX 20.1 Sensitivity of Neoplastic Diseases to Chemotherapy

High Sensitivity
Acute lymphocytic leukemia
Acute myelocytic leukemia
Breast cancer
Burkitt lymphoma
Ewing sarcoma
Hodgkin disease
Oat cell
Wilms' tumor

Moderate Sensitivity
Head and neck, squamous
Endometrial
Neuroblastoma
Prostate
Bladder
Chronic lymphocytic leukemia
Colorectal
Chronic myelocytic leukemia
Cervix
Kaposi sarcoma (acquired immunodeficiency syndrome [AIDS])
Ovary

Little Sensitivity
Liver
Pancreatic
Lung
Renal
Melanoma

cells, thereby destroying them. The reproductive cycle of a cell consists of the following four stages (Fig. 20.2):

G1 ("gap" 1), which is the postmitotic or pre-DNA synthesis phase
S, which is the period of DNA synthesis
G2 ("gap" 2), which is the premitotic or post-DNA synthesis phase
M, which is the period of mitosis

TABLE 20.1	Classification of Antineoplastic Drugs
Cell cycle—specific	Antimetabolites
	Bleomycin
	Vinca alkaloids
	Podophyllin
Cell cycle—nonspecific	Alkylating agents
	Antibiotics
	Cisplatin
	Nitrosoureas

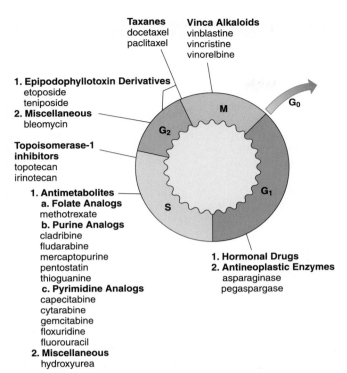

Taxanes
docetaxel
paclitaxel

Vinca Alkaloids
vinblastine
vincristine
vinorelbine

1. Epipodophyllotoxin Derivatives
etoposide
teniposide
2. Miscellaneous
bleomycin

Topoisomerase-1 inhibitors
topotecan
irinotecan

1. Antimetabolites
  a. Folate Analogs
  methotrexate
  b. Purine Analogs
  cladribine
  fludarabine
  mercaptopurine
  pentostatin
  thioguanine
  c. Pyrimidine Analogs
  capecitabine
  cytarabine
  gemcitabine
  floxuridine
  fluorouracil
2. Miscellaneous
  hydroxyurea

1. Hormonal Drugs
2. Antineoplastic Enzymes
  asparaginase
  pegaspargase

Fig. 20.3 General phases of the cell cycle in which the various cell-cycle–specific chemotherapeutic drugs have their greatest proportionate kills of cancer cells. See text for explanation of phases. (From Lilley LL, Harrington S, Snyder JS. *Pharmacology and the Nursing Process.* 7th ed. St. Louis: Mosby; 2014.)

CLASSIFICATION

> Groups divided by how they work.

The antineoplastic agents are divided into groups depending on their mechanisms and sites of action (Fig. 20.4). Box 20.2 lists some antineoplastic agents by classification.

The alkylating agents contain alkyl radicals that react with DNA in all cycles of the cell, preventing reproduction. The antimetabolites attack the cells in the S period of reproduction by interfering with purine or pyrimidine synthesis. These agents incorporate the drug into a compound or inhibit an enzyme from functioning and are more effective against rapidly proliferating neoplasms. Plant alkaloids are mitotic inhibitors that act by arresting cells in metaphase. Because of their low bone marrow toxicity, they are often used in combination with other agents

with more bone marrow toxicity. Antibiotics are cell cycle–nonspecific and are effective for solid tumors. Other agents include hormones, such as prednisone, which interrupt the cell cycle at the G stage. Steroids are used to suppress lymphocytes in leukemias and lymphomas and in combination therapies. Estrogens are used for palliation in inoperable breast cancer. Tamoxifen, an antiestrogenic substance, is used to manage breast cancer. It has also been shown to prevent breast cancer when used in women who have a high risk for breast cancer. Cisplatin, a heavy metal complex of platinum, is cell cycle–nonspecific. Hydroxyurea inhibits ribonucleoside diphosphate reductase, which would otherwise interfere with the conversion of ribonucleoside diphosphates to deoxyribonucleoside diphosphates. Procarbazine produces chromosomal breakage.

ADVERSE DRUG EFFECTS

Rapidly growing cells, such as neoplastic cells, are more susceptible to inhibition or destruction by antineoplastic agents. The most serious difficulty encountered in antineoplastic therapy stems from the lack of selectivity between tumor tissue and normal tissue. Some normal cells exhibit a faster reproduction cycle than slowly growing tumor cells. In an effort to eradicate a malignancy, certain normal cells are also destroyed, resulting in adverse effects. Because the cells of the gastrointestinal tract, bone marrow, and hair follicles are among the faster growing normal cells, the early side effects are associated with these tissues.

Table 20.2 lists the most common adverse reactions associated with some antineoplastic agents. These are the more common or agent-specific reactions associated with the drugs listed. The principal adverse effects are as follows.

Bone Marrow Suppression

The bone marrow is suppressed because it is a tissue that is rapidly turning over. Inhibition of the bone marrow results in **leukopenia** or agranulocytosis, thrombocytopenia, and anemia. The degree of resulting cytopenia depends on the drugs being used, the condition of the bone marrow at the time of administration, and other contributing factors. Symptoms of this adverse reaction may include susceptibility to infection, bleeding, and fatigue. The rise and fall in hematologic effects are related to location in the cycle of administering the drug.

Osteonecrosis

Bisphosphonates work by binding tightly to the bone directly beneath the bone cells known as osteoclasts which actively dissolve bone. The binding of bisphosphonates to the osteoclasts prevents the dissolving of the bone. This allows bone production to continue, bone density to improve and reduces the incidence of bone fractures. However, the drugs can cause osteonecrosis of the jaw bone. About 94% of all cases of osteonecrosis have been reported in cancer patients receiving intravenous bisphosphonates, in particular pamidronate and zoledronic acid,

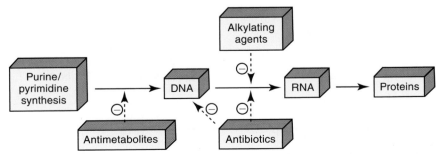

Fig. 20.4 Locations of action (−) of some antineoplastic agents. The synthesis of proteins can be interfered with at the purine/pyrimidine, DNA, or RNA level.

BOX 20.2   Antineoplastic Agents by Group

Alkylating Agents
Nitrogen Mustards
Mechlorethamine (Mustargen)
Cyclophosphamide (Leukeran)
Chlorambucil (Leukeran)
Melphalan (Alkeran)
Uramustine (Uracil mustard)
Ifosfamide (Ifex)
Bendamustine (TREANDA)

Nitrosoureas
Carmustine (BCNU, BiCNU)
Lomustine (CCNU, CeeNU)
Streptozocin (Zanosar)
Estramustine (Emcyt)

Alkylating-like
Busulfan (Myleran)
Pipobroman (Vercyte)
Thiotepa
Cisplatin (Platinol)
Carboplatin (Paraplatin)
Nedaplatin (Aqupla)
Oxaliplatin

Antimetabolites
Folic Acid Analog
Methotrexate (Amethopterin)

Pyrimidine Analog
Fluorouracil (5-FU)
Floxuridine (FUDR)
Cytosine arabinoside (ARA-C, Cytosar-U)
Azacytidine (Vidaza)

Purine Analog
Mercaptopurine (6-MP, Purinethol)
Thioguanine (6-TG)
Cladribine (Leustatin)
Fludarabine (Fludara)
Pentostatin (Nipent)

Miscellaneous Antineoplastics
Plant Alkaloids
Vinblastine (Velban)
Vincristine (Oncovin)

Antibiotics
Dactinomycin (actinomycin-D) (Cosmegen)
Doxorubicin (Adriamycin)
Bleomycin (Blenoxane)
Mitomycin-C (Mutamycin)
Plicamycin (mithramycin) (Mithracin)
Daunorubicin (Cerubidine)
Pirarubicin
Aclarubicin

Hormones
Adrenocorticosteroids (prednisone)
Androgen:
   Testolactone (Teslac)
   Fluoxymesterone (Halotestin)
Antiandrogen:
   Flutamide (Eulexin)
   Nilutamide (Nilandron)
   Bicalutamide (Casodex)
Estrogen:
   Diethylstilbestrol
   Ethinyl estradiol (Estinyl)
Antiestrogen:
   Tamoxifen (Nolvadex)
   Raloxifene (Evista)
   Fulvestrant (Faslodex)
   Toremifene (Fareston)
Aromatase inhibitors:
   Anastrozole (Arimidex)
   Exemestane (Aromasin)
   Letrozole (Femara)
Progestin:
   Medroxyprogesterone
   Megestrol (Megace)
Goserelin (Zoladex)
Leuprolide (Lupron)

Immune Modulators
Levamisole (Ergamisol)
Interferon alpha-n3 (Alferon N)
Interferon alpha-2b (Intron A)
Interferon alpha-2a (Roferon-A)

Podophyllotoxin Derivatives
Etoposide (VePesid)
Teniposide (Vumon)

Aminobisphosphonates
Alendronate (Fosamax)
Ibandronate (Boniva)
Pamidronate (Aredia)
Risedronate (Actonel)
Zoledronate (Zometa)

Other
l-Asparaginase (Elspar)
Hydroxyurea (Hydrea)
Procarbazine (Matulane)
Paclitaxel (Taxol)
Altretamine (Hexalen)
Trastuzumab (Herceptin)
Imatinib mesylate (Gleevec)

Selected Monoclonal Antibodies
Nivolumab (Opdivo)
Pembrolizumab (Keytruda)
Rituximab (Rituxan)

TABLE 20.2 Selected Adverse Reactions of Some Antineoplastic Agents

Drug	Uses/Adverse Reactions
Methotrexate (MTX)	GI, BMS
5-Fluorouracil	GI, BMS
Dactinomycin	GI, **BMS**
Doxorubicin	GI, BMS, **cardiotoxicity**
Mechlorethamine	Vomiting, BMS, bifunctional (binds at two sites)
Cyclophosphamide	BMS, **hemorrhagic cystitis** (Tx: ↑H_2O + mannitol + topical in bladder [mesna]), ↑antidiuretic hormone (Tx: furosemide)
Nitrosoureas	**Hematopoietic depression**, BMS
Vinblastine	**BMS**, peripheral neuropathy
Vincristine	**Peripheral neuropathy** (numbness and tingling of extremities; foot drop)
Tamoxifen	Increased bone and tumor pain
Cisplatin	Platin complex, persistent vomiting, **nephrotoxicity** (Tx: ↑H_2O + mannitol); electrolyte disturbances, ototoxicity, paresthesias, BMS
Procarbazine	**BMS**, psychic disturbances, procarbazine possesses monoamine oxidase inhibitor activity and has potential for severe drug and food interactions
Asparaginase	**Hypersensitivity**, bleeding/clotting abnormalities, liver toxicity, pancreatitis, seizures
Anastrozole	Nausea, vomiting, diarrhea, abdominal pain, constipation, Leukopenia
Exemestane	Nausea, vomiting, abdominal pain, dyspepsia, diarrhea, anorexia, constipation, increase in appetite, lymphocytopenia
Letrozole	Nausea, vomiting, constipation, anorexia, abdominal pain, dyspepsia, diarrhea
Trastuzumab	Nausea, vomiting, diarrhea, anorexia, neutropenia
Paclitaxel	Nausea, vomiting, diarrhea, mucositis, BMS

Boldface indicates that toxicity is usually dose limiting.
BMS, Bone marrow suppression; *GI*, gastrointestinal tract toxicity; *Tx*, treatment.

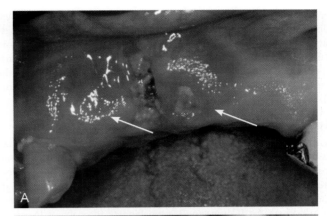

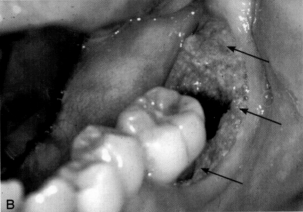

Fig. 20.5 (A) Lesions from bisphosphonate-related osteonecrosis of the jaw at extraction sites of upper central incisors (teeth #8 and #9). Note the inflamed gingivae at the site of infection; (B) Bisphosphonate-related osteonecrosis of the jaw at extraction site of tooth #18. Necrotic, non-healing exposed bone extends up the ramus and to the buccal aspect of tooth #19. (Reprinted with permission from Editorials Bisphosphonate-Related Osteonecrosis of the Jaw in Patients with Osteoporosis, June 15, 2012, Vol 85, No 12, American Family Physician Copyright © 2012 American Academy of Family Physicians, All Rights Reserved.)

for multiple myeloma or metastatic carcinoma. The incidence is much lower for patients taking oral bisphosphonates for osteoporosis with less than 1 case per 100,000 patients per year.

Bisphosphonate-related osteonecrosis of the jaw, now referred to as Medication-Related Osteonecrosis of the Jaw (MRONJ), is that area of the bone that has died and been exposed in the mouth for more than 8 weeks to a bisphosphonate. The name was changed from BRONJ to MRONJ to include antiresorptive (denosumab) and antiangiogenic therapies that are now associated with this condition. The exact mechanism of action of this problem is unknown. It has been reported that bisphosphonates can cause microdamage because they alter bone deposition and the repair process. Prolonged use may suppress bone turnover to the point that microdamage persists and accumulates, resulting in hypodynamic bone with decreased biomechanical competence. Symptoms of MRONJ include exposed bone, localized pain, gum tissue swelling and inflammation, and loosening of previously stable teeth (Fig. 20.5). Risk factors for MRONJ include the use and dose form of bisphosphonates, duration or number of treatments of bisphosphonates, and dental procedures. Most of the cases of osteonecrosis of the jaw occur after tooth extractions and other dental procedures that traumatize the jaw.

There are four stages and an at-risk category of MRONJ. The at-risk category includes all patients that have received oral or IV bisphosphonates and have no evidence of necrotic bone. Stage 0 includes patients that have no evidence of necrotic bone but have non-specific clinical findings and symptoms. During stage 1, the patient presents with exposed bone that shows no evidence of disease or inflammation of the soft tissue around it. During stage 2, the patient presents with a painful area of exposed bone that is accompanied by soft tissue or bone inflammation or infection. Lastly, stage 3 is associated with bone fracture. The patient can also present with an extensive amount of exposed bone and soft tissue inflammation and infection.

Unfortunately, MRONJ is very difficult to treat once it occurs. There are several means to help minimize or prevent it. Antibiotics and pain medications are indicated for patients with Stage 0 MRONJ. The dental hygienist should ask if the patient is taking or receiving a bisphosphonate drug. Maintenance oral health examinations and any other dental procedure should be performed before bisphosphonate therapy is started, or within 3 months after the start of therapy, if possible. Dental surgical procedures should be performed with use of minimal bone manipulation and supported with local and systemic antibiotic prophylaxis. In patients with osteonecrosis of the jaw, dead bone should be removed as necessary with minimal trauma to adjacent tissue. Chlorhexidine rinses, systemic antibiotics, and analgesics should be used if clinically necessary. Bisphosphonate-free "holidays" are not recommended before a dental procedure because these drugs stay in the bone for years. Bisphosphonate therapy is often stopped until the bone heals or the patient's cancer progresses to the point that resumption of bisphosphonate therapy is necessary.

Gastrointestinal Effects

Gastrointestinal problems are common because the gastrointestinal tract tissue is rapidly turning over. The sloughing of the gastrointestinal mucosa can produce many symptoms. Clinically, these disturbances are expressed as nausea, stomatitis, oral ulcerations, vomiting, and hemorrhagic diarrhea. Nausea and vomiting may be treated using phenothiazines (prochlorperazine [Compazine]), cannabinoids (dronabinol [Marinol] and nabilone [Cesamet]), metoclopramide (Reglan), and scopolamine.

Dermatologic Effects

Cutaneous reactions vary from mild erythema and maculopapular eruptions to exfoliative dermatitis and Stevens-Johnson syndrome. Alopecia is frequent, but the hair usually regrows when therapy is discontinued.

Hepatotoxicity

Liver problems occur principally with the antimetabolites (e.g., methotrexate [MTX]) but may occur with other agents as well.

Neurologic Effects

Neurotoxic effects, such as peripheral neuropathy, ileus, inappropriate antidiuretic hormone secretion, and convulsions, have been associated primarily with administration of vincristine or vinblastine.

Nephrotoxicity

> Allopurinol prevents hyperuricemia.

The renal tubular impairment that occurs secondary to hyperuricemia is caused by rapid cell destruction and the release of nucleotides. The treatment of leukemias and lymphomas often results in rapid tumor destruction with a consequent high uric acid level. Allopurinol (Zyloprim) is a xanthine oxidase inhibitor used in the management of gout. It blocks the production of uric acid by blocking its synthesis. Before the initiation of a regimen of antineoplastic agents that release purines and pyrimidines, allopurinol is administered to prevent hyperuricemia. Allopurinol can prolong the action and increase the toxicity of cyclophosphamide and the thiopurines (azathioprine and mercaptopurine).

Immunosuppression

Because the antineoplastic agents have an immunosuppressant effect, enhanced susceptibility to infection or a second malignancy may occur after treatment.

Germ Cells

Inhibition of spermatogenesis and oogenesis is frequent, at least temporarily. Mutations within the germ cells may occur. The menstrual cycle may also be inhibited. Recovery occurs after discontinuation of the drug.

Oral Effects

Adverse effects on the oral tissue are primarily those of discomfort, sensitivity of the teeth and gums, mucosal pain and ulceration, gingival hemorrhage, dryness, and impaired taste sensation. Table 20.3 reviews

TABLE 20.3   Oral Side Effects of Selected Cancer Chemotherapeutic Agents

Drug	Oral Side Effect(s)
Cyclophosphamide	Ulceration of the oral mucosa
Doxorubicin	Hyperpigmentation of the oral mucosa, especially the tongue, mucositis
Anastrozole	Dry mouth
Exemestane	None reported
Letrozole	Dry mouth, oral taste changes, metallic taste
Trastuzumab	Mouth sores
Paclitaxel	Mouth sores

some of the oral effects associated with common cancer chemotherapy drugs. Infection of the oral mucosa from leukopenia and bleeding (petechiae on the hard palate) from thrombocytopenia can occur. Appropriate maintenance of the oral cavity (Boxes 20.3 and 20.4) should be undertaken even before, and certainly during, antineoplastic therapy.

Patients taking antineoplastic agents may experience inflammation of the mouth, xerostomia, or glossitis. In these cases, the dental health care worker should not recommend any products containing alcohol (e.g., elixirs) because alcohol is drying to the oral mucosa.

Oral mucositis is one of the most common forms of oral side effects associated with chemotherapy. Oral mucositis refers to the mouth sores on the soft tissues of the tongue and inside the mouth (Fig. 20.6). Typical signs and symptoms include shiny, swollen tissue of the tongue and inside of the mouth, red, inflamed patches, sometimes white spots, and sticky mucus or blood in the mouth. The sores do not start right away. The patient usually begins to feel symptoms (soreness) within about 1 week of starting chemotherapy. The sores usually begin to heal about 1 week after chemotherapy is stopped, and the mouth sores and pain disappear by about 3 weeks after discontinuation of therapy.

The treatment of oral mucositis is based on the patient's symptoms. Treatment options include over-the-counter pain relievers such as ibuprofen and acetaminophen and opioid analgesics. Saline rinses and topical, alcohol-free mouth rinses with an anesthetic are used to treat the pain. The issue with these remedies is that they provide only short-term relief. Ice chips and cryotherapy appear to be effective in treating

BOX 20.3   Oral Care for Patients on Antineoplastic Therapy

Before Chemotherapy
- Eliminate and/or manage infection.
- Control periodontal disease (include prophylaxis).
- Provide oral hygiene instruction.

During Chemotherapy
- Schedule appointment just before next chemotherapy.
- Consult with oncologist before any procedure.
- Document hematologic status (laboratory test).
- Treat only if neutrophil count is >1000 cells/mm.
- Give endocarditis antibiotic prophylaxis if venous catheter present.
- Institute home oral hygiene program
- Culture lesions for infection.

After Chemotherapy
- Follow and maintain oral health.

BOX 20.4 Home Oral Hygiene

- Keep your mouth moist:
  - Drink lots of water.
  - Suck on ice chips.
  - Suck on tart, sugarless gum or candy.
  - Use a saliva substitute.
- Keep your mouth and gums clean:
  - Brush your teeth, gums, and tongue with a soft-bristle toothbrush properly twice a day,
  - Soften the bristles with warm water if your mouth hurts.
  - Use a fluoride toothpaste.
  - Use an alcohol-free mouth rinse.
  - Floss daily, avoiding those areas that are bleeding or sore.
  - Rinse several times a day with a solution of baking soda and salt, especially after emesis.
  - If you have dentures, do not wear dentures at night and make sure that dentures fit properly.
- For a sore mouth:
  - Choose foods that are easy to chew and swallow.
  - Take small bites of food and chew slowly; sip water as you chew.
  - Eat soft, moist foods.
  - Soften foods with gravy, sauces, broth, or yogurt if you have trouble swallowing.
- Avoid the following:
  - Sharp, crunchy foods
  - Sugary beverages
  - Caffeinated beverages
  - Alcoholic beverages
  - Tobacco products
- Call your health care provider if the pain persists.

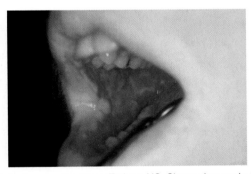

Fig. 20.6 Oral mucositis. (From Treister NS. Chemotherapy-induced oral mucositis; April 23, 2013, Medscape. http://emedicine.medscape.com/article/1079570-overview.)

the pain associated with mucositis. More often than not, patients are treated with 2% viscous lidocaine. Lidocaine is often mixed with equal parts of diphenhydramine and either Maalox or Kaopectate. Patients should also follow the recommendations in Box 20.4.

Some patients may experience hyposalivation or xerostomia as a result of chemotherapy, which will aggravate oral mucositis. Patients should be counseled to sip water to help alleviate the dry mouth. Artificial saliva can be used. The patient can also rinse with a mixture of 1/2 teaspoonful of baking soda and/or 1/4 teaspoonful of salt in 1 cup of warm water several times a day to alleviate dry mouth symptoms. This process will also clean and lubricate the oral tissue and provide a protective barrier for the oral mucosa. Chewing tart, sugarless gum

enhances salivary flow as necessary. Patients should also follow the recommendations in Box 20.4.

COMBINATIONS

Agents of widely differing mechanisms of action are often used together to inhibit the reproduction of neoplastic cells in all phases and to gain therapeutic advantage for the host. Mixtures of these agents may act synergistically, leading to enhanced cytotoxicity with fewer side effects. This is the rationale for combination drug therapy.

Antineoplastic drugs are used in lower doses to manage diseases associated with inflammation or autoimmune conditions and transplantation. Examples are azathioprine (Imuran), methotrexate (Rheumatrex), and cyclosporine (Sandimmune). Diseases that are treated with these agents include rheumatoid arthritis, systemic lupus erythematosus, pemphigus vulgaris, and psoriasis.

The doses of agents used to treat diseases with an autoimmune component are often lower than the doses used to treat cancer. Some drug interactions that would be important with higher doses are often safe in the lower doses used for autoimmune diseases. With organ transplantation, immunosuppressives are used to prevent rejection of the foreign tissue.

DENTAL IMPLICATIONS

Dental patients who are to take cancer chemotherapy agents should optimize their oral health before antineoplastic agents are begun (ideal conditions). However, often the dental health care worker has less than a day in which to attempt to attain this level of dental health.

> Timing important: agranulocytosis—infections; thrombocytopenia—bleeding.

If oral hygiene or dental procedures are to be performed in a patient who is taking antineoplastic agents, the procedures should be planned to coincide with the presence of the highest level of formed blood elements. That time would be either just before treatment or on the first few days of treatment (drug does not immediately depress the bone marrow maximally).

After a cycle of drugs is completed, the effect on the bone marrow increases to maximum. During this time, dental treatment should be avoided. The white blood cell count is often too low (agranulocytosis), and the chance of infection is great. The platelets may also be low (thrombocytopenia), and bleeding can occur. The optimal time to perform dental procedures will vary with each drug or drug regimen. Proper oral management of the patient receiving chemotherapy is described in Boxes 20.3 and 20.4. The general dental implications of the antineoplastic agents are listed in Box 20.5.

BOX 20.5 Management of the Dental Patient Taking Antineoplastic Agents

- Maximize oral hygiene before chemotherapy.
- Match hygiene instructions to patient's symptoms.
- There is potential for infection; watch for symptoms.
- Check neutrophil count before treatment.
- Check thrombocytes for adequate clotting.
- Rinse with soda/saline and/or chlorhexidine.

DENTAL HYGIENE CONSIDERATIONS

- Patients receiving cancer chemotherapeutic drugs must be treated carefully.
- The dental hygienist should meet with the patient prior to beginning chemotherapy in order to outline an optimal oral hygiene plan. The dental hygienist should then meet with the patient during and after chemotherapy in order to adjust the plan as necessary.
- The best defense for the patient is to receive maximum oral hygiene and health care prior to chemotherapy.
- Dental procedures should be avoided during chemotherapy because the patient is at high risk for infection as a result of low white blood cell counts.
- Platelet counts may also be low, putting the patient at increased risk for bleeding.
- Patients should schedule oral hygiene just prior to beginning a chemotherapeutic regimen because this is when they are feeling their best and white blood cell counts are highest.
- Review the information in Boxes 20.3, 20.4, and 20.5.

ACADEMIC SKILLS ASSESSMENT

1. Explain the adverse effects associated with the antineoplastic agents.
2. Explain oral care for patients receiving chemotherapy. Explain the importance of factors such as white blood cell count.
3. How would you counsel a patient on the appropriate oral hygiene program during chemotherapy?
4. Do GI adverse reactions affect oral hygiene? If so, how?

CLINICAL CASE STUDY

Mary Jones is a 55-year-old woman of mixed European descent who has been a patient of yours for close to 15 years. Her daughter came in for her scheduled appointment and told you that Mrs. Jones underwent surgery for breast cancer 2 months ago. Mrs. Jones has an appointment with you next month and plans on keeping it. Her daughter would like to know whether there is anything her mother can do to "get a running start" on preventing or minimizing the oral adverse reactions associated with chemotherapy that she is starting next week.

1. What are the oral adverse reactions associated with cancer chemotherapy agents?

2. What should Mrs. Jones do for oral care prior to chemotherapy and how can you help in the matter?
3. Counsel Mrs. Jones on the importance of good oral hygiene during chemotherapy.
4. What should Mrs. Jones do to maintain good oral hygiene during and after chemotherapy?
5. Why should you be concerned about bone marrow suppression in someone receiving chemotherapy that requires oral health care?
6. Do adverse reactions affect oral hygiene? If so, how?

PART IV

Special Situations

Chapter 21
Emergency Drugs, 234

Chapter 22
Pregnancy and Breastfeeding, 244

Chapter 23
Substance Use Disorders, 252

Chapter 24
Natural/Herbal Products and Dietary Supplements, 265

Chapter 25
Oral Conditions and Their Treatment, 271

Chapter 26
Hygiene-Related Oral Disorders, 282

Emergency Drugs

http://evolve.elsevier.com/Haveles/pharmacology

LEARNING OBJECTIVES

1. Summarize the general measures a dental professional should follow to train for an emergency, including:
   - Describe the necessary preparation for treatment in the event of an emergency.
   - List what can be done to help minimize the occurrence of an emergency in the dental office.
   - List the steps that should be followed if an emergency does occur in the dental office.
2. Name and describe several categories of emergencies and provide common examples within each category.
3. List the critical drugs to include in a dental office emergency kit and several examples of second- or third-level drugs that would be optional.
4. Name several pieces of equipment that would be included in the emergency kit.

A growing number of older patients who are taking multiple drugs seek dental treatment each year. The demographics of our population, the use of fluorides, and management of periodontal disease have increased the age of the average dental patient. Dental offices are administering more complicated drug regimens; dental appointments are taking longer; and dental patients are on average getting sicker. With these changes, the chance that an emergency will occur in the dental office continues to increase. Both the dentist and the dental hygienist should become familiar with the most common emergency situations, their management, and the drugs used to treat them. When an emergency occurs, the dentist and hygienist working together can increase the chance of producing the best outcome. Many emergency situations can be handled correctly with adequate knowledge. Lack of this knowledge during an emergency may cause panic in a dental office. If the dental office and its personnel are prepared for an emergency, handling one will be easier. Before patients who might be at risk for an emergency arrive for dental care, the treatment of a potential emergency related to their disease should be reviewed. It is the responsibility of each dental health care worker to make sure the members of the team can act in a coordinated manner.

GENERAL MEASURES

Steps Indicated

To prepare the dental office for an emergency, the following steps should be taken:

Training: All office personnel should be trained and retrained in emergency procedures before an emergency occurs. Each person should have an assigned role to perform during the emergency. It is up to the individual practice to determine each practitioner's role during an emergency. They should practice for an emergency at least once every 6 months. The following training should be obtained:
- Basic cardiac life support (cardiopulmonary resuscitation [CPR]) training (required)
- Advanced cardiac life support (ACLS) training (optional, unless performing conscious sedation)

Phone number availability: The telephone numbers of the closest physician, emergency room, and ambulance service (often 911) should be posted and should be programmed into the speed dial function of the office phone system.

Emergency kit: The items for the office's emergency kit, including the drugs and the devices (nondrug items) needed should be obtained and assembled. The kit should be checked every 3 months to make sure that the drugs are not out of date. Some companies offer this service by subscription.

To minimize the chances of an office emergency, the procedures listed in Box 21.1 should be performed for each new dental patient. It is easier to prevent than to treat a dental emergency. If an emergency occurs in the dental office, the steps listed in Box 21.2 should be taken.

Preparation for Treatment

C: Chest compression.
A: Airway.
B: Breathing.

BOX 21.1 Methods of Minimizing Emergencies in the Dental Office

- Observe the patient's stature, build, gait, coloring, age, facies, and respiration.
- Observe and record the amount of anxiety; use active listening to determine hidden nervousness.
- Take the patient's blood pressure and pulse rate, and perform any necessary laboratory examination.
- Take a complete patient history, including medication history, past dental and anesthetic experiences, restrictions on physical activity, diseases, and present condition.
- Request medical consultations as needed.
- Prescribe premedication, if appropriate, and avoid drug interactions.

BOX 21.2 Treatment of an Emergency in the Dental Office

- Recognize the abnormal occurrence.
- Make a proper diagnosis.
- Call 911 (or appropriate emergency number).
- Note the time.
- Position the patient properly.
- Maintain an airway.
- Administer oxygen.
- Monitor vital signs.
- Provide symptomatic treatment.
- Administer cardiopulmonary resuscitation (CPR) if there is no pulse.

Before any emergency treatment can be administered, investigation of the patient's signs and symptoms must lead to a diagnosis of the problem. The American Heart Association recommends that patients be assessed as follows: C-A-B: Chest compressions (C) are performed first, followed by assessment of the airway (A), and then breathing (B). Chest compressions, or hands-on-only CPR, are recommended first because people without training can administer them with guidance via telephone from an emergency medical technician or from a 911 dispatcher (Fig. 21.1). The use of drug therapy in these situations is only ancillary to the primary measures of maintaining adequate circulation and respiration. One should remember that drugs are not necessary for the proper management of most emergencies. Whenever there is doubt as to whether to give the drug, it should not be given.

In the dental office, each health care worker should be certified for both CPR and ACLS. The legal implications of lack of CPR training could be serious. ACLS training can be helpful in certain rural situations or if the technique of preoperative sedation or conscious sedation is used in the dental office.

The categories of emergencies are discussed in the next section. The most commonly used drugs and the choice of drugs and equipment for a dental office emergency kit are addressed.

CATEGORIES OF EMERGENCIES

This section discusses the signs, symptoms, and treatment of the most common emergency situations, dividing them into change in consciousness; respiratory, cardiovascular, and other emergencies; and drug-related emergencies.

Lost or Altered Consciousness

Many common dental emergencies involve either unconsciousness or altered consciousness. Dental office personnel should be ready to handle such an emergency and determine the best course of treatment.

Syncope

> Syncope most common.

The emergency most often encountered in the dental office is simple **syncope** (**fainting**, also known as **vasomotor collapse**) or transient unconsciousness. The skin takes on an ashen-gray color, and **diaphoresis** occurs. The release of excessive epinephrine results in a pooling of the blood in the peripheral muscles (β-adrenergic effect, vasodilation), a decrease in total peripheral resistance, and a sudden fall in blood pressure. A reflex tachycardia follows, but soon, decompensation results in severe bradycardia. These effects are brought about by anxiety, fear, or apprehension, all of which are common in a dental situation. Treatment involves placing the patient in the Trendelenburg position (head down) (Fig. 21.2), causing blood to rush to the head, which has the effect of giving the patient a transfusion of whole blood.

The most important component in the treatment of syncope is for the dental health care worker to exhibit confidence in action and voice. If the hygienist shows control over the situation, the patient will be less anxious and apprehensive and less likely to repeat the syncopal attack.

Spirits of ammonia can be administered by inhalation. The old practice of putting the head between the legs should be avoided because venous return is cut off by the slumped position.

Hypoglycemia

The most common cause of hypoglycemia is an excessive dose of insulin in a patient with diabetes. The medical history in this case is

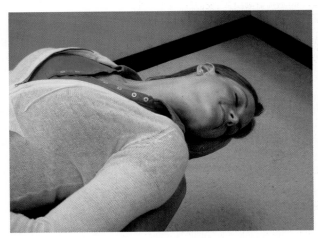

Fig. 21.2 For the Trendelenburg position, the individual should be tilted back even further in the dental chair so that the head is below the level of the heart and turned to one side. (From Malamed SF. *Medical Emergencies in the Dental Office.* 7th ed. St. Louis: Mosby; 2015.)

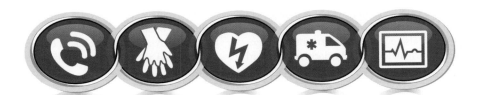

Fig. 21.1 Chain of survival. The links in this chain are as follows: Immediate recognition and activation, early cardiopulmonary resuscitation, rapid defibrillation, effective advanced life support and integrated post-cardiac arrest care. (Reprinted with permission Web-based Integrated 2010 & 2015 American Heart Association Guidelines for CPR & ECC Part 4: Systems of Care and Continuous Quality Improvement © 2015 American Heart Association, Inc.)

important, so the dental health care worker can determine the dose and type of insulin and food intake before the appointment. Often, patients inject their usual daily dose of insulin but fail to eat before coming to the dental office. If this is the case, then patients should be asked to eat before any dental procedures are begun. The time of the hypoglycemia can be estimated from knowledge of the peak effect of the particular insulins used (see Chapter 18).

The patient with hypoglycemia has a rapid pulse and decreased respiration and is very talkative. Hunger, dizziness, weakness, and occasionally tremor of the hands can occur. Diaphoresis, nausea, and mental confusion are other signs of hypoglycemia. If the signs of hypoglycemia are recognized before they become severe, the patient can be given a sugary drink or oral glucose. If the patient lapses into unconsciousness and has no swallowing reflex, dextrose must be given intravenously.

Diabetic Coma

Less common than hypoglycemia, the diabetic coma is caused by elevated blood sugar. The symptoms frequent urination, loss of appetite, nausea, vomiting, and thirst are seen. Acetone breath, hypercapnia, warm dry skin, rapid pulse, and a decrease in blood pressure can occur. Treatment is undertaken only in a hospital setting and involves administration of insulin after proper laboratory results are obtained (blood glucose).

Seizures

> Seizures/epilepsy.

Seizures are most commonly associated with epilepsy, especially the grand mal type (see Chapter 14), but they can also result from a toxic reaction to a local anesthetic agent. *Seizures* are abnormal movements of parts of the body in clonic and/or tonic contractions and relaxations. The patient may become unconscious. Generally, seizures are self-limiting, and treatment should consist of protecting the patient from self-harm, moving any sharp objects out of the patient's reach, and turning the patient's head to the side to prevent aspiration. In some situations, diazepam may be administered intravenously, but observation of the patient is often sufficient.

Respiratory Emergencies

Respiratory emergencies involve difficulty in breathing and exchange of oxygen. They include hyperventilation, asthma, anaphylactic shock, apnea, and acute airway obstruction.

Hyperventilation

Hyperventilation is one of the most common dental emergency situations. The increased respiratory rate is often brought on by emotional upset associated with dental treatment. Tachypnea, tachycardia, and paresthesia (tingling of the fingers and around the mouth) have been reported. Nausea, faintness, perspiration, acute anxiety, lightheadedness, and shortness of breath can also occur. The treatment is calm reassurance. Position the patient upright, loosen tight clothing, and work with the patient to control breathing.

Asthma

Normally, patients who have acute asthmatic attacks have a history of previous attacks and carry their own medication. The most common sign of an asthmatic attack is wheezing with prolonged expiration (squeak). The patient's own medication (multidose inhalers containing β_2-agonist such as albuterol) should be used first. The dose should be

repeated two times. If there is no response to these, hospitalization for administration of aminophylline (parenteral or oral) and parenteral corticosteroids and epinephrine should be considered. Oxygen should also be administered.

Anaphylactic Shock

> Anaphylaxis: emergency; 4 minutes to treat.

The most common cause of anaphylactic shock is an injection of penicillin, although anaphylactic reactions have also been caused by many other agents. Examples are eating peanuts and being exposed to latex rubber items. The reaction usually begins within 5 to 30 minutes after ingestion or administration of the antigen. Usually, a weak, rapid pulse and a profound decrease in blood pressure occur. There is dyspnea and severe bronchial constriction.

Parenteral epinephrine is the drug of choice for anaphylaxis and must be administered immediately in cases of severe anaphylactic shock. It may be given in the deltoid muscle or injected under the tongue. If bronchoconstriction is predominant, albuterol administered by inhalation or nebulization may suffice. After the life-threatening symptoms have been controlled, intravenous corticosteroids, intramuscular diphenhydramine, and aminophylline may also be used.

Acute Airway Obstruction

Acute airway obstruction or aspiration (e.g., aspiration of vomitus) is usually a result of a foreign body (e.g., a crown) in the pharynx or larynx; laryngospasm may be drug induced. Gasping for breath, coughing, gagging, acute anxiety, and cyanosis are signs and symptoms of acute airway obstruction. If the patient is conscious, position them in a semisupine position, clear their throat with a finger sweep or suction, and remove the object if possible. Perform the Heimlich maneuver (abdominal thrusts). If there is concern that they may swallow the object, place the patient in the Trendelenburg position on the right side and encouraging coughing. One should not allow the patient to sit up. Clearing the pharynx and pulling the tongue forward before performing the Heimlich maneuver (external subdiaphragmatic compression) should be attempted next. Finally, the Heimlich maneuver should be performed and repeated if needed (Fig. 21.3). Patients that are unconscious should be placed in the Trendelenburg position on the right side. Tilt the head so that the jaw is thrust forward. Sweep or suction the patient's mouth to remove the object. Perform CPR. A cricothyrotomy, or tracheotomy, which is hardly a dental office maneuver, is indicated if the object cannot be dislodged by the other methods. For aspiration, the use of suction, intubation, and ventilatory assistance is suggested. Steroids, antibiotics, and aminophylline are also administered. When drug-induced laryngospasm is present, succinylcholine, a neuromuscular blocking agent, and positive pressure oxygen are the agents of choice. The operator must have training and equipment to artificially breathe for the patient before succinylcholine is administered. The swallowing of objects during a dental procedure can best be prevented with the use of a rubber dam and throat packing, when appropriate.

Cardiovascular System Emergencies

Emergency situations involving the cardiovascular system include angina pectoris, myocardial infarction (MI), cardiac arrest, acute congestive heart failure, arrhythmias, and hypertensive crisis. The primary concern in any cardiovascular emergency is the maintenance of adequate circulation. Performing CPR, calling emergency personnel, and

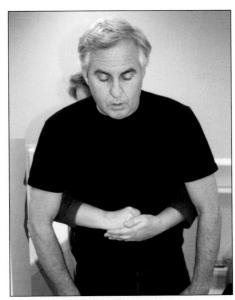

Fig. 21.3 The proper technique for an abdominal thrust (Heimlich maneuver). (From Bird DL, Robinson DS. *Modern Dental Assisting.* 11th ed. St. Louis: Saunders; 2015.)

administering oxygen are appropriate for most emergencies. The drugs used in cardiovascular emergencies are discussed individually later in the chapter.

Angina Pectoris

Without a previous history of angina, diagnosis of this condition can be difficult. It often begins as substernal chest pain that radiates across the chest, to the left arm, or to the mandible. It may also produce a feeling of heaviness in the chest. The pulse becomes rapid, and tachypnea can occur. An anginal attack can be brought on by stress from pain, trauma, or fear, especially in a dental situation.

Premedication with sublingual nitroglycerin before a stressful dental situation may prevent an acute anginal attack. Treatment of an acute anginal attack is with sublingual nitroglycerin (see Chapter 12). Opioids or diazepam is used in hospitalized patients. One should always check

to make sure that the patient has not taken a medication used to treat erectile dysfunction within 24 hours of receiving nitroglycerin. If the patient has taken a medication to treat erectile dysfunction, he should not receive nitroglycerin but should be treated in a hospital for the acute angina attack. Nitroglycerin also should not be used to prevent an acute attack if an erectile dysfunction drug has been used within 24 hours of the scheduled appointment. If the patient does not respond to sublingual nitroglycerin, a call should be placed for emergency services.

Acute Myocardial Infarction

An acute MI (heart attack) often begins as severe pain, pressure, or heaviness in the chest that radiates to other parts of the body. Sweating, nausea, and vomiting can occur. The pain is persistent and is unrelieved by rest or nitroglycerin (three doses). In this way, an MI can be differentiated from an anginal attack. An irregular rapid pulse, shortness of breath, diaphoresis, and indigestion can occur. Treatment includes administration of oxygen, an aspirin tablet, and an opioid analgesic agent and transfer to a hospital. The risk of death is greatest within the first 6 hours after an MI.

Hospitalized patients who have suffered an MI are given lidocaine for arrhythmias and vasopressor agents to maintain an adequate blood pressure. New drugs that can dissolve clots are administered soon after the event and may reverse the clot.

Cardiac Arrest

When cardiac arrest occurs, generally there is sudden circulatory and respiratory collapse. Without immediate therapy, cardiac arrest is fatal. Permanent brain damage occurs in 4 minutes. Pulse is absent, and blood pressure is unobtainable. After a few minutes, the patient becomes cyanotic and the pupils are fixed and dilated. The first and most important treatment is to immediately recognize that cardiac arrest is occurring and activate the emergency response system. Early CPR with an emphasis on chest compressions should be initiated, followed by rapid defibrillation, effective advanced life support measures, and integrated postcardiac arrest procedures (Figs. 21.4 and 21.5).

Today, every dental practice should have an automated external defibrillator (AED). An AED, if used within the first 5 minutes of cardiac arrest, can save up to 50% of those experiencing cardiac arrest. The American Dental Association (ADA) Council on Scientific Affairs recommends that dentists consider purchasing an AED for their dental

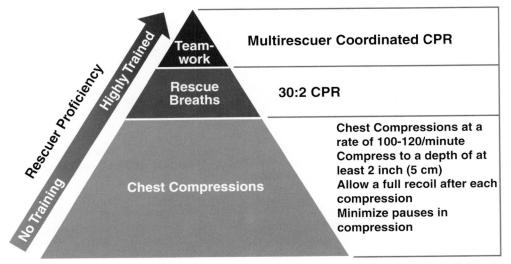

Fig. 21.4 Building blocks of cardiopulmonary resuscitation *(CPR)*. *(Circulation.* 2017;137:e7–e13. © American Heart Association, Inc.)

BLS Healthcare Provider
Adult Cardiac Arrest Algorithm—2015 Update

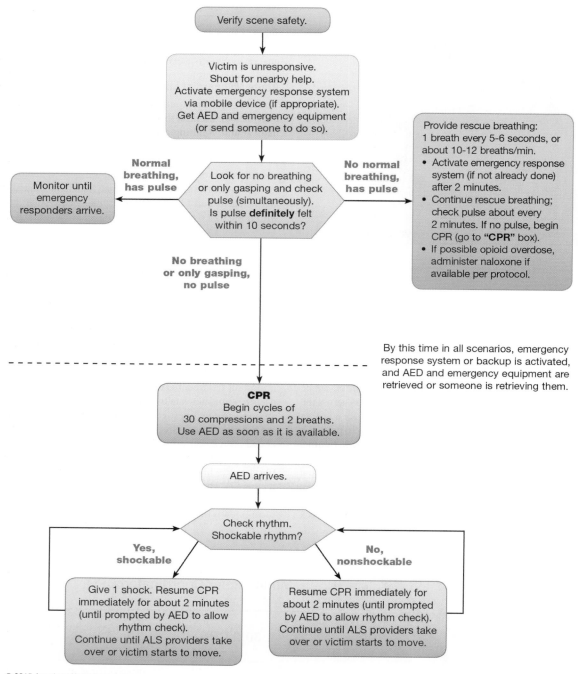

© 2015 American Heart Association

Fig. 21.5 Simplified adult basic life support (*BLS*) algorithm. (Reprinted with permission Web-based Integrated 2010 & 2015 American Heart Association Guidelines for CPR & ECC Part 5: Adult Basic Life Support and Cardiopulmonary Resuscitation Quality © 2015 American Heart Association, Inc.)

offices if emergency medical services personnel with defibrillation skills and equipment are not available within a reasonable time. Most states require AEDs for dental practices that use general anesthesia, and many require them for the use of conscious sedation. Several states require AEDs, or full-function defibrillators, for all dental practices.

Other medications used in a hospital setting for cardiac arrest include epinephrine for cardiac stimulation and lidocaine for arrhythmias. Parenteral opioid analgesics are given for the pain. Defibrillation is used to treat asystole.

Other Cardiovascular Emergencies

Arrhythmias, another cardiovascular emergency, depend on an electrocardiogram for diagnosis before treatment. A cerebrovascular accident (CVA, stroke), resulting in weakness on one side of the body or speech defects, is treated with oxygen administration and immediate hospitalization so "clot busters" can be administered. Hypertensive crisis is treated with antihypertensive agents given intravenously (see Chapter 12). Treatment of these cardiovascular emergencies is undertaken in a hospital setting.

Other Emergency Situations

Some emergency situations involve symptoms that do not fit into the other categories.

Extrapyramidal Reactions

The antipsychotic agents (see Chapter 15) can produce extrapyramidal reactions. Parkinson-like movements, such as uncoordinated tongue and muscular movements and grimacing, can occur. Prochlorperazine (Compazine), which is used for nausea and vomiting, can produce this type of reaction. Intravenous diphenhydramine (Benadryl) is the treatment of choice.

Acute Adrenocortical Insufficiency

Adrenal crisis usually occurs in a patient who is taking enough steroids to suppress the adrenal gland. When the patient is subjected to acute severe stress without increasing the steroid dose, his or her body may be unable to respond to the stress, and adrenal crisis occurs. Nausea, vomiting, abdominal pain, and confusion may result. Cardiovascular collapse and irreversible shock may lead to death. The treatment for adrenal crisis is parenteral hydrocortisone and oxygen by inhalation. After hospitalization, patients receive fluid replacement and vasopressor agents if symptoms dictate.

Thyroid Storm

Thyroid storm is a condition in which hyperthyroidism is out of control. Signs and symptoms include hyperpyrexia, increased sweating, hyperactivity, mental agitation, shaking, nervousness, and tachycardia. Heart failure and cardiovascular collapse may follow. Temperature is controlled by tepid baths and aspirin. β-Blockers are given to control the cardiovascular symptoms. Another agent that may be used is hydrocortisone. Aspirin should be avoided in these patients (displaces thyroxine [T_4] from binding sites). Sodium iodide and propylthiouracil are given to inhibit the action of the thyroid gland. Untreated severely hyperthyroid patients should not be given atropine or epinephrine because these agents may precipitate a thyroid storm.

Malignant Hyperthermia

Malignant hyperthermia is a genetically determined reaction that is triggered by inhalation general anesthetics or neuromuscular blocking agents such as succinylcholine. The most notable symptom is a rapidly rising temperature. Baths and aspirin are used to control the elevated temperature. Prompt treatment with dantrolene (Dantrium) can control acidosis and body temperature by reducing calcium released into the muscles during the contractile response. Before dantrolene, death was a common outcome. Fluid replacement, steroids, and sodium bicarbonate may be used.

Drug-Related Emergencies

Opioid Overdose

Opioids, administered in the dental office or prescribed by the dentist, can cause overdose symptoms. Respiration can be depressed, or respiratory arrest may occur. Illegitimate use of street drugs (e.g., heroin) or prescription opioids can produce overdose symptoms. The most common symptoms of overdose from the opioids are shallow and slow respiration and pinpoint pupils. The drug of choice for opioid overdose is naloxone (Narcan), an opioid antagonist (see Chapter 6). If the dental health practitioner suspects an opioid overdose, whether from illegal use of a prescription opioid, heroin, or one administered in the office, or the patient is alert enough to state this, then naloxone should be administered to the patient.

Reaction to Local Anesthetic Agents

Toxic reactions to local anesthetic agents usually result from excessive plasma levels of the anesthetic. Both central nervous system (CNS) stimulation, and CNS depression can occur. The stimulation is exhibited as excitement or convulsions (see Chapter 9). Following stimulation, depression can occur, with symptoms such as drowsiness, unconsciousness, or cardiac and respiratory arrest. The treatment of this toxic reaction is symptomatic. If convulsions are a predominant feature, diazepam can be administered. If hypotension is predominant, a pressor agent can be given. In the presence of reflex bradycardia, atropine may be administered. Usually, patients who have a toxic reaction to local anesthetics must be watched closely, but drug administration is rarely necessary. This reaction does not occur unless a dose of local anesthetic above the maximum dental dose has been given.

Epinephrine

Toxic reactions to epinephrine occur most often after the placement of the gingival retraction cord used before taking impressions. The symptoms range from nervousness to frank shaking and can also include tachycardia. Because epinephrine is quickly metabolized, the main treatment is to remove the cord and reassure the patient. Becoming panicky would cause the patient to release endogenous epinephrine, and the reaction would continue. Above all else, the dental health care worker must remain calm.

EMERGENCY KIT FOR THE DENTAL OFFICE

Although the choice of drugs for a dental office emergency kit depends on individual circumstances, experience, and personal preference, the dental health care worker should make sure there is an emergency kit in the dental office (Fig. 21.6). Table 21.1 lists some emergency drugs, their therapeutic uses, and their usual adult doses. Other drugs that may be included if the office personnel are trained in ACLS include the level 2 drugs atropine and lidocaine as well as calcium chloride.

Drugs

Table 21.1 lists the drugs that should be considered for inclusion in a simple emergency dental kit. These may vary, depending on the preference and experience of the practitioner. Some equipment and drugs that are not used by dental office personnel are kept in the emergency kit for use by a physician or for people with ACLS training in an emergency.

Obtaining small quantities of these medications may be difficult because they are often sold in packages of 12. A hospital pharmacy may be able to help the practitioner because the pharmacy buys in large quantities and could sell the few ampules that are needed for the dental office emergency kit. The security of the kit should be ensured by the use of a "breakable" lock that can be used to determine whether tampering has occurred. The kit should be stored in a prominent place in the dental office, but control of the drugs, such as the diazepam or an opioid, if included, should be ensured.

Level 1 (Critical) Drugs

Epinephrine. Epinephrine (Fig. 21.7) must be included in the dental office emergency kit for treatment of cardiac arrest, anaphylaxis, or acute asthmatic attack. It should not be used in treatment of shock because it can cause decreased venous return with increased ischemia and can precipitate ventricular fibrillation. The rationale for the use of epinephrine for cardiac arrest is β-stimulation of the myocardium. In the

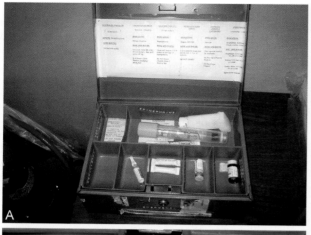

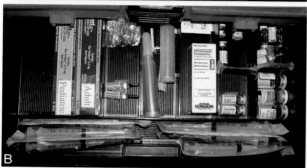

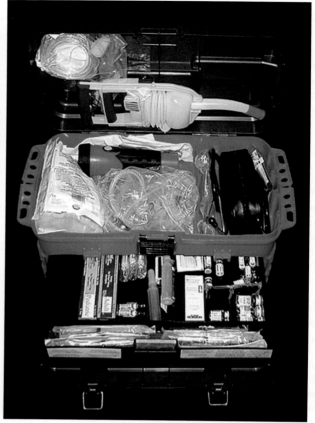

Fig. 21.6 Examples of self-made emergency kits. (A) Simple version with basic items only. (B) Large version with many drugs and additional equipment. (From Malamed SF. *Medical Emergencies in the Dental Office*. 7th ed. St. Louis: Mosby; 2015.)

TABLE 21.1 Emergency Drugs and Their Indications

Drug	Indication(s)
Level 1: Critical Drugs	
Albuterol (inhaled; Ventolin)	Treatment of an acute asthma attack
Diphenhydramine	Treatment of allergic reaction
Epinephrine	Treatment of cardiac arrest, anaphylaxis, or acute asthma attack
Glucose, oral (usually in the form of a tube of cake frosting)	Treatment of hypoglycemia
Nitroglycerin	Treatment of an acute anginal attack
Oxygen	Treatment of emergency situations in which the individual is having difficulty breathing
Level 2: Secondary Drugs	
Atropine	Increase in cardiac rate
β-Blockers	Reduction in blood pressure
Dextrose 50%	Intravenous solution for hypoglycemic patients who cannot swallow
Diazepam/alprazolam	Initial treatment of status epilepticus
Glucagon	Management of severe hypoglycemic reactions
Hydrocortisone	Treatment of allergic reactions, anaphylaxis, or adrenal crisis
Morphine	Opioid analgesic used to treat the pain associated with myocardial infarction
Spirits of ammonia	Treatment of syncope
Other Drugs	
Bretylium	Treatment of arrhythmias
Procainamide	Treatment of arrhythmias
Verapamil	Treatment of arrhythmias
Lidocaine	Treatment of arrhythmias
Flumazenil	Treatment of benzodiazepine overdose
Naloxone	Treatment of opioid overdose

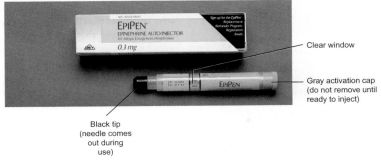

Fig. 21.7 The EpiPen is an emergency preloaded supply of epinephrine. (From Proctor DB, Adams, AP. *Kinn's the Medical Assistant: An Applied Learning Approach.* 12th ed. St. Louis: Saunders; 2014.)

treatment of severe anaphylaxis and acute asthmatic attacks, it acts as a physiologic antagonist to the massive release of mediators that occurs in these conditions. Without epinephrine, these chemicals cause bronchoconstriction and decreased oxygen exchange. Because epinephrine's cardiac effects are diminished in the presence of acidosis, adequate mechanical resuscitation and external cardiac massage accompany its administration. Epinephrine may be administered by intravenous or intracardiac routes (by trained personnel). Dental personnel may find injection into the frenulum under the tongue more convenient.

Diphenhydramine. Diphenhydramine (Benadryl), an antihistamine, is used in the treatment of some allergic reactions. Because antihistamines compete with histamine for tissue receptor sites, a rapid reversal of allergic symptoms cannot be expected. For this reason, epinephrine and diphenhydramine are used together in severe allergic reactions or anaphylaxis.

Oxygen. Oxygen is indicated in most emergencies, especially if respiratory difficulty is a problem. Patients with chronic obstructive pulmonary disease (COPD) should be given oxygen with caution because it may cause apnea. All dental office personnel should know the procedure for administering inhalation oxygen. All potential members of the dental team should review the procedure on a regular basis.

Nitroglycerin. Sublingual nitroglycerin tablets or nitroglycerin spray (see Chapter 12) should be kept in the dental office emergency kit to manage an acute anginal attack. The sublingual spray may be used in place of the tablets (Fig. 21.8).

Glucose. Oral glucose (Fig. 21.9), or any available liquid carbohydrate, is used to manage hypoglycemia in the conscious or semiconscious patient with diabetes. If the patient can swallow, then the oral route is preferable. A small amount may be placed in the buccal pouch, where it can be slowly swallowed. Tubes of glucose for this purpose are available, or cake frosting in tubes may be used.

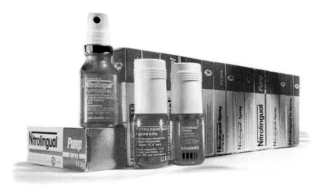

Fig. 21.8 Nitrolingual spray. (From Malamed SF. *Medical Emergencies in the Dental Office.* 7th ed. St. Louis: Mosby; 2015.)

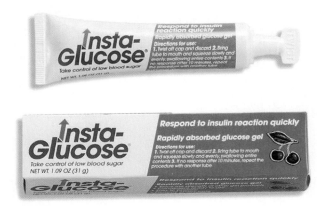

Fig. 21.9 Oral glucose gels. (Courtesy Valeant Pharmaceuticals, Montreal, Canada.)

Albuterol. Albuterol is a short-acting β_2-adrenergic agonist that produces bronchodilation. It is used in the management of an acute attack of asthma or respiratory distress accompanying anaphylaxis. If used properly, albuterol can produce bronchodilation in a few seconds.

Level 2 Drugs

Benzodiazepines. Diazepam (Valium) and midazolam (Versed) are the drugs of choice for the treatment of most seizures if a drug is needed. However, in the majority of cases, seizures are self-limiting and require only supportive care in the form of protecting the patient from physical harm and administering oxygen.

One cause of seizures in the dental office is a toxic reaction to a local anesthetic from an overdose or an idiosyncrasy (see Chapter 9). Antiepileptic drugs should be used conservatively because they may enhance the CNS depression from the local anesthetic.

Aromatic ammonia spirits. Containers of aromatic ammonia spirits, designed to be crushed, can be used to treat syncope (Fig. 21.10). Aromatic ammonia acts by irritating the membranes of the upper respiratory tract, resulting in stimulation of respiration and blood pressure. A dental office should have one (unexpired) container near each dental chair for easy access.

Morphine. Morphine and meperidine are opioid analgesics administered to a patient who has suffered an acute MI. These agents relieve pain and allay apprehension. They are used for cases of pulmonary embolism and angina for the same reasons.

Hydrocortisone. A corticosteroid used for allergic reactions, anaphylaxis, and adrenal crisis is hydrocortisone sodium. Even given intravenously, hydrocortisone has a slow onset of action. Epinephrine is still the drug of choice for anaphylaxis and serious allergic reactions

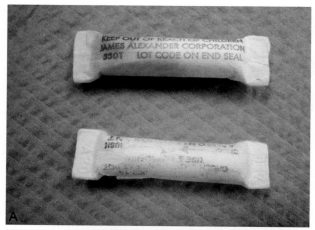

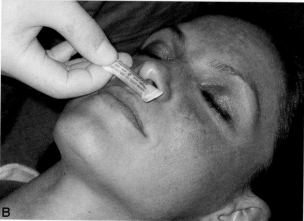

Fig. 21.10 (A) Aromatic ammonia Vaporole, used *(top)* and unused *(bottom.)* (B) Vaporole crushed and being held under the patient's nose. (From Malamed SF. *Medical Emergencies in the Dental Office.* 7th ed. St. Louis: Mosby; 2015.)

because it acts immediately as a physiologic antagonist. The use of epinephrine should be followed by administration of hydrocortisone, which may be given intramuscularly or intravenously.

Dextrose. Intravenous dextrose is used to manage hypoglycemic episodes when a patient with diabetes is unconscious and cannot swallow. Hypoglycemia occurs most commonly when the patient's insulin, exercise, and food intake are out of balance. In the dental office, all patients with hypoglycemia should be recognized before unconsciousness occurs.

Glucagon. Glucagon is used for the management of severe hypoglycemic reactions. It can be given intramuscularly, intravenously, or subcutaneously. If the patient does not show a response to the subcutaneous or IM glucagon, intravenous glucose should be considered.

Atropine. Atropine is used as a preoperative antisialagogue and to increase the cardiac rate when it has been slowed by vagal stimulation. It is administered intramuscularly, intravenously, and subcutaneously.

β-Blockers. β-Blockers, such as esmolol and labetalol, are administered by intravenous infusion to manage intraoperative or postoperative tachycardia or hypertension.

Other Drugs

Naloxone. Naloxone (Narcan), a pure opioid antagonist, is the drug of choice for opioid-induced apnea or overdose. There are four different kits that can used. Its use is extremely safe, but more than one administration may be needed because of its short duration of action. The first kit is an intravenous dose form. The initial dose is 0.4 mg (1 mL)

intravenously, but it can also be given subcutaneously or intramuscularly. The onset of action is approximately 2 minutes by the intravenous route. This dose should be repeated several times in case the dose of opioid was high (sometimes a combination of self-administered plus dentist-administered opioids).

The second is an autoinjector with audio prompts that administers a 0.4 mg dose intramuscularly via a retractable needle. The third dose form is given via a single-step nasal spray that administers a dose concentration of 4 mg/0.1 mL into one nostril the fourth naloxone product is a multistep nasal spray assembled by combining a prefilled Luer-Lok syringe with a nasal atomizer, that administers a dose concentration of 2 mg/2 mL, where 1 mL is administered to each nostril. As with the intravenous dose forms, additional doses may be necessary. A potential problem with giving naloxone is precipitating withdrawal in an addict (see Chapter 6). Naloxone is effective in reversing the respiratory depression caused by opioid drugs; if no response occurs, other causes of respiratory depression must be considered. Naloxone should be in the dental practice emergency kit if its patients are given opioids preoperatively or intraoperatively and because of the high numbers of patients abusing opioids. The dental practitioner may need to administer naloxone if a patient is experiencing overdose symptoms as a result of self-administration of an opioid.

Flumazenil. Flumazenil (Romazicon) is a benzodiazepine antagonist used for reversing most of the effects of the benzodiazepines. It may be used after conscious sedation with diazepam or lorazepam. It should be in the emergency kit only if parenteral benzodiazepines are administered in the dental office.

Antiarrhythmics. Procainamide, lidocaine, verapamil, and bretylium are used for their antiarrhythmic effect. The specific arrhythmia should be identified before an antiarrhythmic agent is selected. Arrhythmias are not problems that most dental offices are equipped to treat.

Equipment

An oxygen mask, a manual resuscitation bag, and an oxygen tank with a flow gauge are needed to administer positive pressure oxygen. A sphygmomanometer and stethoscope are used to take a patient's blood pressure. Disposable syringes, needles, and a tourniquet are used to administer medications. A laryngeal suction cannula is used to suction the throat if aspiration occurs. All dental practices should have an AED in case a patient goes into cardiac arrest. Box 21.3 lists essential equipment for a dental office emergency.

With ACLS training, a more advanced emergency kit can be prepared. Nasal and oral airways are used to maintain an unobstructed airway. Endotracheal tubes and a laryngoscope are required for intubation. Intravenous solutions, tubing, butterfly needles, and adhesive

---

BOX 21.3   Emergency Devices

Level 1 (Critical Devices)
- Syringes/needles
- Tourniquets
- System to administer oxygen*
- Automated external defibrillator (AED)

Level 2 (Secondary Devices)
- Cricothyrotomy device
- Endotracheal tube
- Laryngoscope
- System to administer intravenous (IV) infusions

*Oxygen cylinder with pressure regulator, flowmeter, and means of delivery (e.g., Ambu bag).

tape are used for intravenously administering drugs. A cricothyrotomy (incision through skin and cricothyroid membrane before a tracheotomy is performed) kit can be used for acute airway obstruction when other measures fail.

Many dental offices do not have staff trained to use the more advanced equipment. Without training, attempts to use this equipment may be more harmful than using simple measures. If untrained, personnel should stick to CPR.

DENTAL HYGIENE CONSIDERATIONS

- The best way to treat a medical emergency is to prevent one from occurring.
- Well-trained dental hygienists can treat emergencies that do occur.
- Make sure that patients have brought their rescue medication with them and have placed the medication within easy reach.
- Monitor vital signs.
- Always check and make sure that the drugs in the emergency kit are within their expiration dates.
- Keep oxygen close by.
- Be able to assess a patient if an emergency occurs and to relay that information to the dentist and emergency medical personnel.
- Review Boxes 21.1 and 21.2.

ACADEMIC SKILLS ASSESSMENT

1. State what general measures the dental health care worker should be familiar with to respond to any emergency situation.
2. For each of the following common emergencies, state the signs, symptoms, and treatment (including drugs):
   a. Cardiac arrest
   b. Angina pectoris
   c. Acute MI
   d. Convulsions
   e. Syncope
   f. Asthma
   g. Anaphylactic shock
   h. Hypoglycemia
3. List the equipment required to treat the emergencies in question 2, and explain the rationale for the inclusion of each item.
4. Give the names of the drugs required in an emergency kit for the dental office.
5. What drugs should be included in an ideal emergency kit?
6. What are the indications for the drugs most commonly found in an emergency kit for the dental office?

CLINICAL CASE STUDY

Kirsty Bellows is 16 years old and new to your practice. During the medication/health history, you learn that she has type 1 diabetes mellitus that was diagnosed when she was 3 years old. Miss Bellows is treated with a combination of regular and NPH insulin via an insulin pump and maintains good control of her plasma glucose levels. During the oral examination, Miss Bellows starts to feel weak and dizzy, and appears to be somewhat confused.

1. What is happening to Miss Bellows, and what is the cause?
2. How can this condition be treated?
3. What are the different ways to prevent this situation from happening again?
4. What would happen if Miss Bellows's plasma glucose levels became too low?
5. What would happen if Miss Bellows's plasma glucose levels became too high?
6. What are the signs and symptoms of elevated plasma glucose values?
7. How could this situation be prevented?

Pregnancy and Breastfeeding

LEARNING OBJECTIVES

1. List the two main concerns in the administration of drugs during pregnancy.
2. Describe the pregnancy trimesters in relation to dental treatment, define teratogenicity, outline the US Food and Drug Administration's prescription drug use in special populations, including pregnancy,

lactation and females and males of reproductive potential, and discuss how breastfeeding affects dental drug use.

3. Name several types of local anesthetic, antiinfective, and antianxiety agents, and state their indications or contraindications for pregnant women.

Dental treatment of the pregnant or nursing woman is always of special concern to dental hygienists. Pregnant women often need additional dental treatment during their pregnancies, and, in addition, that treatment must be carefully planned. Many questions about drug therapy for the pregnant or breastfeeding woman arise. The literature, unfortunately, does not provide all the answers. This chapter attempts to offer guidelines for determining the relative risk when drugs are prescribed for the pregnant woman or nursing mother. No unnecessary drug should be administered to the pregnant woman. If a drug is to be administered, the risk to the fetus must be weighed against the benefit to the woman. An adequate health history, including whether a woman might be pregnant (puberty to menopause), should be taken at each dental appointment. Close coordination with the patient's obstetric health care professional is recommended when questions about her potential use of drugs arise. Consultations should be documented in the patient's chart. Box 22.1 lists the dental implications involved in managing a pregnant dental patient.

GENERAL PRINCIPLES

Two Main Concerns

Two main concerns must be addressed when considering whether to

> Teratogenic: produces abnormal fetus.

give a drug to a pregnant woman. The first is that the drug may be teratogenic. The term *teratogen* is derived from the Greek prefix *terato-,* meaning "monster," and the suffix *-gen,* meaning "producing." These two combine to give rise to the meaning of *teratogen*: "producing a monster." The second is that the drug can affect the near-term fetus, causing the newborn infant to have an adverse reaction, such as respiratory depression or jaundice. A relatively new concern is the long-term (physiologic and psychological) consequences of in utero drug exposure that are not evident at birth.

History

In 1941, a relationship between getting German measles during pregnancy and blindness, deafness, and death of the offspring was noted. Scientists recognized that exogenous agents could affect the unborn fetus, producing congenital abnormalities. In 1961, a "harmless" sedative, thalidomide, available over-the-counter (OTC) in Europe, was taken by pregnant women. An increase in the rare birth defect phocomelia (shortness or absence of limbs) occurred shortly thereafter. Thalidomide was later implicated in these birth defects. Environmental factors are also thought to contribute to birth defects.

PREGNANCY

Pregnancy Trimesters

Pregnancy involves three trimesters, each 3 months long. During the first trimester, the organs in the fetus are forming. This is considered the most critical time for teratogenicity. If abnormalities occur very early in development, spontaneous abortion is the usual outcome. With later exposure, abnormalities occur in the fetus. Often, a woman is unaware that she is pregnant for at least half of this trimester. Dental prophylaxis with detailed instructions and a visual examination of the oral cavity without X-rays should be performed if the patient is pregnant. Because the woman in the first trimester of pregnancy may feel nauseated at any time during the day or night (often referred to as morning sickness), other elective dental treatment should be avoided at this time.

The second trimester is an excellent time for the patient to receive both oral health instructions and another dental prophylaxis treatment, if needed. The patient's periodontal status should be carefully evaluated. The patient is most comfortable during this trimester.

The third trimester is closest to delivery. The woman is beginning to feel uncomfortable, and it is difficult for her to lie prone for any length of time. If dental treatment is needed, she may feel more comfortable sitting or with the right hip elevated. In addition, this is the time when premature labor is most likely to begin. Drugs that may affect the newborn child should not be given during this trimester.

BOX 22.1 Management of the Pregnant Dental Patient

- Avoid elective dental treatment except in the second trimester.
- Avoid any unnecessary drugs, especially during the first trimester.
- If drugs are needed, check the US Food and Drug Administration (FDA) categories to choose the safest.
- Minimize periodontal problems; perform oral prophylaxis before pregnancy or during second trimester; monitor for periodontal conditions.
- Avoid radiographs unless absolutely necessary; use lead apron.
- Pay particular attention to periodontal disease because it has been associated with low-birth-weight newborns.
- Position patient in recumbent position in last trimester with right hip elevated (not Trendelenburg position).
- If morning sickness is a problem, schedule an afternoon appointment.
- Give frequent breaks for urination, especially during the first trimester.

Teratogenicity

> Teratogenicity difficult to identify.

It is difficult to prove that a drug is teratogenic in humans (Box 22.2).

Drugs that are known teratogens include thalidomide, certain vitamin A analogs (isotretinoin), antineoplastic agents (busulfan, cyclophosphamide), oral anticoagulants (warfarin), lithium, methimazole, penicillamine, some antiepileptic agents (phenytoin, trimethadione, valproic acid), the tetracyclines, certain steroids (diethylstilbestrol, androgens), and ethyl alcohol. Table 22.1 lists selected drugs with adverse effects on the fetus.

US Food and Drug Administration Pregnancy Categories

> US Food and Drug Administration pregnancy "grades."

In 2015, the US Food and Drug Administration (FDA) eliminated the pregnancy categories A, B, C, D, and X for drugs with new information that is more meaningful to both the practitioner and patient. The old system has been replaced with narrative sections and subsections that allow for better patient-specific counseling and informed decision-making for pregnant women that require medication. Fig. 22.1 gives a summary of the new system compared to the old system. The "Pregnancy" subsection provides information regarding dosing and potential risk to the developing fetus, pregnancy exposure registry, clinical considerations, and data on how women are affected when using medication. The "Lactation" subsection replaces the "Nursing Mothers" section and provides information about drugs that should not be used during breastfeeding, clinical considerations, risk benefits,

BOX 22.2 Reasons It Is Difficult to Prove a Drug Is Teratogenic

- Different animal species and humans vary among themselves in their responses to drugs.
- Timing of the drug exposure varies with each drug.
- One drug can produce a variety of abnormalities, and different drugs can produce the same abnormality.
- Drugs that are teratogenic are not uniformly so.
- A drug's effect on the fetus may be different from its effect on the mother.
- The teratogenic effects of a certain drug on the fetus may not be evident for many years.

TABLE 22.1 Selected Drugs With Adverse Effects on the Fetus

Drug	Trimester(s)	Effect(s)
Angiotensin-converting enzyme inhibitors (ACEIs)	All	Renal damage, congenital malformations
Amphetamines	All	Abnormal development patterns, neonatal withdrawal symptoms
Androgens	All	Masculinization of female fetus
Antidepressants, tricyclic	Third	Neonatal withdrawal symptoms
Antineoplastics	All	Congenital malformation
Barbiturates	All	Neonatal dependence
Carbamazepine	All	Neural tube defects; congenital malformations
Chlorpropamide	All	Neonatal hypoglycemia, prolonged
Clomipramine	First, third	Neonatal lethargy, hypotonia, cyanosis, hypothermia
Cocaine	All	Increased spontaneous abortion, abruptio placentae, premature labor, abnormal development, decreased school performance, seizure
Diazepam	All	Neonatal dependence, sedation; congenital malformations during first trimester
Diethylstilbestrol	All	Vaginal adenosis, vaginal adenocarcinoma, genital abnormalities, testicular cancer
Ethanol	All	Fetal alcohol syndrome
Etretinate	All	Multiple congenital malformations
Heroin	All	Neonatal dependence
Iodide	All	Congenital goiter, hypothyroidism
Isotretinoin	All	Extremely high risk of congenital anomalies
Lithium	First	Ebstein's anomaly
Methadone	All	Neonatal dependence, neonatal withdrawal symptoms
Methylthiouracil	All	Hypothyroidism
Metronidazole	First	May be mutagenic
Penicillamine	All	Cutis laxa, connective tissue defects, other congenital malformations
Phencyclidine	All	Abnormal neurologic findings, poor suck reflex and feeding
Phenytoin	All	Fetal hydantoin syndrome
Propylthiouracil	All	Hypothyroidism
Smoking	All	Intrauterine growth retardation, sudden infant death syndrome
Streptomycin	All	Eighth nerve toxicity, fetal ototoxicity
Tamoxifen	All	Increased spontaneous abortion and fetal damage
Tetracycline	All	Discolored teeth, altered bone growth
Thalidomide	All	Phocomelia, severe birth defects
Valproic acid	All	Neural tube defects, congenital malformations

Continued

TABLE 22.1 Selected Drugs With Adverse Effects on the Fetus—cont'd

Drug	Trimester(s)	Effect(s)
Warfarin	First	Hypoplastic nasal bridge, chondrodysplasia
	Second	Central nervous system malformations
	Third	Risk of bleeding; discontinue 1 month before delivery

Boldface indicates dental drug.
Data from Katzung BG. *Basic & Clinical Pharmacology*. 7th ed. Stamford, CT: Appleton & Lange; 2012.

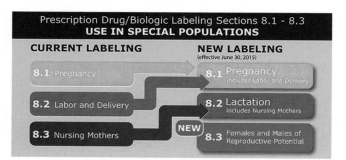

Fig. 22.1 US Food and Drug Administration pregnancy categories. (From https://www.fda.gov/BiologicsBloodVaccines/GuidanceCompliance RegulatoryInformation/ActsRulesRegulations/ucm445102.htm. Accessed 05/15/2018.)

timing of drug use and nursing, and the effects of all drugs on the nursing child. The final subsection, "Females and Males of Reproductive Potential," provides information regarding pregnancy testing, birth control, infertility, and the effects of medication on reproductive potential.

BREASTFEEDING

Questions about the safety of certain drugs given to a nursing mother are appearing more often because nursing has become more popular. As during pregnancy, the risk-to-benefit ratio should be carefully considered before drugs are given to the nursing mother. Drugs without strong indications for use should not be taken. Almost all drugs given to the mother can pass into the breast milk in varying concentrations. The amount of drug that appears in the milk depends on the plasma concentration of the drug, lipid solubility, degree of ionization, and binding to plasma proteins. While nursing, the baby ingests the drug, which may affect him or her.

For a few drugs, nursing is clearly contraindicated. If these drugs must be given, breastfeeding should be discontinued or the milk expressed and discarded until the mother stops taking the drug. For drugs that do not contraindicate breastfeeding, the timing of nursing can further reduce the dose to which an infant is exposed.

DENTAL DRUGS

Questions relating to drug administration in conjunction with dental treatment refer to whether a specific drug may be safely given to the pregnant woman. In general, a drug should be used in a pregnant woman only if the benefits to the pregnant woman outweigh the risks

to the fetus and a definite indication exists. Table 22.2 summarizes the information about which dental drugs can be used in pregnant women.

Local Anesthetic Agents

No drug is used more often in the dental office than a local anesthetic agent. Local anesthetic amides have been reported to cause fetal bradycardia and neonatal depression when given in very large doses to a pregnant woman near term. High doses may produce uterine vascular constriction, leading to fetal heart rate changes. Lidocaine, prilocaine, and etidocaine have been tested in animals without teratogenic effects. Bupivacaine has been shown to be teratogenic in rats and rabbits, whereas mepivacaine has not been tested. Low doses of a local anesthetic given by careful, slow injection have not been associated with any problems in the fetus. Lidocaine is the local anesthetic of choice for the pregnant woman because of its low risk for both the mother and developing fetus, and it is not associated with methemoglobinemia (as is prilocaine) and is not highly lipid soluble (as is etidocaine), which would prolong its effect.

Epinephrine

Small doses of epinephrine, administered with appropriate care, are similar to those produced endogenously. Large doses could have adverse effects in the fetus, including anoxia from vasoconstriction. If procedures are to be short, then local anesthetics without epinephrine are preferred. These comments also apply to other vasoconstrictor substances contained in local anesthetic solutions.

Analgesics

Analgesics should be given in the lowest possible dose and for the shortest duration possible to control pain. In dentistry, adjunctive therapy (incision, drainage, and curettage) should be used first.

Aspirin

> Acetylsalicylic acid: No.

Studies in animals have shown that aspirin (acetylsalicylic acid [ASA]) can cause a variety of birth defects involving the eyes, central nervous system (CNS), gastrointestinal tract, and skeleton. In humans, controlled studies have not been able to demonstrate that aspirin use during pregnancy increases the incidence of birth defects. During the third trimester, aspirin can prolong gestation, complicate delivery, decrease placental function, or increase the risk of maternal or fetal hemorrhage. Premature closure of the patent ductus arteriosus may occur (see Chapter 5). These effects have been reported with long-term use of high doses of aspirin. Abuse of aspirin may increase the risk of stillbirth or neonatal death.

Nonsteroidal Antiinflammatory Drugs

> Nonsteroidal antiinflammatory drugs: No.

The effects of nonsteroidal antiinflammatory agents (NSAIDs) are similar to those of aspirin; therefore, if they are given near term, the outcome for the fetus would be expected to be the same. NSAIDs can delay delivery and make it more difficult and can constrict the ductus arteriosus. NSAIDs also potentiate vasoconstriction in a patient with hypoxia. All NSAIDs carry a warning to avoid use during pregnancy. For ibuprofen and naproxen, studies in animals have not shown adverse effects on the fetus; however, they should be used with caution because they carry the same risks as aspirin. Ibuprofen is the NSAID of choice for the nursing mother.

TABLE 22.2 Dental Drug Use During Pregnancy*

Dental Drug	Use ok? First Trimester	Second/Third Trimester	Comment(s)	Nursing Use Ok?	Comment(s)
Local Anesthetics					
Bupivacaine	No	No	Embryocidal in rabbits; high lipid solubility	No	CNS changes
Lidocaine	Yes	Yes	First-choice anesthetic; fetal bradycardia near term	Yes	Central nervous system (CNS) changes
Mepivacaine	Yes	Yes	Fetal bradycardia near term; no animal testing	Yes	CNS changes
Vasoconstrictors					
Epinephrine	Yes	Yes	Vasoconstriction can produce hypoxia; limit to cardiac dose	Yes	Hyperactivity or irritability
Analgesics					
Acetaminophen	Yes	Yes	Teratogenic at overdose levels	Yes	Present in milk in small amounts (peak 1–2 hr); no documented problems
Aspirin	No	No	Bleeding; near-term dystocia and prolonged gestation, delayed parturition, premature closure of patent ductus arteriosus; treatment of certain pregnancy problems	Yes, caution	Occasional low dose poses minimal hazard; chronic high dose may present problems; infant may have inhibition of prostaglandins
Nonsteroidal antiinflammatory drugs (NSAIDs)	No	No	All NSAIDs should be avoided during pregnancy	No	Avoid NSAIDs; ibuprofen may be used when more information is available
Opioids	Yes	Yes	Respiratory depression near term; use low doses, short duration; high doses contraindicated	Yes	Small doses: no problem; large doses (addiction): sedation, poor feeding, constipation
Penicillines/Cephalosporins					
Amoxicillin, ampicillin	Yes	Yes	Safe	Yes	Allergy, diarrhea
Augmentin†	Yes	Yes	Safe	Yes	Allergy, diarrhea
Cephalosporins	Yes	Yes	Safe	Yes	Allergy, diarrhea
Penicillin V	Yes	Yes	Safe, especially penicillin V	Yes	Allergy, diarrhea
Macrolides					
Azithromycin	Avoid	Yes	Unlikely to be needed in dentistry	Yes	Insufficient information
Clarithromycin	Avoid	Yes	Teratogenic in mice and monkeys	Yes	Insufficient information
Erythromycin	Yes	Yes	Safe, except estolate form (cholestatic jaundice)	Yes‡c	Present in milk; diarrhea
Tetracyclines					
Doxycycline	No	No	Stains teeth; affects bones	No	Tooth staining questionable
Minocycline	No	No	Stains teeth; affects bones	No	Tooth staining questionable
Tetracycline	No	No	Stains teeth; affects bones	No	Tooth staining questionable

Continued

TABLE 22.2   Dental Drug Use During Pregnancy—cont'd

Dental Drug	Use ok? First Trimester	Use ok? Second/Third Trimester	Use ok? Comment(s)	Nursing Use Ok?	Nursing Comment(s)
Others					
Clindamycin	Yes	Yes	Very low risk of pseudomembranous colitis	Yes/No[‡]	Diarrhea; pseudomembranous colitis
Metronidazole	No	Yes, caution	Only if alternatives do not exist	No	Express and discard milk
Antifungals					
Clotrimazole, topical	No	Yes, caution	Poorly absorbed topically, abnormal liver function	Yes	No proof of problems
Ketoconazole, systemic	No	No	Embryotoxic in rats	Yes	No proof of problems
Miconazole, topical			No link with fetal abnormalities	Yes	No proof of problems
Nystatin	Yes	Yes	Not absorbed into systemic circulation from gastrointestinal tract	Yes	Not absorbed into systemic circulation from mouth or gastrointestinal tract
Antivirals					
Acyclovir	No	No	Limited experience	No	Concentrated in milk
Penciclovir	Probably		Topical		Insufficient information
Antianxiety Agents					
Alprazolam	No	No	Floppy infant syndrome; cleft lip; neural tube defects; do not use in dentistry	No	Long-term use by nursing mother can lead to infant lethargy and weight loss; slower metabolism may lead to accumulation of drug and its metabolites
Benzodiazepines[¶]					
Diazepam	No	No	Floppy infant syndrome; cleft lip; neural tube defects; withdrawal syndrome	No	Long-term use by nursing mother can lead to infant lethargy and weight loss; slower metabolism may lead to accumulation of drug and its metabolites
Estazolam	No	No		No	
Halazepam	No	No		No	
Lorazepam	No	No	Floppy infant syndrome; anal atresia	No	
Midazolam	No	No		No	
Nitrous oxide (with oxygen)	No	Yes, caution	Ensure adequate oxygen intake; female operators should avoid long-term or frequent exposure[§]	Yes	Nitrous oxide excreted via the lungs; amount in milk is negligible
Quazepam	No	No		No	
Temazepam	No	No	Cleft lip	No	
Triazolam	No	No		No	

*Do not administer any drug that is not absolutely necessary; potential risk to the fetus must be weighed against the benefit to the mother; consult the patient's health care provider before using drugs.

[†]Augmentin = amoxicillin + clavulanic acid.

[‡]References differ.

[§]Check levels in the dental operatory; minimize risk; increase ventilation exchanges.

[¶]Clorazepate, flurazepam, oxazepam—no category.

Acetaminophen

> Acetaminophen: Yes.

Although no controlled studies in humans have been done, acetaminophen (APAP) is generally considered to be safe in pregnancy. In large doses, it may be associated with renal changes in the fetus similar to those that occur in adults.

Opioids

Doses of opioids used by addicts have been demonstrated to cause problems in the fetus. The opioids, with the exception of codeine, have not been associated with teratogenicity. Retrospective studies have associated the use of codeine during the first trimester with fetal abnormalities involving the respiratory, gastrointestinal, cardiac, and circulatory systems and with inguinal hernia and cleft lip and palate (Fig. 22.2). These studies suggest that codeine or other opioids should not be used indiscriminately during the first trimester. Its near-term administration can produce respiratory depression in the infant. If the mother is addicted, the infant will experience withdrawal symptoms after birth. The use of codeine in limited quantities for a limited duration is common in clinical practice. Although opioids appear in breast milk when analgesic doses are administered, the small amounts appear to be insignificant. Proper timing of the doses of analgesic further reduces the dose the infant receives. The infant should be observed for signs of sedation and constipation.

Antiinfective Agents

Antiinfective agents should be used during pregnancy only when a definite indication for their use exists. Their prophylactic use, use when no indication exists, and use when an infection can be locally treated are inappropriate.

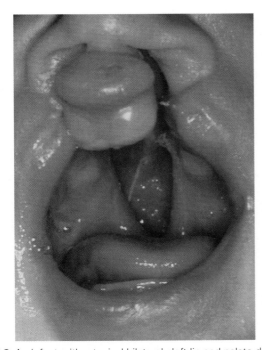

Fig. 22.2 An infant with a typical bilateral cleft lip and palate deformity. Certain drugs used during pregnancy, including opioids and benzodiazepines, have been known to cause this deformity. (From Zitelli BJ, McIntire SC, Nowalk AJ. *Zitelli and Davis' Atlas of Pediatric Physical Diagnosis.* 6th ed. St. Louis: Saunders; 2012.)

Amoxicillin

The most common antiinfective agent used in dentistry is amoxicillin. It is generally agreed that amoxicillin is safe to use during pregnancy. Using amoxicillin for a dental infection that is not controlled by local measures would be acceptable. Amoxicillin appears in breast milk, and infants exposed to it should be observed for signs of diarrhea, candidiasis, and allergic reactions.

Erythromycin

Erythromycins, other than the estolate form, also appear to be safe for use during pregnancy. The estolate form (Ilosone) should not be used in pregnant women, in whom it has been associated with reversible hepatic toxicity. Erythromycin is concentrated in breast milk but has not been documented to cause problems in infants.

Cephalosporins

The first- and second-generation cephalosporins have not been associated with teratogenicity. These cephalosporins should be used in dentistry only for a specific indication.

Tetracyclines

All tetracyclines, including tetracycline and doxycycline, are contraindicated during pregnancy because of the potential for adversely affecting the fetus. They cross the placenta and are deposited in the fetal teeth and bones. Deciduous teeth may become stained (see Fig. 7.4), and fetal bone growth inhibited. Hepatotoxicity can occur in the pregnant woman treated with large doses of tetracycline. Whether the amount excreted in milk, after it is complexed with the calcium in milk, can cause problems in the nursing infant is not known.

Clindamycin

Clindamycin should be used for dental infections during pregnancy for susceptible anaerobic infections not sensitive to penicillin. It is also indicated for prophylaxis of endocarditis in penicillin-allergic patients. No adverse fetal effects have been reported with its use. Because clindamycin is excreted in breast milk if it is given to nursing mothers, the exposed infant should be monitored for diarrhea.

Metronidazole

In animals, metronidazole can produce birth defects, so it should be used carefully during the first trimester. It would be difficult to encounter a dental situation in which the risk to the fetus from metronidazole would not be greater than the benefit to the mother. Because animal studies have shown metronidazole to be carcinogenic, the nursing mother should be given metronidazole only if she expresses and discards her milk during treatment and for 48 hours after the last dose.

Nystatin

Nystatin is safe to use during pregnancy to treat oral *Candida* infections. When applied topically or taken orally, it is not absorbed into the systemic circulation. This agent may also be used to treat thrush in either the pregnant woman or the nursing infant.

Clotrimazole

Small amounts of clotrimazole are absorbed from topical administration of this agent. No occurrences of abnormality have been reported, but nystatin is safer.

Ketoconazole

Ketoconazole is classified by the FDA as a category C drug. It has been shown to be teratogenic in rats, producing an abnormal number of digits (syndactyly [Fig. 22.3] and oligodactyly). Dystocia during delivery has been demonstrated in animals. Ketoconazole appears in breast milk and may increase the chance that kernicterus (jaundice) will occur in the nursing infant. If ketoconazole must be used, breast milk must be expressed and discarded during therapy and for 72 hours after cessation of therapy. Fluconazole, like ketoconazole, is also classified as a category C drug.

Antianxiety Agents

Nitrous Oxide-Oxygen Mixture

Operating room personnel, both male and female, who are exposed to trace amounts of nitrous oxide (N_2O) have a significantly higher incidence of spontaneous abortion and birth defects in their children. These data suggest that methods for reducing the environmental exposure, especially long term, should be explored and implemented. Pregnant dental health care workers should have knowledge of the levels of N_2O present in the dental offices in which they practice.

Benzodiazepines

First-trimester use of the benzodiazepines (chlordiazepoxide and diazepam) has been reported to increase the risk of congenital malformations. Cleft palate and lip and neural tube defects (Fig. 22.4) have been seen. Other benzodiazepines may also be associated with this increase in risk. Benzodiazepines are indicated during pregnancy only for the treatment of status epilepticus (no dental use).

Long-term ingestion of the benzodiazepines by a pregnant woman can produce physical dependence in her infant. Floppy infant syndrome, or neonatal flaccidity, has been seen at birth after such exposure, with inadequate sucking reflex or apnea. Use of benzodiazepines in the nursing mother, which may accumulate in the neonate because of slower metabolism, may cause sedation and feeding difficulties. Therefore, if any of these agents is needed, the exposed infant should be monitored for sedation.

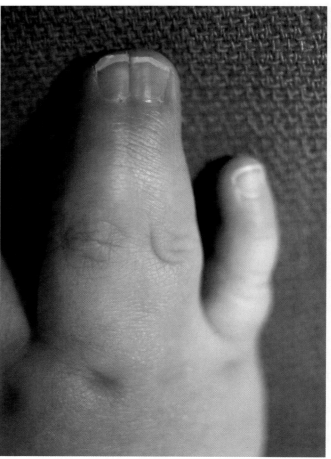

Fig. 22.3 Complete simple syndactyly. Administration of the drug ketoconazole to pregnant women has been shown to cause this deformity. (From Canale ST, Beaty JH. *Campbell's Operative Orthopaedics*. 12th ed. St. Louis: Mosby; 2013.)

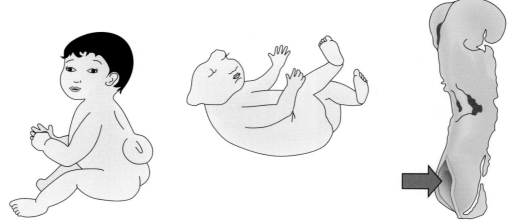

Fig. 22.4 Neural tube defects include spina bifida *(left)* and anencephaly *(middle)*. Administration of benzodiazepines during pregnancy can cause neural tube defects. (From Schlenker E, Long S. *Williams' Essentials of Nutrition & Diet Therapy*. 10th ed. St. Louis: Mosby; 2011. Redrawn from Centers for Disease Control and Prevention, Atlanta.)

Alcohol

Pregnancy + alcohol = **fetal alcohol syndrome.**

Although alcohol is not a dental drug, it is mentioned here because the evidence for the teratogenicity of alcohol is strong. Fetal alcohol syndrome (FAS) is the syndrome associated with the changes that occur in an infant exposed to excessive alcohol intake by the mother. FAS involves abnormalities in three areas: growth retardation (prenatal or postnatal), CNS abnormalities (neurologic or intellectual), and facial dysmorphology (e.g., microcephaly, microphthalmia, or short palpebral fissures, and flat maxillary area or a thin lip [Fig. 22.5]). Infants born to mothers who drank throughout pregnancy show more tremors, hypertonia, restlessness, crying, and abnormal reflexes after birth than control infants.

Pregnant dental patients should be encouraged to abstain from the ingestion of alcohol. No safe threshold level for the pregnant woman is known. Well-documented studies show that adverse effects on the fetus are dose related and can extend for years after the birth of the baby. The dental health care worker, as a health care professional, is in a position to remind the pregnant woman to care for her oral cavity and also her baby's development.

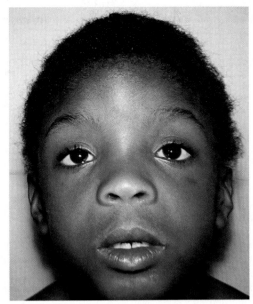

Fig. 22.5 A child with fetal alcohol syndrome. (From Zitelli BJ, Davis HW. *Atlas of Pediatric Physical Diagnosis.* 6th ed. St. Louis: Mosby; 2012.)

DENTAL HYGIENE CONSIDERATIONS

- The dental hygienist should ask appropriate questions during the medication/health history regarding pregnancy and lactation.
- The information that the dental hygienist obtains will help avoid the use of specific drugs if the patient is pregnant or lactating.
- Pregnant women should not be x-rayed because x-rays are harmful to the developing fetus.
- The dental hygienist should consult with the appropriate reference to determine the FDA pregnancy category of a drug before it is prescribed to a pregnant or nursing mother.

- Pregnant women may require a semi-supine position in the dental treatment chair. The dental hygienist should work with the patient to determine the best position.
- Mothers who are nursing should nurse just prior to receiving medication if medication is necessary.
- Always check blood pressure and pulse.
- Appointments should be planned for the second trimester when there is less risk for nausea and vomiting.
- Stress the importance of oral health care because pregnancy can lead to gingival inflammation.
- Review the information in Box 22.1.

ACADEMIC SKILLS ASSESSMENT

1. Describe the proper method for the dental hygienist to obtain information about possible pregnancy or breastfeeding patients. State the information to be obtained.
2. Explain the three trimesters and the special risks for each one.
3. Define *teratogenicity* and describe why identifying drugs that produce it is so difficult.
4. Explain the FDA pregnancy categories and state their significance.

5. Determine the factors that are important when a woman who is breastfeeding is to receive drugs.
6. For the commonly used dental drugs, such as local anesthetics, antibiotics, and analgesics, state the agents in each group that are the least safe.
7. Describe two activities that the dental health care worker should perform before giving a pregnant woman any medications to minimize future legal problems.

CLINICAL CASE STUDY

Lynn Watson is a 32-year-old woman who has been coming to your practice for about 3 years. She is 8 months pregnant and feeling rather "large." She is in today for her scheduled oral examination and cleaning. During the examination, both you and the dentist note several cavities. All three of you agree that the cavities can wait until the baby is about 6 weeks post-postpartum. Mrs. Watson has been reading up on breastfeeding and formula feeding and has decided to breastfeed. She wants you to know this because she is concerned about the use of a local anesthetic if she is nursing the baby.

1. When would be the more appropriate time to perform an elective procedure on Mrs. Watson?
2. What are the concerns associated with medications and breastfeeding?
3. What factors determine the amount of drug that is absorbed in breast milk?
4. Can local anesthetics with vasoconstrictors be given to lactating women? Why or why not?
5. What would you tell Mrs. Watson about the use of a local anesthetic with a vasoconstrictor?

Substance Use Disorders

LEARNING OBJECTIVES

1. Define substance use disorder.
2. Name several types of central nervous system depressants that are commonly abused, and outline the typical pattern of abuse, treatment, adverse reactions, management of overdose and withdrawal, and dental treatment implications of each.
3. Identify several types of central nervous system stimulants that are commonly abused.
4. Describe the pattern of abuse and the withdrawal and treatment options associated with tobacco use, and summarize the role of the dental hygienist in tobacco cessation.
5. Discuss several psychedelic hallucinogens, and recognize the symptoms produced by their use.
6. Discuss ways in which the dental hygienist can identify patients or colleagues who may be abusing drugs.

Dental hygienists may become involved with substance use disorder in a variety of ways. Both legal and illegal drugs can be abused. Patients seen in the dental office may be abusing drugs. Another interaction with the abusing patient involves the "potential" patient. Potential patients call the dental office, complain of pain, and request a prescription. Employees working in the dental office, including the dentist, dental hygienist, dental assistant, receptionist, and bookkeeper may abuse drugs. Friends and relatives, along with their friends and relatives, may abuse drugs. In our society, substance use disorder, especially in adolescents, is epidemic. Wherever there are people, substance use disorder can occur. Therefore, the dental hygienist should become familiar with the various types of drugs commonly abused and their patterns of abuse. It is important to be able to recognize the problem in others. Because substance use disorder is also a community issue, the dental hygienist should have a heightened awareness of the potential for patients to present with abuse problems (a high index of suspicion, but not one unrealistically high). The proper awareness is only learned with experience.

> Alcohol and tobacco: worst public health problems.

Alcohol and tobacco abuse cause more medical problems than all the other drugs of abuse combined. If no one in the United States used tobacco or drank alcohol, half of the filled hospital beds would be empty.

The idea of using drugs for profound effects on mood, thought, and feeling is as old as civilization. Only the kinds of substances used for this purpose have changed. Abuse has assumed a much bigger role in society because the forms of drugs used today are much stronger and have a much faster onset of action. This quick reinforcement produces abuse more quickly. For example, natives in Colombia have chewed coca leaves for many years as part of their culture, with little inappropriate use. Purifying cocaine and making it into a powder form to be "snorted" increased its abuse. When cocaine was "free based," it became easier to abuse, but the chemical reaction was dangerous. The more recent adaptation of cocaine, making it into "rocks," has increased abuse of the drug even more by making it available to smoke in convenient, small, reasonably priced doses. As is common with drugs of abuse, the potential for abuse is greatly increased when a drug is very potent, has a quick onset of action, is inexpensive, and is easy to distribute, making it the perfect drug of abuse.

Agents used for their psychoactive properties (capable of changing behavior or inducing psychosis-like reactions or both) can be divided into those that also have therapeutic value (opioids and sedative-hypnotics) and those that have no proven therapeutic value (psychedelics). Some agents may move from one category to the other. For example, marijuana, an agent previously considered to be worthless, is now claimed to be useful in the treatment of the nausea associated with cancer chemotherapy and for glaucoma. However, more controlled studies are needed to determine whether this claim is true.

GENERAL CONSIDERATIONS

Abuse of a drug is defined as its use for nonmedical purposes, almost always for altering consciousness. Both legitimate and illegitimate drugs may be abused. Whether a drug has an abuse potential is determined by the drug's pharmacologic effect. In contrast, *misusing* a drug means using it in the wrong dose or for a longer period than prescribed. The difference between these two uses is subtle.

Definitions

Terms relating to abuse that are used in this chapter are defined as follows:

Abstinence syndrome: A constellation of physiologic changes undergone by people who have become physically dependent on a drug or chemical who are abruptly deprived of that substance. The intensity of the syndrome varies with the individual drug.

Addiction: Addiction is a chronic, relapsing brain disease that is characterized by compulsive drug-seeking use despite complications or negative consequences (medical or social).

Substance use disorders: According to *The Diagnostic and Statistical Manual of Mental Disorders, Fifth Edition (DSM-5)*, Substance use disorders occur when the recurrent use of alcohol and/or drugs causes clinically and functionally significant impairment, such as health problems, disability, and failure to meet major responsibilities at work, school, or home. According to the DSM-5, a diagnosis of substance use disorder is based on evidence of impaired control, social impairment, risky use, and pharmacological criteria. Substance use disorders are defined as mild, moderate, or severe, which is determined by the number of criteria that the person demonstrates.

Enabling: The behavior of family or friends who associate with the addict that results in continued substance use disorder. This inappropriate coping mechanism requires family therapy.

Habituation: Physiologic tolerance to or psychological dependence on a drug.

Misuse: Use of the drug for a disease state in a way considered inappropriate.

Physical/physiologic dependence: The state in which the drug is necessary for continued functioning of certain body processes. In a dependent person, discontinuing the drug produces the abstinence syndrome, sometimes called withdrawal (physiologic reactions).

Psychologic dependence: The state in which, following withdrawal of the drug, there are manifestations of emotional abnormalities and drug-seeking behavior. Craving is present, but there is no physiologic dependence.

Relapse: Relapse is the return to drug use after an attempt to stop. Relapse indicates the need for more or different treatment.

Tolerance: With repeated dosing, the dose of a drug must be increased to obtain the same effect. Or the same dose of a drug, with consecutive dosing, has less effect.

Withdrawal: The constellation of symptoms, as specified in the DSM-5, that occurs when a physically dependent person stops taking the drug.

Psychological Dependence

Psychological dependence is a state of mind in which a person believes that he or she is unable to maintain optimal performance without having taken a drug. Psychological dependence can vary in severity from mild desire (e.g., for a morning cup of coffee) to compulsive obsession (e.g., for the next dose of cocaine). Although some highly abused drugs have only psychological dependence, the "need" to use them can be as strong as or stronger than that for drugs with a physical dependence. Other examples are benzodiazepines, opioids, and amphetamines.

Physical Dependence

Physical dependence refers to the altered physiologic state that results from constantly rising drug concentrations. The presence of physical dependence is established by withdrawal or abstinence syndrome, a combination of many drug-specific symptoms that occur upon abrupt discontinuation of drug administration. Withdrawal symptoms are often the opposite of the symptoms of use of the drug, for example, excessive parasympathetic action (e.g., diarrhea, lacrimation, and piloerection ["goose flesh"]) when withdrawing from opioids.

Tolerance

Tolerance: body gets "used to" drug.

Tolerance is characterized by the need to increase the dose continually to achieve the desired effect or the diminishing effect of taking the same dose. Tolerance can also be defined as a markedly diminished effect with the continued use of the same amount of drug. The type of tolerance referred to in this discussion of misuse of psychoactive drugs is *central* (functional or behavioral) *tolerance,* that is, a definite decrease in the response of brain tissue to constantly increasing amounts

of a drug. (One can think of the brain becoming "stronger" [less responsive] to "withstand" the large doses it must tolerate.)

Addiction and Habituation

Addiction and *habituation* are terms that have been misused almost as much as the drugs they attempt to characterize. Any use of these terms must be preceded by an adequate definition. In both addiction and habituation, the desire to continue using the drug is present, but in addiction, dependence is also present. Habituation and addiction are only degrees of misuse or abuse of drugs. Drugs that produce tolerance and physical dependence are grouped according to their ability to be substituted for one another. For example, if a person is addicted to heroin, an opioid, then other opioids, such as morphine, can prevent withdrawal. However, a barbiturate cannot be substituted for an opioid, and vice versa. Therefore, the opioids and barbiturates are separate groups of dependence-producing drugs. The phenomenon of substitution to suppress withdrawal between different drugs is called *cross-tolerance* or *cross-dependence.* It is observed among members of the same drug group but not among different drug groups. Cross-tolerance may be either partial or complete and is determined more by the pharmacologic effect of the drug than by its chemical structure.

Most characteristics of substance use disorders are determined by the individual drug involved, but the following generalizations can be made:

- For comparison of drugs in the same group, the time required to produce physical dependence is shortest with a rapidly metabolized drug and longest with a slowly metabolized drug.
- The time course of withdrawal reactions is related to the half-life of the drug. The shorter the half-life, the quicker the withdrawal.

Approximately 80% of incarcerated (jailed) individuals are there because of substance use disorders.

Many drugs have been abused extensively, and whether abuse can occur is a function of a particular drug's effects on neurotransmitters (combined with some genetic component within the user). At various times, sniffing airplane glue, inhaling propellant, smoking banana peels, smoking **peyote** (contains **mescaline**), and ingesting morning glory seeds have been attempted. The problems and treatment of substance use disorder are less related to the drugs themselves, although they can cause definite problems, than to the "inner person" of the patient involved in this type of behavior and his or her genetic predisposition. To treat abuse, a multifactorial approach is needed: counseling, education, self-help groups, and an intense desire to stop.

"Huffing": abusing volatile substances.

Propellant that is included in paint cans is preferred. The procedure is called "huffing" because the contents are sprayed into a plastic bag and fumes are repeatedly inhaled. Abuse of paint can easily produce irreversible damage to the liver and brain.

This chapter discusses the properties of the specific groups of agents abused and the differences among the groups. The abusable drugs are divided into the following groups: central nervous system (CNS) depressants ("downers"), CNS stimulants ("uppers"), and hallucinogens. Some drugs, depending on the dose, may belong to more than one group. For example, marijuana may be classified as either a CNS depressant or a hallucinogen. Table 23.1 lists the common drugs of abuse by category.

TABLE 23.1 | Drugs of Abuse by Category

Drug Group	Most Common Examples	Other Examples
Opioids	Heroin	Morphine Codeine Meperidine Hydromorphone
Stimulants	Cocaine Methamphetamine Bath Salts	Amphetamines Methylphenidate Nicotine
Depressants (sedative-hypnotics)	Ethanol Benzodiazepines Inhalants Nitrous oxide*	Barbiturates Nonbarbiturate sedatives
Hallucinogens	Lysergic acid diethylamide (LSD)	Mescaline Phencyclidine (PCP)
Other	Marijuana Spice K-2	Caffeine

*In dentistry because of availability.

CENTRAL NERVOUS SYSTEM DEPRESSANTS

CNS depressants include alcohol, opioids, barbiturates, benzodiazepines, volatile solvents (glue and gasoline), and nitrous oxide (abused mainly in dentistry).

Ethyl Alcohol

> Alcohol use disorder affects 8.4% of men and 4.2% of women in the United States.

Ethyl alcohol, or ethanol (ETH-an-ol), is a sedative agent used socially. Because it is legal, its availability makes it the most often abused drug. Abuse of alcohol, called *alcohol use disorder,* is the number one public health problem in the United States and is associated with many major medical problems. Data from the National Survey on Drug Use and Health 2014 showed that 52.4% of all Americans age 12 and older reported drinking alcohol. Most drink in moderation; however, more than 17 million Americans who drink alcohol have alcohol use disorder. Many accidental deaths are associated with the use of alcohol. More than 88,000 people die from alcohol-related causes annually, and 31% of traffic fatalities are alcohol-related. In 2010, alcohol misuse cost the United States 249 billion dollars. Three-quarters of the total cost of alcohol misuse is related to binge drinking.

Pharmacokinetics

Ethyl alcohol is rapidly and completely absorbed from the gastrointestinal tract. Peak levels during fasting occur in less than 40 minutes. Food delays absorption and reduces the peak levels. Alcohol is oxidized in the liver to acetaldehyde, which is then metabolized to carbon dioxide (CO_2) and water (H_2O) (Fig. 23.1).

Its metabolism follows zero-order kinetics, so a constant amount of alcohol is metabolized per unit of time regardless of the amount ingested. Because of zero-order kinetics, excessive intake of alcohol can have a prolonged effect. It is also excreted from the lungs (alcohol breath) and in urine.

Acute Intoxication

With mild alcohol intoxication, impairment of judgment, emotional lability, and nystagmus occur. When intoxication is moderate, dilated pupils, slurred speech, ataxia, and a staggering gait are noted. If intoxication is severe, seizures, coma, and death can occur. Treatment involves fluids and electrolytes, thiamine (vitamin B$_6$), sodium bicarbonate, and magnesium.

Withdrawal

> Delirium tremens.

Withdrawal from alcohol use occurs after the use of alcohol. The more alcohol consumed and the more time spent consuming it, the more violent the withdrawal syndrome (Fig. 23.2). Stage 1 withdrawal usually begins 6 to 8 hours after drinking has stopped and includes psychomotor agitation and autonomic nervous system hyperactivity. Stage 2 withdrawal includes hallucinations, paranoid behavior, and amnesia. Stage 3 includes disorientation, delusions, and grand mal seizures. It takes 3 to 5 days after cessation of drinking alcohol for stage 3 to occur. A cross-tolerant benzodiazepine (e.g., chlordiazepoxide; see Chapter 11) may be used to prevent withdrawal symptoms. Withdrawal from alcohol is termed *delirium tremens (DTs)* because the patient often experiences shaky (tremor) movements. Alcohol withdrawal can be life threatening if not properly treated.

Long-Term Effects

The long-term medical effects of alcohol use disorder can include deficiency of proteins, minerals, and water-soluble vitamins. Impotence, gastritis, esophageal varices, arrhythmias, and hypertension have also been reported. If a pregnant woman is using ethanol chronically, fetal alcohol syndrome can occur (see Fig. 22.4). The infant is retarded in body growth and has a small head (microencephaly), poor coordination, underdevelopment of the midface, and joint anomalies. In more severe cases, cardiac abnormalities and mental retardation are present. Chronic alcohol use increases the risk of cancer of the mouth, pharynx, larynx, esophagus, and liver, which may also occur with tobacco use, making the risk higher than with alcohol alone. The liver can be affected with alcoholic hepatitis and amnesic syndrome (Wernicke-Korsakoff syndrome), and peripheral neuropathy can occur.

Alcohol Use Disorder

Alcoholism or alcohol use disorder is a disease in which the alcoholic continues to drink despite the knowledge that drinking is causing a variety of problems (Box 23.1). Most Americans are moderate drinkers, which is defined as one drink per day for women and up to two drinks per day for men. However, more than 17 million Americans have alcohol use disorder because of binge drinking or heavy drinking. According to the Substance Abuse and Mental Health Administration, binge drinking is defined as drinking five or more drinks on the same occasion at least once in a 30-day time period. The National Institute on Alcohol Abuse and Alcoholism defines binge drinking as a pattern of drinking that produces blood alcohol levels greater than 0.8 gm/dL. This usually occurs after four drinks for women and five drinks for men in a 2-hour time span. Heavy drinking is defined as drinking five or more drinks on the same occasion on at least five or more days in a 30-day time period. There is a genetic link for alcoholism; children of alcoholics are at a much greater risk for becoming alcoholic. In the future, genetic testing may be able to identify at-risk children and target that population for intense educational and social intervention for prevention.

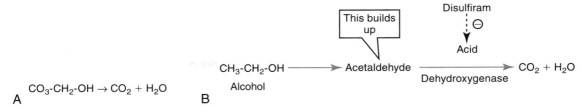

Fig. 23.1 (A) Metabolism of alcohol. (B) Effects of disulfiram on alcohol metabolism.

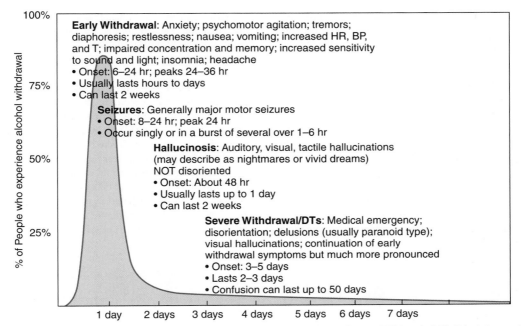

Fig. 23.2 Alcohol withdrawal syndrome. *DTs,* Delirium tremens. (From Stuart GW, Laraia MT. *Principles and Practice of Psychiatric Nursing.* 10th ed. St. Louis: Mosby; 2013.)

BOX 23.1   CAGE: A Self-Test for Alcoholism

- Have you ever felt you ought to Cut down on your drinking?
- Have people Annoyed you by criticizing your drinking?
- Have you ever felt bad or Guilty about your drinking?
- Have you ever had a drink first thing in the morning to steady your nerves or get rid of a hangover (Eye-opener)?

More information on CAGE can be obtained by reading Ewing JA. Detecting alcoholism: the CAGE. *JAMA.* 1984;262:1905–1907.

"Red flags" for alcohol abuse include drinking at an inappropriately early time, shaking when not drinking, blackouts when drinking, and being told that you drink too much. Missing work and problems in personal relationships are also strong warning signs.

Treatment

> Alcoholics Anonymous has the best results.

Alcoholics Anonymous. Alcoholics Anonymous, the most successful group for treating alcoholism, is a self-help organization made up of recovering alcoholics. The members (who are recovering alcoholics) give support to alcoholics who are attempting recovery. For most alcoholics, inpatient detoxification is usually not required. In fact, inpatient treatment does not give the alcoholic any experience in recovery in the "real world." Outpatient psychiatric treatment can help provide some insight for alcoholics.

Drug treatment. Alcoholics who are motivated and socially stable can be given disulfiram (dye-SUL-fi-ram; Antabuse). Occasionally, employers insist on the ingestion of disulfiram as a condition of employment of an alcoholic person.

Because disulfiram inhibits the metabolism of aldehyde dehydrogenase, a buildup of acetaldehyde occurs. Acetaldehyde produces significant side effects if alcohol is ingested. They include vasodilation, flushing, tachycardia, dyspnea, throbbing headache, vomiting, and thirst. The reaction may last from 30 minutes to several hours. Certain drugs that produce the disulfiram-like reaction (e.g., metronidazole) may cause a minor version of these symptoms with alcohol intake.

Naltrexone (ReVia), an oral opioid antagonist, is an old drug with a new use. Originally, it was indicated to prevent relapse in the opioid-dependent patient. Its new use is to reduce alcohol craving. Because naltrexone is partially effective in decreasing craving for alcohol, the logical conclusion is that alcohol stimulates some of the opioid receptors (among other receptors). More detailed knowledge of the receptors affected by alcohol may improve the chance of developing other agents to manage this disease. Other agents that might be useful are related to other neurotransmitters such as dopamine and serotonin.

Acamprosate (Campral) is the newest drug approved by the Food and Drug Administration to treat alcohol use disorder. Acamprosate appears to work by modulating/normalizing alcohol-disrupted brain activity, particularly in the GABA (gamma aminobutyric acid) and glutamate neurotransmitter systems that would otherwise stimulate withdrawal. It reduces alcohol cravings and does not cause sickness if alcohol is ingested.

Psychotropic agents may be helpful in managing the alcoholic patient because of the high incidence of comorbidity of psychiatric conditions.

Dental Treatment of the Alcoholic Patient

The dental hygienist must have an index of suspicion for alcoholism in patients treated in the dental office. The great majority of alcoholics look exactly like our neighbors, not like those characterized in old movies (e.g., unshaven, shaky). All health care workers have been given the charge to identify alcoholic patients and help them obtain treatment.

The dental treatment of the alcoholic patient involves some modifications, depending on the severity of the disease process. Most alcoholic patients have poor oral hygiene. Check for the sweet musty breath and painless bilateral hypertrophy of parotid glands characteristic of alcoholism. Cirrhosis of the liver can occur when alcoholics continue to abuse alcohol (Fig. 23.3). The major problem in these patients is a failure of the liver to perform adequately. Because of hepatic failure, the liver is able to store less vitamin K and the conversion of vitamin K to the coagulation factors is reduced. The outcome of these effects is a deficiency in coagulation factors II, VII, IX, and X (vitamin K–dependent factors) with resulting bleeding tendencies.

The patient's **international normalized ratio** (INR) can be elevated to 6 or more without the presence of other concomitant medications. Thrombocytopenia secondary to portal hypertension and bone marrow depression magnifies the hemostatic deficiency, sometimes resulting in spontaneous gingival bleeding. With the presence of esophageal varices, spontaneous bleeding can occur. Later in liver failure, the abdomen becomes distended with fluid (the patient appears to be 9 months pregnant).

Oral complications of alcoholism include glossitis, loss of tongue papillae, angular/labial cheilosis, and *Candida* infection. Healing after surgery may be slow, and bleeding may be difficult to stop.

Because alcohol and tobacco use and abuse predispose a patient to oral squamous cell carcinoma, the dental hygienist should check any oral lesions carefully. Special attention should be paid to leukoplakia and ulceration (especially on the lateral border of the tongue or the floor of the mouth).

With reduced liver function, the liver has difficulty metabolizing drugs usually metabolized in the liver. The levels of drugs metabolized by the liver, such as amide local anesthetics and oxidized benzodiazepines, will not fall as rapidly as in normal patients. Dose reductions are necessary because of diminished liver function. The signs of potential advanced alcoholic liver disease are listed in Box 23.2.

The dental hygienist should maintain an index of suspicion to be able to identify alcoholic patients. The dental hygienist should smell the patient's breath, palpate the parotid glands, expect poor oral hygiene, and evaluate the patient's bleeding tendency. Patients with cirrhosis and severe hepatic disease have greatly prolonged prothrombin

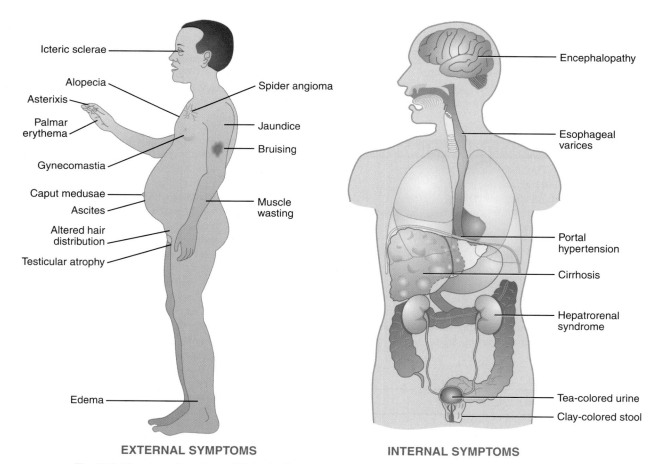

EXTERNAL SYMPTOMS   **INTERNAL SYMPTOMS**

Fig. 23.3 Clinical manifestations of cirrhosis. (From Mahan LK, Escott-Stump S. *Krause's Food, Nutrition, & Diet Therapy.* 13th ed. St. Louis: Saunders; 2012.)

times and may require vitamin K a few days before a surgical procedure in which bleeding is expected. Table 23.2 lists the dental management of the alcoholic patient.

BOX 23.2   Signs of Advanced Alcoholic Liver Disease

Head Area
Edema/puffy face
Parotid gland enlargement
Advanced periodontal disease
Sweet, musty breath odor
Ecchymoses, petechiae, bleeding

Rest of the Body
Memory deficit
A lot of injuries
Spider angiomas
Jaundice
Ankle edema
Ascites
Palmar erythema
White nails
Transverse pale band on nails

Modified from Little JW, Falace D, Miller C, et al. *Dental Management of the Medically Compromised Patient.* 7th ed. St. Louis: Mosby; 2008.

Nitrous Oxide

Nitrous oxide (N_2O) is an incomplete general anesthetic readily available in many dental offices (see Chapter 10). It is abused primarily by dentists, dental hygienists, and dental assistants. Food service employees sometimes become N_2O abusers because it is available in the aerosol in canned whipping cream products. Misuse often begins as therapeutic use only, progressing to abusive or recreational use at a later stage.

Abuse Pattern

N_2O is available in the dental office in tanks and as a propellant for whipping cream (Fig. 23.4). The availability of this gas to dental office personnel probably accounts for its unique abuse pattern.

Abuse of N_2O can result in psychological but not physical dependence. Inhalation of a 50% to 75% concentration produces a "high" for 30 seconds, followed by a sense of euphoria and detachment for 2 to 3 minutes. Tingling or warmth around the face, auditory illusions, slurred speech, and a stumbling gait can occur. The typical chemically dependent dentist (with N_2O as the drug of choice) is a 40-year-old white man who has often abused illicit drugs and primarily uses alone.

Adverse Reactions

General. Adverse reactions include dizziness, headache, tachycardia, syncope, and hypotension. N_2O impairs the ability to drive or operate heavy machinery. Other effects of N_2O use include hallucinations and religious experiences. Equilibrium, balance, and gait are affected. Long-term use of N_2O can produce chronic mental dysfunction and infertility.

TABLE 23.2   Dental Management of the Alcoholic Patient

Condition	Comment(s)	Management
Bleeding abnormalities		Platelet administration during and after chronic alcohol abuse
		Thrombocytopenia secondary to congestive splenomegaly, folate deficiency, bone marrow ethyl alcohol toxicity; quickly reverse if patient stops drinking; platelet reversal begins up to 2–3 days and increases 20,000–60,000/day
		Impaired aggregation decreased thromboxane A_2, increased bleeding time (like ASA or NSAIDs); improves 2–3 weeks after stopping
		Decreased hemostasis: vitamin K-dependent clotting factors missing
If cirrhosis and decreased liver function, clotting factors not being made (vitamin K-dependent)	Perform liver function test—aspartate aminotransferase (AST)	Give vitamin K, give whole blood (fresh clotting factors)
		Prothrombin time prolonged
		Use local hemostatic procedure
Gastrointestinal Tract Problems		
Stomach bleeding (varices)	Avoid NSAIDs, ASA	Use a topical dose form instead.
Drug interactions		Acute intake—high levels
		Chronic intake—increased metabolism
Acute Alcohol Use		
Enzyme-induced drugs metabolized by liver are metabolized at a slower rate with acute ingestion resulting in higher blood levels of such drugs.		Drug dose may need to be decreased.
Chronic Alcohol Use		
Chronic alcohol use can slow down drug metabolism.	Lower drug dose	This may be necessary for up to several weeks after alcohol cessation.
Acetaminophen	Dose should be no more than 4 g over 24 hours	Alcohol damages the liver leaving less area for acetaminophen to be metabolized, resulting in toxic metabolites of acetaminophen.

ASA, Aspirin; *NSAIDs,* nonsteroidal antiinflammatory drugs.
Data from Glick M. Medical considerations for dental care of patients with alcohol-related liver disease. *J Am Dent Assoc.* 1997;128:61–72; and Mandel L, Hamele-Bena D. Alcoholic parotid sialadenosis. *J Am Dent Assoc.* 1997;128(10):1411–1415.

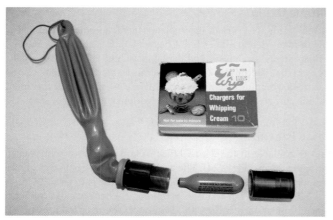

Fig. 23.4 Whippet assembly for recreational misuse of nitrous oxide (N₂O). (From Clark MS, Brunick AL. *Handbook of Nitrous Oxide and Oxygen Sedation.* 4th ed. St. Louis: Mosby; 2015.)

If 100% N₂O is inhaled, nausea, cyanosis, and falling may occur. Without oxygen, pure N₂O can produce hypoxia that results in death. Dentists who have self-administered N₂O have been found dead in their dental chairs with the mask still attached to the face.

Myeloneuropathy

> Myelopathy with abuse may be irreversible.

Chronic use or abuse can lead to myelopathy (sensory and motor) resulting in a combination of symptoms pathognomonic for N₂O abuse. Initial symptoms include loss of finger dexterity and numbness or paresthesia of the extremities. Position and vibration sensory neurons are lost. Other sensations, such as of pain, light touch, and temperature, may be lost. Later, Lhermitte's sign, clumsiness, and weakness can be demonstrated. Neurologic deficiencies include extensor plantar reflex and polyneuropathy (slow conduction velocity in nerves). The neurologic deficiency is similar to that of spinal cord degeneration in pernicious anemia. The neurologic problems from vitamin B_{12} deficiency are improved by parenteral vitamin B_{12}. Whether B_{12} improves N₂O myelopathy is controversial. If the abuse of N₂O is discontinued soon enough, clinical improvement can occur. However, with continued abuse, the myelopathy is often irreversible.

Opioid Analgesics

Heroin, methadone (Dolophine), morphine, hydromorphone (Dilaudid), meperidine (Demerol), fentanyl, oxycodone (Percodan), and oxycodone sustained-release (OxyContin) are currently the most popular abused opioids. In 2014, an estimated 1.9 million people had opioid use disorder related to prescription pain relievers, and more than 586,000 had opioid use disorder related to heroin. Since 1999, opioid overdose has increased 265% for men and more than 400% for women. Opioids used as analgesics are discussed in Chapter 6, which focuses on the pharmacology of the opioids themselves. It should be noted that opioids sold illegally on the street may be adulterated; that is, they may contain other unknown agents or diluents and often contain inactive filler so the doses can be more easily divided.

In addition to being analgesics, opioids produce a state described as complete satiation of all drives in some people. The opioids elevate the user's mood, cause euphoria, relieve fear and apprehension, and produce a feeling of peace and tranquility. They also suppress hunger, reduce sexual desire, and diminish the response to provocation.

Undoubtedly, initial abuse is reinforced by this "positive" experience. Other side effects include slowed respiration, constipation, urinary retention, and peripheral vasodilation.

With the development of physical dependence, however, the driving motivation to obtain the drug becomes more and more negative. Fear of withdrawal syndrome begins to override other motivations. At this point, the addict may resort to criminal activity and violence to support the drug habit. These activities are not direct actions of the drug but are related to opioid dependence.

Pattern of Abuse

Heroin is a highly addictive opioid that is illegal and has no accepted medical use in the United States. In 2014, about 435,000 people over the age of 12 were current heroin users. The incidence of heroin use has increased dramatically in the United States because of an intense crackdown on the availability of prescription opioid drugs. Also, heroin is cheaper than opioid analgesics. Another major concern is that today's heroin is being laced with fentanyl, making it even more dangerous for those who abuse it. The signs and symptoms of an acute overdose are fixed, pinpoint pupils (P^3), depressed respiration, hypotension and shock, slowing or absence of reflexes, and drowsiness or coma. Tolerance develops to most of the pharmacologic effects of the opioids, including the euphoric, analgesic, sedative, and respiratory depressant actions. However, tolerance does not develop to miosis or constipation.

The symptoms and time course of the withdrawal syndrome are determined by the specific drug used and the dose of drug used. Withdrawal usually begins at the time of the user's next scheduled dose. The first signs of withdrawal from heroin are yawning, lacrimation, rhinorrhea, and diaphoresis, followed by a restless sleep. With further abstinence, anorexia, tremors, irritability, weakness, and excessive gastrointestinal activity occur. The heart rate is rapid, the blood pressure is elevated, and chills alternate with excessive sweating. Without treatment, symptoms disappear by about the eighth day after the last dose of heroin.

Management of Acute Overdose and Withdrawal

> Triad: respiratory depression, pinpoint pupils, and coma.

If the triad of **narcotic** overdose (respiratory depression, P^3, and coma) is present, naloxone (Narcan) should be administered immediately. Chapter 6 reviews the most current guidelines regarding naloxone for a narcotic overdose. Chapter 21 reviews the different naloxone dose forms. If there is no response, it is unlikely that the depressed respiration is caused by opioid overdose.

In the past, immediate withdrawal reaction from an opioid sold on the street was only moderately distressing to the patient because of the poor quality and dilution of such a drug. Recently, high-quality heroin has reached the streets, and overdoses are more common and the withdrawal more intense. These people require naloxone immediately as their only chance for survival.

Patients in withdrawal can be made comfortable with methadone, a long-acting opioid that can replace heroin and then be gradually withdrawn. A phenothiazine or benzodiazepine is often administered for relief of tension. Long-term rehabilitation programs use several treatment approaches, such as **methadone maintenance**. These include substitution of a physiologically equivalent drug (e.g., methadone) in high doses, gradual weaning from methadone, and use of a long-acting opioid antagonist (e.g., naltrexone) (see Chapter 6).

Dental Implications

The following should be considered when treating a dental patient who abuses or has in the past abused opioids (narcotics).

Pain control. Because an opioid abuser develops tolerance to the analgesic effects of any opioid, treating pain with opioids is ineffective and can cause a recovering addict to begin using opioids again. It is best to alleviate the cause of the pain first and then to prescribe nonsteroidal antiinflammatory drugs (NSAIDs) for analgesia.

Prescriptions for opioids

> Be alert for "shoppers."

Opioid users often come to the dental office requesting an opioid for severe pain ("shopping"). Often, the substance user suggests the name or partial name of a specific opioid or claims to have allergies to several less potent agents.

Increased incidence of disease. Certain diseases that can be transmitted by use of needles for injections have a higher incidence in opioid abusers. These include hepatitis B, human immunodeficiency virus (HIV) producing acquired immune deficiency syndrome (AIDS), and sexually transmitted diseases (STDs). Infections caused by the use of nonsterile solutions and instruments can produce osteomyelitis and abscesses in the kidneys and heart valves. Intravenous substance users have about a 30% chance of development of cardiac valve damage over a 3-year period.

Chronic pain. The dental hygienist occasionally encounters dental patients with chronic pain. There are two ways in which these patients present to the dental office: a patient with symptoms of chronic dental-related pain (temporomandibular joint disorder or trigeminal neuralgia) and a patient reporting an elongation of the period of pain related to normal dental treatment (e.g., patient gets several refills of opioids for a root canal and no pathology can be identified). Patients who have pain for a much longer time than normal deserve a workup for chronic pain. Opioids are usually not effective in the management of chronic pain. If the dentist begins providing prescriptions for opioids to some patients, it is difficult to stop writing these prescriptions. The patients may state, "I hurt real bad." Another subtle lever that may improve the chance that the dentist would prescribe more opioids is the unsettling feeling that he or she has not performed some dental treatment correctly. Sometimes mild references to malpractice can magnify this worry. One should not be blackmailed into prescribing opioids if one feels uncomfortable. One should just state the office policy; for example, "The policy of this office is that no refills for an opioid (narcotic) analgesic are given without an additional office visit. It is important to identify the cause of the pain so it can be alleviated."

Prescription Opioids

Prescription opioids include hydrocodone, oxycodone, morphine, meperidine, and codeine. While the vast majority of patients take these drugs to manage pain, many others improperly use them. The 2014 report of the National Survey on Drug Use and Health reported that 50.5% of individuals who misused opioid pain medication got them from a friend or relative, and 22.1% got them from a doctor. This survey also reported that 4.3 million Americans engaged in misuse of opioid medications for more than 1 month. Approximately 1.9 million Americans met the criteria for opioid use disorder. As with heroin, the acute overdose of prescription opioids is treated with naloxone (Chapter 21).

Opioid Street Drug

Opioids available on the street change with time and are different in different parts of the country. The dental hygienist should be aware that most substance users misuse more than one substance and that street drugs are often adulterated.

An illicitly produced meperidine derivative that had classic opioid effects contained 1-methyl-4-phenyl-1,2,3,6-tetrahydropyridine (MPTP). This powerful neurotoxic agent is now known to have a toxicity unrelated to its opioid effects. It causes classic and permanent (irreversible) Parkinson's disease by destroying the cells in the substantia nigra (they make dopamine) within a very short period. This contaminant has become a valuable research tool because it can induce Parkinson's disease in animals, providing an animal model for research of drugs for treatment of Parkinson's disease.

SEDATIVE-HYPNOTICS

Sedative-hypnotics include barbiturates; alcohol; meprobamate (Miltown); benzodiazepines, such as chlordiazepoxide (Librium) and diazepam (Valium); and N_2O. Although their chemical structures vary greatly, their pharmacologic actions and patterns of abuse are similar.

Initial symptoms resemble the well-known symptoms of alcohol intoxication: loss of inhibition, euphoria, emotional instability, belligerence, difficulty thinking, poor memory and judgment, slurred speech, and ataxia. With increasing doses, drowsiness and sleep occur, respiration is depressed, cardiac output is decreased, and gastrointestinal activity and urine output are diminished. Paradoxic reactions can range from elation to excessive stimulation. The mechanism of excitement with a CNS depressant is related to an increased sensitivity to blocking of the inhibitor fibers, leaving the excitatory fibers unopposed. With additional CNS depression, the excitatory fibers are also depressed, resulting in sedation.

Pattern of Abuse

> Addict's usual dose becomes closer to fatal dose with growing tolerance.

The CNS depressant drugs are generally taken orally, often in a combination with some of the other drugs of abuse. With an acute overdose, respiratory and cardiovascular depression occurs, leading to coma and hypotension. The pupils may be unchanged or small, and lateral nystagmus is seen. Confusion, slurred speech, and ataxia are always present. Compared with opioids, the CNS depressants have a slower onset of tolerance and physical dependence. Tolerance to the sedative effect is not accompanied by a comparable tolerance to the lethal dose. With prolonged misuse, emotional instability, hostile and paranoid ideations, and suicidal tendencies are common.

Although the withdrawal syndrome for all CNS depressants is similar, its time course depends on the half-life of the substance used. The first signs of withdrawal are insomnia, weakness, tremulousness, restlessness, and perspiration. Often nausea and vomiting, together with hyperthermia and agitation, occur. Delirium and convulsions may culminate in cardiovascular collapse and loss of the temperature-regulating mechanism.

Another troubling abuse of the sedative-hypnotics involves administering them to other people to control them. Old movies have demonstrated the "slipping of a Mickey Finn" (chloral hydrate) to knock a person out ("knock-out drops"). A recent similar practice involves using a short-acting benzodiazepine, flunitrazepam, or Rohypnol (nickname is "Ruffies" or "Roofies") to make an unsuspecting young woman excessively sedated. After the woman becomes semiconscious, her partner takes sexual advantage of her and commits rape. This is often referred to as "date rape." Because of the excessive sedation and the amnesia produced by the flunitrazepam, recounting or even remembering what happened is difficult for the victim. Therefore prosecution would be unlikely because it would be difficult to prove whether the action was consensual.

Management of Acute Overdose and Withdrawal

The most important consideration with an acute overdose of a CNS depressant is support of the cardiovascular and respiratory systems. An airway must always be established and maintained. Patients that overdose on a benzodiazepine should be treated with flumenazil (Chapter 11). Early gastric lavage after intubation and dialysis can assist in removal of some drugs. CNS stimulants are harmful and should not be given.

In contrast to withdrawal from opioids, withdrawal from CNS depressants can be life threatening, and the patient should be hospitalized. The treatment of withdrawal from any CNS depressant involves (1) replacement of the abused drug with an equivalent drug and (2) gradual withdrawal of the equivalent drug.

The drug usually substituted for the abused drug is a long-acting benzodiazepine such as chlordiazepoxide or diazepam. The substitute drug is then gradually withdrawn over a period of weeks; during this time, the patient receives psychotherapy.

CENTRAL NERVOUS SYSTEM STIMULANTS

The CNS stimulants include cocaine, the amphetamines, caffeine, and nicotine. In 2014, an estimated 913,000 people age 12 and older had stimulant use disorder because of cocaine, and another 476,000 had stimulant use disorder because of methamphetamines. Also, another 569,000 people age 12 and older reported using methamphetamine in the past month.

CNS stimulants are taken orally, parenterally (intravenously or "skin popping"), intranasally, or by inhalation (smoking). With prolonged use, tolerance develops to the euphorigenic effect and toxic symptoms appear, including anxiety, aggressiveness, stereotyped behavior, hallucinations, and paranoid fears.

Although tolerance develops to the central sympathomimetic effect, no tolerance develops to the tendency to induce toxic psychoses at higher doses. Modest levels of abuse over a long period do not produce withdrawal reactions except fatigue and prolonged sleep, but large doses can precipitate a withdrawal syndrome consisting of aching muscles, a ravenous appetite with abdominal pain, and long periods of sleep. This is followed by profound psychological depression and sometimes even suicide. During this period, abnormal electroencephalographic (EEG) results have been recorded.

Cocaine

Cocaine is a CNS stimulant with local anesthetic properties when applied topically. It is used primarily for its stimulant action by "sniffing," "snorting," or intravenous injection. The latest variant, as previously described, is a free-base form that is smoked and goes by the street name of "crack" or "rock." It is purer and more potent, and the resulting intoxication is far more intense than that from snorted cocaine. Crack or rock cocaine acts much quicker and is much more euphoric and addicting. Cocaine induces intense euphoria, a sense of total self-confidence, and anorexia. Because of its short duration of action, the effects of cocaine last only a few minutes. Paranoia and extreme excitability cause some cocaine users to perform violent acts while under its influence. The paranoia produced by cocaine makes abusers unpredictable. The senseless violent acts sometimes committed by cocaine users cause society to fear cocaine abusers.

Unpredictable actions are feared the most. Psychological dependence becomes intense, but neither tolerance nor withdrawal has been shown. Cocaine's medical use is on mucous membranes (the inside of the nose) in which it produces local anesthesia and vasoconstriction to reduce hemorrhage. There is no appropriate dental use for cocaine. Although cocaine abuse is greatly publicized, the proportion of the population using cocaine is relatively small (in comparison with those using alcohol and tobacco).

Amphetamines
Pattern of Abuse

Drugs in the amphetamine class include methamphetamine (Desoxyn), dextroamphetamine (Dexedrine), diethylpropion (Tenuate), and methylphenidate (Ritalin). Because methamphetamine produces a much longer duration of effect than cocaine, "meth" use is spreading across the nation. The sympathomimetic CNS stimulants are abused for their ability to produce a euphoric mood, a sense of increased energy and alertness, and a feeling of omnipotence and self-confidence. Other effects include mydriasis, increased blood pressure and heart rate, anorexia, and increased sweating.

Crystal meth. Methamphetamine in its crystalline form is known as "crystal meth," which is illegal and made in illegal meth laboratories. Many meth laboratories (labs) have been raided, but more pop up immediately. The manufacturing of methamphetamine can be carried out with common chemistry lab equipment and a precursor drug (ephedrine) that can be bought over the counter. Because of this, ephedrine is no longer available for purchase, and products containing pseudoephedrine are now stocked in the actual pharmacy. Persons over the age of 18 can only purchase a limited quantity of pseudoephedrine each year and must sign a log verifying the purchase. Unfortunately, these meth labs are explosive, smell bad (distinctive odor), and have been found in many residential neighborhoods.

Oral adverse reactions of methamphetamine include xerostomia and bruxism. Xerostomia and bruxism, in combination with poor nutrition, increased sugar consumption, and poor oral hygiene, can result in a condition known as "meth mouth" (Fig. 23.5). Patients with meth mouth suffer from severe tooth decay and loss, tooth fractures, and enamel erosion. Treatment can be dangerous with active meth users because local anesthetics may be necessary. The cardiac effects associated with local anesthetics and vasoconstrictors can intensify the cardiac effects of meth. To treat patients, the dentist or dental hygienist should prescribe fluoride to fight tooth decay and prevent caries and drugs to treat xerostomia. Patients should be counseled on proper nutrition and good oral-hygiene techniques.

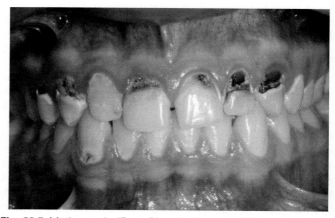

Fig. 23.5 Meth mouth. (From Bird DL, Robinson DS. *Modern Dental Assisting.* 11th ed. St. Louis: Saunders; 2015.)

Bath salts. "Bath salts" refer to a growing group of drugs containing one or more synthetic chemicals related to cathinone, an amphetamine-like substance found in the Khat plant. This synthetic amphetamine-like substance is called "bath salts' because its crystalline powder dose form looks like bath salts. They were first introduced on the US market as a legal "high." In 2012, legislation was signed making mephedrone and 4-methylenedioxypyrovalerone (MDPV) illegal in the United States. They are sold in small plastic or foil packages labeled "not for human consumption." However, they can be taken orally, injected, or inhaled. The inhaled and injected dose forms have demonstrated the worst outcomes. Its energizing and agitating effects are similar to cocaine and amphetamine, in that they elevate dopamine levels in the brain circuits that regulate reward and movement. Bath salts can cause euphoria, increased sociability, increased heart rate, and elevated blood pressure. Bath salts also cause hallucinations, paranoia, agitation, delirium, psychosis, and violent behavior. Deaths have been reported.

Bath salts have resulted in an alarming number of emergency room visits across the country. Patients are being seen for cardiac symptoms (racing heart, high blood pressure, and chest pain) and psychiatric symptoms, including paranoia, hallucinations, and panic attacks. Some patients present with "excited delirium," which also includes dehydration, breakdown of skeletal muscle tissue, and renal failure. Bath salt users report that the drug triggers intense cravings and that they are highly addicted. Frequent consumption may lead to tolerance, dependence, and strong withdrawal symptoms.

Management of Acute Overdose and Withdrawal

Signs and symptoms of an acute overdose include dilated pupils (sympathetic autonomic nervous system stimulation), elevated blood pressure, rapid pulse, and cardiac arrhythmias. The patient may exhibit diaphoresis, hyperthermia, fine tremors, and hyperactive behavior.

Treatment of an overdose of a CNS stimulant is symptomatic. It may include a phenothiazine for psychotic symptoms, a short-acting sympathomimetic blocking agent if hypertension is severe, and a tricyclic antidepressant if severe depression occurs.

The most serious sociologic problem with stimulant abuse is the induction of mental abnormalities, especially in young abusers. Experimental evidence suggests that amphetamine psychoses can be induced in previously unaffected volunteer subjects. The psychoses are dose related, and repeated dosing can reproduce the psychoses.

Caffeine

Caffeine, the most widely used social drug in the world, is contained in coffee, tea, soft drinks, sports drinks, energy drinks, and other drinks named to reflect the effect of their contents. Its action on the CNS is stimulation, which is why many people use these beverages. Caffeine toxicity can occur with as little as 300 mg of caffeine (contained in two to three cups of coffee). With five cups or more of caffeine daily, physical dependence can occur. Although many people do not consider caffeine a drug, a withdrawal syndrome can be identified that begins around 24 hours after the last cup of coffee. It consists of headache, lethargy, irritability, and anxiety. Tolerance develops to the effects of caffeine, and some people continue to use caffeine even when it causes harm. Table 23.3 lists the caffeine content of several beverages.

Tobacco
Nicotine

Awareness of the toxicity from chronic smoking and chewing tobacco has increased dramatically over the past 2 decades. The CNS-active component of tobacco is nicotine, but a large number of components of the gaseous phase of tobacco smoke contribute to its undesirable effects: carbon monoxide, nitrogen oxides, volatile nitrosamines, hydrogen cyanide, volatile hydrocarbons, and many others.

TABLE 23.3 Caffeine Content of Selected Caffeine-Containing Beverages

Beverage	Caffeine (mg)
Coffee:	
Espresso restaurant style	40–75/1 oz
Espresso restaurant style, decaffeinated	0–15/1 oz
Generic brewed	95–200/8 oz
Generic, decaffeinated	2–12/8 oz
McDonald's brewed	100/16 oz
Starbucks Latte	150/16 oz
Pike Place brewed	330/16 oz
Pike Place brewed, decaffeinated	25/16 oz
Tea, brewed	14–61/8 oz
Green tea	24–40/8 oz
Cola drink	30–40/12 oz
Mountain Dew	46–55/12 oz
5-Hour Energy Drink	207/2 oz
Cran•Energy	70/8 oz
Monster	80/8 oz
Red Bull	76–80/8 oz
Vault, regular or sugar free	47/8 oz
Chocolate, milk	3–6/oz
Chocolate chips, semisweet	104/1 cup
Hershey Kisses	9 mg/9 pieces
No-Doz, maximum strength	100 mg/tablet
Excedrin, extra-strength	130 mg/2 tablets

oz, Ounce.

Pattern of Abuse

Cigars are the new "dumb craze."

Approximately 26% of Americans over the age of 12 smoke. Young adults aged 18 to 25 had the highest rate of current use of a tobacco product (35%), followed by adults aged 26 or older (25.8%), and by youths aged 12 to 17 (7%) based upon 2014 data. Children commonly begin smoking between 11 and 14 years of age. In some geographic areas, more teenage girls than teenage boys smoke. The newest craze is cigar smoking; it is portrayed as glamorous, and famous movie stars are observed doing it. Smokers claim that the most desirable effects of smoking are greater alertness, muscle relaxation, facilitation of concentration and memory, and decreases in appetite and irritability. These are consistent with the effect of nicotine on the CNS. In addition, nicotine produces an increase in blood pressure and pulse rate and induces nausea, vomiting, and dizziness through stimulation of the chemoreceptor trigger zone. Smokers are tolerant to these latter effects, but such tolerance does not last long. The first cigarette of the day may induce a certain degree of dizziness and nausea. Chronic use of tobacco is causally related to many serious diseases, including coronary artery disease and oral and lung cancers.

Smokeless Tobacco

In some communities, more than one-fourth of high school males use chewing tobacco. Oral mucosal changes caused by tobacco include chronic gingivitis, leukoplakia, and precancerous lesions. In these patients, an extremely thorough oral examination should be done at each prophylaxis. Education concerning the oral health hazards that smokeless tobacco poses should also be included.

Electronic cigarettes. Electronic (e)-cigarettes are an electronic nicotine delivery system that uses a liquid that contains nicotine and numerous flavorings, propylene glycol, vegetable glycerin, and other ingredients that are heated into an aerosol that the user inhales. Other electronic nicotine-delivery systems include vapes, vaporizing, hookah pens, and e-pipes. They are often manufactured to look like cigarettes, pipes, and cigars. e-cigarettes were developed to provide an alternative to conventional cigarettes because of their harmful added ingredients. A person that uses an e-cigarette only inhales nicotine and not the tars and other substances found in regular cigarettes. The number of persons using e-cigarettes is high, especially among young adults and children. According to 2016 statistics, 2 million middle and high school students used e-cigarettes. Also, 11% of high school students and 4.3% of middle school students were current users of e-cigarettes. The use of e-cigarettes rose from 1.5% to 16% among high school students and 0.6% to 5.3% among middle school students. Of these students, 81% stated that the different flavorings was the primary reason for use.

Like conventional cigarettes, e-cigarettes contain nicotine, which is harmful to the developing brain. Children, teenagers, and pregnant women should not use them. Little is known at this time regarding the long-term use of e-cigarettes. The US Food and Drug Administration now regulates the electronic nicotine-delivery systems. Also, manufacturers of electronic delivery systems must bear the required nicotine addictiveness warning statement.

Management and Withdrawal

The withdrawal syndrome that occurs after cessation of chronic tobacco smoking or chewing varies greatly from person to person. The most consistent symptoms are anxiety, irritability, difficulty in concentrating, and cravings for cigarettes. Drowsiness, headaches, increased appetite, and sleep disturbances are also common. The syndrome is rapid in onset (within 24 hours after the last cigarette) and can persist for months.

The syndrome of withdrawal from tobacco can be suppressed to some extent by administration of nicotine chewing gum (Nicorette, Nicorette DS) or nicotine patches (NicoDerm, Nicotrol, and Habitrol; Table 23.4). These products do reduce the irritability and difficulty concentrating but appear to be less effective in controlling insomnia, hunger, and the craving for tobacco. The most important dental side effect of the use of nicotine gum is dislodgment of dental fillings. Another form of nicotine replacement is the nasal spray Nicotrol NS. A potential problem with the nasal spray is that the rapid rise in blood level it causes more closely mimics the effect of using tobacco.

Bupropion

Another approach to treating tobacco cessation involves the use of bupropion (Wellbutrin, Zyban), which is an antidepressant, to reduce craving. Dentists can prescribe bupropion, but should encourage concomitant treatment modalities (e.g., behavior modification). The recommended dosage schedule is 150 mg daily (qd) for 3 days, followed by

TABLE 23.4	Nicotine-Containing Products
Vehicle	**Product**
Patch	Habitrol, NicoDerm, Nicotrol, ProStep
Gum	Nicorette
Nasal spray	Nicotrol NS

150 mg twice a day (bid) for 2 to 3 months if the patient is experiencing success. Refills should not be indicated on the original prescription because the dental hygienist should talk with the patient by phone before authorizing a refill (see Chapter 15).

Varenicline

Varenicline (CHANTIX) is a nicotine-receptor blocker that binds to the receptor to prevent the nicotine from reaching it. By binding to this receptor, varenicline limits the amount of dopamine that is released in the brain. It is thought that stimulation of nicotinic receptors releases dopamine, which accounts for the feeling of pleasure that is often associated with tobacco use. Varenicline is taken daily for the first 3 days of therapy and is then used twice daily for the remaining course of therapy. This agent is taken after meals with a full glass of water. A normal course of therapy is 12 weeks. The most common side effects include nausea, sleep problems, constipation, gas, vomiting, and changes in mood and behavior. It cannot be used in conjunction with other smoking cessation drug products.

It should be noted that varenicline carries a Black Box warning regarding serious neuropsychiatric events. Persons using varenicline have reported behavioral changes, including hostility, agitation, depression, and suicidal ideation. Symptoms were reported almost immediately after starting the drug to several weeks into therapy. Any changes should be reported to the patient's physician.

The Dental Hygienist's Role in Tobacco Cessation

Dental hygienists are especially situated to be helpful in promoting tobacco cessation because of their role in encouraging patients to change habits (e.g., floss, brush teeth, and use fluoride). Smoking cessation is another habit change (behavior modification). The dental hygienist is in a position to point out some of the oral manifestations of nicotine and tobacco abuse firsthand in the patient's own mouth. The National Cancer Institute currently has a program for dental personnel that include a variety of patient education devices (available by calling the Institute at 800-4-CANCER) or at Smokefree.gov. Every dental office should offer its patients help in smoking cessation.

PSYCHEDELICS (HALLUCINOGENS)

According to the National Survey on Drug Use and Health, first-time users of hallucinogens has remained steady since 2002 at 1.2 million people.

The psychedelic agents are capable of inducing states of altered perception and generally do not have any medically acceptable therapeutic use. The drugs in this section include lysergic acid diethylamide (LSD) and phencyclidine (PCP), but many other agents, including psilocybin, dimethyltryptamine (DMT), 2,5-dimethoxy-4-methylamphetamine (STP), methylenedioxyamphetamine (MDMA), Ecstasy (now known as Molly), and mescaline (peyote), also belong to this class. Clearly, the agents discussed in this section represent only a fraction of those released on the illicit drug market. These hallucinogens are often mislabeled or adulterated with substances such as strychnine.

Psychedelic agents affect perceptions in such a way that all sensory input is perceived with heightened awareness; sounds are brighter and clearer, colors are more brilliant, and taste, smell, and touch are more acute. Psychedelic-induced dependence is psychological, and tolerance develops within a short time. These two characteristics, combined with the unpredictable nature of the response, favor periodic rather than continuous abuse of psychedelic drugs. Prolonged use can cause long-lasting mental disturbances varying from panic reactions to depression to schizophrenic reactions.

Lysergic Acid Diethylamide

LSD is the most potent hallucinogen; only micrograms are required for an effect. In addition to its psychogenic actions, LSD has sympathomimetic effects, including tachycardia, rise in blood pressure, hyperreflexia, nausea, and increased body temperature.

An overdose of LSD produces symptoms that include widely dilated pupils, flushed face, elevated blood pressure, visual and temporal distortions, hallucinations, derealization, panic reaction, and paranoia. Because the user does not lose consciousness and is highly suggestible, treatment is to provide reassurance ("talking the user down"). In rare cases, chlorpromazine has been used to treat the situation in an emergency. Flashbacks, commonly precipitated by marijuana use, can occur years after ingestion of LSD. This agent is currently making another comeback.

Phencyclidine

PCP (or angel dust), originally developed as an animal tranquilizer, was popular in the 1970s. It inhibits the reuptake of dopamine, serotonin, and norepinephrine. Although it has anticholinergic properties, hypersalivation is produced. It is a powerful CNS stimulant with dissociative properties. Users may exhibit sweating and a blank stare. Changes in body image and disorganized thought have led to bizarre behavior and psychosis. Elevation of blood pressure and pulse and muscle movement and rigidity occur. PCP is abused alone or as an adulterant in other street drugs.

Marijuana

Marijuana is the most used drug, after alcohol and tobacco, in the United States. According to 2014 data from the Substance Abuse and Mental Health Services Administration, about 22.2 million people age 12 and older used marijuana during the past month. Data also show that 4.2 million Americans meet the criteria for substance use disorder with cannabis.

Marijuana (marihuana, cannabis) is derived from the hemp plant, and its active ingredient is tetrahydrocannabinol (tet-ra-hi-dro-can-NAB-i-nol; THC). Recreational marijuana use is illegal in the United States except in Colorado, Washington State, California, Massachusetts, Maine, Nevada, Alaska, Oregon, and Washington, DC. However, it remains an illegal substance under federal law. Marijuana can be administered orally or by inhalation (smoking), and its effects include an increase in pulse rate, reddening of the conjunctivae (bloodshot eyes), and behavioral changes. Slight changes in blood pressure and pupil size and hand tremors have been noted. With normal doses, euphoria and enhanced sensory perception occur. This stage is followed by sedation and altered consciousness (a dreamlike state). Signs of use and dependence include a heightened sense of visual, auditory, and taste perception, poor memory, increased heart rate and blood pressure, red eyes, decreased coordination, difficulty concentrating, increased appetite, slowed reaction time, and paranoid thinking.

Studies of the influence of marijuana on driving have concluded that the drug impairs the motor and mental abilities required for safe driving. For example, the perception of time and distance is distorted, and reflexes are reduced. A more common adverse reaction is apprehensive, nervous, and panic-stricken feelings that the user is losing his or her mind. This reaction responds to friendly reassurance. Psychological dependence on marijuana is determined by the frequency of use. Physical dependence, tolerance, and withdrawal symptoms are rare.

Of particular interest to the dental hygienist is the fact that a high level of marijuana abuse may cause xerostomia. It has been noted anecdotally that some marijuana users have gingivitis. Heavy marijuana smoking can lead to chronic bronchitis and precancerous changes in the bronchioles.

Medical Marijuana

Medical marijuana refers to the use of cannabis and its constituents, THC and cannabidiol, for the treatment of disease and the alleviation of disease symptoms. THC is known to reduce intraocular pressure and has been used in the treatment of resistant glaucoma. It is also effective as an antiemetic to treat the nausea associated with cancer chemotherapy. Dronabinol (Marinol), synthetic THC, is a schedule III drug because it has some potential for abuse, and nabilone (Cesamet), synthetic cannabinoid, is a schedule II drug because of its high potential for abuse. Both drugs are usually used when conventional treatment of nausea and vomiting associated with chemotherapy fail to work. They are also used as appetite stimulants in HIV/AIDs patients and cancer chemotherapy patients.

Currently, 29 states and the District of Columbia have passed medical marijuana laws legalizing the use and production of medical marijuana for qualifying patients under state law. However, its use remains illegal under federal law.

Synthetic Marijuana

Synthetic marijuana or cannabis is a designer drug created by spraying natural herbs with synthetic chemicals that have psychoactive effects similar to those of cannabis. This product is known as "Spice" and "K-2." These drugs are marketed as "safe," legal alternatives to marijuana. For several years, these products could be purchased in gas stations and head shops. Because the chemicals used to create these products have a high potential for abuse and no accepted medical use in the United States, the US Drug Enforcement Administration has declared the five active chemical substances used most frequently to make synthetic marijuana products as schedule I drugs. This makes it illegal to sell, buy, or possess the products. The products are very popular among high school students and even in elementary school students because they are touted as natural products. Synthetic marijuana is abused by smoking, though some users may prepare it as an herbal infusion for drinking.

Patients report experiences similar to those with marijuana, including elevated mood, relaxation, and altered perception. In many cases, the effects are even stronger than those of marijuana. Many children have been treated in emergency rooms or via Poison Control Centers because of elevated heart rate, vomiting, agitation, confusion, and hallucinations brought on by this drug. In a few cases, users have experienced heart attacks.

IDENTIFYING THE SUBSTANCE USER

"Shoppers," as previously discussed, interact with many health care workers in an attempt to obtain controlled substances for illegitimate uses. Some references suggest that shoppers can be identified by the presence of poor hygiene, long-sleeved shirts, scars along veins, sunglasses, abrupt changes in behavior, moodiness, and behaving as though they were under the influence of an intoxicant, although usually this is not the case.

Most shoppers are excellent storytellers and actors with convincing histories and the presence of a pathologic dental condition. They look and behave like typical patients. They may suggest specific drugs or give a history of allergy to analgesics they do not want. One should note the patient's response to the mention of drugs that the dental provider is going to prescribe. This can be a tip-off that the patient is hoping for a more potent drug.

Abusers have more sexually transmitted diseases and blood-borne infections.

Intravenous substance users are more likely to have STDs, to have hepatitis (hepatitis B virus [HBV] and hepatitis C virus [HCV]) or be hepatitis carriers, to be HIV positive or have AIDS, to be infected with multidrug-resistant tuberculosis, and to have altered heart valves.

The dental office should not stock many controlled substances so as not to become the target of robberies and burglaries. Addicts searching for drugs can be violent. The supply of controlled substances must be under lock and key and located in an inconspicuous place.

THE IMPAIRED DENTAL HYGIENIST

When dental hygienists abuse drugs, they can present a danger to the patients being treated.

A professional who is abusing drugs, like most abusers, is in denial, and confrontation by staff, relatives, and friends is often ineffective. The dentist's dental practice deteriorates, and mood swings, including depression, occur. Often, suicide is thought to be the only recourse.

Any dental hygienist who observes or suspects that another worker is abusing drugs should report the person to the appropriate "impaired professional committee" for their profession. Most state boards currently have committees to work with any impaired dental professional (those that have abused alcohol or drugs). The committee's goal is to help the dental hygienist become a functioning practitioner again. The objective of these committees is not to punish the worker or to make the person lose his or her license. These committees can also investigate a suspicion of abuse. The difficulty in self-regulation lies with the silent practitioners who do not want to get involved.

DENTAL HYGIENE CONSIDERATIONS

- Conduct a detailed medication and health history and an extraoral and clinical examination for evidence of substance abuse.
- Monitor the patient's blood pressure and heart rate at each visit.
- Perform an oral cancer screening, evaluate salivary flow, and recommend anticaries agents as necessary.
- Monitor for caffeine stains and educate the patient about the high risk for stains with caffeine consumption.
- Educate the patient regarding the risks of tobacco, especially smokeless tobacco.
- Avoid aspirin and NSAIDs in patients with alcohol abuse issues.

- Acetaminophen should be avoided if there is liver damage due to alcohol abuse.
- Opioid analgesics should be avoided in patients recovering from substance abuse.
- Vasoconstrictors should not be used in patients who are actively using cocaine.
- Recommend nonalcoholic mouth rinses.
- Always be on the lookout for the substance user or "shopper."
- Monitor methamphetamine users for meth mouth.

ACADEMIC SKILLS ASSESSMENT

1. Define the following terms:
   a. Psychological dependence
   b. Tolerance
   c. Physical dependence
   d. Withdrawal syndrome
   e. Addiction
   f. Abstinence
   g. Abuse
2. What physical effects occur at low and high doses of caffeine consumption?
3. Can one build tolerance to or become "addicted" to caffeine?
4. What are the symptoms associated with caffeine withdrawal?
5. What is caffeine toxicity, and what are its signs and symptoms?
6. What factors influence the metabolism of alcohol?
7. What are the physiologic effects of alcohol?
8. What are the long-term effects of chronic alcohol consumption?
9. Is caffeine effective in treating acute alcohol intoxication? What should be done?

10. Describe the long-term problems associated with cigarette smoking. Mention several organs that are affected.
11. Discuss the use of smokeless tobacco in adolescents and their idols (think baseball).
12. State oral changes that can occur with smokeless tobacco.
13. Describe the increased use of cigars and hypothesize about probable causes.
14. Describe the dental hygienist's role, if any, in a dental office tobacco cessation program. Could a community role for the dental hygienist be planned?
15. What are some of the products available to people to help them stop smoking or using other smokeless tobacco products?
16. What is "meth mouth," and how can it be treated?
17. What are some concerns of Spice and K-2 that could be of concern to the dental hygienist?
18. Why would the dental hygienist be concerned if the patient was abusing bath salts.

CLINICAL CASE STUDY

Thirty-two-year-old Sam Raphael has been coming to your practice for about 7 years. Lately, he has been very nervous and anxious. His caffeine consumption has increased to the point that he is consuming 10 cups of coffee per day in addition to two espresso-like coffees each afternoon. Work has been rather stressful, and he has taken to smoking one or two cigarettes with each espresso drink. He is also in the middle of relationship problems. Unfortunately, he finds himself having several beers each evening to relax after all the coffee and cigarettes. He tells you all of this as you review his medication/health history.

1. What physical effects occur at low and high doses of caffeine consumption?
2. Can one build tolerance or become "addicted" to caffeine?

3. What are the symptoms associated with caffeine withdrawal?
4. Is Mr. Raphael suffering from caffeine toxicity? Is so, what is this, and what are its signs and symptoms?
5. What factors influence the metabolism of alcohol?
6. What are the physiologic effects of alcohol?
7. What are the, long-term effects of chronic alcohol consumption?
8. Is caffeine effective in treating acute alcohol intoxication? What should be done?
9. Mr. Raphael is upset that he started smoking and would like to stop. What would you recommend and why?
10. What are the oral effects associated with tobacco use?

24

Natural/Herbal Products and Dietary Supplements

ℯ http://evolve.elsevier.com/Haveles/pharmacology

LEARNING OBJECTIVES

1. Discuss why people choose herbal products over traditional medicine.
2. Discuss the federal legislation governing herbal and dietary products.
3. Discuss the safety of herbal and nutritional products, and explain the adverse effects associated with their use and their impact on oral health care.
4. Explain the drug interactions associated with herbal products and their impact on oral health care.
5. Discuss the standardization of herbal products and the Good Manufacturing Practice standard introduced by the US Food and Drug Administration.
6. Discuss the herbal supplements that are used in oral health care.

Herbal medicine, also called *botanical medicine* and *phytomedicine,* refers to the use of a plant's seeds, berries, roots, leaves, bark, or flowers for medicinal purposes. Long practiced outside conventional medicine, herbalism is becoming much more commonplace in Western medicine. More aggressive marketing of the purported health benefits of herbal and dietary supplements has dramatically increased their use during the last decade. Some people use herbal supplements because they are available without a prescription, eliminating the cost and time of visiting a health care professional whose prescription is needed for conventional agents (Fig. 24.1). Others have turned to herbal supplements because of cultural influences, a sense of taking control of one's own health, distrust of physicians, and a lack of health insurance. Also, improvements in analysis and quality control, along with advances in clinical research, show the value of these supplements in the treatment and prevention of disease.

> Patients do not always report supplement use.

The recent trend in the use of natural or herbal substances has seen an exponential rise in the use of these products and the number of people using them. As a result, dental hygienists need to inquire about the use of these products as part of the health history/medication review.

During this growth period, concerns have been raised about adequate safety and efficacy research and about a lack of uniform product standardization. Because they are considered to be natural products or dietary supplements, manufacturers do not have to prove efficacy in treating or preventing a specific disease, nor can they make that claim. However, they can state that herbal or natural products can be used for general health and well-being. Because they are considered natural products or dietary supplements, most patients do not consider them medicine, especially since a prescription is not necessary for their use. Dental hygienists should make it a point to ask about herbal or dietary supplement use because many patients fail to mention them.

Much of what is known about herbal products or supplements has been compiled by the German Commission E, an expert panel composed of physicians, pharmacists, pharmacologists, and biostatisticians. This commission was originally established by the German Federal Health Agency (equivalent to the US Food and Drug Administration [FDA]) to review and analyze the world literature on plant-based products. Commission E monographs contain information regarding the chemistry, pharmacology, toxicology, traditional uses, and, if available, data on clinical trials, epidemiologic studies, and patient case records on herbal products. These monographs are regarded as the most authoritative guide to herbal therapy available today. An English translation is available and is titled *The Complete German Commission E Monographs: Therapeutic Guide to Herbal Medicines.*

LIMITED REGULATION

Dietary Supplement Health and Education Act

More than 20,000 herbal (botanical) and other natural products are available in the United States. The term *natural* has been associated with herbal products because they are primarily derived from plant sources. Herbal products are marketed as dietary supplements in the United States and are not required to comply with safety and efficacy regulations imposed on drug products. Manufacturers cannot make claims of curing conditions, but they can make claims of improving structure or function. The FDA will allow a qualified health claim if there is scientific evidence to support it. Before 1994, the FDA attempted to propose stricter regulations for the herbal supplement industry. However, aggressive lobbying by the dietary supplement industry and thousands of letters from the general public to Congress blocked the proposed regulations.

> US Food and Drug Administration must prove a product is unsafe.

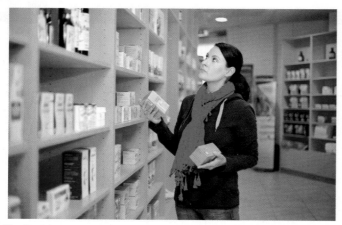

Fig. 24.1 Herbal supplements are widely available without a prescription—in grocery stores, drug stores, and health food stores. (Copyright JupiterImages Corporation.)

Today, herbal products are regulated by the Dietary Supplement Health and Education Act (DSHEA), which exempts vitamins, minerals, and botanical products from meaningful FDA regulation. Before this act, the manufacturer had to prove that an herbal product was safe and effective. Today, the FDA must prove that the product is unsafe. The manufacturer needs only to notify the FDA of any efficacy claims. Changes in the Federal Food, Drug and Cosmetic Act in 2006 now require the supplement industry to report all serious dietary supplement-related adverse drug effects to the FDA. In 2007, the FDA drafted regulations that would require supplement manufacturers to test for purity and to ensure that their products do not contain contaminants and to verify that the contents within the package matched the labeling information. These regulations were approved in August 2007 and were to be phased in during the next 3 years, to be completely in place by the end of 2010. However, when the final bill, the Dietary Supplement Full Implementation and Enforcement Act of 2010, was introduced it was referred back to committee twice. Many in Congress felt that the bill was over regulating the dietary supplement industry. However, the proposed legislation is needed to regulate this growing industry. In 2011, the FDA Food Safety and Modernization Act of 2010 was signed. This provides the FDA with mandatory recall authority for all foods, including dietary supplements, expands facility registration obligations, and requires the FDA to issue new dietary ingredients' guidance.

Package Labeling

Other aspects of the DSHEA prevent the use of therapeutic claims on the label. All herbal products must be labeled as dietary supplements. These products cannot have labels such as "for treatment of hypertension." However, the labels can contain claims of effects on the structure or function of the body. Thus, a natural product could be said to "increase immunity" without a comment about what that might mean to a person's health. Another rule is that information may be provided that may not be necessarily scientific, but it cannot be false or misleading. Again, the responsibility for proof of misleading labeling is in the hands of the FDA.

The DSHEA requires that the following phrase must be included on each natural product's label: "This product is not intended to diagnose, treat, cure, or prevent any disease." This phrase is also required in the advertising of such herbal products. (It is said really quickly in television and radio ads.) Another requirement is that information about the product must be physically separate from the natural product. The product would be on one shelf and the information would be placed in another aisle. It is unclear what benefit separating the information from the product would serve other than having gotten the act passed. Health food store employees help customers obtain the literature and associate it with the products to determine their purchase choices.

SAFETY OF HERBAL AND NUTRITIONAL PRODUCTS

Many consumers consider herbal products to be nontoxic or free of side effects because they are often called "natural" remedies. Most of the herbal products available contain ingredients that have profound pharmacologic effects. Some products may have potential therapeutic effects, and the vast majority have adverse effects and drug interactions. Since 1994, the FDA has investigated more than 800 reports of adverse reactions with more than 100 different ephedra alkaloid-containing products. Adverse effects included insomnia, nervousness, tremor, headaches, hypertension, seizures, arrhythmias, heart attack, stroke, and death. More than 50% of the adverse effects were reported in people younger than 40 years, and another 25% occurred in people 40 to 49 years of age. In 2004, following reports of cardiovascular events with ephedra (ma huang), the FDA issued a regulation prohibiting the sale of all dietary supplements containing ephedrine alkaloids and warned consumers to stop taking the product. In December 2007, the Adverse Events Reporting Law amended the federal Food, Drug and Cosmetic Act to require the reporting of "serious" adverse events for both over-the-counter (OTC) drugs and dietary supplements.

> Treat herbal products as drugs.

Because some herbal products have pharmacologically active ingredients, the dental health professional should acknowledge this fact and treat any herbal product as a drug. Any use of herbal products by the patient should be noted in the patient's chart. Table 24.1 lists examples of selected herbal products, their adverse effects, and implications for the dental hygienist.

Oral Adverse Effects

The most common adverse oral and dental effects of herbal medications are many and include dysgeusia, gingival hyperplasia, intraoral hemorrhage, necrosis, oral candidiasis, oral ulceration, stomatitis, tooth discoloration, and xerostomia, according to research conducted at the Case Western Reserve University School of Medicine. St. John's wort, an herbal supplement used to treat mild depression, causes xerostomia, just as prescribed antidepressants do. Oral ulcers, lip irritation, swelling, and gingival bleeding have been reported with the use of feverfew. There have been reports of increased gingival bleeding with ginkgo, and oral and lingual dyskinesia with the use of kava. Other reports include tongue numbness and taste changes with the use of echinacea.

DRUG INTERACTIONS

Herbal products can interact with conventional drugs, leading to disastrous results. The principal concerns associated with these interactions are increased risk for toxicity and a reduced therapeutic effect. The dental health professional should be aware of this possibility. Several drug-herbal product interactions have been identified and validated. Garlic, Gingko biloba, and feverfew can increase the risk for bleeding when taken in conjunction with antiplatelet drugs or anticoagulants (Fig. 24.2). Ma huang contains ephedrine and can

TABLE 24.1 Selected Natural Herbs: Adverse Effects and Dental Hygiene Implications

Herbal Supplement(s)	Adverse Effect(s)	Dental Hygiene Implications
Feverfew	Oral mucosal irritation, ulcerations	Potential to cause ulcerations. Check oral cavity for ulcerations.
Ephedra (ma-huang)	Tachycardia, hypertension	Monitor blood pressure and pulse rate.
Niacin, yohimbe	Postural hypotension	Raise the chair to the sitting position slowly. Have the patient dangle the legs over the side of the treatment chair for a few minutes and then slowly get out of the treatment chair.
Chaparral, comfrey, kava (oral dose forms)	Hepatotoxicity, bleeding	Reduce the metabolism of many drugs. Patient may require lower doses of those drugs because of the potential for increased bleeding during procedures. Monitor the patient for clotting.
Angelica, clove, feverfew, garlic, ginkgo, ginseng, red clover, high doses of vitamin E	Bleeding	Potential for increased bleeding during procedures. Monitor the patient for clotting.
Coenzyme Q_{10}, echinacea, milk thistle, pomegranate, wormwood	Allergic reactions	Watch for and alert the patient to the possibility of skin rash, stomatitis, angioedema, shortness of breath.

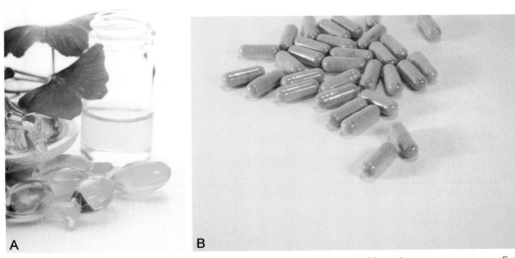

Fig. 24.2 Herbal products can interact with more conventional drugs, with serious consequences. For example, both *Ginkgo biloba* (A) and ginseng (B) can increase the risk of bleeding when taken in conjunction with antiplatelet or anticoagulant agents. (Copyright JupiterImages Corporation.)

increase the heart rate when given with sympathomimetic drugs. St. John's wort can induce the 3A/4 isoenzyme of the cytochrome P-450 system and can increase the metabolism of many different drugs; it can also increase or decrease the effects of local and general anesthetics used in oral health care. Table 24.2 lists examples of drug-herbal product interactions and implications for the dental hygienist.

The most common negative result of drug interactions between traditional drugs used in dentistry and herbal supplements is bleeding. Increased bleeding during dental procedures can lead to a variety of complications and sometimes hospitalization. Dental procedures that can result in bleeding include tooth extractions, periodontal surgeries, root planing, and biopsy. Bleeding can also complicate routine procedures, such as prophylaxis, examinations, and restorations. It is recommended that dentists and dental hygienists counsel their patients to stop using certain herbal supplements prior to any type of dental procedure (Table 24.3).

Unfortunately, there is little information regarding drug interactions with herbal supplements, mostly as a result of the inherent uncertainties regarding herbal products. In many instances, the purity and potency of a product is unknown, the dose is not standardized, package labeling is incomplete or inaccurate, or the product may contain more than one active ingredient. If a patient is taking conventional drugs and herbal supplements and a perceived drug interaction occurs (toxicity or decreased therapeutic effect), it is difficult to determine what was actually responsible for the effect. Until herbal products are standardized and labeling is accurate and comprehensive, it will be difficult to obtain accurate information on possible interactions.

Reliable scientific sources of information regarding herbal supplements are available and are reviewed in Box 24.1.

STANDARDIZATION OF HERBAL PRODUCTS

Standardization is the process by which one or more active ingredients of an herb are identified, and all batches of the herbs produced by a single manufacturer contain the same amount of active ingredient specified on the label. Consumers expect that all prescription

TABLE 24.2 Selected Herbal Supplements and Dental Hygiene Implications

Herbal Supplement(s)	Interacting Drug	Dental Hygiene Implications
Cranberry	Opioid analgesics, antidepressants, some antibiotics	Large amounts of cranberries can reduce urinary pH and potentially increase the excretion of these drugs.
Black cohosh, butterbur, *Echinacea purpurea*	Acetaminophen, NSAIDs, macrolide antibiotics, azole antifungals	Additive hepatotoxicity. Avoid the use of herbal supplements with these drugs.
Coleus forskolin, goldenseal, gotu kola, hawthorn, melatonin, nettle root, passion flower, valerian root	Benzodiazepines, barbiturates, CNS depressants, opioids	Potential to lower blood pressure. Monitor blood pressure at each visit. Watch for orthostatic hypotension. Potential to increase the risk for sedation. Remind the patient of this risk.
Dong quai	Antihypertensives, opioids, benzodiazepines, CNS depressants, barbiturates, aspirin, warfarin	Increased risk for postural hypotension. Monitor blood pressure. Raise the patient slowly from the supine to sitting position. Have the patient dangle the legs over the side of the treatment chair for several minutes before getting up. Increased bleeding. Monitor the patient for clotting.
Bilberry fruit, bromelain, chamomile, Cordyceps, coenzyme Q_{10}, evening primrose, garlic, ginger, ginseng, ginkgo, feverfew, guggul, horse chestnut, kava, licorice, oil of cloves, turmeric	Warfarin, heparin products, aspirin, clopidogrel, NSAIDs	Increased bleeding. Monitor the patient for clotting. Advise the patient to stop the herbal supplements 2 weeks before procedures that result in bleeding.
Guar gum	Penicillins	Decrease absorption of the penicillins. Use the gum 1 hr after taking the penicillin product.
St John's wort	Induces the cytochrome P-450 isoenzymes CYP3A/4, CYP1A2, and CYP2 Many drug interactions	Advise the patient of enhanced sedation with CNS depressants. Increased potential for photosensitivity when used with tetracycline. Advise patients to use sunblock and stay out of the sun. Increased use for serotonin syndrome if used with tramadol or meperidine.
Yohimbe	Indirect-acting sympathomimetics	Risk for hypertension. Monitor blood pressure and pulse.

CNS, Central nervous system; *NSAIDs*, nonsteroidal antiinflammatory drugs.

TABLE 24.3 Recommendations for Discontinuing Herbal Supplements Prior to a Dental Procedure

Herbal Supplement	Recommendation
Garlic and ginseng	Stop at least 7 days prior to procedure.
St John's wort	Stop at least 5 days prior to procedure.
Ginkgo	Stop at least 36 hr prior to procedure.
Kava and ephedra	Stop at least 24 hr prior to procedure.

and nonprescription drug products are standardized and that what is printed on the label is actually in the drug in the container. However, consumers may not expect the same level of standardization with an herbal supplement because herbal supplements are considered food products, or they may just assume that such standardization has taken place. A major consequence of a lack of standardization is the variability of the quantity of the known or supposed active ingredient. In a study of 44 feverfew products, 32% contained less than the minimum 0.2% of parthenolide, which is proposed as the necessary primary active ingredient and concentration. Another 23% did not contain any detectable levels of parthenolide.

GOOD MANUFACTURING PRACTICE

Good Manufacturing Practice (GMP) standards were introduced by the FDA in 2003 to ensure that dietary supplements are devoid of adulterants, contaminants, and impurities and that package labels accurately reflect the identity, purity, quality, and strength of what is actually inside the packages. Package labeling should also include both active and all inactive ingredients present in the formulation. It was not until 2007 that GMP standards mandated that manufacturers establish quality-control procedures that would prevent mislabeled or underfilled bottles; variations in tablet size, color, and potency; and the prevention of contamination with drugs, bacteria, pesticides, glass, lead, and other potential contaminates. These regulations require manufacturers of herbal supplements to test their products for purity and provide accurate labeling information for consumers. However, testing is left to the discretion of the manufacturer, and the FDA does not inspect all manufacturing facilities for compliance. Only those manufacturers that have demonstrated unsafe practices are subject to more frequent inspections. If a supplement is found to be contaminated or mislabeled, the FDA considers it to be adulterated or misbranded. Larger companies were to comply with these regulations by 2008, and companies with less than 20 employees had until 2010. Despite these much-needed standards, manufacturers are not obligated to prove that their products are safe or effective.

BOX 24.1   Scientific Sources of Information for Herbal Supplements

Journals
- *American Journal of Chinese Medicine*
- *Journal of Alternative and Complementary Medicine: Research on Paradigm, Practice, and Policy*
- *Alternative Therapies in Clinical Practice*
- *Alternative Therapies in Health and Medicine*
- *Alternative Medicine Review*
- *Focus on Alternative and Complementary Therapies*
- *Journal of Herbal Pharmacotherapy*

Databases
- Alternative and Allied Medicine Database
- Centralized Information Services for Complementary Medicine
- Cochrane Complementary Medicine Field
- Natural Products Alert
- Natural Medicines Comprehensive Database

Websites
- Research Council for Complementary Medicine: www.rccm.org.uk
- American Botanical Council: www.herbalgram.org
- National Institute of Health, National Center for Complementary and Alternative Medicine: http://nccam.nih.gov
- The Cochrane Library: www.cochrane.co.uk
- Center for Food Safety and Applied Nutrition: http://vm.cfsan.fda.gov
- International Bibliographic Information on Dietary Supplements: http://dietary-supplements.info.nih.gov/databases/ibids.html
- Micromedex Internet Healthcare Services: www.micromedex.com/products/hcs/
- National Institutes of Health's Office of Dietary Supplements: http://.ods.od.nih.gov/databases/ibids/html
- American Herbal Products Association: www.ahpa.org
- Facts and Comparisons: http://www.factsandcomparisons.com/
- healthfinder: http://healthfinder.gov

Manufacturers are not required to prove that their products are safe or effective.

Rather than wait for the GMP standards to be implemented, the United States Pharmacopeia Convention (usually called USP like its publication) began testing herbal supplements for quality. A "seal of approval" is given to products that meet their standards, which are very similar to those of the GMP. The USP requires that manufacturers pay for the testing. The Federal Trade Commission (FTC) has forced some herbal supplement manufacturers to remove advertisements with false or unsubstantiated claims.

HERBAL SUPPLEMENTS USED IN ORAL HEALTH CARE

Herbal supplements are used in several different oral health care products. They include essential oils (EOs) that are used in mouth rinses (thymol, eucalyptol, or menthol), xylitol, acemannan, oil of cloves, and triclosan.

Acemannan

Acemannan hydrogel is an extract of the aloe vera plant leaf that has immunomodulating properties. It is available as an OTC topical patch to reduce the healing time of aphthous ulcerations. It is thought to cause the ulceration to heal at a faster rate. Acemannan hydrogel was found to be as effective as both prescription and nonprescription products in healing aphthous ulcerations.

Essential Oil Mouth Rinse

More than 20 mouth rinses that contain the EOs thymol, eucalyptol, and menthol have been approved by the American Dental Association (ADA). EOs are proposed to have a bacteriostatic effect on oral pathogens known to cause plaque and gingivitis. Clinical trials have shown that EOs are effective in protecting against plaque and gingivitis.

Oil of Cloves (Eugenol)

Oil of cloves has been used for many years as a topical analgesic for dental pain. This nonprescription product is used empirically by dental professionals. There are no published trials that confirm its efficacy. The proposed mechanism of action of oil of cloves is unclear, but it is thought to affect pulpal nerves in some way to deaden pain.

Triclosan

Triclosan is an herbal-based product that has been shown to significantly reduce plaque and gingivitis in comparison with placebo dentifrice. One triclosan-containing product has received the ADA's Seal of Acceptance for its antigingivitis effect.

Xylitol

Xylitol is a naturally occurring sweetener derived from plants that can be extracted from birch bark, raspberries, plums, and corn fiber. Its sweetness is comparable to that of sucrose, but it has one fewer carbon than sucrose and cannot be metabolized by *Streptococcus mutans* to form acids. As a result, xylitol consumption reduces *S. mutans* levels, yielding antibacterial and cariostatic effects (Fig. 24.3). Xylitol's antibacterial effects inhibit the ability of microbes to adhere to and grow in plaque.

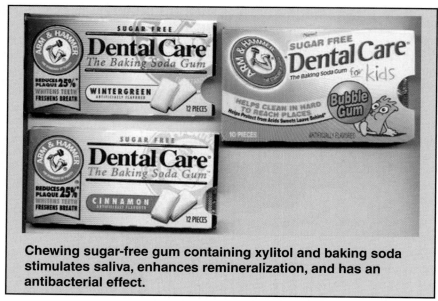

Chewing sugar-free gum containing xylitol and baking soda stimulates saliva, enhances remineralization, and has an antibacterial effect.

Fig. 24.3 Xylitol-containing products, such as sugar-free gum with xylitol, can help prevent caries. (From Darby ML, Walsh MM. *Dental Hygiene: Theory and Practice*. 4th ed. St. Louis: Saunders; 2015.)

DENTAL HYGIENE CONSIDERATIONS

Dental hygienists need to know about these products to:
- Identify clinical considerations for commonly used herbal products.
- Make personal choices in the use of herbal products on the basis of evidence.
- Find out about undisclosed medical conditions that the patient may be self-treating with herbal products. By knowing the indication(s)

for the herb, the dental health care worker can be alerted to the presence of unreported diseases. (For example, if a patient is taking St. John's wort, he or she may be treating depression.)
- Identify adverse effects associated with herbal products.
- Identify drug interactions with drugs that might affect the patient.
- Identify sources of oral health care implications of herbal products.

ACADEMIC SKILLS ASSESSMENT

1. What is the Dietary and Supplement Health and Education Act, and how does it regulate herbal products?
2. List four herbal supplement-drug interactions and their impact on oral health care.
3. What is the process of standardization of herbal products?
4. What is GMP, and how does it relate to herbal supplements?
5. What is acemannan, and how is it used in oral health care?
6. What is the role of EO mouth rinse in oral health care?
7. What is the role of triclosan in oral health care?
8. What is the role of xylitol in oral health care?

CLINICAL CASE STUDY

Martha Smith-Lewis is a 67-year-old woman who has been coming to your practice for close to 20 years. She has been a healthy woman with no chronic health problems. Today she comes in for her scheduled oral health maintenance examination. She tells you that she has been having problems remembering things lately and that she has been feeling down. Mrs. Smith-Lewis did some research on her own and has chosen to self-treat her low mood with St. John's wort and has started taking a multivitamin with ginkgo to help with her memory problems. During her oral examination, you and the dentist both note a cavity that needs to be filled. That tooth was bothering Mrs. Smith-Lewis prior to her visit, so she self-treated with ibuprofen.
1. What is St. John's wort, and what is it used to treat?

2. What are some of the dental hygiene implications associated with St. John's wort, central nervous depressant drugs, and tetracycline?
3. What is ginkgo used to treat? Is there FDA approval for its treatment?
4. What are some of the adverse dental effects associated with ginkgo?
5. What drugs does gingko interact with?
6. Should either of these drugs be discontinued before Mrs. Smith-Lewis undergoes a dental procedure? Why or why not?
7. If these drugs should be discontinued before a dental procedure, how soon before the procedure should Mrs. Smith-Lewis be told to stop taking them?
8. How would you counsel Mrs. Smith-Lewis about using herbal supplements without her physician's knowledge?

25

Oral Conditions and Their Treatment

http://evolve.elsevier.com/Haveles/pharmacology

LEARNING OBJECTIVES

1. Name several common infectious lesions of the oral cavity and summarize the treatments for each.
2. Describe immune reactions resulting in canker sores and lichen planus and discuss the treatments for each.
3. Name several oral conditions that result from inflammation and the measures used to treat them.
4. Discuss treatment options for xerostomia and name several other possible drug-induced oral side effects.
5. Discuss the pharmacologic agents most commonly used to treat oral lesions.

The dental hygienist is the first professional that patients visit when they notice a lesion in the oral cavity. Patients often ask the dental hygienist and dentist, "What is this? How do I get rid of it? How long will it take to go away? Why do I have it? Is it cancer?" Patients who have even visited several physicians may appear at the office with commonly seen oral lesions. The first step is the diagnosis. Obtaining an in-depth history of the problem (by listening and asking open-ended questions) and examining the lesion can often result in a diagnosis or potential diagnoses. Depending on the diagnosis, the lesion may require only reassurance, palliative treatment, specific treatment, or even surgical intervention.

This chapter discusses a few of the more common oral lesions and the medications used for their treatment. Before individual oral lesions are discussed, commonly used treatments for several types of lesions are described.

INFECTIOUS LESIONS

Acute Necrotizing Ulcerative Gingivitis

Acute necrotizing ulcerative gingivitis: Vincent infection.

Acute necrotizing ulcerative gingivitis (ANUG), which is also called *Vincent infection* and *trench mouth,* has both bacteriologic (spirochetes) and environmental (stress, debilitation) factors (Fig. 25.1). ANUG is a spreading ulcer associated with a distinctive odor; the ulcerated area begins at the interdental papillae. The main symptoms are painful bleeding gums and ulceration of the interdental papillae. It is classified as a necrotizing periodontal disease along with necrotizing ulcerative periodontitis. The severe gingival pain that occurs with ANUG distinguishes it from the more common chronic periodontitis, which is not painful. ANUG is the acute form of necrotizing ulcerative gingivitis (NUG), which is the usual course of the disease. If not properly treated, or if neglected, it can become chronic and/or recurrent.

Good oral hygiene is the cornerstone of treatment, but other modalities have been recommended. Mouthwashes, such as hydrogen peroxide, or saline rinses assist through their flushing action. If pain or an elevated temperature accompanies ANUG, aspirin, nonsteroidal antiinflammatory drugs, or acetaminophen can be recommended. If eating is difficult, food supplements, such as Meritene, Sustacal, or Sustagen, may be used instead of meals. Vitamin supplementation is useful only if the patient has a vitamin deficiency. The food supplements mentioned contain the required vitamins and minerals. Antibiotics should be considered only if the patient is immunosuppressed or there is evidence of systemic involvement (see Table 7.1). Antibiotics useful for the immunosuppressed patient with ANUG include penicillin VK and metronidazole. Topical chlorhexidine gluconate, which is active against gram-positive and gram-negative organisms and *Candida* organisms, is used as a rinse for ANUG. The majority of ANUG cases respond dramatically to local treatment (oral prophylaxis with scaling).

Herpes Infections

Herpes simplex herpes labialis: fever blister or cold sore.

Primary herpetic gingivostomatitis (Fig. 25.2), or primary herpes, is the manifestation of the initial herpes infection. Occurring principally in infants and children, it is caused by the **herpes simplex** virus (HSV). Because it is often associated with or follows other infections, it is also known as a *fever blister* or *cold sore.* The painful lesions may appear throughout the oral mucosa. Beginning as an erythematous area, numerous ulcers with a circumscribed area of erythema appear. The ulcers can coalesce to form larger irregular ulcers with gray centers. Other signs of herpes include the formation of vesicles that become scabbed. Systemic symptoms that are more severe in infants can develop and, in some cases, can be life threatening.

Without treatment, herpes is self-limiting in the patient with normal immunity. Approximately 80% to 90% of the adult population has been exposed to HSV. HSV-1 is involved in most oral lesions, and transmission is usually not sexual. HSV-2 is usually responsible for genital herpes and is transmitted sexually. Both HSV-1 and HSV-2 can spread to other parts of the body, for example, the eyes, genitals, and fingers (herpetic whitlow). When the lesions are in the vesicle stage, they are contagious, and the virus can survive for several hours on surfaces (one should think about possibilities in the dental office).

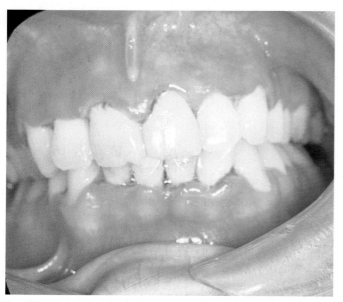

Fig. 25.1 Necrotizing ulcerative gingivitis. (From Ibsen OAC, Phelan JA. *Oral Pathology for the Dental Hygienist.* 6th ed. St. Louis: Saunders; 2014.)

After the primary episode, the patient may experience recurrent outbreaks (cold sores or fever blisters) that occur at irregular and variable intervals. Events that may precipitate a herpetic outbreak include sunlight (ultraviolet light), hormonal changes such as menstruation, lip pulling, a rubber dam, biting an anesthetized lip, emotional stress, and other infections (e.g., a viral respiratory infection). According to the Centers for Disease Control and Prevention, patients with active herpetic lesions receive dental treatment provided that either emergency dental care is required or the treatment is for the lesions only. All other care should be delayed until the lesions have healed. If the patient requires care, one should repeatedly apply a nonpetroleum lubricant to the lips and should be careful when manipulating the lips to minimize the trauma from a dental appointment. The effectiveness of the antiviral drugs varies depending on whether the outbreak is a primary episode or recurrence and whether the patient is immunocompromised or not.

Treatment

The treatment of herpes may include an antiviral agent, depending on the patient and the episode. Most instances of herpes simplex can be treated with symptomatic measures.

Symptomatic treatment of lesions includes swishing the mouth with topical diphenhydramine (DPH) (Benadryl) elixir or viscous lidocaine and spitting it out. Antiviral agents, such as acyclovir,

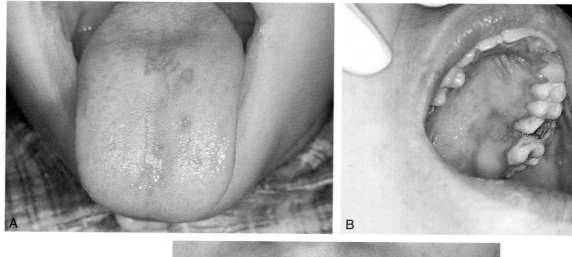

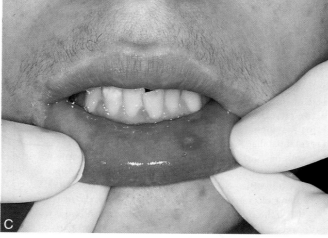

Fig. 25.2 (A) Primary herpetic gingivostomatitis in a child. (B) Primary herpetic gingivostomatitis in an adolescent. Note the painful swollen gingiva. (C) Primary herpetic gingivostomatitis in an adolescent. (From Ibsen OAC, Phelan JA. *Oral Pathology for the Dental Hygienist.* 6th ed. St. Louis: Saunders; 2014.)

TABLE 25.1   Dosing of US Food and Drug Administration-Approved Antiviral Agents in the Management of Herpes Labialis

Drug	Indication	Dosing
Acyclovir topical cream (Zovirax)	Treatment of recurrent herpes labialis in adults and adolescents 12 years and older	Apply 5 times a day for 4 days
Acyclovir systemic ointment (Zovirax)	Treatment of herpes labialis in immunocompromised patients	Apply q3h, for a total of 6 times a day while awake, for 7 days
Valacyclovir systemic (Valtrex)	Treatment of herpes labialis	2 g orally every 12 hours for 1 day
Famciclovir (Famvir)	Treatment of herpes labialis in adults	1500 mg oral in a single dose
Penciclovir topical (Denavir)	Recurrent herpes labialis in immunocompetent patients	Apply every 2 hours while awake for 4 days
Docosanol 10% topical cream (Abreva)	Nonprescription treatment for herpes labialis	Apply 5 times daily

valacyclovir, and penciclovir, are useful in certain herpes simplex infections (Table 25.1). Docosanol is another antiviral that is available without a prescription.

Acyclovir

Acyclovir is available in tablet, capsule, oral suspension, ointment, cream, and parenteral forms. This discussion is limited to the oral and topical products; parenteral products are not discussed in depth.

The approved indications for oral acyclovir include the treatment of primary and recurrent HSV in the immunocompromised patient. In the nonimmunocompromised patient, oral acyclovir is indicated for both treatment of the primary (first episode) outbreak and prophylaxis. Used prophylactically, it reduces the number and severity of recurrent outbreaks. Acyclovir should not be used prophylactically to prevent minor outbreaks because excessive use may lead to resistant strains of herpes.

> Oral acyclovir proved effective when taken prophylactically.

Administration of oral acyclovir can be used before situations known to precipitate herpes lesions, such as a ski trip or wedding (stress), or a dental appointment that will produce trauma. The usual prophylactic dose of acyclovir is 400 mg twice a day (bid). It has yet to be shown that oral acyclovir has a significant clinical effect in the treatment of recurrent lesions in the immunocompetent patient. It may shorten the time to healing or the pain by a small amount.

Topical acyclovir ointment does not affect the course of recurrent herpes in the immunocompetent patient. This may be a result of poor penetration or delay in applying the ointment. Cell damage may be irreversible by the time symptoms are noticed. Topical acyclovir cream was recently approved to treat herpes labialis in immunocompetent patients.

The incidence of resistance of the herpes organisms to acyclovir is increasing. If herpes lesions fail to respond to therapy, the virus should be tested for susceptibility to acyclovir. Resistant strains have been identified, especially in patients who test positive for human immunodeficiency virus (HIV) are on long-term acyclovir therapy. This is the same principle that produces antibiotic resistance in the general population.

Penciclovir

> Penciclovir: reduces lesion duration and viral shedding by 0.7 days.

Penciclovir (Denavir), which is available only topically, has been shown to reduce by one-half day the duration and pain of lesions on the lips and face associated with both primary and recurrent herpes simplex. The advantages of penciclovir over acyclovir are that penciclovir can achieve

a higher concentration within the cell and that it remains in the cells longer. Table 25.1 summarizes the indications for the antiviral agents.

Docosanol (Abreva). Docosanol is the only antiviral drug available without a prescription to treat recurrent HSV. It is available as a topical 10% cream and should be applied at the first sign of symptoms. It has been shown to reduce the duration by about one half day in patients with recurrent HSV.

Famciclovir and valacyclovir. Both famciclovir and valacyclovir are prodrugs that are converted to active antiviral agents. They are indicated in the treatment of acute localized varicella-zoster infections and recurrent genital herpes in immunocompetent adults. Valacyclovir is also indicated for the treatment of herpes labialis. Ganciclovir is indicated for serious cytomegalovirus retinitis in immunocompromised patients. It may be effective in some acyclovir-resistant organisms.

Treatment of symptoms

> Diphenhydramine or lidocaine topically.

Palliative treatment involves treating the patient's symptoms. In a primary episode of herpes, fever may be managed by the administration of acetaminophen or by sponging the affected area with tepid water. The discomfort associated with herpes may be relieved by swishing DPH. This product is available under many trade names, for example, Diphen Cough, Diphenhist, Genahist, and Siladryl. All of these products are alcohol-free liquids. Perhaps the most commonly available proprietary product is Benadryl. The strength of all the products is 12.5 mg of the active ingredient per 5 mL (1 teaspoonful). Other agents, such as viscous lidocaine (Xylocaine) and combinations of DPH with kaolin (Kaopectate), calcium carbonate (Maalox Quick Dissolve), and simethicone (Mylanta Gas), are recommended for use in the oral cavity. Because antihistamines, such as DPH, are similar in structure to local anesthetics, they have some local anesthetic action and can therefore reduce the pain.

Sodium carboxymethylcellulose paste (Orabase plain or with benzocaine) may reduce discomfort. Food supplements may be used if intake of food is impossible (because of oral discomfort). These remedies are the same as those used for patients receiving cancer chemotherapy agents. Corticosteroids are contraindicated because they suppress the cellular immunity that inhibits viral infections.

Candidiasis (Moniliasis)

> Candidiasis often secondary to the use of broad-spectrum antibiotics.

Candidiasis, a fungal infection caused by *Candida albicans,* often affects the oral and vaginal mucosa. Candidiasis occurs when the organisms multiply and predominate. Because *Candida* is part of the normal oral flora, it is always present in small numbers. When other flora are suppressed, *Candida* can predominate.

When a patient presents with oral candidiasis, it is important that the dental health care worker search exhaustively for potential predisposing factors. Systemic antibiotic treatment, especially with broad-spectrum antibiotics such as tetracycline, can predispose a patient to candidiasis. A dental health care worker may be the first professional to diagnose HIV-positive patients or those with acquired immunodeficiency syndrome (AIDS) (Fig. 25.3).

Although candidiasis can appear in several different forms, the lesions are typical and can usually be diagnosed from their clinical appearance. They may be confirmed by culture. Topical products available to treat oral candidiasis include nystatin products (aqueous suspension, vaginal tablets [used as lozenges], and lozenges [pastilles]), and clotrimazole troches (see Chapter 8).

With chronic candidiasis (Fig. 25.4), ketoconazole tablets taken orally once daily can be used. Systemic alternatives include either fluconazole or itraconazole. All are effective, but they should be continued for at least 2 weeks and/or at least 2 or 3 days past the time when the symptoms have disappeared.

Angular Cheilitis/Cheilosis

> Angular cheilitis: cracks in corners of mouth.

Angular cheilitis appears as simple redness, fissures, erosion, ulcers, and crusting located at the angles of the mouth, which may or may not be painful (Fig. 25.5). Most cases of cheilitis are associated with a mixed infection. Often *C. albicans* infection is present, and not uncommonly both *Candida* and gram-positive bacteria, such as streptococci and/or staphylococci, also invade the lesion.

Predisposing factors include moisture from drooling (moist areas are more likely to be infected with fungus). In the past, a decrease in vertical dimension of occlusion was thought to contribute to angular cheilitis, but later evidence has not shown this to be true.

Depending on the presentation of the patient's lesion, therapy is addressed toward treating the secondary infection(s). If *Candida* organisms are present, treatment with an antifungal agent (see Chapter 8) is indicated. Examples of topical antifungal agents are nystatin, clotrimazole, and miconazole. If inflammation is present, some practitioners prescribe a combination of an antifungal agent mixed with a topical steroid (e.g., Mycolog [nystatin (Mycostatin) plus triamcinolone acetonide (TAC; Kenalog)]). One concern, which may or may not be clinically significant, about using steroids with a fungal infection is that steroids inhibit the inflammatory reaction associated with cellular immunity (this is the reaction that normally fights fungal infections).

If a bacterial overgrowth is suspected, the organisms responsible are usually similar to staphylococci and streptococci. To treat this bacterial infection, systemic penicillinase-resistant penicillins, such as dicloxacillin, are indicated (see Chapter 7). Mupirocin (Bactroban) is a topical antibacterial useful in the treatment of staphylococcal and streptococcal infections. Using mupirocin decreases the likelihood of adverse reactions, and mupirocin is as effective as

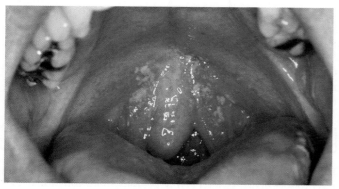

Fig. 25.3 Candidiasis in a patient with human immunodeficiency virus infection. (From Ibsen OAC, Phelan JA. *Oral Pathology for the Dental Hygienist.* 6th ed. St. Louis: Saunders; 2014.)

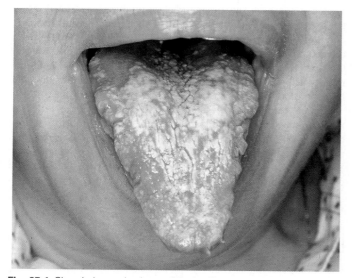

Fig. 25.4 Chronic hyperplastic candidiasis. (From Ibsen OAC, Phelan JA. *Oral Pathology for the Dental Hygienist.* 6th ed. St. Louis: Saunders; 2014.)

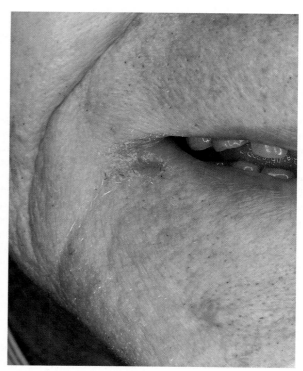

Fig. 25.5 Angular cheilitis. (From Ibsen OAC, Phelan JA. *Oral Pathology for the Dental Hygienist.* 6th ed. St. Louis: Saunders; 2014.)

systemic penicillinase-resistant penicillins (see Chapter 7). A topical antifungal agent and mupirocin can be used concomitantly if both are indicated.

Although rarely produced by a deficiency of vitamin B$_6$ (pyridoxine) or B$_2$ (riboflavin), cheilosis can result from deficiencies of these vitamins. Vitamin B supplements would be useful, but only if a vitamin deficiency exists.

Alveolar Osteitis

> Dry socket increases with birth control pills, smoking, and diabetes.

Alveolar osteitis, or "dry socket," occurs in 2% to 3% of all tooth extractions, most commonly in the lower molar region, where the incidence is considerably higher than in other areas. Alveolar osteitis is thought to be caused by loss or necrosis of the blood clot that has formed in the extraction site, exposing the underlying bone. The exposed bone is severely painful. Predisposing factors include oral contraceptive use and menstrual cycle phase. Smoking, especially after extraction, can increase the likelihood of dry socket. Inhaling on a cigarette produces a negative pressure in the oral cavity that may dislodge the clot.

Infection, swelling, elevated temperature, lymphadenopathy, and a foul odor may be present. Treatment consists of rinsing with saline water and debridement, placement of a pack, analgesics, and supportive therapy. There is some indication that local placement of antibiotics may reduce the incidence of dry socket, but aseptic techniques, proper suturing techniques, and minimal trauma should be used as prophylactic measures. Most literature does not recommend the use of prophylactic antibiotics. If infection is present, antibiotics are indicated (as treatment not prophylaxis). Antibiotics may be indicated in patients at high risk for infection.

IMMUNE REACTIONS

Recurrent Aphthous Stomatitis

> Recurrent aphthous stomatitis: canker sore.

Recurrent aphthous stomatitis (RAS), which is sometimes referred to as a canker sore, is a common oral lesion occurring in about 20% of the population. It is seen in patients older than 20 years and has an unknown etiology, although an involvement of the immune system is suspected.

RAS manifests clinically as a few small to many large ulcers. The ulcers can even coalesce into giant ulcers. Although three distinct types have been clinically identified—minor, major, and herpetiforme—the most common form of aphthous ulcers is the minor type (Fig. 25.6).

The etiology of aphthous stomatitis involves an immunologic component and may be associated with a focal immune dysfunction in which T lymphocytes play a significant role. The ratio of T-helper (CD4$^+$) cells to T-suppressor/cytotoxic (CD8$^+$) cells is decreased. An increase in the CD8$^+$ cells is seen. The oral mucosa is destroyed by lymphocytes.

Many hypotheses have been advanced concerning the etiology of RAS, including the following: an allergenic/hypersensitivity reaction (endogenous [autoimmune], exogenous [hyperimmune]), genetic, hematologic, hormones, infection, nutrition, and nonspecific events such as trauma and stress. Another hypothesis is that it is a hypersensitivity reaction to the sodium lauryl sulfate present in many over-the-counter (OTC) products, including most toothpastes Table 25.2 contains a list of several sodium lauryl sulfate free toothpastes which have been developed as a result of the concern with sodium lauryl sulfate.

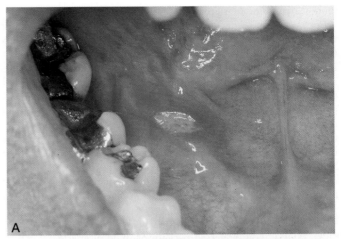

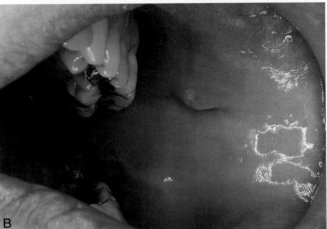

Fig. 25.6 (A) Example of a minor aphthous ulcer. (B) Minor aphthous ulcer on the buccal mucosa on the papilla of Stensen duct. (From Ibsen OAC, Phelan JA. *Oral Pathology for the Dental Hygienist*. 6th ed. St. Louis: Saunders; 2014.)

TABLE 25.2 Toothpastes (Dentifrices) That Do Not Contain Sodium Lauryl Sulfate

Dentifrice	American Dental Association Approved?
CloSYS	Yes
Sensodyne Fresh Mint, Fresh Impact	Yes
Sensodyne-Proenamel	No
Tom's of Maine Botanically Bright	No
Uncle Harrys's Natural Toothpaste, Cinnamon	No

Many products with almost identical names made by the same company do contain sodium lauryl sulfate. Several Tom's of Maine products contain sodium lauryl sulfate. The ingredients are listed on toothpaste tubes.

Corticosteroids

Corticosteroids have been the mainstay of therapy for RAS for many years. Topical steroids, such as fluocinonide and betamethasone, are used to reduce the inflammation associated with the lesions. Topical corticosteroids are available in different strengths and potencies (see Chapter 16). The amount of antiinflammatory action present depends on the strength of the steroid; however, the possibility for adverse reactions associated with the corticosteroids rises with the strength of the steroid. Creams or gels are more easily applied than ointments (greasy base), but gels, because they contain alcohol, can cause burning. Examples of topical steroids are TAC, clobetasol, and fluocinonide.

Another base, carboxymethylcellulose paste (Orabase), is a plasticized base that hardens into a plastic-like plaster. Steroids are incorporated into this paste, which is applied after the area is dried. Patient opinions differ with respect to this base. Some like its plastic consistency and covering of the lesion, but others dislike the soft, shell-like inflexible lump of base. Orabase is available plain or mixed with either hydrocortisone or TAC.

In severe cases of RAS, a short course of systemic steroids (40 mg/day) may be indicated.

Diphenhydramine

DPH alone is now preferred because of its local anesthetic action. Tetracycline suspension mixed with nystatin and DPH has been advocated.

Immunosuppressives

> Immunosuppressives: last resort.

As a last resort, immunosuppressive agents, such as azathioprine (Imuran), methotrexate (Rheumatrex), and cyclosporine (Sandimmune), have been used to treat severe aphthous ulcers. Other immunomodulating agents, such as thalidomide and interferon, also have been used. Thalidomide use is only approved for those patients that also have HIV infection.

Tetracycline has been used in the past, but current thinking is that adding tetracycline suspension to mixtures does not increase the therapeutic effect. Chlorhexidine (Peridex) has been used to manage this condition.

Lichen Planus

Lichen planus is a skin condition that often involves lesions on the oral mucous membranes (Fig. 25.7). The oral lesions are present without the skin lesions in 65% of cases. Lichen planus can manifest in three forms: striated, plaquelike, and erosive (contains the atrophic and bullous subtypes). The most characteristic type is hypertrophic lichen planus; this lesion has a white lacelike pattern that intersects to form a reticular pattern.

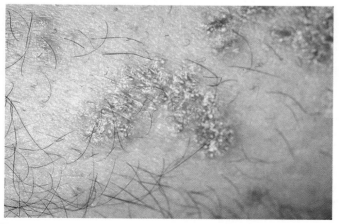

Fig. 25.7 Skin lesions of lichen planus. (From Ibsen OAC, Phelan JA. *Oral Pathology for the Dental Hygienist*. 6th ed. St. Louis: Saunders; 2014.)

Symptoms of pain vary between no pain and extreme pain, depending on the presence of ulceration. The etiology of lichen planus is unknown, but current hypotheses include viral infection, autoimmune disease, and hypersensitivity reaction to an unknown agent. The treatment for lichen planus depends on symptoms and involves oral and topical steroids, oral retinoids, and immunosuppressants.

MISCELLANEOUS ORAL CONDITIONS

Geographic Tongue

With geographic tongue, the tongue may have lesions that typically appear to be a "map of the world" with the lesions appearing to be the continents. Usually, the lesions have red centers with a white hyperkeratotic margin. There are changes in the patterns over time, and they may even disappear. The lesions are typically asymptomatic. However, some patients may complain of soreness and burning, which could be attributed to spicy foods or alcohol. The etiology of geographic tongue is unknown, but the condition may be related to hormonal changes, stress, infection, psoriasis, or autoimmune diseases. Treatment includes reassurance and avoidance of irritating food and alcohol.

Burning Mouth or Tongue Syndrome

Burning mouth or tongue syndrome has been called glossodynia and glossopyrosis (*pyro*, burn). With this syndrome, the oral cavity commonly appears normal, but the patient gives a history of experiencing a discomfort described as pain or a burning sensation that increases in severity through the day.

Glossodynia, painful tongue, is divided into two types: with and without observable alterations on the tongue. It can be caused by many conditions, both local and systemic. Because the tongue is sensitive, small inflammation of fungiform papillae or small trauma from a tooth can be extremely painful. Other visible changes in the tongue are atrophy of the filiform papillae and generalized redness. Burning, stinging, or itching may occur.

The nature of the psychological component of this disease is unclear, but it is known that the presence of chronic disease can lead to depression and anxiety. Patients often are concerned that the cause of their problem may be related to malignancy. Scientific study must be done to determine its cause.

The etiology of burning tongue has not been elucidated, but numerous hypotheses have been proposed, including xerostomia, candidiasis, acid reflux, nutritional deficiency (B_{12}, folate, or iron), immunologic reaction, hormonal changes, allergic reaction, inflammatory process, psychogenic reaction, and idiopathic reaction. (The variety of hypotheses indicates that the cause of burning tongue has not yet been determined.)

The treatment of burning tongue syndrome depends on the particular etiology the practitioner believes in. Some clinicians treat the patient as they would if the patient had candidiasis. Others test for vitamin deficiencies. Palliative therapy involves using topical DPH to relieve the symptoms. Tricyclic antidepressants, such as amitriptyline, can be used on a trial basis, beginning with a dose of 10 mg at bedtime and slowly raising the amount until an effective dose is achieved (up to 150 mg/day). Amitriptyline is used for two effects. It is thought that depression may play a role in this syndrome, and the amitriptyline may treat the depression. However, this is unlikely because the dose used is not antidepressant and the onset of action against the tongue problem is much quicker than the antidepressant effect of amitriptyline. The second mechanism of amitriptyline's proposed effect is that the agent is acting as an adjunct in the management of chronic pain. Amitriptyline has been shown to be effective in chronic pain. Additional studies are needed to determine whether any psychotropic agents might be effective in treating burning tongue.

INFLAMMATION

Pericoronitis

Pericoronitis is inflammation of the tissue around the crown of the tooth. This term, most commonly applied to partially erupted third molars, refers to an inflammatory response that is produced when food and bacteria become trapped between the operculum and the tooth. Periodontal pockets can become painful and swell. If the condition is observed early in its course, debridement with saline irrigation and the use of warm saline rinses will rectify the situation. In severe pericoronitis, debridement is still the primary treatment. If the affected tooth is to be extracted, extraction can prevent further episodes of pericoronitis. With erupting third molars, repeated episodes may occur. Analgesics can be used for the discomfort. Infection, usually managed by local treatment, may rapidly spread in debilitated patients and should be aggressively treated with antibiotics.

Postirradiation Caries

Changes in saliva after radiation therapy and lack of proper plaque control can rapidly accelerate the rate of dental caries. Generalized cervical decay within the first year after radiation therapy can result. Meticulous oral hygiene, reinforced by the hygienist, short duration between subsequent recall appointments, use of artificial salivas, and self-application of sodium fluoride gel four times daily in a bite guard are recommended.

Root Sensitivity

Sensitivity of exposed root surfaces may be precipitated by heat, cold, and sweet or sour foods. Occlusal trauma may produce irritation to the exposed dentinal tubules; occlusal adjustment is the treatment. Roots exposed by periodontal surgery, extensive root planing, or accumulation of plaque and its byproducts are more difficult to manage. Applications of glycerin with burnishing, sodium fluoride, stannous fluoride, fluoride varnish, and adrenal steroids have been used in the dental office in an attempt to reduce root sensitivity.

Adequate clinical trials for these products are lacking. The patient may use home brushing with concentrated sodium chloride and 0.4% stannous fluoride. Sodium fluoride gel may also be self-applied in a bite guard. Desensitizing toothpastes have helped some patients, but controlled clinical trials with sufficient patient populations are lacking. Current research indicates that root sensitivity due to recession, bleaching, or abrasion may be successfully treated with amorphous calcium phosphate.

Actinic Lip Changes

Long-term exposure of the lip to the sun can cause irreversible tissue changes known as actinic cheilitis. These sun-related changes occur near the vermilion border of the lips and can progress to malignancy. Sunscreen preparations with higher (>15) sun protective factors should be applied before sun exposure and reapplied as needed. If keratotic changes have occurred, treatment is topical 5-fluorouracil (5-FU), an antineoplastic agent that promotes sloughing of the skin (bad layers of cells are sloughed off). A topical steroid (see Chapter 20) may be used to relieve the irritation produced by 5-FU.

Stomatitis

Stomatitis is an inflammation of the mucus lining the cheeks, gums, tongue, lips, throat, and roof or floor of the mouth. Stomatitis is caused by poor oral hygiene, by poorly fitted dentures, by mouth burns from hot food or drinks, or by conditions that affect the entire body, such as medications, allergic reactions, radiation therapy, and infections. Treatment is based on its cause and usually includes good oral hygiene. If stomatitis is a result of mouth burns, it should resolve on its own.

DRUG-INDUCED ORAL SIDE EFFECTS

Drug-induced oral side effects can be produced by a wide variety of agents. Different kinds of lesions can be produced by the same drug, and the same kind of lesion can be produced by different agents. Some drugs that can cause changes in the oral cavity are listed in Box 25.1. Common oral side effects include xerostomia, drug-induced lichenoid-like reaction, and hypersensitivity reactions.

The most commonly listed oral side effect of drugs is xerostomia. Many drugs have been stated to cause xerostomia, but the effect is variable, depending on the patient and the dose of the drug. An extensive list of xerostomia-producing drugs is available in Appendix D.

Xerostomia

Xerostomia, or dryness of the mouth, may result from a drug (e.g., atropine), a disease (e.g., Sjögren syndrome [Fig. 25.8]), age, or irradiation. Radiation therapy to the head and neck affects the salivary glands so that the consistency of saliva is altered and its volume is reduced substantially.

Many different groups of drugs produce xerostomia (see Appendix D). For example, the anticholinergics and other drugs with anticholinergic side effects are likely to cause it. With xerostomia, the patient has a dry mouth. Saliva washes the teeth; xerostomia produces an increase in the incidence of caries, especially class V lesions.

Treatment of xerostomia consists of the following:

Caries prevention: The use of fluoride trays and gels and other topical agents to counteract the formation of caries should be recommended and demonstrated.

Artificial saliva: Artificial saliva may be suggested for use in patients with xerostomia. Table 25.3 lists selected drug groups and examples most likely to produce dry mouth.

Home care: The use of fluoride rinses or trays containing fluoride to deliver fluoride should be recommended before extensive caries occurs. Drinking water or chewing sugarless gum should be encouraged in place of gum and candies containing sugar.

Change in medication or reduction in dose: With some drug groups, such as antidepressants, there are drugs that produce significant xerostomia and others that produce much less xerostomia. For example, the antidepressant amitriptyline produces a significant amount of xerostomia, whereas a different antidepressant, sertraline, produces much less. Any medication change must be coordinated with the patient's physician and would depend on many factors.

Pilocarpine: Cholinergic agents such as pilocarpine can stimulate an increase in saliva in patients with functioning parotid glands. Chapter 4 discusses its dose and adverse effects.

Cevimeline hydrochloride (Evoxac): Cholinergic agonist that binds to muscarinic receptors and increases the secretion of salivary glands. This drug is approved by the US Food and Drug Administration (FDA) for the treatment of dry mouth in persons with Sjögren syndrome. Adverse effects include excessive salivation, lacrimation, urination, and defecation.

Sialorrhea

Certain drugs may produce an increase in saliva termed *sialosis, sialism,* or *sialorrhea.* One example is the cholinergic agent pilocarpine.

BOX 25.1 Oral Side Effects of Drugs

Discoloration

Intrinsic

Tetracycline/doxycycline
Minocycline
Excessive fluoride (fluorosis)

Extrinsic

Stannous fluoride (extrinsic)
Chlorhexidine (extrinsic)
Liquid iron (extrinsic)

Sialorrhea (Ptyalism)

Cholinergics:
  Pilocarpine
Cholinesterase inhibitors:
  Neostigmine
Ethionamide
Iodides
Ketamine
Lithium
Aldosterone
Apomorphine
Mercurials
Niridazole
Nitrazepam

Sialosis

Propylthiouracil (PTU)
Methimazole
Iodides
Isoprenaline
Methyldopa
Oxyphenbutazone
Sulfonamides

Gingival Bleeding

Warfarin (Coumadin)
Ticlopidine (Ticlid)
Quinidine
Aspirin

Xerostomia*

Antihypertensives:
  Clonidine—centrally acting
  Diuretics
Psychotropic:
  Antipsychotics
  Antidepressants
Antihistamines
Anticholinergics
Anticonvulsants
Laxatives

Muscle relaxants:
  Cyclobenzaprine

Taste Changes*

Metronidazole
Angiotensin-converting enzyme (ACE) inhibitors
Penicillamine
Griseofulvin
Gold salts

Gingival Enlargement

Anticonvulsants:
  Phenytoin
  Sodium valproate
  Phenobarbital
Cyclosporine
Calcium channel blockers:
  Nifedipine
  Diltiazem
Verapamil

Systemic Lupus Erythematosus

Antiarrhythmics:
  Procainamide
  Quinidine
Hydralazine
Isoniazid
Anticonvulsants:
  Hydantoins
  Ethosuximide
Lithium
Thiouracil

Parotitis

Cardiovascular drugs:
  Methyldopa
  Guanethidine
  Clonidine
  Bretylium
  Carisoprodol
  Methocarbamol
  Orphenadrine
Opioids
Sedative-hypnotics

Erythema Multiforme

Antiinfectives:
  Penicillins
  Tetracyclines
  Sulfonamides
  Clindamycin
Anticonvulsants

Stomatitis

Antineoplastic agents:
  Nitrogen mustard
  Methotrexate
  5-Fluorouracil
  6-Mercaptopurine
  Chlorambucil
  Doxorubicin
  Daunorubicin
  Bleomycin
Antiarthritics:
  Penicillamine
  Gold salts
Local application:
  Aspirin
  Valproic acid (inside capsule)
Gentian violet

Pigmentation

Amalgam (e.g., tattoo)
Antineoplastics:
  Cisplatin
  Doxorubicin
Oral contraceptives
Minocycline
Antimalarials

Candidiasis

Broad-spectrum antibiotics
Corticosteroids

Sialoadenitis

Phenylbutazone
Oxyphenbutazone
Nitrofurantoin
Isoproterenol
Iodine (iodides)
α-Methyldopa

Caries

Xerostomia-producing agents
Sugar-containing medications

Muscle-Related Effects

Dystonic reactions
Antipsychotic agents
Metoclopramide
Cisapride
Bruxism:
  Amphetamines

*Additional information can be located in Appendix D.

Hypersensitivity-Type Reactions

Hypersensitivity reactions may be hyperimmune responses triggered by an antigenic component of the drug or its metabolite. Contact stomatitis is more localized when gum and candy are responsible and is more diffuse with toothpaste use. The buccal mucosa and the lateral borders of the tongue are often involved. Even cinnamon-flavored products have been implicated in hypersensitivity reactions. The potential for a hypersensitivity reaction is determined by the particular drug, the frequency of administration, the route of administration (antibiotics administered topically are more likely to produce hypersensitivity reactions than those given parenterally), and the patient's immune system (immunoglobulin E [IgE]).

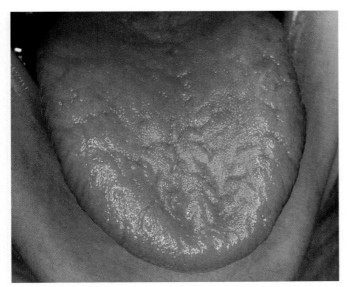

Fig. 25.8 Sjögren syndrome. The patient had severe xerostomia. (From Ibsen OAC, Phelan JA. *Oral Pathology for the Dental Hygienist.* 6th ed. St. Louis: Saunders; 2014.)

TABLE 25.3 Agents That Produce Xerostomia (Dry Mouth)

Drug Group	Examples
Anticholinergics*	Dicyclomine, hyoscyamine sulfate, trihexyphenidyl
Antihypertensives*	Methyldopa, clonidine, prazosin
Antipsychotics*	Haloperidol, thiothixene, phenothiazines, thioridazine
Tricyclic antidepressants*	Amitriptyline, desipramine
Antihistamines	Diphenhydramine, chlorpheniramine maleate, hydroxyzine
Adrenergic agents	Phenylpropanolamine, pseudoephedrine
Diuretics	Dyazide, hydrochlorothiazide
Benzodiazepines	Alprazolam, diazepam, triazolam

*Most likely to produce xerostomia.

Oral Lesions That Resemble Autoimmune-Type Reactions

Lichenoid-Like Eruptions

Many drugs are associated with eruptions that resemble lichen planus. Box 25.2 lists some drugs that have been associated with this type of reaction. The most common drug implicated is hydrochlorothiazide (HCTZ). Others are β-blockers and antimalarials.

Lupus-Like Reactions

Oral manifestations can occur with systemic lupus erythematosus. These lesions may also be produced by a variety of drugs, including antiarrhythmic agents and anticonvulsants.

Erythema Multiforme–Like Lesions

Some drugs (e.g., anticonvulsants) can produce lesions that resemble those of erythema multiforme.

Stains

Staining of teeth may occur either as the teeth are formed or, in a few cases, in adult teeth. The tetracyclines are incorporated into forming teeth and thereby stain them (Fig. 25.9). Today, this adverse reaction is well known, and pregnant women or very small children are not given tetracycline. With adults, both intrinsic and extrinsic stains may occur. Minocycline is thought to produce a blue-gray discoloration in fully mineralized adult teeth. Chlorhexidine rinse and liquid iron preparations can also cause extrinsic staining.

Gingival Enlargement

Gingival hyperplasia, now known as *gingival enlargement* (Fig. 25.10), has been renamed because hyperplasia is not the sole process that occurs in the gums. Gingival enlargement can occur in relation to several drug groups; the most common three are the following:

- *Phenytoin (Dilantin):* Chapter 15 discusses phenytoin and gingival enlargement. The rate of occurrence varies with the patient population, but almost half of the patients exhibit this reaction. Occurrence of gingival enlargement in patients taking phenytoin may be dose related. Oral hygiene practices affect its incidence and severity.
- *Cyclosporine:* Cyclosporine is the antirejection drug used for every patient who has had a kidney transplant and for patients receiving many other transplants. Cyclosporine is associated with gingival enlargement.
- *Calcium channel blockers (CCBs):* CCBs are used for hypertension and congestive heart failure and have been associated with gingival enlargement.
- *Others:* Other implicated drugs include some anticonvulsants such as carbamazepine (Tegretol) and valproic acid (Depakene).

Osteonecrosis of the Jaw

Osteonecrosis of the jaw (ONJ) occurs when the jaw bone is exposed and begins to starve because of a lack of blood flow to the area. The bone begins to weaken and die, a process that is usually associated with pain. ONJ is associated with cancer therapy, including irradiation, infection, steroid use, and bisphosphonate therapy. The vast majority of cases occur with intravenous bisphosphonate therapy. Fewer cases are reported in patients taking bisphosphonates for the treatment of osteoporosis. ONJ is treated conservatively with rinses, antibiotics, and oral analgesics. The best way to treat it is to prevent it or minimize the risk for it. Chapter 20 discusses this topic in greater detail.

AGENTS COMMONLY USED TO TREAT ORAL LESIONS

Corticosteroids

For many oral lesions, especially those with a component of inflammation or immune response, corticosteroids are used. Depending on the severity of the lesions, the topical corticosteroids would be selected according to potency. Weak, intermediate, and potent corticosteroids are used in turn until an agent is effective. The proper strength of steroid is the least potent that will ameliorate the lesion (see the steroid topical chart in Chapter 16). Hydrocortisone cream 1% is a low-potency topical steroid available OTC. The 2.5% hydrocortisone cream is available by prescription. TAC is more potent than hydrocortisone and is in the middle range of potency of the steroids. It is available as 0.025%, 0.1%, and 0.5 %; the first two strengths are classified as moderate, and 0.5% is stronger. Fluocinonide (Lidex) is more potent than TAC and is available as a 0.05% cream or solution. Clobetasol (Temovate), 0.05% cream or solution, is in the most potent group. The latter would be used only if the other agents were ineffective.

BOX 25.2   Drugs Associated With Lichenoid Eruptions

Heavy Metals
Arsenic
Bismuth
Gold salts
Mercury (in amalgam)
Palladium

Antihypertensives
Methyldopa

β-Blockers
Labetalol
Oxprenolol
Practolol
Propranolol

Diuretics
Thiazides
Furosemide
Spironolactone

Antiarrhythmics
Quinidine
Procainamide

Angiotensin-Converting Enzyme (ACE) inhibitors
Captopril
Enalapril

Calcium Channel Blockers
Nifedipine

Ulcerative Colitis Agents
Sulfasalazine
Mesalazine

Antimalarials
Chloroquine

Hydroxychloroquine
Quinacrine (Atabrine)
Quinine
Levamisole

Antitubercular Agents
Streptomycin
Pyrimethamine
p-Aminosalicylic acid (PAS)
Ethambutol
Isoniazid

Antiinfectives
Tetracycline
Demeclocycline
Ketoconazole

Antineoplastic Agents
Hydroxyurea
5-Fluorouracil

Sulfonylureas
Chlorpropamide
Tolbutamide
Tolazamide

Psychotropics
Phenothiazines
Chlorpromazine
Lithium

Others
Nonsteroidal antiinflammatory agents (NSAIDs)
Carbamazepine
Allopurinol
Triprolidine
Penicillamine
Dapsone

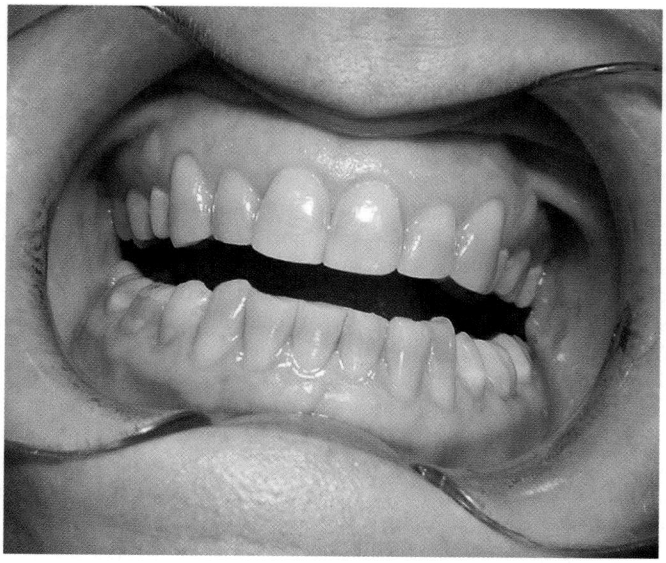

Fig. 25.9 Discoloration of teeth caused by tetracycline ingestion. (From Ibsen OAC, Phelan JA. *Oral Pathology for the Dental Hygienist.* 6th ed. St. Louis: Saunders; 2014.)

If topical corticosteroid therapy is ineffective or if the condition is severe, systemic corticosteroids may be indicated. Of the systemic steroids, prednisone is most common. There is little reason to use other agents because all corticosteroids have virtually the same effect. With systemic steroids, the dose begins high (usually 40 of prednisone per day) and is then tapered, depending on the progress of the lesions. In some cases, long-term systemic corticosteroid therapy is required to control the oral lesion. When systemic steroids are used long term, their adverse reactions must be managed (i.e., osteoporosis, fluid retention, diabetes, hypertension, and the manifestations moon face, buffalo hump, and abdominal striae).

Palliative Treatment

Palliative treatment is treatment designed to make the patient more comfortable. Agents that reduce the pain of the oral cavity can be topical and systemic. Topical agents are applied by swishing the liquid around in the mouth. These agents include a local anesthetic agent (viscous lidocaine) (see Chapter 9) and an antihistamine with local anesthetic properties (DPH elixir) (see Chapter 17).

Many combination products have been prescribed, but their benefit over plain DPH elixir is controversial. Mixtures of DPH, lidocaine, and magnesium-aluminum hydroxide have been advocated. Systemic analgesics can often provide relief from a painful oral lesion. Topical

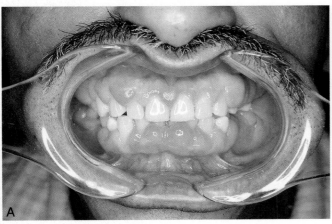 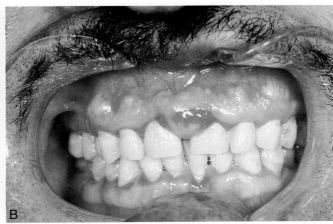

Fig. 25.10 (A) Fibrous gingival enlargement. (B) Inflamed gingival enlargement. (From Ibsen OAC, Phelan JA. *Oral Pathology for the Dental Hygienist*. 6th ed. St. Louis: Saunders; 2014.)

and systemic agents may be used together for an additive effect. One concern with the use of topical local anesthetics is that reduction in the sensations from the throat could lead to choking. This possibility can be minimized by having the patient avoid eating directly after application. If isolated lesions are present, the anesthetic can be painted on the lesion using a cotton-tipped swab.

DENTAL HYGIENE CONSIDERATIONS

- Recognize the clinical manifestations of the various oral conditions.
- Conduct a thorough medication/health history because many drugs and physical disorders can cause or aggravate oral conditions.
- Be familiar with the therapies for the various oral conditions.

- Educate the patient about the appropriate therapy once the dentist has made the diagnosis and prescribed the appropriate therapy.
- Educate the patient about appropriate ways to avoid offending causes of some of the oral conditions.

ACADEMIC SKILLS ASSESSMENT

1. Name two ways to reduce alveolar osteitis.
2. Describe three causes of xerostomia and name several drugs that can cause it.
3. Explain the management of xerostomia, including preventive measures.
4. State the best way to prevent actinic lip changes.
5. Describe the treatment of a patient with ANUG.
6. Describe two appropriate treatments for RAS.

CLINICAL CASE STUDY

Malcom Smith is 52 years old and has been a long-time patient of this dental practice. His medication/health history is significant for lung cancer, stage two. He was fortunate because the oncologist was able to remove the tumor. However, one of his lymph nodes tested positive for cancer cells, and he is now undergoing chemotherapy. His chief complaint today is a constant dry mouth that is not relieved by drinking water or juices or sucking on sugarless candy. He would like some help with this issue.

1. What are some of the causes of xerostomia?
2. Which drugs can cause xerostomia?
3. How can xerostomia be treated?
4. What is Salagen and what is its role in treating xerostomia?
5. How is Salagen different from other drugs used to treat xerostomia?

26

Hygiene-Related Oral Disorders

ⓔ http://evolve.elsevier.com/Haveles/pharmacology

LEARNING OBJECTIVES

1. Discuss how improper oral hygiene can lead to dental caries and describe the general background of carious lesions.
2. Discuss the importance of caries prevention and the nonpharmacologic therapies that are available to aid in this effort.
3. Discuss the proper methods that patients should use when brushing and flossing.
4. Discuss pharmacologic therapies and the role of fluoride in preventing caries.
5. Discuss the possibility of toxicity with the use of fluoride, differentiate between acute and chronic fluoride toxicity, and discuss treatments for both types.
6. Compare and contrast both professionally applied and at-home fluoride preparations.
7. Discuss the proper method for administering professionally applied fluoride preparations and identify various professionally applied topical agents.
8. Discuss the general types of patient-applied fluoride preparations and the proper methods that patients should use regarding at-home fluoride treatments.
9. Discuss the importance of Xylitol and Chlorhexidine in relation to dental hygiene.
10. Discuss gingivitis: its pathophysiology, incidence, and available treatments.
11. Discuss tooth hypersensitivity: its pathophysiology and available treatments, both at-home and in-office.

Oral disorders or diseases are among the most prevalent diseases in American society. Each year, dental disorders result in a loss of more than 164 million hours from work. Nearly one-third of adult Americans have untreated tooth decay and one in every seven adults 35 to 44 years of age have gum disease. Severe gum disease affects 14% of Americans aged 45 to 54 years. The rate of gum disease increases to one in four Americans age 65 years and older. Less than 60% of adults older than 65 years visit an oral health care provider during a given year. Almost 25% of Americans 60 years and older have lost all of their permanent teeth. The growing number of older persons with their own natural teeth has many dental implications.[1]

Poor or improper oral hygiene is a direct cause of dental caries, gingivitis, and halitosis. Nonprescription products for preventing and treating hygiene-related oral disorders are available in pharmacies, food stores, and other retail outlets. Dental hygienists are in the forefront on educating the public about the proper use of these products and their role in preventing hygiene-related oral disorders.

DENTAL CARIES

> Highest caries risk: persons with poor oral hygiene.

Approximately 20% of the general population has experienced dental caries. The incidence of dental caries in children decreased from the 1970s until the mid-1990s. This decrease has been attributed to fluoridation of public water supplies, dentifrices, and mouth rinses, not improved oral hygiene. Despite improvements in these areas, the incidence of dental caries in primary teeth of children 2 to11 years of age appears to be on the rise. Currently, 42% of children 2 to 11 years of age have caries in their primary teeth. Of these children, 23%
have untreated caries. Also, 21% of children 6 to11 years of age have caries in their permanent teeth, and 8% have untreated decay. The incidence of tooth decay in adolescents aged 12 to 19 years is 59%. Patients at highest risk for caries are those with poor oral hygiene. Patients at increased risk include those with orthodontic appliances, xerostomia, or gum recession, those who are living at or below the poverty level, black non-Hispanic, or of Hispanic origin, and those who use tobacco. Box 26.1 gives a more detailed overview of the risk criteria for caries.

Dental caries is considered an infectious disease that affects the calcified tissue of the teeth. Certain plaque bacteria generate acid from dietary carbohydrates, causing acid demineralization of tooth enamel, which then leads to the formation of carious lesions. Plaque buildup is directly related to the incidence of oral disease. If left untreated, these lesions can destroy the tooth.

Carious lesions start slowly on the enamel surface and initially produce no clinical symptoms. Once demineralization of the tooth progresses through the enamel to the soft dentin, the destruction proceeds at a much faster pace. At this point, the patient becomes aware of the problem either by directly noticing the carious lesion or by experiencing sensitivity to hot and cold stimuli. If left untreated, the lesion can damage the dental pulp and lead to necrosis of vital pulp tissue.

Prevention

The key to preventing dental caries is good dental plaque control. Reduction in the amount and frequency of refined carbohydrate intake, plaque removal, and fluoride use can lower the incidence of dental caries. Antiplaque products aid in the mechanical removal of plaque and slow or inhibit its buildup on teeth. Two methods are available to remove plaque from the teeth: mechanical and chemical. Mechanical methods include brushing and flossing, and chemical methods include

BOX 26.1 Risk Categories for Dental Caries

Low Risk: All Age Groups
- No risk factors for caries*
- No incipient or cavitated primary or secondary carious lesions during the past 3 years

Moderate Risk: <6 Years of Age
- No incipient or cavitated primary or secondary carious lesions during the past 3 years; however, the patient has at least one risk factor for caries*
- One or two incipient or cavitated primary or secondary carious lesions during the past 3 years

Moderate Risk: >Years of Age
- One or two incipient or cavitated primary or secondary carious lesions in the last 3 years
- No incipient or cavitated primary or secondary carious lesions in the last 3 years; however, the patient has at least one factor for caries*

High Risk: <6 Years of Age
- Any incipient or cavitated primary or secondary carious lesions during the past 3 years, or the patient has multiple risk factors for caries*
- Low socioeconomic background, suboptimal fluoride exposure, xerostomia

High Risk: >6 Years of Age
- Three or more incipient or cavitated primary or secondary carious lesions during the past 3 years
- Presence of multiple risk factors for caries*
- Suboptimal fluoride exposure, xerostomia

*High titers of cariogenic bacteria, poor oral hygiene, prolonged nursing (bottle or breast), developmental or acquired defects in enamel, genetic abnormality of the teeth, multisurface restorations, chemotherapy, radiation therapy, eating disorders, alcohol or drug abuse, irregular dental care, orthodontic appliances, and cariogenic diet all increase the risk for development of caries.

From ADA Council on Scientific Affairs. Professionally applied topical fluoride: evidence-based clinical recommendations. *J Am Dent Assoc.* 2006;137(8):1151. Copyright © 2006 American Dental Association. All rights reserved. Modified 2009 with permission.

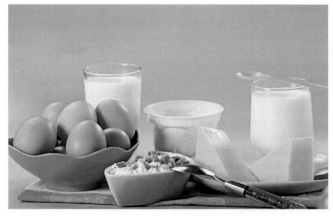

Fig. 26.1 Dairy products can have a cariostatic effect. Proteins in these foods raise pH levels and can inhibit bacterial growth. (Courtesy Teresa Kasprzycka, Image from www.BigStockPhoto.com.)

BOX 26.2 Guidelines for Proper Toothbrushing

- Brush at least twice daily.
- Place a small amount of toothpaste on the toothbrush.
- If using powder, apply the powder to a wet toothbrush, making sure to cover all bristles.
- Powder must be applied twice.
- Use a gentle scrubbing motion and place the toothbrush at a 45-degree angle against the gumline to make sure that the tips of the bristles do the work.
- Do not use excessive force. Excessive force can lead to gingival recession and tooth hypersensitivity.
- Brush for at least 1 minute.
- Gently brush the tongue to reduce debris, plaque, and bacteria, which can cause oral hygiene problems.
- Do not swallow paste or powder.
- Rinse the mouth and expectorate the water.

BOX 26.3 Guidelines for Proper Use of Dental Floss

- Pull out approximately 18 inches of floss from its container and wrap most of it around your middle finger.
- Wrap the remaining floss around the middle finger of the other hand until approximately 1 inch of floss remains visible.
- Using a gentle gliding motion, place the floss between two teeth until it reaches the gumline.
- When at the gumline, curve the floss into a C-shaped curve against one tooth and gently slide the floss into the space between the gum and tooth until you feel resistance.
- Hold the floss tightly against one tooth and gently scrape the side of the tooth while moving the floss away from the gumline.
- Repeat this process until all teeth have been flossed.

specific drug products to prevent or remove plaque buildup. The dental hygienist should teach the patient that the best way to ensure healthy teeth and gingival tissues is to mechanically remove plaque by brushing at least twice daily and by flossing at least once a day.

Nonpharmacologic Therapies

Dietary measures. One of the easiest ways, although in some ways the most difficult, to prevent caries is to avoid highly cariogenic foods. Foods with higher water content, those that stimulate saliva flow, and foods high in protein are less cariogenic. Proteins in dairy products raise pH levels and can inhibit bacterial growth (Fig. 26.1). Noncariogenic sugar substitutes, such as sorbitol, xylitol, and aspartame, can help reduce the risk for development of caries.

Mechanical measures. Toothbrushes, floss, oral irrigating devices, and specialty aids are the primary types of plaque removal devices.

Toothbrushes. Both manual and electric toothbrushes are available for plaque removal. The proper frequency and method of brushing often vary from patient to patient. Although there are no definite guidelines as to how often patients should replace a toothbrush, it is recommended that the average life of a toothbrush is 3 months. Wear and tear and bacterial accumulation lead to increased plaque buildup instead of plaque removal. Box 26.2 describes the proper method of brushing.

Dental floss. Interdental plaque removal can help decrease the incidence of proximal caries, gingival inflammation, and periodontal pocketing. Proper flossing techniques require some finger dexterity and practice. Box 26.3 describes the proper method of flossing.

Pharmacologic Therapies

Pharmacologic management of plaque and calculus enhances the mechanical removal by either acting directly on plaque bacteria or disrupting plaque so that it can be removed mechanically.

Fluoride. Fluoride is the agent most commonly used to reduce demineralization and remineralize decalcified areas. The type and amount of fluoride that a person receives depend on his or her risk for development of caries (see Box 26.1). Those with a low risk for caries require only fluoridated dentifrices. Additional, professionally applied fluoride is not recommended in this group because of insufficient evidence for any benefit. Patients considered to have a moderate-to-high risk for caries benefit from professionally applied fluoride products. According to the American Dental Association (ADA), only adults who have had active caries in the last 3 years and have risk factors for caries should receive professionally applied fluoride products.

Mechanism of action. Fluoride is thought to work by two different means. Fluoride ions interact with mineralized tissue, including bones and teeth. Once incorporated into developing teeth, fluoride systemically reduces the solubility of dental enamel by enhancing the development of fluoridated hydroxyapatite, thereby forming the stable compound calcium fluoride at the enamel surface. This chemical structure facilitates the remineralization of early carious lesions during repeated cycles of demineralization and remineralization. This same action is thought to occur when topical fluoride is administered. The second action of the fluoride ion is thought to occur on the individual microorganisms in biofilm. Topically applied stannous fluoride (SnF) inhibits bacterial enzyme systems and alters the acid production that would result in demineralization of tooth structure.

Toxicity. As with any drug, side effects can occur with fluoride. Nausea and vomiting have been reported in children who have swallowed some of their fluoride treatment. Both acute and chronic toxicity can occur with fluoride use. Acute toxicity is a result of fluoride overdose and is a medical emergency. Chronic fluoride toxicity occurs over time and is treated medically.

Acute toxicity

> Acute toxicity: medical emergency.

Acute toxicity of fluoride occurs with a single overdose of fluoride. Signs and symptoms of acute toxicity are nausea, vomiting, diarrhea, intestinal cramping, profuse salivation, black stools, progressive hypotension, and cardiac abnormalities. Death can occur as the result of cardiovascular and respiratory collapse.

Immediate treatment is necessary; it involves giving the patient calcium. Milk should be given because it will bind to fluoride and prevent systemic absorption. A designated member of the oral health care team should call 911 for emergency medical treatment. Other team members should induce emesis to get the fluoride out of the stomach if the patient does not spontaneously vomit. Monitor patient vital signs and prepare for cardiopulmonary resuscitation (CPR) until emergency help arrives.

Chronic toxicity

> Chronic toxicity is treated esthetically.

Drinking water with more than 2 ppm of fluoride can lead to fluorosis of tooth enamel during the period of tooth mineralization. Dental fluorosis or mottled tooth enamel is the most common sign of chronic fluoride toxicity during tooth development. The color changes in tooth enamel are a result of hypomineralization of the outer third of the tooth enamel. Children who drink water with at least 1 ppm of fluoride and ingest fluoride supplements are at risk for chronic toxicity. Table 26.1 reviews the current recommendations of the American Academy of Pediatrics, American Academy of Pediatric Dentistry, and the ADA Council on Access, Prevention, and Interpersonal Relations regarding fluoride supplementation and drinking water fluoridation. The treatment of chronic toxicity, which is one of esthetics, consists of bleaching the anterior teeth and covering the anterior teeth with porcelain restorations.

TABLE 26.1 Dosing Schedule for Fluoride Supplement Dependent on Water Fluoride Ion Concentrations In Drinking Water

Child's Age	DOSING SCHEDULE FOR FLUORIDE SUPPLEMENTS (MG/DAY)* BASED ON FLUORIDATION CONCENTRATION IN DRINKING WATER (PPM)		
	<0.3 ppm	0.3–0.6 ppm	>0.6 ppm
6 months to 3 years	0.25	0	0
3–6 years	0.5	0.25	0
6–16 years	1	0.5	0

*2.2 mg of NaF (sodium fluoride) = 1 mg fluoride ion.
Data from Council on Scientific Affairs, American Dental Association: Intervention: fluoride supplementation. In ADA Council on Access, Prevention and Interprofessional Relations: Caries diagnosis and risk assessment. *J Am Dent Assoc.* 1995:126(6 suppl):19-S.

Fluoride preparations. Fluoride preparations can be organized into two groups: those applied by the dental hygienist and those applied by the patient.

Professionally applied fluoride topical agents. Currently accepted agents for professional application are sodium fluoride (NaF) and acidulated phosphate fluoride (APF). The two types are equally efficacious in preventing caries. NaF is recommended when restorations are present because of the damage caused by acids. Topically administered fluoride products must remain in contact with the tooth surface for a specified time to allow the chemical change to develop. It is recommended that fluoride applications remain in place for 4 minutes. The ionic exchange lasts for about 30 minutes, which is why the patient is instructed to refrain from eating or drinking for at least 30 minutes after fluoride applications. Topical fluoride applications last for only 5 to 8 weeks because fluoride leaches from the enamel and returns to preapplication levels. Daily applications of low concentration–fluoride dentifrices help maintain fluoride levels in tooth structure.

Annual 4-minute in-office topical fluoride applications reduce tooth decay in permanent teeth of children living in nonfluoridated areas by 26%. Some topical fluoride products are marketed as 1-minute in-office applications. However, clinical trials have not proved that they are as effective as the 4-minute applications. The ADA has given its Seal of Acceptance only to the 4-minute application products.

The concentration of fluoride products varies, and selected products are listed in Table 26.2 and shown in Figs. 26.2 and 26.3. Box 26.4 reviews the administration of professionally applied fluoride products. The higher the fluoride concentration, the better the anticariogenic

TABLE 26.2 Fluoride Concentrations of Professionally Applied Preparations

Preparation	Fluoride Concentration (ppm)
Solution, Foam, Gels, and Varnish: In-Office Applications	
Sodium 2%	9,050
Sodium varnish 5%	22,600
Acidulated phosphate fluoride (APF) 1.23%	12,300
Prescription Gels: Daily Home Use	
Sodium 1.1%	5,000
0.4% stannous fluoride and 1.1% sodium fluoride in APF	5,000

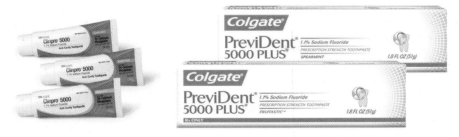

High concentration 5000 ppm fluoride
toothpaste/gel for caries high-risk
clients from age 6 years and older

Fig. 26.2 Sample prescription fluoride products. (Courtesy Dr. Mark Dillenges. From Darby ML, Walsh MM. *Dental Hygiene: Theory and Practice.* 4th ed. St. Louis: Saunders; 2015.)

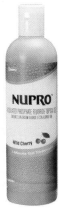

Fig. 26.3 Examples of topical fluoride gels for professional application. (Courtesy Dentsply International, York, PA.)

effect. Products with higher fluoride concentrations are recommended for patients who have widespread decay or are at increased risk for caries. Patients undergoing head and neck radiation therapy often require higher concentrations of fluoride.

The following are summaries of various professionally applied topical agents:

NaF varnish with a 5% NaF concentration is currently available for use in the United States as a dentin-desensitizing agent and as a cavity liner. The US Food and Drug Administration (FDA) has not approved the varnish for its anticaries effect. However, the use of fluoride varnish for caries prevention has been endorsed by the ADA. It is the recommended method of fluoride application for those at high risk for caries.

NaF varnish has several advantages over the 4-minute in-office application. The varnish can be applied without prior oral prophylaxis, stays on the enamel longer than topical fluorides, and can be applied if saliva is present. It dries quickly (within 10 seconds) and is slowly released into saliva so there is less systemic absorption, which reduces the risk of toxicity. Finally, application time is short, well tolerated, and safe. NaF varnish is applied to the occlusals or the smooth surface of teeth and leaves a yellow color on the occlusal surface. Varnish is available as a one-time application formulation and must be mixed in the dispensing cup. It is applied with a small brush and dries quickly so the patient does not gag. The patient should not eat for 2 hours after the application and should not brush his or her teeth for 1 day after the varnish has been applied. Toothbrushing can remove the newly applied varnish. Varnishes are applied two to four times a year. In high-risk individuals, the varnish should be applied every 3 to 6 months. NaF is a relatively safe product. The product dries quickly, and over time, small amounts are released into the systemic circulation. Preschool and school-aged children treated with NaF varnish had no adverse effects on renal function or increased plasma fluoride levels.

Topical NaF is available as a viscous gel or foam and is stable in a 2% solution. It comes in several different flavors, is nonirritating to surrounding tissue, and does not stain teeth or restorations. All NaF agents have a neutral pH of 7.0 and are ideal for porcelain or composite restorations or sealants. NaF is applied twice yearly for 4 minutes. A concentrated 2% NaF rinse is available for in-office use. Patients swish the product for 30 seconds and then expectorate. This treatment is applied four times a year.

BOX 26.4 In-Office Administration of Topical Fluoride Products

- Keep the patient in an upright, seated position.
- Place a properly functioning saliva ejector in the floor of the mouth.
- Use the right size tray for the patient.
- Provide the patient with a napkin to catch oral fluids during fluoride application.
- Use a ribbon of gel or foam to cover no more than half the tray's depth.
- Advise the patient to not swallow the fluoride.
- Have the patient lean his or her head forward so fluids will flow to the front of the mouth.
- After the manufacturer's recommended time period of application, remove the tray and suction oral fluids and excess fluoride; wipe the teeth, tongue, and mucosa thoroughly with gauze; and have the patient expectorate for 1 minute.
- Advise the patient to refrain from eating or drinking for at least 30 minutes after the applications.

APF 1.23%: The pH of this product is 3.5, which makes it acidic. Raising the acidity of the fluoride increases the uptake of fluoride by the tooth enamel. APF products are applied every 6 to 12 months following oral prophylaxis. APF is stable, does not irritate surrounding tissue, does not discolor teeth or restorations, and causes a slight astringent taste in the mouth. This product is indicated for patients taking medications on a long-term basis that contain sugar. APF is contraindicated in patients with porcelain, composite, or glass ionomer restorations, or sealants.

SnF is available only in a two-part rinse that contains SnF 1.64% and APF 0.3%. The manufacturer recommends a 60-second pretreatment rinse with APF to enhance stannous uptake, followed by a 60-second rinse with SnF. It should be noted that this product is not endorsed by the ADA.

Patient-applied topical fluoride preparations. Patient-applied topical fluoride preparations help maintain the fluoride applied during oral prophylaxis as well as prevent, stop, and reverse the caries process. Home fluoride products should be used daily at low concentrations. With the exception of dentifrices, rinses and gels come with the warning to expectorate after using them and should not be used in children younger than 6 years.

Following are summaries of the general types of patient-applied fluoride preparations.

Dentifrices: Almost 98% of all dentifrices or toothpastes available in the United States contain some form of fluoride. Table 26.3 lists several of them (Fig. 26.4). The vast majority of fluoridated dentifrices

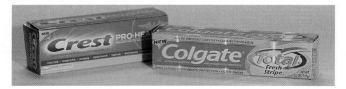

Fig. 26.4 Sample sodium fluoride dentifrices that have the American Dental Association Seal of Acceptance for dental caries prevention. (Courtesy Dr. Mark Dillenges. From Darby ML, Walsh MM. *Dental Hygiene: Theory and Practice.* 4th ed. St. Louis: Saunders; 2015.)

with ADA acceptance for their anticaries effect contain 0.243% NaF, which provides 1100 ppm fluoride. Products that also contain triclosan 0.3% carry ADA approval for its effects against gingivitis. Patients should brush at least twice daily. Studies have shown that children between the ages of 10 to 15 years who brush three times daily with a fluoride dentifrice have a 46% lower decayed-missing-filled rate compared to only 21% for those who only brush once a day. Children should use a pea-sized amount of toothpaste to minimize fluoride ingestion.

Gels: Fluoride gels are prescription gels that the patient self-applies at home (see Table 26.2). The gels are applied for 1 to 2 minutes with a toothbrush or they can be placed in a custom-fitted tray. The gels are intended for adults at high risk for caries, although they can be used in school-aged children. They are often recommended for people undergoing head and neck irradiation.

TABLE 26.3 Selected Dentifrices

Trade Name	Primary Ingredients	Fluoride Concentration (ppm)
Fluoride Toothpastes		
Aquafresh Extra Fresh Toothpaste	Calcium carbonate, hydrated silica, sodium monofluorophosphate (fluoride 0.15%)	850–1150
Colgate Toothpaste	Dicalcium phosphate dehydrate, sodium monofluorophosphate (fluoride 0.15%)	850–1150
Crest Cavity Protection Gel	Hydrated silica, sodium fluoride (0.15%)	850–1150
Tartar-Control Toothpastes		
Colgate Baking Soda and Peroxide Tartar Control Toothpaste	Hydrated silica, sodium monofluorophosphate (fluoride 0.15%), pentasodium triphosphate, tetrasodium pyrophosphate	850–1150
Crest Tartar Protection Gel/Toothpaste	Silica, sodium fluoride (fluoride 0.15%), tetrapotassium pyrophosphate, disodium pyrophosphate, tetrasodium pyrophosphate	850–1150
Antiplaque/Antigingivitis Toothpastes		
Colgate Total Toothpaste	Hydrated silica, sodium bicarbonate, sodium fluoride (fluoride 0.14%), triclosan 0.3%	850–1150
Crest Multicare Toothpaste	Hydrated silica, sodium fluoride (fluoride 0.15%), sodium bicarbonate, tetrasodium pyrophosphate	—
Sodium Laurel Sulfate–Free Toothpastes		
Biotène Dry Mouth Toothpaste	Lactoperoxidase, glucose oxidase, lysozyme, sodium monofluorophosphate 0.15%	850–1150
Sensodyne Original Flavor Toothpaste	Potassium nitrate 5%, sodium fluoride (fluoride 0.13%)	850–1150
Botanical-Based Toothpastes		
Tom's of Maine Toothpastes	Peppermint, spearmint, orange, mango, fennel, carrageenan, propolis, cassia, myrrh, cinnamon	—
Viadent Original Toothpaste	Zinc citrate trihydrate (2%), sodium monofluorophosphate (0.13% w/v fluoride ion)	—

Rinses: Mouthrinses are indicated as adjunct to proper brushing and flossing, and can be classified as either cosmetic or therapeutic (Table 26.4 and Fig. 26.5). Therapeutic mouthrinses contain an active ingredient, typically fluoride salt for cavity protection or antibacterial ingredients, such as chlorhexidine, cetylpyridinium chloride, or essential oils to help prevent plaque build-up and gingivitis. Cosmetic mouthrinses are focused on maintaining fresh breath and removal of debris. Most mouthrinses contain similar ingredients such as glycerin or sorbitol (have a sweet taste and adjusts mouthfeel to be more mild), surfactants for foaming and mouth cleansing, zinc salts (astringent that helps neutralize bad breath and reduce tartar build-up), and flavor components. Flavors are important components to indicate mouth freshness and can include mint, spicy, or medicinal, with some regional flavors and variations. Flavor selection is also key to drive compliance based on consumer preferences. Alcohol can be added to provide a stronger and longer lasting mouthfeel, enhance flavor, and solubilize other mouthrinse ingredients..

TABLE 26.4   Selected Mouth Rinses

Trade Name	Primary Ingredients
Cosmetic Mouth Rinses	
Biotène	Lysozyme, lactoferrin, glucose oxidase, lactoperoxidase
Lavoris	Zantate, clove oil, zinc chloride
Targon	Polyethylene glycol 40, hydrogenated castor oil
Therapeutic Mouth Rinses	
Crest Pro-Health Rinse	Cetylpyridinium chloride 0.07%
Listerine Tartar Control Antiseptic	Sodium lauryl sulfate, tetrasodium pyrophosphate
Scope	Cetylpyridinium chloride, domiphen
Fluoridated Mouth Rinses	
ACT for Kids	Sodium fluoride 0.05%, cetylpyridinium chloride
Oral-B Anti-Cavity Rinse	Sodium fluoride 0.05%
Botanical-Based Mouthwashes	
Glyoxide	Carbamide peroxide
Listerine	Thymol, eucalyptol, methyl salicylates, menthol
Tom's of Maine	Peppermint, spearmint, cinnamon, fennel, aloe vera, witch hazel

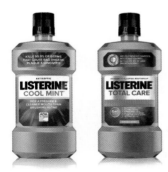

Fig. 26.5 Sample over-the-counter 0.05% sodium fluoride rinses with the American Dental Association ADA Seal of Acceptance. (© J&JCI. Used with permission.)

Dental hygienists should be aware that mouth rinses may mask pathologic conditions.

A concern with cosmetic mouth rinses is that they may mask pathologic conditions. Patients may mistake oral malodor associated with periodontal disease, oral infections, or respiratory infections as simple bad breath. Patients should be instructed that if bad breath persists after proper toothbrushing and rinsing, they should contact their oral health care provider.

Since the 1990s, the number of mouth rinses promoted for their antiplaque activity has increased dramatically. Ingredients for plaque control include aromatic oils, such as thymol, eucalyptol, menthol, and methyl salicylates, and agents with antimicrobial activity, such as quaternary ammonium compounds. Phenols control plaque by destroying bacterial cell walls, inhibiting bacterial enzymes, and extracting bacterial lipopolysaccharides. Cetylpyridinium chloride is a cationic surfactant capable of bactericidal activity, although it does not penetrate plaque well. Domiphen bromide is similar to cetylpyridinium.

Mouth rinses are generally safe when used as directed. A burning sensation and oral irritation have been reported. Unsupervised use is contraindicated in persons with mouth irritations or ulcers. These products should be kept out of the reach of children. The alcohol content in mouth rinses ranges from 0% to 27%, with most products containing 14% to 27% alcohol. Ingestion of alcohol-containing mouth rinses poses a great danger for children. In case of accidental ingestion, the caregiver should seek professional assistance or contact a poison control center. Children's products also contain fluoride. Box 26.5 reviews the proper guidelines for using home topical fluoride treatments.

Xylitol. Xylitol is a natural product found in plants that looks and tastes like sucrose but is not fermented by cariogenic bacteria. Xylitol has been found to reduce the levels of *Streptococcus mutans* in plaque and saliva, inhibit the attachment of biofilm to teeth, and prevent the transmission of oral bacteria from mother to child. A five-carbon sugar alcohol, xylitol cannot be digested by bacteria. It interferes with the metabolism of *S. mutans* as it is transported into the cell. Once

BOX 26.5   Guidelines for Using At-Home Topical Fluoride Preparations

- Use the topical fluoride rinse no more than once per day.
- Brush teeth with a fluoride dentifrice before rinsing.
- For a fluoride rinse:
  Pour 10 mL into a calibrated measuring cup and then place it in the mouth.
  Rinse vigorously for approximately 60 seconds.
  Spit out the fluoride rinse. Do not swallow it.
- For fluoride gel:
- Brush the teeth with the gel and allow the gel to remain on the teeth for 60 seconds then expectorate.
- Do not eat or drink for 30 minutes after the treatment.
- Supervise children as necessary to make sure that they do not swallow the fluoride preparation.
- Instruct children younger than 12 years of age on the importance of good rinsing techniques.

Data from Fairbrother KJ, Heasman PA. Anticalculus agents. *J Clin Periodontol.* 2000;27:285–301; and Whitaker AL. Prevention of hygiene-related oral disorders. In: Berardi RR, Ferris SP, Hume AL et al., eds. *Handbook of Nonprescription Drugs.* 16th ed. Washington, DC: American Pharmacists Association; 2009.

in the cell, it may stay bound to the transport protein. The degree of antibacterial effect depends on the amount of xylitol ingested and the frequency of use. More often than not, chewing gum is the delivery vehicle. Several clinical trials have demonstrated the beneficial effects of chewing xylitol-based gum. Box 26.6 lists available products that contain xylitol.

Chlorhexidine. Chlorhexidine gluconate 0.12% is a bis-biguanide local antiinfective that is used to kill *S. mutans* bacteria and reduce the harmful effects of biofilm. Chlorhexidine mouth rinse, when used 15 mL twice daily for 1 week and is repeated every month for 6 months is effective in reducing the incidence of caries (Fig. 26.6).

GINGIVITIS

Gingivitis is the result of the accumulation of supragingival bacterial plaque. If this plaque buildup is not controlled, the plaque grows and invades subgingival spaces. If left untreated, chronic gingivitis can lead to severe periodontal disease or periodontitis. Gingivitis is the mildest form of periodontal disease and the most common.

Prevention

Preventive measures against gingivitis are similar to those against caries. The prevention of gingivitis depends on plaque control. Therefore many of the same products used to prevent caries are also used to prevent gingivitis. Active antigingivitis ingredients in dentifrices, mouth rinses, and other plaque removal products include SnF, triclosan, cetylpyridinium chloride, and stabilized SnF.

Brushing and flossing are the first line of defense in treating and preventing gingivitis. Brushing, flossing, and rinsing twice a day dramatically reduce plaque buildup.

Chlorhexidine

Chlorhexidine: adjunct therapy used for a limited time.

Chlorhexidine is active against both gram-positive and gram-negative bacteria and has some antifungal activity. It is a safe product that does not appear to succumb to bacterial resistance. Chlorhexidine binds to the bacterial cell membrane and increases its permeability, resulting in cell death. Chlorhexidine rinse is used in persons with periodontal disease. It is used not prophylactically but as an adjunct therapy for up to 6 months. It is discontinued when the periodontal disease is under control. Chlorhexidine rinse 0.12% is used twice daily. Patients rinse for 30 seconds with 15 mL of chlorhexidine twice a day. The most common adverse effects include tooth and mucosal staining, bitter taste, taste alteration, increased calculus formation, and mucosal irritation. It is best for the patient to rinse after eating in the morning and before bedtime because of the taste changes. Sodium laurel sulfate reduces the antimicrobial effect of chlorhexidine, and the two should be administered at least 30 minutes apart. Chlorhexidine gluconate is now available as an alcohol-free rinse.

Essential Oils

The antigingivitis mouth rinse that contains thymol, menthol, and eucalyptol has been shown to reduce gingivitis and plaque. In a recent clinical trial, use of an essential oil mouth rinse plus brushing and flossing was found to be effective in reducing interproximal bleeding. The essential oil mouth rinse produced results to similar to those of chlorhexidine at the end of 6 months of therapy, whereas chlorhexidine showed improvements at the end of the first 3 months.

Triclosan

Triclosan is a natural substance with antibacterial efficacy that reduces plaque and gingivitis. Research has shown that triclosan is more effective than fluoridated products in reducing gingivitis. Triclosan carries the ADA Seal of Acceptance as an antigingivitis agent. The only dentifrice product in the United States containing 0.3% triclosan, copolymer, and 0.243% NaF is Colgate Total. It has no side effects and is safe to use. Most recently, the FDA has stated that there is no evidence that triclosan in personal care items provides any additional benefits beyond the antigingivitis effects found in toothpaste.

TOOTH HYPERSENSITIVITY

Oral pain and discomfort are among the most common oral health disorders in the United States. Tooth hypersensitivity, or dentinal hyperalgesia (DH), is characterized by a short, sharp pain that comes from exposed dentin in response to thermal, chemical, or physical stimuli and that that cannot be attributed to any other type of dental defect or

Antibacterial Therapy: Age 6 Years and Older

Chlorhexidine gluconate 0.12%
- Rinse 15 mL twice daily for 1 week
- Repeat every month for 6 months and reassess
- Recommended use is morning and evening after toothbrushing
- Patients should be instructed to not rinse with water or other mouthwashes, brush teeth, or eat immediately after use.

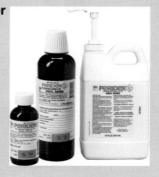

Fig. 26.6 Example of a 0.12% chlorhexidine gluconate mouth rinse. (Courtesy 3 M ESPE, St Paul, MN.)

disease. Severe attrition and gingival recession as a result of abrasions, erosions, abfraction, and abnormal tooth development can lead to tooth hypersensitivity. Tooth hypersensitivity can occur after teeth whitening treatments if the root surfaces are exposed. Bleaching can increase the risk for sensitivity.

Pathophysiology

Two processes are necessary for the development of DH: the dentin must become exposed through the loss of gingival recession or enamel and the dentin tubules must be open to the oral cavity and the pulp (Fig. 26.7). This occurs when the smear layer of the dentin tubular plugs is removed and the outer orifice of the tubule is opened and exposed to stimuli. When heat, cold, pressure, or acid touch exposed dentin or reach an open tubule, fluid flow in the dentinal tubule increases, causing greater stimulation of the nerves and resulting in pain.

> Both internal (reflux) and external (drugs, foods, or drinks) acids lead to dental erosion.

Dental erosion, which affects tooth enamel, is a result of both intrinsic and extrinsic acids. Extrinsic sources of acid include medication, foods, and drink. Citrus juices, carbonated drinks, wines, and ciders put the patient at risk for tooth hypersensitivity. The most common cause of intrinsic acid production is gastric reflux.

Treatment

The goals of treating tooth hypersensitivity are to alter the damage to the tooth surface using the appropriate dentifrice and to stop abrasive toothbrushing practices. The choice of therapeutic agent should be based on effectiveness, caries risk, amount of tooth structure present, patient acceptance, cost, and esthetics. Treatment for acute DH includes placing a barrier between the exposed nerve at the area where the pulp interfaces with the dentin tubule and the opening of the exposed dentin tubules that opens to the oral cavity. Desensitizing agents seal the dentin tubules and prevent irritants from stimulating the nerves when topically applied to the dentin.

At-Home Therapies

The most common therapy for at-home use is desensitizing toothpaste (Table 26.5 and Fig. 26.8). The vast majority of desensitizing toothpastes contain 5% potassium nitrate. Potassium ions are thought to diffuse along dentin tubules and decrease the excitability of intradental nerves by altering their membrane potential and reducing repolarization.

In-Office Therapies

Professionally applied products include fluorides (NaF, SnF), potassium oxalate, and adhesives and resins (Fig. 26.9). Their effects are temporary because they do not adhere to the dentin surface.

Fluorides. NaF is thought to work through the formation of insoluble calcium fluoride within the dentin tubules. ADA-accepted products for desensitization include 33.3% SnF applied as a paste or solution and burnished over the sensitive dental area. NaF therapy is not permanent and must be repeated for an extended effect.

Oxalates. Oxalate products reduce dentin permeability and occlude the tubules. Several clinical trials have demonstrated their efficacy, but other trials have found that they are no better than placebo.

Adhesives and resins. Adhesive products differ from other in-office therapies in that they provide longer-lasting desensitization. They include cavity varnishes, bonding agents, and restorative resin materials. Cavity varnishes provide a protective barrier between the dentin tubules and the oral environment. However, acids dissolve them and they need to be reapplied. Restorations seal the tubule, providing an opportunity for permanent protection.

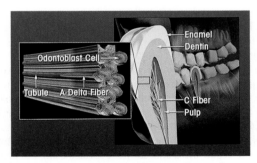

Fig. 26.7 Structure of a dentinal tubule. (Courtesy Osprey Communications, Inc., Stamford, CT.)

TABLE 26.5 Selected Desensitizing Toothpastes	
Trade Name	**Active Ingredients**
Crest Pro-Health	Stannous fluoride 0.454%, sodium hexametaphosphate
Orajel Sensitive Pain-Relieving Toothpaste for Adults	Potassium nitrate 5%, sodium monofluorophosphate 0.20%
Crest Sensitivity Protection	Potassium nitrate 5%, sodium fluoride 0.243%

These toothpastes have earned the American Dental Association Seal of Acceptance for Desensitization.

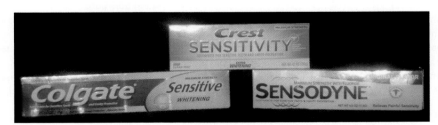

Fig. 26.8 Examples of desensitizing dentifrices. (From Darby ML, Walsh MM. *Dental Hygiene: Theory and Practice.* 4th ed. St. Louis: Saunders; 2015.)

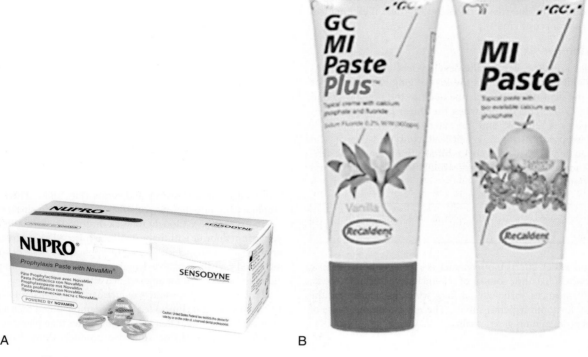

A

B

Fig. 26.9 Examples of professionally applied desensitizing agents. (Part A: Courtesy Dentsply International, York, PA; Part B: Copyright Statement: © GC America, Inc., all rights reserved, courtesy of GC America, Inc.)

DENTAL HYGIENE CONSIDERATIONS

The primary objective of patient-centered oral health care is the removal of plaque to prevent caries and gingivitis. Most patients need only follow product instructions and self-care measures provided by the dental hygienist.

Patient Education for Caries and Gingivitis
Nondrug Therapies
- Avoid cariogenic foods that contain more than 15% sugar.
- Eat low-cariogenic foods such as foods with high water content (fresh fruit), foods that stimulate saliva flow, and foods high in protein.
- Alcohol and tobacco use can cause caries and gingivitis.
- Hormonal changes during pregnancy exaggerate the inflammatory effect of plaque, which can lead to gingivitis. Consider incorporating gum massage as an antigingivitis measure.

Plaque Removal
- Mechanically remove plaque buildup by brushing teeth at least twice daily (see Box 26.2).
- Use a toothbrush with nylon bristles.
- Replace the toothbrush when the bristles show signs of wear and tear.
- For children younger than 2 years, apply a tiny dollop of fluoride paste, about the size of a grain of rice, once the first tooth appears.
- Children less than 3 years of age should just get a "smear" of toothpaste.
- Use only regular strength fluoride toothpastes in children ages 2 to 6 years.
- For preschool children (3–6 years of age), place a pea-size amount of toothpaste on the toothbrush and brush the child's teeth until they can do it themselves.

- Teach children how to rinse the mouth and spit out toothpaste or mouth rinse and to avoid swallowing fluoride.

Flossing Teeth
- Floss teeth at least once a day (see Box 26.3).

Mouth Rinse and Gels
- Teach children how to rinse with mouth rinses and to avoid swallowing fluoride (see Boxes 26.4 and 26 5).
- Teach adults and children not to swallow mouth rinses.

Patient Education for Tooth Hypersensitivity
The objectives for the patient regarding self-care for tooth hypersensitivity are to repair the damaged tooth surface using the appropriate home or in-office therapy and to stop abrasive brushing. Most patients obtain positive results by following product instructions and the dental hygienist's recommendations.

Patient Self-Care
- Use soft-bristled toothbrushes and brush by applying light pressure to the teeth and gums.
- Use a toothpaste for sensitive teeth and brush at or near the receding gumline.
- Note that relief may not be observed for several days to weeks.
- The better the plaque removal, the more quickly the sensitivity will resolve.
- Use prescription and nonprescription products as directed by the oral health care provider.

ACADEMIC SKILLS ASSESSMENT

1. Describe the two ways to minimize the risk for dental caries.
2. Describe the mechanism of action of fluoride in preventing caries.
3. Describe the signs of acute fluoride toxicity and chronic fluoride toxicity.
4. How is acute fluoride toxicity managed?
5. What directions should be given to the patient for topical home-use fluoride products?
6. What directions should be given to the patient following fluoride varnish applications?
7. How is xylitol used to prevent dental caries?
8. How should 0.2% chlorhexidine be used?
9. What are the adverse effects of chlorhexidine rinse?
10. What are the contributing factors to dentin hypersensitivity?
11. Compare and contrast in-office and home-use desensitization products.

CLINICAL CASE STUDY

Annie Lin, 6 years old, has been coming to your practice for 3 years. She is in today for her scheduled oral health maintenance examination. So far so good; she has been very good about brushing her teeth, flossing, and rinsing with help from her parents. During today's examination, you will clean her teeth and review good brushing techniques.

1. How much toothpaste should a 6-year-old child place on his or her toothbrush?
2. Mrs. Lin has brought Annie's baby brother, who is now 6 months old. He is getting ready to cut his first tooth. When should the Lins start oral health care with him?
3. Why kind of mouth rinse should Annie be using? Why?
4. Many of the toothpastes geared for children taste very good. What is the concern regarding the ingestion of too much toothpaste in young children?

REFERENCE

1. Harris NO, Garcia-Godoy F. *Primary Preventive Dentistry*. 6th ed. Stamford, CT: Appleton & Lange; 2004.

BIBLIOGRAPHY

Weck Marciniak M. Oral and pain discomfort. In: Beredi RR, Ferreri SP, Hume AL, et al., eds. *Handbook of Nonprescription Drugs*. 16th ed.Washington, DC: American Pharmaceutical Association; 2009:602–623.

Whitaker AL. Prevention of hygiene-related disorders. In: Beredi RR, Ferreri SP, Hume AL, et al., eds. *Handbook of Nonprescription Drugs*. 16th ed.Washington, DC: American Pharmaceutical Association; 2009:581–600.

A | APPENDIX

Medical Acronyms

Term	Meaning
2-PAM	pralidoxime
5-FU	5-fluorouracil
5-HT	serotonin (5-hydroxytryptamine)
AAC	antibiotic-associated colitis
ACE	angiotensin-converting enzyme
ACEI	angiotensin-converting enzyme inhibitor
ACTH	adrenocorticotropic hormone
AD(H)D	attention deficit (hyperactivity) disorder
ADA	American Dental Association
ADHA	American Dental Hygiene Association
ADP	adenosine diphosphate
AHA	American Heart Association
AHF	antihemophilic factor
AIDS	acquired immunodeficiency syndrome
AII	angiotensin II
ALG	antilymphocyte globulin
ALL	acute lymphocytic leukemia
ALT	alanine aminotransferase (formerly called SGPT)
APAP	acetaminophen
APTT	activated partial thromboplastin time
ARA	angiotensin receptor antagonist
ARB	angiotensin receptor blocker
ASA	aspirin
ASA I, II, III, IV	American Society of Anesthesiology planes of anesthesia
ASCVD	atherosclerotic cardiovascular disease
AST	aspartate aminotransferase (formerly called SGOT)
ATG	antithymocyte globulin
ATP	adenosine triphosphate
AV	atrioventricular
AZT	zidovudine, azidothymidine
BCG	bacillus Calmette-Guérin (vaccine)
BCP	birth control pill
BE	bacterial endocarditis
BMS	bone marrow suppression
BMT	bone marrow transplant
BNDD	Bureau of Narcotics and Dangerous Drugs (now DEA)
BP	blood pressure

Term	Meaning
BPH	benign prostatic hypertrophy
BT	bleeding time
BUN	blood urea nitrogen
CABG	coronary artery bypass graft
CAD	coronary artery disease
CAT	computed axial tomography
C & S	culture and sensitivity (testing)
CBC	complete blood count
CDC	US Centers for Disease Control and Prevention
c-GMP	cyclic guanosine monophosphate
CIS	carcinoma in situ
CK	creatine phosphokinase
CLL	chronic lymphocytic leukemia
CML	chronic myelocytic leukemia
CNS	central nervous system
COM	catecholamine-O-methyl transferase
COPD	chronic obstructive pulmonary disease
CRH	corticotropin-releasing hormone
CSF	corticotropin-stimulating factor or cerebrospinal fluid
CVA	cerebral vascular accident
CVS	cardiovascular system
D/C	discontinue
DDAVP	1-deamio-8-D-arginine vasopressin, desmopressin
ddC	zalcitabine
ddI	didanosine
DEA	Drug Enforcement Administration
DIC	disseminated intravascular coagulation
DIP	distal interphalangeal (joints)
DM	diabetes mellitus, dextromethorphan
DMARD	disease-modifying antirheumatic drug
DNA	deoxyribonucleic acid
DTs	delirium tremens
EACA	ε-aminocaproic acid
EBV	Epstein-Barr virus
ECG	electrocardiogram
ED50	effective dose in 50% of patients
EEG	electroencephalogram
ENL	erythema nodosum leprosum
EPA	Environmental Protection Agency
EPS	extrapyramidal syndrome
ESRD	end-stage renal disease

Term	Meaning
EtOH	ethanol (alcohol)
FAD	flavin adenine dinucleotide
FDA	US Food and Drug Administration
FMN	flavin mononucleotide
FTAs	fluorescent treponema antibodies
G6PD	glucose-6-phosphate dehydrogenase ($NADP^+$)
GABA	γ-aminobutyric acid
GBV	hepatitis G virus
GCF	gingival crevicular fluid
GI(T)	gastrointestinal (tract)
GU	genitourinary
GVHD	graft-versus-host disease
HAV	hepatitis A virus
HBcAg	hepatitis B core antigen
HBcAb	hepatitis B core antibody
HBIG	hepatitis B immune globulin
HBP	high blood pressure
HBsAg	hepatitis B surface antigen
HBV	hepatitis B virus
HCTZ	hydrochlorothiazide
HCV	hepatitis C virus, parenteral non-A, non-B hepatitis
HDL	high-density lipoprotein (cholesterol)
HDV	hepatitis D virus, delta hepatitis virus
HER2	human epidermal growth factor receptor 2 protein
HEV	hepatitis E virus, epidemic non-A, non-B hepatitis
HF	heart failure
HGBV-C	hepatitis GB virus C
HGV	hepatitis G virus
HIV	human immunodeficiency virus
HPA	hypothalamic-pituitary-adrenal (axis)
HPV	human papillomavirus
HR	heart rate
HRT	hormone replacement therapy
HSV	herpes simplex virus
HSV-1	herpes simplex virus, type I
HSV-2	herpes simplex virus, type II
HTN	hypertension
HZV	herpes zoster virus
I & D	incision and drainage
IBD	inflammatory bowel disease
IBS	irritable bowel syndrome
ID	intradermal
IDDM	insulin-dependent diabetes mellitus
IDU	idoxuridine
IE	infective endocarditis
IgE	immunoglobulin E
IgG	immunoglobulin G
IgM	immunoglobulin M
IM	intramuscular
IND	investigational new drug
INH	isoniazid
INR	international normalized ratio
ISI	international sensitivity index
IV	intravenous

Term	Meaning
IVF	in vitro fertilization
IUD	intrauterine device
LD50	lethal dose in 50% of subjects
LDH	lactic acid dehydrogenase
LDL	low-density lipoprotein (cholesterol)
LFT	liver function test
LH	luteinizing hormone
LJP	localized juvenile periodontitis
LSD	lysergic acid diethylamide
MAC	*Mycobacterium avium* (intracellulare) complex
MAO	monoamine oxidase
MAOI	monoamine oxidase inhibitor
MCA	monoclonal antibody
MD	multiple dystrophy
MDM	minor determinate mixture
MDR	multidrug-resistant
MHC	major histocompatibility complex
MI	myocardial infarction
MRI	magnetic resonance imaging
MS	multiple sclerosis, morphine sulfate
MTX	methotrexate
N_2O	nitrous oxide
NDA	new drug application
NHL	non-Hodgkin's lymphoma
NIDDM	non-insulin-dependent diabetes mellitus
NMS	neuromalignant syndrome
NNRTI	nonnucleoside reverse transcriptase inhibitor
NPH	neutral protein Hagedorn (insulin)
NPO	nil per os (nothing by mouth)
NREM	non-rapid eye movement
NS	normal saline
NSAIAs	nonsteroidal antiinflammatory agents
NSAIDs	nonsteroidal antiinflammatory drugs
NTG	nitroglycerin
NTX	naltrexone
N&V	nausea and vomiting
O_2	oxygen
OA	osteoarthritis
OB	obstetrics
OCs	oral contraceptives
OCD	obsessive-compulsive disorder
OD	overdose
O & E	observation and examination
OGTT	oral glucose tolerance test
OPV	oral poliovirus vaccine
OSHA	Occupational Safety and Health Administration
OTC	over-the counter
PABA	*p*-aminobenzoic acid
PANS	parasympathetic autonomic nervous system
para 1	unipara (1 child)
PAS	para-aminosalicylic acid
PAT	paroxysmal atrial tachycardia
PBP	penicillin-binding protein
PCN	penicillin

Term	Meaning
PCP	*Pneumocystis carinii,* phencyclidine
PCR	polymerase chain reaction
PD	Parkinson's disease
P/D	packs per day
PDE5	phosphodiesterase type 5
PDT	photodynamic therapy
PG	pregnant, prostaglandin
pH	function of amount of hydrogen ion (log 1/[H +])
PID	pelvic inflammatory disease
PMC	pseudomembranous colitis
PMS	premenstrual syndrome
PO	per os (by mouth)
PPD	purified protein derivative
PPL	penicilloyl polylysine
PT	prothrombin time
PTCA	percutaneous transluminal coronary angioplasty
PTH	parathyroid hormone
PTT	partial thromboplastin time
PTU	propylthiouracil
PUD	peptic ulcer disease
PVD	peripheral vascular disease
PVT	paroxysmal ventricular tachycardia
QRS	ECG effects of cardiac muscle depolarization
RA	rheumatoid arthritis
RAS	recurrent aphthous stomatitis
RBC	red blood cell
RHD	rheumatic heart disease
RNA	ribonucleic acid
R/O	rule out
RPR	rapid plasma reagin
RSV	respiratory syncytial virus
SA	sinoatrial (node)
SANS	sympathetic autonomic nervous system
SAR	structure-activity relationship
SC	subcutaneous

Term	Meaning
SGOT	serum glutamic oxaloacetate transferase (AST)
SGPT	serum glutamic pyruvate transferase (ALT)
SL	sublingual
SLE	systemic lupus erythematosus
SMP-TMX	sulfamethoxazole-trimethoprim
SOB	shortness of breath
SQ	subcutaneous
SSRI	selective serotonin reuptake inhibitor
STD	sexually transmitted disease
STS	serologic test for syphilis
SVT	supraventricular tachycardia
T_3	triiodothyronine
T_4	levothyroxine
TB	tuberculosis
TBG	thyroid-binding globulin
TCA	tricyclic antidepressant
TCN	tetracycline
THC	tetrahydrocannabinol
TI	therapeutic index
TIA	transient ischemic attack
TMD	temporomandibular disease
TMJ	temporomandibular joint
TNF	tumor necrosis factor
TNM	tumor node metastasis
tPA	tissue plasminogen activator
TPP	thiamine pyrophosphate
TPR	total peripheral resistance
TRH	thyroid-releasing hormone
TSH	thyroid-stimulating hormone
TT	thrombin time
Tx	treatment
TXA	thromboxane
VLDL	very-low-density lipoprotein (cholesterol)
VZV	varicella-zoster virus
WBC	white blood cell

Medical Terminology

This appendix does not attempt to provide a course in medical terminology. To cover that subject completely would require an entire book. However, there are many medical vocabulary words in pharmacology needed to discuss drugs and their effects. In fact, many of these words that sound strange now will seem familiar later. Without this vocabulary, one will find it difficult to comprehend drug reference sources. Because some of the words will be unfamiliar, one should have an opportunity to learn these and other new terms.

When one sees a medical terminology word that one does not know, one should approach the word like a puzzle and attempt to identify any pieces that are known. One should consider whether one has seen a piece before and what it might mean. One should guess what those few letters might mean. Then one should "look up" the drug in a database, medical dictionary, or even the glossary in the appendix. One should write the word on a small card (one-third of a 3 × 5 card) and write the definition on the other side. After one has written the definition on the card, one should consider the word parts and identify the little pieces that make up the word. These pieces may be beginning pieces (prefixes), middle pieces (word roots [=core]), or end pieces (suffixes). There are also pieces that mean no or not or that reverse the word's meaning. These little pieces come from Greek and/or Latin word parts. Now one should look at a couple of words.

- *Hypertension: Hyper-:* One may have heard someone say "That person is 'hyper-.'" It means a lot of, or more of, or too much of. Therefore, the *hyper-* piece of the word means excessive. *Tension* refers to tension or blood pressure. So *hypertension* means excessive blood pressure. What would be the definition of hypotension?
- Dysmenorrhea: *Dys-* means bad, difficult, or abnormal; *Men-* is a root word meaning monthly and is associated with menstruation. The suffix *-rhea* refers to flow. From these parts, the definition of this word is "painful menstrual flow."
- The prefix *a-* refers to less or lack of. What is the definition of *amenorrhea*?
- If the prefix for the nose is *rhin-* (as in rhinoceros nose horns, wild animal, charge), then what does *rhinorrhea* mean?
- If the suffix *-itis* means inflammation, then what does *rhinitis* mean?
- *Thyroidectomy: Thyroid* refers to the thyroid gland, whereas *-ectomy* means surgical removal. So the word means "surgical removal of the thyroid gland." How about *tonsillectomy*?

Box B.1 lists a few prefixes, Box B.2 a few core words, and Box B.3 a few suffixes. One can add new word parts as one learns them.

When a new drug group is named, a generic name and a trade name are given. The generic name is longer, and the trade name is short and easier to remember. Sometimes, when more members of a drug group are discovered and marketed, the subsequent drugs in the group are given the same suffix. A few drug suffixes—drug names ending in the same letters that belong to the same group—are listed in Box B.4.

BOX B.1 A Few Prefixes

without, absent
brady- slow
hemi- half
hyper- above, excessive
intra- within
lith- stone, calculus
pan- all
qua- four; quarter (one-fourth of a dollar); *qid* (Latin *quater in die*) means "4 times a day"
sub- under (submarine?)
tachy- fast
tri- tricycle (3-wheeled); *tid* means "3 times a day"

BOX B.2 A Few Root or Core Words

bronch- bronchus
cardi- heart
cephal- head
chol- gall, bile
col- colon
cyan- blue
derm- skin
epitheli- epithelium (outside of skin)
gast- stomach
hem- blood
hepat- liver
leuk- white
lingu- tongue
lip- fat
my- muscle
neph- kidney
neuro- nerve
path- disease
pneum- lungs, air
post- back, behind
proct- rectum
prostat- prostate
stenosis- narrowing
stomat- mouth
thrombo- blood clot
vertebr- spine

BOX B.3   A Few Suffixes

-*algia* pain
-*dynia* pain
-*ectomy* surgical removal
-*itis* inflammation
-*lysis* destruction, loosening
-*malacia* softening
-*megaly* enlargement
-*ologist* specialist
-*oma* tumor
-*otomy* incision into
-*penia* fewer (abnormal)
-*plasty* surgical repair
-*ptosis* droopy or falling down
-*rrhea* flow
-*scopy* visual examination ("scope it out")
-*thorax* chest

BOX B.4   Suffixes for Drugs

-*azolam* benzodiazepines
-*clovir* antiviral agents
-*cycline* antibiotics
-*dipine* calcium channel blockers
-*ecoxib* cyclooxygenase (COX) II–specific antiinflammatories
-*floxacin* antiinfectives, quinolones
-*glinide* hypoglycemics, oral
-*glitazone* thiazolidinediones (antidiabetic)
-*ifene* antiestrogens
-*lukast* leukotriene inhibitors
-*mycin* antibiotics
-*olol* β-blockers
-*prazole* proton pump inhibitors
-*pril* angiotensin-converting enzyme (ACE) inhibitors
-*sartan* angiotensin II receptor antagonists
-*stigmine* cholinergic agents
-*triptan* serotonin agonists, for migraine
-*tron* serotonin antagonists
-*[con]azole* antifungals, azoles
-*[va]statin* 3-hydroxy-3-methylglutaryl (HMG)-CoA reductase inhibitors

What If...

This appendix addresses a number of patient-related questions that are among the most common the dental practitioner will encounter in daily practice. The "decision trees" in this appendix help guide the practitioner through the steps involved in assessing clinical situations quickly and making related treatment decisions.

Topics covered in "What If" include drugs safe to use in pregnancy, allergy management, infective endocarditis prophylaxis, and a summary of the relationship between dental treatment, warfarin, and the international normalized ratio.

Allergies discussed include those to codeine, aspirin, penicillin, sulfites, and latex.

WHAT IF ... THE PATIENT IS PREGNANT?*

Drug Group	Drug Name	OK to Use?
Local anesthetics	Lidocaine with epinephrine	Yes
Analgesics	Aspirin	No
	Acetaminophen	Yes
	Nonsteroidal antiinflammatory drugs	No
	Opioids	Yes
Antiinfective agents/antibiotics	Penicillin	Yes
	Erythromycin	Yes*
	Tetracycline	No
	Doxycycline	No
	Clindamycin	Yes
	Metronidazole	No

*Avoid erythromycin estolate in pregnancy.

WHAT IF ... THE PATIENT IS ALLERGIC TO ASPIRIN?

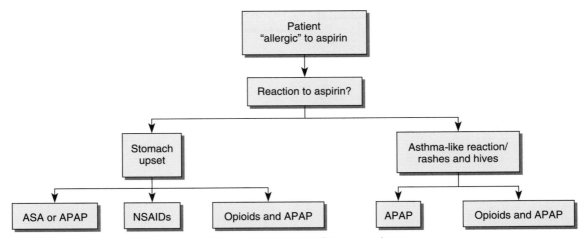

APAP, Acetaminophen; ASA, aspirin; NSAIDs, nonsteroidal antiinflammatory drugs.

*For more details see Chapter 22.

WHAT IF ... THE PATIENT IS ALLERGIC TO PENICILLIN?

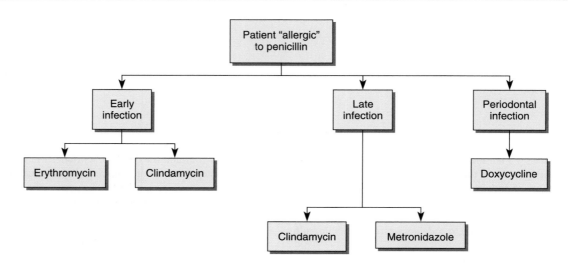

WHAT IF ... THE PATIENT IS ALLERGIC TO SULFITES?

There is a lack of cross-hypersensitivity among the following: "sulfa" drugs, sulfites, sulfur, sulfate, and sulfide. "Sulfa drugs" are used to treat urinary tract infections, and the allergic reaction to any of them is usually a rash. Dental patients allergic to "sulfa" drugs may safely be given local anesthetics or a vasoconstrictor that contains sulfites.

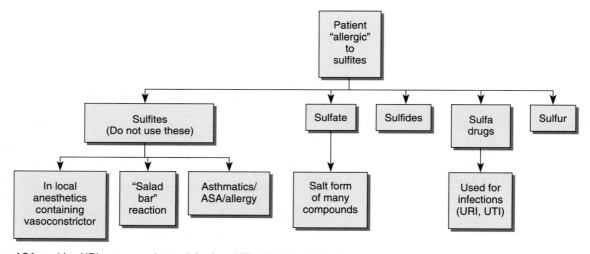

ASA, aspirin; URI, upper respiratory infection; UTI, urinary tract infection.

WHAT IF ... THE PATIENT IS ALLERGIC TO CODEINE?

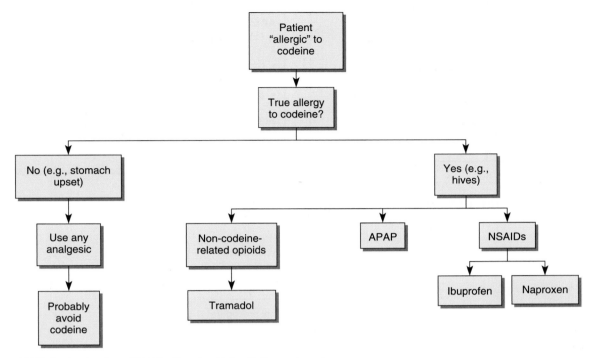

APAP, Acetaminophen; *NSAIDs*, Nonsteroidal antiinflammatory drugs.

WHAT IF ... THE PATIENT IS ALLERGIC TO LATEX?

The increased use of latex-containing products has exposed more people with increasing frequency to latex allergens. Latex comes from the rubber tree and contains natural latex. Patients who are frequently exposed to latex-containing products (e.g., patients with spina bifida) and health care workers who use latex products (e.g., dental professionals) have a greater likelihood of development of allergies.

The extent of the reactions to latex ranges from contact dermatitis to severe anaphylactic reaction with death in a few minutes. If a dental practitioner uses any latex materials in his or her office, then parenteral epinephrine should be readily available.

There is also a cross-hypersensitivity between the foods listed in Box C.1 and latex allergy. If a patient is allergic to the listed fruits, then the dental health care worker should carefully question the patient regarding any reactions to latex-containing products (e.g., balloons, condoms). The patient should also be informed about cross-hypersensitivity that may occur between these fruits and latex. When powdered gloves are used, the latex can be absorbed into the powder and circulated around the room. This airborne latex can float around rooms and can even be stirred up with cleaning. Airborne latex can produce respiratory reactions such as asthma and anaphylaxis.

If a patient has an allergy to latex, he or she should be given the first appointment so that the latex particles have not contaminated the operatory air. The ventilation should be checked and measured for the complete replacement of room air to make sure that the particles are removed overnight. One should be aware of the occupants of the building because use of latex in another office could inject latex particles into the central heating or cooling.

Manufactured latex products may contain a small amount of natural latex proteins, a very large amount, or somewhere in between. Asking for more information on the latex gloves used in the dental office may enable the switch to a different brand to the reduce the exposure to allergenic proteins.

When a latex-allergic patient is treated, non-latex equipment should be substituted for any products that contain latex (Box C.2). Newer product catalogs contain a wide range of dental-related products (e.g., non-latex bite blocks, dams, and adhesives for bandages). Books that contain additional information about latex allergy may include infection-control topics.

BOX C.1   Foods Having Potential for Cross-Hypersensitivity With Latex Hypersensitivity

- Apples
- Avocados
- Bananas
- Carrots
- Celery
- Cherries
- Chestnuts
- Hazelnuts
- Kiwis
- Melons
- Papayas
- Peaches
- Pears
- Pineapples
- Potatoes
- Rye
- Strawberries
- Tomatoes
- Wheat

BOX C.2   Dental Objects Composed of Latex

All Commonly Used Brands Contain Latex
- Gloves
- Rubber dam
- Local anesthetic cartridges (stopper)
- Syringes (black rubber inside)
- Bite block

Some Brands May Contain Latex
- Strings that hold mask on
- Strings that hold gown on
- Glasses bridges

WHAT IF ... THE CARDIAC PATIENT NEEDS ANTIBIOTICS? (SEE CHAPTER 7)

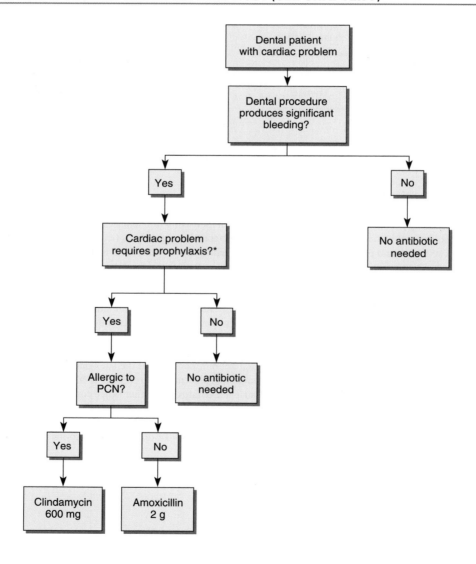

*See Box 7.6.
PCN, Penicillin.

WHAT IF ...THE PATIENT WITH PRIMARY TOTAL JOINT REPLACEMENT NEEDS ANTIBIOTICS? (SEE CHAPTER 7)

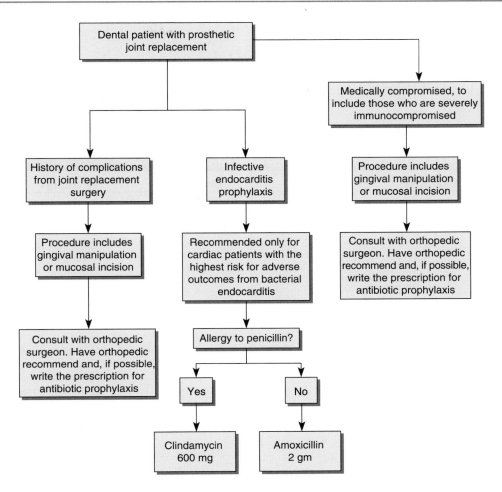

WHAT IF ... THE PATIENT IS TAKING WARFARIN (COUMADIN)? (SEE CHAPTER 12)

Dental Procedure	OK to Treat if INR <
Periodontal probing	<4
Restorative, simple scaling/root planning endodontics	3.5
Extraction, simple	2.5–3.5
Extraction, multiple	2–3.5
Periodontal surgery	2.5

INR, International normalized ratio.

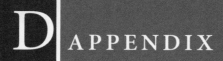

Oral Manifestations: Xerostomia and Taste Changes

TABLE D.1 Agents That Produce Xerostomia (Dry Mouth)*

Drug Group	Examples	Drug Group	Examples
β₂-agonist adrenergic agents (decongestants, anoretics)	Albuterol (Proventil, Ventolin) Dextroamphetamine (Dexedrine) Dopamine (Intropin) Ephedrine Epinephrine (Adrenalin) Isoproterenol (Isuprel) Metaproterenol (Alupent) Methylphenidate (Ritalin) Phenylephrine (Neo-Synephrine) Pseudoephedrine (Sudafed)	Antidepressants, tricyclic	Amitriptyline (Elavil) Amoxapine (Asendin) Clomipramine (Anafranil) Desipramine (Norpramin, Pertofrane) Doxepin (Sinequan, Adapin) Imipramine (Tofranil) Nortriptyline (Aventyl) Protriptyline (Vivactil) Trimipramine (Surmontil)
Serotonin amplifiers	Dexfenfluramine (Redux)	Antidepressants, other	Bupropion (Wellbutrin, Zyban) Maprotiline (Ludiomil) Mirtazapine (Remeron) Nefazodone (Serzone)‡ Sibutramine (Meridia) Trazodone (Desyrel) Venlafaxine (Effexor)‡
Antiarrhythmics	Disopyramide Procainamide Quinidine		
Anticholinergics†	Atropine Belladonna Belladonna alkaloids with phenobarbital (Donnatal) Clidinium (in Librax, in Clindex) Dicyclomine (Bentyl) Flavoxate (Urispas) Glycopyrrolate (Robinul [Forte]) Homatropine (Isopto Homatropine) Ipratropium (IH) (Atrovent) Hyoscyamine (Anaspaz, Levsin) Meclizine (Antivert) Methantheline (Banthine) Methscopolamine (Pamine) Oxybutynin (Ditropan) Propantheline (Pro-Banthine) Scopolamine (hyoscine)	Antidepressants, selective serotonin reuptake inhibitors	Fluoxetine (Prozac) Fluvoxamine (Luvox) Paroxetine (Paxil) Sertraline (Zoloft)
		Antidepressants, monoamine oxide inhibitors	Isocarboxazid (Marplan) Phenelzine (Nardil) Tranylcypromine (Parnate)
Antiparkinsonian agents	Amantadine (Symmetrel) Benztropine (Cogentin) Biperiden (Akineton) Ethopropazine (Parsidol) Levodopa + carbidopa (Sinemet) Pergolide (Permax) Procyclidine (Kemadrin) Selegiline (Eldepryl) [AKA deprenil and deprenyl] Trihexyphenidyl (Artane)	Antihistamines	Azatadine (Optimine) (ophthalmic) Brompheniramine (Dimetane) Carbinoxamine (Clistin) Chlorpheniramine (Chlor-Trimeton) Clemastine (Tavist) Cyclizine Cyproheptadine (Periactin) Dexchlorpheniramine (Polaramine) Dimenhydrinate (Dramamine) Diphenhydramine (Benadryl) Hydroxyzine (Atarax, Vistaril) Levocabastine (Livostin) (ophthalmic) Meclizine (Antivert) Methdilazine Olopatadine (Patanol) (ophthalmic) Phenindamine Promethazine (Phenergan) Tripelennamine (PBZ) Triprolidine (Actidil)
Anticonvulsants	Carbamazepine (Tegretol) Gabapentin (Neurontin)		

Continued

TABLE D.1   Agents That Produce Xerostomia (Dry Mouth)—cont'd

Drug Group	Examples
Antihistamines, nonsedating	Acrivastine (in Semprex-D) Cetirizine (Zyrtec) Fexofenadine (Allegra) Loratadine (Claritin)

Antihypertensives	Calcium channel blockers
	    Bepridil (Vascor)
	α_1-antagonists
	    Prazosin (Minipress)
	    Doxazosin (Cardura)
	    Terazosin (Hytrin)
	α_2-agonists
	    Clonidine (Catapres)[§]
	    Guanabenz (Wytensin)
	    Guanfacine (Tenex)
	    Methyldopa (Aldomet)
	Peripheral α antagonists
	    Guanethidine (Ismelin)
	    Guanadrel (Hylorel)
	Reserpines

Antipsychotics[†]	Chlorpromazine (Thorazine) Clozapine (Clozaril) Droperidol (Inapsine) Fluphenazine (Prolixin) Haloperidol (Haldol) Loxapine (Loxitane) Mesoridazine (Serentil) Methdilazine (Tacaryl) Molindone (Moban) Pimozide (Orap) Prochlorperazine (Compazine) Promazine (Sparine) Promethazine (Phenergan) Quetiapine (Seroquel) Risperidone (Risperdal)[‡] Thioridazine (Mellaril) Thioxanthenes Trifluoperazine (Stelazine) Triflupromazine (Vesprin)

Benzodiazepines/ sedative-hypnotics	Benzodiazepines
	    Alprazolam (Xanax)
	    Chlordiazepoxide (Librium)
	    Clonazepam (Klonopin)
	    Clorazepate (Tranxene)
	    Diazepam (Valium)
	    Estazolam (ProSom)
	    Flurazepam (Dalmane)
	    Halazepam (Paxipam)

Drug Group	Examples
	Lorazepam (Ativan) Midazolam (Versed) Oxazepam (Serax) Prazepam (Centrax) Quazepam (Doral) Temazepam (Restoril) Triazolam (Halcion)
Others	Phenobarbital Zolpidem (Ambien)
Cardiac glycoside	Digoxin

Diuretics	Thiazides
	    Hydrochlorothiazide (HCTZ)
	Loop
	    Bumetanide (Bumex)
	    Furosemide (Lasix)
	Combinations
	    Dyazide
	    Maxzide

Antiemetics	Metoclopramide (Reglan) Dronabinol (Marinol) Ondansetron (Zofran) Oxybutynin (Ditropan)
Miscellaneous	Caffeine Cromolyn (Intal) Ergotamine (Ergostat, in Cafergot) Nicotine (smoking cessation) Vitamin A analogs Isotretinoin (Accutane)
Muscle relaxants	Carisoprodol (Soma) Chlorzoxazone (Parafon Forte) Cyclobenzaprine (Flexeril) Methocarbamol (Robaxin) Orphenadrine (Norflex)
Opioids	Codeine Meperidine Morphine Oxycodone Pentazocine Propoxyphene Tramadol

[*]See Boxes 25.1 and 25.2 for other oral effects of drugs.
[†]More likely than others to produce xerostomia.
[‡]Less likely to cause xerostomia.
[§]Most likely to produce xerostomia.

TABLE D.2   Agents That Alter Taste

Drug	Taste Effects
ACE inhibitors	
Aceon	
Acetazolamide	M
Adenosine	M
Albuterol	C

Drug	Taste Effects
Allopurinol	N
Al(OH)$_3$	Chalky
Amiodarone	U
Amoxapine	U, A
Ampicillin	N

TABLE D.2   Agents That Alter Taste—cont'd

Drug	Taste Effects	Drug	Taste Effects
Antineoplastics	N	Moexipril (ACE inhibitor)	A
Antithrombin III	F	Moricizine	B
Aspirin	N	Nedocromil	U
Auranofin	M	Norfloxacin	B
Aurothioglucose	M	Nortriptyline	U
Aztreonam	A	Ofloxacin	A
Benazepril	C	Omeprazole	A
Benzocaine	N	Pamidronate	L
Bepridil	A	Penicillamine	N
Bitolterol	A	Pentamidine	B, M
Budesonide	B, L	Perindopril	D
Calcifediol	M	Perindopril erbumine	A
Calcitriol	M	Phytonadione	C
Carboprost tromethamine	A	Pirbuterol (Maxair)	C
Ceftriaxone	A	Pravastatin	A
Chlorhexidines	C, L	Propafenone	L
Cidofovir	A	Protirelin	B
Clarithromycin	A	Protriptyline	U
Clofazimine	A	Propylthiouracil	L
Clofibrate	N	Quinapril	C
Clomipramine	U	Quinidine	B
Cyclophosphamide	N	Quinine	B
Gold salts	N	Ramipril	A
Griseofulvin	N	Ranitidine/bismuth	D
Interferon alfa-2a	M, C	Rifabutin	P
Interferon alfa-n3	M, C	Ritonavir	A
Iodinated glycerol	M	Simvastatin	U
Iron dextran complex	M	Sodium phenylbutyrate	A
Potassium iodide	M	Succimer	B
Labetalol	A	Terbinafine	A
Levamisole	P	Terbutaline	B
Lithium	A	Tetracycline	N
Lomefloxacin	A	Trazodone	B
Losartan	A	Triazolam	A
Lovastatin	A	Tricyclic antidepressants	N
Mechlorethamine	M	Ursodiol	U, M
Mesna	B	Valsartan	A
Metaproterenol	B	Vinblastine	M
Methazolamide	M	Vinorelbine	M
Methimazole	A		
Methylergonovine	F		
Metronidazole	M, C		

A, Abnormal; *ACE,* angiotensin-converting enzyme; *B,* bad; *C,* change; *D,* disturbance; *F,* foul; *L,* loss; *M,* metallic; *N,* not specified; *P,* perversion; *U,* unpleasant.

Children's Dose Calculations

CALCULATION OF CHILDREN'S DOSE

The patient's weight is the usual basis for determining drug dose, although not the ideal method. This appendix lists various methods for determining a child's dose on the basis of an adult dose.

Clark's Rule

$$\frac{\text{Weight}(\text{lb}) \times \text{Adult dose}}{150} = \text{Infant dose}$$

Fried's Rule

$$\frac{\text{Age}(\text{mo}) \times \text{Adult dose}}{150} = \text{Infant dose}$$

Young's Rule

$$\frac{\text{Age}(\text{yr}) \times \text{Adult dose}}{\text{Age}(\text{yr}) + 12} = \text{Child dose}$$

Cowling's Rule

$$\frac{\text{Age}(\text{at next birthday}) \times \text{Adult dose}}{24} = \text{Child dose}$$

Surface Area Rule

$$(0.7 \times \text{Weight in lb}) + 10 = \% \text{Adult dose}$$

$$(1.5 \times \text{Weight in kg}) + 10 = \% \text{Adult dose}$$

DISCUSSION

Because weight may vary in children of the same age, a better method of calculating a child's or an infant's dose is based on body surface area. This method requires the use of a table or nomogram from which the body surface of the child can be determined. The child's body surface is a function of the height and weight of the child. The surface area formula is a convenient and more accurate formula than those based on the age or weight of the child.

Another method used to determine the child's dose is to follow a suggested pediatric dosage schedule prepared by the manufacturer. These doses are usually given in terms of milligrams of drug per kilogram of body weight per 24 hours (occasionally dose to give every 6 hours). This practice is especially common for antibiotic agents. It is important to note that the 24 hours dose calculated must be divided into the number of doses to be given daily. The manufacturer's recommendations probably provide the most accurate suggestions.

EXAMPLE

What is the dose of amoxicillin for rheumatic heart disease prophylaxis for a 50-lb child? (See Chapter 7.)

$$\text{Dose} = 50 \, \text{mg} / \text{kg of body weight}$$

Change pounds to kilograms: Divide by ≈ 2 equals 25 kg for a 50-lb child

$$\frac{2.2 \, \text{lb}}{1 \, \text{kg}} = \frac{50 \, \text{lb}}{x \, \text{kg}}$$

$$x = \frac{50 \, \text{lb}}{2.2} = 23 \, \text{kg}$$

Multiply dose in milligrams per kilograms by number of kg = mg = dose

$$\frac{50 \, \text{mg}}{\text{kg}} = \frac{x \, \text{mg}}{23 \, \text{kg}}$$

$$x = (50 \times 23) \, \text{mg}$$

GLOSSARY

A

abscess   accumulation of pus in a body tissue, usually caused by a bacterial infection

acetic acid   substance produced when acetylcholine is broken down

acetylcholinesterase   enzyme that destroys acetylcholine; inactivates effect

acromegaly   enlargement of peripheral body parts such as head, face, hands, feet; secondary to metabolic disorder

active transport   movement of ions or molecules across cell membrane; uses energy to accomplish; can be against a gradient

addiction   dependence on a substance (e.g., alcohol or other drugs) or an activity to the point that stopping is very difficult and causes severe physical and mental reactions

adrenal medulla   center portion of the adrenal gland; secretes epinephrine

adverse effect   unwanted effects of a drug

adverse reaction   unwanted effects of a drug

affective disorder   mental disorder involving abnormal moods and emotions, includes depression and bipolar affective disorder (manic-depressive disorder)

afferent   coming back to center; for example, nerves from periphery to CNS

afterload   load against which the heart beats

agranulocytosis   sudden drop in white blood cell count that is accompanied with a high fever

akathisia   motor restlessness; muscular quivering

akinesia   loss (or difficulty) of voluntary movement

allergy   hypersensitivity reaction caused by an antigen-antibody reaction

alopecia   baldness or loss of hair, mainly on the head

amblyopia   dimness of vision without apparent physical deficit or disease

ampules   sterile sealed glass containers, broken before use

anabolic steroid   drug similar to testosterone that builds muscles and strengthens bones

anaphylactic shock   serious allergic reaction resulting in difficulty breathing, low blood pressure, and death

anaphylaxis   hypersensitivity reaction that produces difficulty breathing; life threatening

anesthesia   loss of sensation in a certain part of the body (local/general)

angiotensin-converting enzyme inhibitor (ACEI)   drug group used to treat high blood pressure

anorexia   reduced appetite, not hungry; food aversion

antacid   drug that neutralizes stomach acids; used to treat indigestion, heartburn, and acid reflux

anticoagulant   prevents blood coagulation

antiemetic   prevents vomiting

antisialagogue   a treatment for excessive salivation

antithyroglobulin   antibodies to thyroglobulin

anxiolytic   action of antianxiety agents; reduces anxiety

apnea   breathing stops, for either a short or a long period; drug- or disease-induced

arachidonic acid   precursor of prostaglandins and leukotrienes

arrhythmia   loss of rhythm; refers to irregular heartbeat

arteriosclerosis   thickening and hardening of artery walls; atherosclerosis

artery   a large blood vessel that carries oxygenated blood from the heart to tissues and organs in the body

arthralgia   pain in joint

arthritis   osteoarthritis: inflamed joints with pain and stiffness; rheumatoid arthritis: autoimmune disease of joints characterized by inflammation, pain, stiffness, and redness

Arthus   type of immediate hypersensitivity produced when an antigen is administered to a previously sensitized rabbit

ascorbic acid   chemical term for vitamin C

asthma   disorder characterized by bronchial constriction and inflamed airways; difficulty breathing

ataxia   cannot coordinate voluntary muscle activity; caused by disorders in the brain or drugs such as alcohol or CNS depressants

atherosclerosis   lipid deposits inside arteries; location of clogging of blood vessels

atony   lack of tone; relaxation

atrial fibrillation   the atria beat rapidly and inconsistently; irregular heartbeat

attention deficit disorder (ADD)   a disorder present in children and adults, characterized by learning and behavior problems, inability to pay attention, and sometimes hyperactivity

aura   a sensation that sometimes comes before a migraine headache or seizure; may include sensations of movement or discomfort or emotions

autocoids   substances produced by some cells that change the function of other cells (e.g., histamine)

autoimmune   reaction that consists of destruction that occurs because of the immune response of the body to itself

B

bacillus   any bacteria that is rod shaped; responsible for many diseases, such as diphtheria, tetanus, and tuberculosis

bacillus Calmette-Guérin   vaccine used to protect against tuberculosis

bacteremia   condition in which bacteria are present in the bloodstream; may occur after minor surgery or infection and may be dangerous for people with a weakened immune system or abnormal heart valves

bacteriostatic   term used to describe a substance that stops the growth of bacteria, such as an antibiotic

barbiturates   group of sedative-hypnotic drugs that reduce activity in the brain; are habit-forming and possibly fatal when taken with alcohol

bile   fluid made in the liver and stored in the gallbladder; aids in digestion

bipolar disorder   illness in which the patient goes back and forth between opposite extremes; the most notable bipolar disorder is manic-depressive disorder, which is characterized by extreme highs and lows in mood

bladder   organ to collect and store urine until it is expelled

blood clot   semisolid mass of blood that forms to help seal and prevent bleeding from a damaged vessel

bradycardia   slow heart rate, usually below 60 beats per minute in adults

bronchodilator   drug that increases the diameter of the bronchioles, improves breathing, and relieves muscle contraction or build-up of mucus

bronchospasm   temporary narrowing of the airways in the lungs, either as a result of muscle contraction or inflammation; may be caused by asthma, infection, lung disease, or an allergic reaction

bundle of His   bundle of conduction tissue located between the atrium and the ventricles

C

calcium   mineral in the body that is the basic component of teeth and bones; essential for cell function, muscle contraction, transmission of nerve impulses, and blood clotting

calcium channel blocker (CCB)   drug used to treat chest pain, high blood pressure, and irregular heartbeat by preventing the movement of calcium into the muscle

cancer   group of diseases in which cells grow unrestrained in an organ or tissue in the body; can spread to tissues around it and destroy them or be transported through blood or lymph pathways to other parts of the body

candidiasis   yeast infection caused by the fungus Candida albicans; occurs vaginally and orally

canker sore   small, painful sore, usually occurs on the inside of the lip or cheek or sometimes under the tongue; most likely an autoimmune reaction, many triggers; aphthous stomatitis

cardiac arrest   cessation of the heart beat; results from a heart attack, respiratory arrest, electrical shock, drug overdose, or a severe allergic reaction

cardiopulmonary resuscitation (CPR)   administration of heart compression and artificial respiration to restore circulation and breathing

cardiovascular system   the heart and blood vessels that are responsible for circulating blood throughout the body

cellulitis   skin infection caused by bacteria (usually streptococci); characterized by fever, chills, heat, tenderness, and redness; if dental, treat aggressively

cerebrospinal fluid   clear, watery fluid circulating in and around the brain and spinal column

cerebrovascular disease   disease affecting any artery supplying blood to the brain; may cause blockage or rupture of a blood vessel, leading to a stroke

chemotherapy   treatment of infections or cancer with drugs that act on disease-producing organisms or cancerous tissue; may also affect normal cells; antibiotics or antineoplastics

cholesterol   substance in body cells that plays a role in the production of hormones and bile salts and in the transport of fats in the bloodstream

cholinergic   stimulated, activated, or transmitted by choline

chronic obstructive pulmonary disease (COPD)   combination of the lung diseases emphysema and bronchitis; characterized by blockage of airflow in and out of the lungs

cleft lip   birth defect in which the upper lip is split vertically, often associated with cleft palate

cleft palate   birth defect in which the roof of the mouth is split, extending from behind the teeth to the nasal cavity; often occurs with other birth defects such as cleft lip and partial deafness

colitis   inflammation of the large intestine (the colon), which usually leads to abdominal pain, fever, and diarrhea with blood and mucus

congenital   present or existing at the time of birth

conjugation   the addition of glucuronic or sulfuric acid to certain toxic substances to terminate their biological activity and prepare them for excretion

contraindication   an aspect of a patient's condition that makes the use of a certain drug or therapy an unwise or dangerous decision

cretinism   congenital disease due to the absence or deficiency of normal thyroid secretion; characterized by physical deformity, dwarfism, mental retardation, and goiter

cycloplegia   spasm of accommodation

D

defibrillation   short electric shock to the chest to normalize an irregular heartbeat

delusions   false beliefs; remain even when evidence to the contrary exists

dependence   reliance on drug to feel "normal"

depolarization   change in polarity (e.g., positive to negative)

depression   feelings of hopelessness, sadness, and a general disinterest in life; in most cases, there is no known cause; may be a result of neurotransmitter abnormality

dermatitis   inflammation of skin

diabetes insipidus   output of large amounts of dilute urine; results from lack of antidiuretic hormone

diabetes mellitus (DM)   disease with abnormal glucose use; insulin lacking or does not work properly; many complications (e.g., periodontal disease)

diaphoresis   perspiration (sweating)

dietary fiber   constituent of plants that cannot be digested, which helps maintain healthy functioning of the bowels (e.g., bran flakes)

diffusion   random movement of molecules in solution or suspension, distributes molecules to different compartments (parts of body); moves from a higher concentration to a lower concentration

direct-acting   acts by stimulation of the receptor

distribution   how a drug moves around the body (where it goes)

diuretic   drug that increases the amount of water in the urine, removing excess water from the body; used in treating high blood pressure and fluid retention

DNA (deoxyribonucleic acid)   responsible for passing genetic information in nearly all organisms

drug   substance that affects the body; used to treat diseases

duration   the time it takes for a drug's effect to cease

dwarfism   undersized, abnormal; body parts not in proportion

dynorphin   endogenous opioid ligand; stimulates kappa receptor

dysgeusia   impairment and/or perversion of taste

dysmorphology   study of abnormal tissue development

dyspepsia   "upset stomach"

dysphoria   unpleasant feeling

dyspnea   difficulty breathing

dysrhythmia   abnormal rhythm

dystocia   difficult childbirth

dystonia   abnormal tone of tissue; can be hyper- or hypo-

dysuria   difficult or painful urination

E

ectopic   out of place (e.g., heart beats from outside the conduction tissues)

ectopic foci   location where ectopic events occur

edematous   edema (fluid retention) present

efferent   conveying or conducting away from an organ or part

efficacy   maximal amount of beneficial effect resulting from a treatment

electrocardiogram (ECG)   graphic record of heart's nerve action potential

electroconvulsive therapy (ECT)   sending electricity through patient's brain; treatment of depressed patient, neuromuscular blockers prevent convulsions

emboli   a mass, such as an air bubble, a detached blood clot, or a foreign body, that travels through the bloodstream and lodges so as to obstruct or occlude a blood vessel

embolism   blockage of a blood vessel by an embolus—something previously circulating in the blood (e.g., blood clot, gas bubble, tissue, bacteria, bone marrow, cholesterol, or fat)

emphysema   chronic disease in which the small air sacs in the lungs (the alveoli) become damaged; characterized by difficulty breathing

endocarditis   inflammation of the inner lining of the heart, usually the heart valves; typically caused by an infection

endocrine gland   gland that secretes hormones into the bloodstream

endorphin   group of chemicals produced in the brain; reduce pain and positively affect mood

endothelium   smooth muscle lining blood vessels and heart

enkephalin   endogenous opioid ligand; stimulates delta receptor

enteral   by way of the gastrointestinal tract

enuresis   involuntary urine release

enzyme   chemical, originating in a cell, that regulates reactions in the body

epilepsy   disorder of the nervous system in which abnormal electrical activity in the brain causes involuntary effects (e.g., seizures)

epinephrine   hormone produced by the adrenal glands in response to stress, exercise, or fear; increases heart rate and opens airways to improve breathing; also called adrenaline

epinephrine reversal   with high doses of epinephrine, the α effect predominates and leads to an increase in blood pressure and a reflex decrease in heart rate (like norepinephrine); when the dose is lower, β effects predominate (α receptors are less sensitive), β1 increases heart rate, β2 produces vasodilation and reflex tachycardia

erythema   redness of skin

estrogens   a group of hormones (produced mainly in the ovaries) that are necessary for female sexual development and reproductive functioning

estrogen replacement therapy   treatment with synthetic estrogen drugs to relieve symptoms of menopause and to help protect women against osteoporosis and heart disease

ethanol   ethyl alcohol

ethyl alcohol   alcohol with two carbons (ethyl); form of alcohol in alcoholic beverages

euthyroid   normal thyroid

excretion   removal of wastes from the body

exophthalmos   eyeballs that protrude, caused by hyperthyroidism

expectorant   medication used to promote the coughing up of phlegm from the respiratory tract

extrapyramidal   refers to part of brain outside the nerve tracks (shaped like pyramids); related to adverse reactions of the antipsychotics; parkinsonian-like

F

facilitated diffusion   movement of agent across cell membranes mediated via a protein

fetal alcohol syndrome   combination of defects in a fetus as a result of the mother drinking alcohol during pregnancy

fibrillation   rapid, inefficient contraction of muscle fibers of the heart caused by disruption of nerve impulses

fight or flight   effects that occur when the sympathetic autonomic nervous system is stimulated

fluoride   halogen added to municipal water to decrease caries; mineral that helps protect teeth against decay

flushing   transient erythema

folic acid   a water-soluble vitamin that is converted to a coenzyme essential to purine and thymine biosynthesis

Food and Drug Administration (FDA)   government organization responsible for approval of prescription drugs

free base   releasing base from salt form, used to change one form of cocaine into another more desirable form (before rock cocaine)

friable   easily breakable, easy to crumble

fungus   group of organisms that include yeasts and molds, toadstools, and Candida

G

gagging reflex   gagging that occurs when a foreign body touches the mucous membranes in the back of mouth; sometimes occurs with alginate impressions or fluoride trays

gastritis   inflammation of the mucous membrane lining of the stomach; causes include viruses, bacteria, and use of alcohol and other drugs

gastroparesis   some paralysis of stomach muscles; common with diabetes

generic drug   nonproprietary name (not trade name)

genital herpes   an infection caused by the herpes simplex virus, which causes a painful rash of fluid-filled blisters on the genitals; transmitted through sexual contact

geographic tongue   disorder of tongue, different colored patches visible, lesions move; lesions look like continents on a world map

gestation   period between fertilization of an egg by a sperm and birth of a baby

giantism (gigantism)   abnormal growth of body or its parts

gingivitis   inflammation of the gums; typically caused by a build-up of plaque resulting from poor oral hygiene

gland   group of cells or an organ that produces substances that are secreted or excreted

glaucoma (wide angle)   disease with elevated pressure in eye; treated with ophthalmic drops; 95% of glaucoma cases

glaucoma (narrow-angle)   disease with elevated pressure in eye because of narrow angle; treated with emergency surgery; 5% of glaucoma cases

glossitis   tongue inflammation

glossodynia   painful (or burning) tongue

glossopyrosis   same as glossodynia

gluconeogenesis   hydrolysis of glycogen to glucose (make glucose)

glucose   sugar that is the main source of energy for the body

glucuronidation   process of combining a drug with glucuronic acid; product is more water soluble, more easily excreted

glutamate   form produced by adding glutamic acid; inhibitor neurotransmitter in central nervous system

glycogenolysis   breaking down glycogen

glycoside   structure produced when sugar condenses with other radicals

goiter   enlargement of the thyroid gland, which produces a swelling on the neck

gout   disorder marked by high levels of uric acid in the blood; usually experienced as arthritis in one joint

gradient   rate of change of variable, especially concentration of drug in two different places

grand mal   type of seizure occurring with epilepsy, producing loss of consciousness, involuntary jerking movements

Graves disease   hyperplasia of thyroid gland; exophthalmos common

gynecomastia   swelling of male breasts; can be side effect of drug

H

H₂ (histamine) blocker   blocks acid production produced by histamine; used to treat acid reflux and ulcers

hallucination   perception that occurs when there is actually nothing there to cause it (e.g., hearing voices when there are none)

hapten   substance that cannot cause antibody production alone; combines with larger molecule that acts as a carrier to stimulate formation of antibodies

Hashimoto's Disease or Thyroiditis   lymphocytes enter thyroid, diffuse goiter; over time, the inflamed thyroid (thyroiditis) causes hypothyroidism

heart attack   see "Myocardial infarction"

heart block   disorder of the heart caused by a blockage of the nerve impulses throughout the heart that alters heartbeat; may lead to dizziness, fainting, or stroke

heart failure   the heart cannot pump effectively

heart rate   rate at which the heart pumps blood; units = heartbeats per minute

heart valve   structure at each exit of the four chambers of the heart that allows blood to exit but not to flow back in

heartburn   burning sensation experienced in the center of the chest up to the throat; caused by gastroesophageal reflux disease (GERD)

Heimlich maneuver   maneuver in which fist of treating person is placed on abdomen of choking person above navel and is forcefully pushed; used to remove object lodged in throat

hematuria   blood in the urine; can be caused by kidney infection

hemoglobin   pigment in red blood cells that is responsible for carrying oxygen; hemoglobin bound to oxygen gives blood its red color

hemolysis   breakdown of red blood cells in the spleen; can cause jaundice and anemia if the red blood cells are broken down too quickly

hemolytic   destruction of blood cells; liberates hemoglobin

hemophilia   inherited disorder; blood lacks a protein needed to form blood clots, leads to excessive bleeding

hemorrhage   blood loss through broken vessel wall

hemorrhoid   bulging vein near the anus; often caused by childbirth or straining during bowel movements

hemostasis   stop bleeding

hepatic microsomal enzymes   enzymes in the liver that are responsible for metabolizing drugs; mixed function oxidases

hepatic   related to the liver

hepatitis   inflammation of the liver, which may or may not be caused by a viral infection; can be caused by poisons, drugs, or alcohol

hepatitis A   caused by the hepatitis A virus; usually transmitted by contact with contaminated food or water

hepatitis B   caused by the hepatitis B virus; transmitted through sexual contact or contact with infected blood or body fluids

hepatitis C   transmitted through sexual contact or contact with infected blood or body fluids

hepatitis D   causes symptoms when hepatitis B is present

hernia   bulging of an organ or tissue through a weakened area in the muscle wall

heroin   a white, bitter, crystalline compound that is derived from morphine and is a highly addictive narcotic

herpes simplex   infection that causes blisterlike sores on the face, lips, mouth, or genitals

hiatal hernia   part of the stomach bulges up into the chest cavity through the diaphragm

high-density lipoprotein (HDL)   protein found in the blood that removes cholesterol from tissues; "good cholesterol"

histamine   chemical released during allergic reactions, causing inflammation; causes production of acid in the stomach and narrowing of the bronchioles

hives   common term for urticaria; an itchy, inflamed rash that results from an allergic reaction

hormone   produced by a gland or tissue; released into the bloodstream; controls body functions such as growth and sexual development (e.g., insulin)

hormone replacement therapy (HRT)   use of natural or artificial hormones to treat hormone deficiencies

huffing   illegal use of hydrocarbon inhalants (e.g., paint, gasoline); inhalant is deposited in a plastic bag and the user breathes in and out

human immunodeficiency virus (HIV)   a retrovirus that attacks helper T cells of the immune system and causes acquired immunodeficiency syndrome (AIDS); transmitted through sexual intercourse or contact with infected blood

hypercalcemia   abnormally high levels of calcium in the blood; can lead to disturbance of cell function in the nerves and muscles

hypercapnia   increase in the arterial level of carbon dioxide; abnormal

hypercholesterolemia   an abnormally high level of cholesterol in the blood, which can be the result of an inherited disorder or a diet that is high in fat

hyperglycemia   abnormally high levels of blood glucose; usually as a result of untreated or improperly controlled diabetes mellitus

hyperlipidemia lipid levels in the blood are abnormally high, including hypercholesterolemia

hyperlipoproteinemia elevation of the lipoproteins in the blood

hyperplasia increase in the number of cells in an organ or tissue

hyperprolactinemia increased level of prolactin in blood; abnormal

hyperpyrexia elevated body temperature; side effect of aspirin overdose

hypertension abnormally high blood pressure, even when at rest

hyperthermia elevated body temperature

hyperthyroidism overactivity of the thyroid gland, causing nervousness, weight loss, hair changes

hyperuricemia elevated blood level of uric acid; associated with gout

hypoglycemia low blood sugar

hypoprothrombinemia low level of prothrombin in blood

hypotension abnormally low blood pressure

hypothyroidism underactivity of the thyroid gland; causing tiredness, cramps, a slowed heart rate, and possibly weight gain

hypoxia reduced level of oxygen in tissues or body

I

iatrogenic term used to describe a disease, disorder, or medical condition that is a direct result of medical treatment

idiopathic something that occurs of an unknown cause

idiosyncratic peculiar characteristic; may be caused by a drug

ileum lowest section of the small intestine, which attaches to the large intestine

immune system cells, substances, and structures in the body that protect against infection and illness

immunity resistance to a specific disease because of the responses of the immune system

immunosuppressant inhibits the activity of the immune system; used to prevent transplant organ rejection and for disorders in which the body's immune system attacks its own tissues (rheumatoid arthritis, psoriasis)

impetigo contagious skin infection caused by bacteria, usually occurring around the nose and mouth; commonly occurring in children; common causative organisms include streptococci and staphylococci

implant organ, tissue, or device surgically inserted and left in the body

impotence inability to acquire or maintain an erection of the penis

incontinence inability to hold urine or feces

incubation period period from when an infectious organism enters the body to when symptoms occur

indirect-acting acts either before or after the receptor (e.g., cause release of neurotransmitter, blocks metabolism of neurotransmitter)

induction increase in production (e.g., enzymes in the liver); time from the start of general anesthesia until surgical anesthesia occurs

infection disease-causing microorganisms that enter the body, multiply, and damage cells or release toxins

inflammation redness, pain, and swelling in an injured or infected tissue

inflammatory bowel disease (IBD) general term for two inflammatory disorders affecting the intestines; also known as Crohn disease and ulcerative colitis

influenza viral infection; characterized by headaches, muscle aches, fever, weakness, and cough; commonly called the "flu"

infusion introduction of a substance, such as a drug or nutrient, into the bloodstream or a body cavity

inhaler device used to introduce a powdered or misted drug into the lungs through the mouth; usually to treat respiratory disorders such as asthma

inhibition reduces an effect (e.g., liver enzymes)

injection use of a syringe and needle to insert a drug into a vein, muscle, or joint or under the skin

innervation nerves that are connected to tissue

inotropic influencing contraction of muscle (especially cardiac)

insomnia inability to sleep, difficulty falling or remaining asleep

insulin shock reaction that occurs when blood sugar is too low; excessive insulin is one factor

insulin hormone made in the pancreas that plays an important role in the absorption of glucose (the body's main source of energy) into muscle cells

interferon protein produced by body cells that fights viral infections and certain cancers

international normalized ratio (INR) laboratory value that adjusts the prothrombin time ratio to take into account the difference in the potency of prothrombin used in different laboratories; used to monitor warfarin use; calculated by taking the PT ratio to the power of the international sensitivity index (ISI):

$$\left(\frac{PT_{text}}{PT_{normal}} \right)^{ISI}$$

international sensitivity index (ISI) factor that is used to convert an individual's PT to an INR; corrects for variability in sensitivity of prothrombin used in different laboratories

intestine long, tubular organ extending from the stomach to the anus; absorbs food and water, passes the waste as feces

intrauterine device plastic device inserted into the uterus that helps to prevent pregnancy

intravascular within blood vessels

intrinsic term used to describe something originating from or located in a tissue or organ

intubation passage of a tube into an organ or structure; used to refer to the passage down trachea for artificial respiration (e.g., during general anesthesia)

invasive describes something that spreads throughout body tissues such as a tumor or microorganism; also describes a medical procedure in which body tissues are penetrated

iodine element for the formation of thyroid hormones

Iodine-131 radioactive iodine; used to treat hyperthyroidism

iron mineral necessary for the formation of important biologic substances such as hemoglobin, myoglobin, and certain enzymes

iron-deficiency anemia type of anemia caused by a greater-than-normal loss of iron resulting from bleeding, problems absorbing iron, or a lack of iron in the diet

ischemia condition in which a tissue or organ does not receive a sufficient supply of blood

J

jaundice yellowing of the skin and whites of the eyes because of the presence of excess bilirubin in the blood; usually a sign of a disorder of the liver

jock itch fungal infection in the groin area

K

Kaposi sarcoma skin cancer that is characterized by purple-red tumors that start at the feet and spread upward on the body; commonly occurs in people who have AIDS

kidney an organ that is part of the urinary tract; responsible for filtering the blood and removing waste products and excess water as urine

L

lacrimation secretion of tears

larynx the voice box; the organ in the throat that produces voice and also prevents food from entering the airway

leukocyte white blood cell

leukopenia abnormally low number of white blood cells in the circulating blood

leukoplakia an abnormal condition characterized by white spots or patches on mucous membranes, especially of the mouth and vulva

lipid-lowering agents drugs taken to lower the levels of specific fats called lipids in the blood to reduce the risk of narrowing of the arteries

lipids group of fats stored in the body and used for energy

lipolysis breakdown of fats

lipoproteins substances containing lipids and proteins; comprising most fats in the blood

liver largest organ in the body, producing many essential chemicals and regulating the levels of most vital substances in the blood

liver failure final stage of liver disease, in which liver function becomes so impaired that other areas of the body are affected, most commonly the brain

low-density lipoprotein (LDL) type of lipoprotein that is the major carrier of cholesterol in the blood, with high levels associated with narrowing of the arteries and heart disease

lumbar spine lower part of the spine between the lowest pair of ribs and the pelvis; made up of five vertebrae

lungs two organs in the chest that take in oxygen from the air and release carbon dioxide

luteinizing hormone (LH)   hormone produced by the pituitary gland that causes the ovaries and testicles to release sex hormones and plays a role in the development of eggs and sperm

lymph   milky fluid-containing white blood cells, proteins, and fats; plays an important role in absorbing fats from the intestine and in the functioning of the immune system

lymphadenopathy   disease that affects lymph nodes; often refers to swelling of lymph nodes; associated with infection

lymphocyte   white blood cell that is an important part of the body's immune system, helping to destroy invading microorganisms

lymphokines   substances that are released by lymphocytes; involved in immune response

lymphomas   group of cancers of the lymph nodes and spleen that can spread to other parts of the body

lysis   destruction of blood cells, bacteria; caused by immune reaction

M

macroangiopathy   disease of larger blood vessels

macrophages   mononuclear cells with phagocytic action

magnesium   mineral that is essential for many body functions, including nerve impulse transmission, formation of bones and teeth, and muscle contraction

malignant   cells that exhibit uncontrolled growth, such as a cancerous tumor

malignant hyperthermia   acute rise in body temperature, muscle rigidity; caused by change in body's muscle metabolism; can be fatal

mandible   lower jaw

mania   mental disorder characterized by extreme excitement, happiness, overactivity, and agitation; usually refers to the high of the highs and lows experienced in manic-depressive disorder

manic-depressive disorder   mental disorder characterized by extreme mood swings, including mania and depression, or a continuing shift between the two extremes

marijuana   plant containing the active ingredient tetrahydrocannabinol; hallucinogen, sedative

mast cell   cell present in most body tissues that releases substances in response to an allergen, which causes symptoms such as inflammation

measles   illness caused by a viral infection, causing a characteristic rash and a fever; primarily affects children

medulla   the soft center part of an organ or body structure (e.g., medulla oblongata [brain], renal medulla [kidney])

megaloblastic anemia   anemia resulting from the lack of vitamin B12 or folic acid

melanoma   skin tumor composed of cells called melanocytes

meningitis   inflammation of the protective membranes that cover the brain, called the meninges; usually caused by infection by a microorganism (meningitis caused by bacteria is life threatening; viral meningitis is milder)

menopause   the period in a woman's life when menstruation stops, resulting in a reduced production of estrogen and cessation of egg production

menstrual cycle   periodic discharge of blood and mucosal tissue from the uterus, occurring from puberty to menopause in a woman who is not pregnant

menstruation   shedding of the lining of the uterus during the menstrual cycle

mescaline   active ingredient in peyote (cactus); a hallucinogen

metabolic tolerance   with chronic use, drug produces less effect because of metabolic change

metabolism   process by which the body changes a drug chemically to make it easier to excrete

metabolite   compound that is produced when a drug is metabolized

metastasis   spreading of a cancerous tumor to another part of the body; through the lymph, blood, or across a cavity; also sometimes refers to a tumor that has been produced in this way

metered-dose inhaler (MDI)   inhaler that gives a specific amount of medication with each use

methadone maintenance   program to treat opioid addicts (heroin) by administering a high dose of oral methadone; usual doses of heroin then cannot produce euphoria

methemoglobinemia   the presence of methemoglobin in the blood due to conversion of part of the hemoglobin to this inactive form

microangiopathy   disease of small capillaries

microcephaly   small head; abnormal

microorganism   any tiny, single-cell organism (e.g., bacterium, virus, or fungus)

microphthalmia   small eyes; abnormal

migraine headache   severe headache, usually accompanied by vision problems and/or nausea and vomiting, that typically recurs

mineral   substance that is a necessary part of a healthy diet (e.g., potassium, calcium, sodium, phosphorus, and magnesium)

minipill   oral contraceptive containing only progesterone (no estrogen)

miosis   constriction of pupil

mitral valve   valve in the heart that allows blood to flow from the left atrium to the left ventricle but prevents blood from flowing back in

mitral valve prolapse   common condition in which the mitral valve in the heart is deformed, may cause blood to leak back across the valve; may be characterized by a heart murmur and sometimes chest pain and disturbed heart rhythm

molecule   smallest unit of a substance that possesses its characteristics

monoamine oxidase   enzyme that destroys single amines

monoamine oxidase inhibitor   substance that works by blocking an enzyme that breaks down stimulating chemicals in the brain; used to treat depression

morbidity   state of being ill or having a disease

mortality   death rate; measured as the number of deaths per a certain population; may describe the population as a whole or a specific group within a population (e.g., infant mortality)

mucous membrane   soft, pink cells that produce mucus; found in respiratory tract (including mouth), eyelids, and urinary tract

mucus   slippery fluid produced by mucous membranes that lubricates and protects the internal surfaces of the body

multiple sclerosis   disease in which the protective coverings (myelin) of nerve fibers in the brain are gradually destroyed; symptoms vary from numbness to paralysis and loss of control of bodily function

muscarinic   receptors that are activated by muscarine, contained in certain mushrooms; anticholinergics block this action

muscle relaxants   group of drugs used to relieve muscle spasm and to treat conditions such as arthritis, back pain, and nervous system disorders such as stroke and cerebral palsy

myalgia   muscle pain

myasthenia gravis   disease in which the muscles, mainly those in the face, eyes, throat, and limbs, become weak and tire quickly; caused by the body's immune system attacking the receptors in the muscles that pick up nerve impulses

mycobacterium   genus of slow-growing bacterium; resistant to the body's defense mechanisms and responsible for diseases such as tuberculosis and leprosy

mydriasis   dilation of the pupils

myeloma   cancerous cells in the bone marrow

myocardial infarction (MI)   heart attack; heart vessel becomes clogged, severe pain in the chest experienced; can be fatal

myocardium   heart muscle

myopathy   a muscle disease

myositis   inflammation of muscle

myxedema   a condition characterized by thickening of the skin, blunting of the senses and intellect, and labored speech, associated with hypothyroidism

N

narcolepsy   frequent and uncontrollable episodes of falling asleep; excessive sleepiness

narcotic analgesics   pain relievers that bind to opioid receptors in the brain; inhibit ascending pain fibers, alter response to pain; often causes tolerance and dependence

narcotic   addictive substance that blunts the senses; with increased doses causes sedation, coma, and death; called opioids

nausea   feeling the need to vomit

necrosis   death of tissue cells

negative feedback   secretion of hormone 1 inhibits the release of hormones 2 and 3 that stimulate the secretion of hormone 1, for example, give prednisone (hormone 1), which inhibits CRF (hormone 2) and ACTH (hormone 3), both of which stimulate release of hydrocortisone

neonate   newborn infant from birth to 1 month of age

neoplasm tumor

nephritis inflammation of kidney(s); caused by an infection, an abnormal immune system response; a metabolic disorder

nerve fibers that transmit electrical messages between the brain and most body areas; convey information both ways

nerve action potential changes in voltage (via ions) that transmits the nerve impulse along the nerve fiber

nerve block preventing transmission of pain from an area of the body by injecting a local anesthetic near a nerve

neuralgia pain along the course of a nerve

neuromuscular junction synapse between the nervous innervation and the somatic (voluntary) muscles

neuropathy disease, inflammation, or damage to the nerves connecting the brain and spinal cord to the rest of the body

neurosis mental illness with anxiety; stimulates useless action (e.g., counting things); relatively mild emotional disorders (e.g., mild depression and phobias)

neurotransmitters chemicals that are released after excitation of the presynaptic neuron; cross synapse to excite the postsynaptic neuron

neutropenia deficiency of white blood cells

neutrophil white blood cell in granulocyte group

nicotinic receptors that are activated by nicotine; contained in cigarettes

nitrates drugs that produce widespread vasodilation; used to treat angina pectoris and heart failure, reduce preload and afterload

nocturnal enuresis bedwetting at night

nonsteroidal antiinflammatory drug (NSAID) drug group that relieves pain and reduces inflammation; not corticosteroids (e.g., ibuprofen)

norepinephrine hormone that regulates blood pressure by causing vasoconstriction of the blood vessels

nystagmus persistent, rapid, rhythmic, involuntary movement of the eyes; used by police to check for the effect of drugs

O

obesity condition in which there is an excess of body fat; used to describe those who weigh at least 20% more than the maximum amount considered normal for age, sex, and height

obsessive-compulsive disorder action that must be repeated to make person comfortable (e.g., hand washing)

oligodactyly fewer than five digits

onset time it takes for a drug's effect to begin

opacities not transparent

opportunistic infection infection by organisms that would be harmless to a healthy person but cause infection in those with a weakened immune system (e.g., persons with AIDS or chemotherapy patients)

optic pertaining to the eyes

oral used in or taken through the mouth

oral contraceptives pills that prevent pregnancy; contain a progesterone and an estrogen

organophosphate organic compounds that combine with acetylcholinesterase, in activating it, called irreversible cholinesterase inhibitors; used as insecticides and war gases

orthopnea breathing difficulty experienced while lying flat; can be a symptom of heart failure or asthma

orthostatic hypotension when a person stands up from the supine position, and the blood pools in the lower extremities and the blood flow to the brain is greatly reduced, causing dizziness and potential fainting; common side effect of some antihypertensives

osteoarthritis disease that breaks down the cartilage that lines joints, especially weight-bearing or malaligned joints; leads to inflammation, pain, and stiffness

osteomalacia loss of minerals and softening of bones because of a lack of vitamin D; called rickets in children

osteoporosis condition in which bones become less dense and more brittle and fracture more easily

otitis media inflammation of the middle ear caused by infection from the nose, sinuses, or throat

ototoxicity harmful effect that some drugs have on the organs or nerves in the ears, which can lead to hearing and balance problems

outpatient treatment medical attention that does not include an overnight stay at a hospital

ovaries two almond-shaped glands located at the opening of the fallopian tubes on both sides of the uterus; produce eggs and the sex hormones estrogen and progesterone

over-the-counter (OTC) medication that can be purchased without a provider's prescription

overdose excessively large dose of a drug; can lead to coma and death; used to commit suicide

ovulation development and release of the egg from the ovary, which usually occurs halfway through a woman's menstrual cycle

oxidation chemical reaction that adds oxygen; can damage cells (free radicals)

oxygen gas that is colorless, odorless, and tasteless; essential to almost all forms of life

oxytocin hormone from the pituitary gland; causes contraction of the uterus and stimulation of milk flow

P

pacemaker small electronic device that is surgically implanted to stimulate the heart muscle to produce a normal heartbeat

palate roof of the mouth

palliative treatment treatment that relieves the symptoms of a disorder without curing it

pallor abnormally pale skin; usually refers to the skin of the face

palpebral fissures eyelid folds

palpitation abnormally rapid and strong heartbeat

pancreas gland that produces enzymes that break down food and hormones (insulin and glucagon) that help to regulate blood glucose levels

pancreatitis inflammation of the pancreas; one cause is alcohol abuse

panic disorder attacks of anxiety, made worse by stress; patient focuses on avoiding situations in which it occurs

paralysis inability to move a muscle

paralytic ileus ilium motility reduced or absent; often caused by general anesthetics

paranoia mental disorder involving delusions (e.g., "the FBI is following me")

parasympathetic pertaining to that part of the autonomic nervous system consisting of nerves and ganglia that function in opposition to the sympathetic system

parathyroid glands small glands located in the neck that produce a hormone that regulates the levels of calcium in the blood

parenteral introduction of a substance into the body by any route other than the digestive tract; often used to mean an injection

Parkinson disease lack of brain dopamine; leads to muscle stiffness, weakness, and trembling

parkinsonism symptoms include restlessness, tremors, rigidity, and lack of facial expression

paroxysmal sudden onset of symptoms (e.g., paroxysmal tachycardia)

partial seizure abnormal electrical discharge in the cortex of the brain, affecting certain functions

pathogen substance capable of causing a disease; usually refers to a disease-causing microorganism

pedal relates to feet (check for pitting edema in feet for congestive heart failure)

peptic ulcer disease (PUD) erosion in the lining of the esophagus, stomach, or small intestine; most related to the presence of *Helicobacter pylori*

perception nerve impulse going to central nervous system

peripheral resistance opposition to flow of blood through the vessels, varies with vessel diameter; total peripheral resistance

peripheral vascular disease (PVD) narrowing of blood vessels in the legs or arms; causing pain and possibly tissue death (gangrene) as a result of a reduced flow of blood to areas supplied by the narrowed vessels

pernicious anemia anemia resulting from deficiency (failure to absorb) of vitamin B12 caused by a deficiency of intrinsic factor (IF) (autoimmune disease); abnormal red blood cells are produced (macrocytic, megaloblastic)

petit mal complete seizure characterized by loss of consciousness for brief periods, posture retained (do not fall)

peyote cactus that contains mescaline; a hallucinogen

pharmacokinetic movement of a drug within the body

pharmacologist specialist in pharmacology

pharmacology science of drugs and their properties

pharyngitis inflammation of the throat (the pharynx); causing sore throat, fever, earache, and swollen glands

pharynx throat; the tube connecting the back of the mouth and nose to the esophagus and windpipe

pheochromocytoma tumor that secretes epinephrine

phobia persisting fear of and desire to avoid something

phocomelia defective development of arms and/or legs; foot or hand connected to body (flipper-like)

photophobia abnormal sensitivity of the eyes to light

pigmentation coloration of the skin, hair, and eyes by melanin

piloerection hair on body standing up

pituitary gland gland located at the base of the brain; releases hormones that control other glands and body processes

placebo inactive substance given in place of a drug; required to adequately test drugs (total effect of the drug equals the effect that a patient taking the drug gets minus the effect that the placebo produces)

placebo effect the positive or negative response to a drug that is caused by a person's expectations of a drug rather than the drug itself

placenta organ formed in the uterus during pregnancy that links the blood of the mother to the blood of the fetus; provides the fetus with nutrients and removes waste

plaque patch of differentiated tissue on body; fatty deposits in an artery cause narrowing of the artery and heart disease; dental plaque: coating on the teeth, consisting of saliva, bacteria, and food debris, which causes tooth decay; demyelinated patch (e.g., multiple sclerosis)

plasma fluid part of the blood (no cells); contains nutrients, salts, and proteins

platelet megakaryocyte fragment shed into blood; plays an important role in blood clotting, contains no nucleus; adhesiveness affected by aspirin

platelet adhesiveness stickiness of platelets; if reduced, retards clotting

Plummer disease hyperthyroidism from nodular toxic goiter

pneumonia inflammation of the lungs, alveoli filled with exudate; most cases are caused by a bacterial or viral infection; symptoms include fever, shortness of breath, and the coughing up of phlegm

polyp mass of tissue that bulges outward from the surface, growth occurs on mucous membranes such as the nose and intestine; bleeds easily and can become cancerous

polyuria excessive production of urine; can be a symptom of a disease, commonly diabetes

posterior describes something that is located in or relates to the back of the body

postural hypotension unusually low blood pressure that occurs after suddenly standing or sitting up

potassium a mineral that plays an important role in the body, helping to maintain water balance, normal heart rhythm, conduction of nerve impulses, and muscle contraction

potency the pharmacological activity or relative strength of a compound

precocity development occurs early; used to refer to early puberty

preganglionic fibers nerve fibers that precede the ganglia, especially in autonomic nervous system

preload force pushing into the heart

priapism penile erection; painful and persistent

progesterone female sex hormone; plays role in reproduction, thickens uterine lining

prostate gland organ located under the bladder that produces a large part of the seminal fluid

prostatic hypertrophy enlarged prostate gland, common in older men

proteins large molecules made up of amino acids that play many major roles in the body, including forming the basis of body structures such as skin and hair, and important chemicals such as enzymes and hormones

prothrombin agent involved in clotting

prothrombin time (PT) time in seconds that it takes for the patient's blood to clot when combined with thromboplastin and calcium

pruritus itching

psoriasis skin disorder characterized by patches of thick, red skin often covered by silvery scales

psychoactive has effect on mood

psychosis mental disorder in which a serious inability to think, perceive, and judge clearly causes loss of touch with reality

pulse changes in diameter of blood vessel caused by the heart beat; synonymous with the heart rate

Purkinje fibers part of the conduction system of the heart located in the ventricles

Q

quinidine-like has effects on cardiac muscle similar to quinidine

R

Raynaud syndrome disease involving constriction of blood vessels of extremities

reaction effect of brain on interpretation of nerve impulse received to central nervous system

rebound congestion vasoconstrictor given, results in vasoconstriction; vasoconstrictor repeated; vasoconstrictor stopped, results in vasodilation (stuffy nose)

receptor structural protein molecule that binds with specific agents (ligands)

retraction cord cord used around tooth to separate tissue from tooth, improves accuracy of impression; many contain epinephrine

S

sacral part of the vertebral column near the pelvis, includes the coccyx

salicylate a salt or ester of salicylic acid

salicylism reaction to an overdose of aspirin

salivation secretion of saliva

schizophrenia category of psychosis

semen fluid containing secretions from the prostate gland and sperm, which is expelled on ejaculation

sialadenitis inflammation of salivary gland

side effect unwanted effect of a drug

silent killer refers to lack of symptoms; hypertension

sinus channels that carry fluid

somatic relating to body or trunk of body

sphygmomanometer instrument that inflates with a gauge to measure blood pressure

Starling's law cardiac output and stroke volume increases with an increase in end-diastolic pressure up to a point, then the heart fails

subdiaphragmatic below the diaphragm

sublingual gland salivary gland located below the tongue

sublingually under the tongue

submaxillary gland salivary gland in lower jaw

supraventricular referring to the atrium (part of heart above ventricles)

synaptic cleft space between nerve cells or between nerve cells and effector organ (space between)

syncope fainting, loss of consciousness

syndactyly fusion or webbing of fingers or toes; fewer digits

T

tachycardia increase in heart rate

tachyphylaxis with repeated administration, the body quickly has a decrease in response

tardive dyskinesia voluntary muscle performance; irreversible; side effect of antipsychotics

temporomandibular joint (TMJ) joint of the lower jaw

teratogenicity abnormal fetus, terato means "monster"

tetraiodothyronine thyroid hormone, T_4

therapeutic effect desired effect of a drug

therapeutic index LD50/ED50; used to compare safety of drugs

thrombocytopenia abnormal decrease in the number of blood platelets

thrombophlebitis inflammation of the venous vessels

thromboplastin substance present in tissues and platelets that is necessary for blood coagulation

thyroidectomy thyroid removal

thyrotoxicosis produced by excessive thyroid hormone

tinnitus ringing of the ears

tolerance process of becoming less responsive to a drug over time; the need for larger amounts of a drug to produce the same effect

toxic of, relating to, or caused by a toxin or other poison

tracheotomy surgical opening of trachea; emergency procedure for choking

transferases enzymes that move one-carbon groups from one substance to another

tremors muscle movement producing shaking; involuntary

trigeminal neuralgia pain in the trigeminal (side of face) nerve

triglycerides type of fat found in blood; risk factor for atherosclerosis

triiodothyronine thyroid hormone; T_3

type I diabetes chronic disease that is caused by a total lack of insulin production and primarily occurs in people less than 20 years of age; can only be treated with insulin

type II diabetes chronic disease that occurs mainly in people older than 40 years, overweight persons; treated with diet changes and oral drugs that reduce glucose levels in the blood; known as type II diabetes; insulin may be needed in some patients

U

unipolar depression mental disorder with only depression as a component (in contrast to bipolar in which there is depression and elation alternating)

urethral refers to urethra, canal between bladder and outside of body

urinary retention retain urine in bladder; associated with prostatic hypertrophy

urination excretion of urine

urticaria itching wheals; hypersensitivity reaction caused by foods, drugs, emotions, or physical agents

V

vagus vagal nerve; parasympathetic autonomic nervous system stimulates vagus (produces bradycardia)

vasoconstriction blood vessels narrow

vasodilation blood vessels widen

vasomotor collapse fainting

ventricular arrhythmia abnormal rhythms originating from ventricles

vesicles sac containing something; in autonomic nervous system vesicles store neurotransmitters

viscous thick

volume depleted amount of water in body (a lot in blood) too low

von Willebrand disease disease with tendency to bleed, prolonged bleeding time; inherited

W

withdrawal the act or process of ceasing to use an addictive drug; the physiological and mental readjustment that accompanies such discontinuation

X

xerostomia reduced saliva (dry mouth)

Note: Page numbers followed by *f* indicate figures, *t* indicate tables and *b* indicate boxes.

A

Abilify, 176*t*
Abreva, 92*t*, 94, 273, 273*t*
acarbose, 211–212*t*, 213
Accupril, 140*b*
acebutolol, 42*t*, 135*t*, 140*b*
acemannan, 269
Aceon, 140*b*
acetaminophen, 46*b*, 50*t*, 54–55, 94, 126*b*, 154, 154*t*, 247–248*t*, 249
    adverse reactions of, 54–55
    doses and preparations of, 55, 56*t*
    drug interactions of, 55
    pharmacokinetics of, 54
    pharmacologic effects of, 54, 54*b*
    in pregnancy, 25
    toxicity of, 55
    uses of, 55, 55*b*
acetic acid, 45–46
acetylsalicylic acid, 45–50
    adverse reactions of, 47–49, 48*t*
    chemistry of, 45–46, 46*f*
    doses and preparations of, 49–50, 50*t*
    drug interactions of, 49
    mechanism of action of, 46, 47*f*
    over-the-counter (OTC) aspirin-containing products, 50*t*
    pharmacokinetics of, 47
    pharmacologic effects of, 47
    toxicity of, 49, 49*b*
    uses of, 49
Activase, 155
Activella, 218*t*
Actos, 211–212*t*, 213
acyclovir, 16, 92–94, 92*t*, 273, 273*t*
Adlyxin, 211–212*t*
α₁-adrenergic blockers, 39, 148
β-adrenergic blockers, 39, 133, 142*t*, 147–148, 148*b*
ADRENOCORTICOSTEROIDS
    Anusol, 185*t*
    Aristocort, 185*t*
    betamethasone valerate, 185*t*, 188, 188*t*
    Cetacort, 185*t*
    clobetasol propionate, 185*t*
    Cortaid, 185*t*
    Deltasone, 194–195*t*
    Dermacort, 185*t*
    dexamethasone, 188*t*
    fluocinolone acetonide, 185*t*
    Flutex, 185*t*
    hydrocortisone, 184, 185*t*, 188, 188*t*
    Hytone, 185*t*
    Kenalog, 185*t*, 188
    Lidex, 185*t*
    methylprednisolone, 188*t*
    Penecort, 185*t*
    prednisone, 188, 188*t*
    Synalar, 185*t*
    Temovate, 185*t*
    triamcinolone acetonide, 185*t*, 188, 188*t*
    Valisone, 185*t*
Advicor, 151*t*
Advil, 51*t*, 53

Aerospan HFA, 194–195*t*
agonist-antagonist opioids, 65
AKTob, 82
albiglutide, 211–212*t*
alcohol, 254–257
Aldactone, 140*b*
Aldomet, 40*t*, 140*b*, 149
aldosterone antagonists, 133, 142*t*
Alfenta, 114, 114*t*
alfentanil, 114, 114*t*
alirocumab, 151*t*
aliskiren, 140*b*
Allerest, 198–199
allopurinol, 53*t*, 56, 230, 280*b*
alogliptin, 211–212*t*
alprazolam, 120*t*, 247–248*t*
Altace, 140*b*
alteplase, 155
amalgam, 278*b*
Amaryl, 210*t*
Ambien, 120*t*, 126
amikacin, 82
Amikin, 82
amiloride, 140*b*
ε-aminocaproic acid, 156
amiodarone, 135*t*
amitriptyline, 179–180*t*, 276
amlodipine, 140*b*
amobarbital, 124*t*
amoxicillin, 68–69, 71*t*, 74–75, 247–248*t*, 249
amphetamines, 40*t*, 260–261, 278*b*
amphotericin B, 94*t*
ampicillins, 73*t*, 74–75, 87*t*
amyl nitrite, 137*t*
amylinomimetic agent, 211–212*t*
Amytal, 124*t*
analgesics
    nonopioid (nonnarcotic) (*see* NONOPIOID (NONNARCOTIC) ANALGESICS)
    opioid (narcotic) (*see* OPIOID (NARCOTIC) ANALGESICS)
Anaprox, 51*t*, 54
Anbesol, 110, 110*t*
androgens, 221–222, 221–222*t*
ANESTHETICS
    GENERAL, 112–118
        Alfenta, 114, 114*t*
        alfentanil, 114, 114*t*
        Amidate, 114*t*
        barbiturates, 114*t*
        benzodiazepines, 114–115, 114*t*
        Brevital, 114*t*
        desflurane, 117
        diazepam, 114–115, 114*t*
        diethyl ether, 114*t*
        Diprivan, 114, 114*t*
        enflurane, 114*t*, 115, 117
        ether, 114*t*
        Ethrane, 114*t*, 117
        etomidate, 114, 114*t*
        fentanyl, 114*t*
        Fluothane, 114*t*, 117
        Forane, 117
        halothane, 117
        isoflurane, 114*t*, 115
        Ketalar, 114, 114*t*
        ketamine, 114, 114*t*
        methohexital, 114*t*

ANESTHETICS (*Continued*)
        methoxyflurane, 114–115*t*, 115
        midazolam, 114, 114*t*
        morphine, 114*t*
        nitrous oxide, 115–117, 115*t*
        opioids, 114, 114*t*
        Penthrane, 114*t*
        Pentothal, 114*t*
        propofol, 114, 114*t*
        sevoflurane, 117
        Sublimaze, 114*t*
        Sufenta, 114, 114*t*
        sufentanil, 114, 114*t*
        Surital, 114*t*
        thiamylal, 114*t*
        thiopental, 114*t*
        Valium, 114, 114*t*
        Versed, 114–115, 114*t*
    LOCAL
        Anbesol, 110, 110*t*
        articaine, 100*t*, 102–103*t*, 105, 108*b*, 109*t*
        benzocaine, 100*t*, 110, 110*t*
        Benzodent, 110
        bupivacaine, 100*t*, 102–103*t*, 104–105, 108*b*, 109*t*
        Carbocaine, 100*t*, 103*t*, 104
        Cetacaine, 110*t*
        Citanest, 100*t*, 103*t*, 104
        cocaine, 98*b*, 100*t*
        Dyclone, 110*t*
        dyclonine, 105, 110*t*
        epinephrine, 107*t*
        ethylaminobenzoate, 100*t*
        Hurricaine, 110, 110*t*
        Isocaine, 103*t*, 104
        levonordefrin, 107*t*
        lidocaine, 100*t*, 102–103*t*, 108*b*, 109–110*t*
        Marcaine, 98, 100*t*, 103*t*, 105
        mepivacaine, 100*t*, 102–103*t*, 108*b*, 109*t*
        Neo-Cobefrin, 107*t*
        Novocain, 100*t*, 105
        Octocaine, 103, 103*t*
        Orabase-B, 110
        Orajel, 110*t*
        Oraqix, 109–110
        Polocaine, 104
        Pontocaine, 100*t*, 105, 110*t*
        prilocaine, 100*t*, 102–103*t*, 108*b*, 109–110, 109*t*
        procaine, 100*t*, 105
        propoxycaine, 100*t*
        Ravocaine, 100*t*
        Septocaine, 100*t*, 103*t*, 105
        tetracaine, 100*t*, 105, 110*t*
        vasoconstrictors, 105–107
        Xylocaine, 98, 100*t*, 103*t*, 109, 110*t*
angiotensin-converting enzyme (ACE) inhibitors, 133, 139, 140*b*, 142*t*, 145–146, 146*b*, 146*f*, 278*b*, 280*b*
angiotensin receptor blockers, 133, 139, 140*b*, 142*t*, 146
Ansaid, 51*t*
Antabuse, 80
antagonists, 65–66
antianginal drugs, 136–139
ANTIANXIETY AGENTS
    alprazolam, 120*t*
    Ambien, 120*t*, 126

ANTIANXIETY AGENTS (Continued)
  amobarbital, 124t
  Amytal, 124t
  analgesic-sedative combinations, 128
  Ativan, 120t
  baclofen, 127–128
  barbiturates, 124–125, 124t, 126b
  Belsomra, 120t
  benzodiazepines, 120–121
  Brevital, 124t
  butabarbital, 124t
  Butisol, 124t
  carisoprodol, 127t
  chlordiazepoxide, 120t
  chlorzoxazone, 127t
  clonazepam, 120t
  clorazepate, 120t
  cyclobenzaprine, 127t
  Dalmane, 120t
  Dantrium, 128
  dantrolene, 128
  diazepam, 120, 120t, 127t
  Doral, 120t
  estazolam, 120t
  eszopiclone, 120t, 126
  Flexeril, 127t
  flurazepam, 120t
  Halcion, 120t
  Klonopin, 120t
  Librium, 120t
  Lioresal, 127–128
  lorazepam, 120t
  Luminal, 124t
  Lunesta, 120t, 126
  melatonin receptor agonist, 120t,
      126–127
  methocarbamol, 127t
  methohexital, 124t
  midazolam, 120–122, 120t
  muscle relaxants, centrally acting, 127,
      127t
  Nembutal, 124t
  nonbenzodiazepine, benzodiazepine receptor
      agonists, 126
  nonbenzodiazepine-nonbarbiturate sedative-
      hypnotics, 126
  Norflex, 127t
  orphenadrine, 127t
  oxazepam, 120t
  Parafon Forte DSC, 127t
  pentobarbital, 124t
  Pentothal, 124t
  phenobarbital, 124t
  ProSom, 120t
  quazepam, 120t
  ramelteon, 120t, 126
  Restoril, 120t
  Robaxin, 127t
  Rozerem, 120t, 126
  secobarbital, 124t
  Seconal, 124t
  Serax, 120t
  Soma, 127t
  Sonata, 120t, 126
  suvorexant, 120t
  temazepam, 120t
  thiopental sodium, 124t
  tizanidine, 128
  Tranxene, 120t
  triazolam, 120t
  Valium, 120t, 127t
  Versed, 120t
  zaleplon, 120t, 126
  Zanaflex, 128
  zolpidem, 120t, 126

antiarrhythmic agents, 135–136, 135–136t, 278b,
    280b
antiarthritics, 278b
antibiotics, 154, 278b
anticholinergic agents, 37, 162
anticoagulants, 152–153
ANTICONVULSANTS
  benzodiazepines, 171–172
  carbamazepine, 168–170, 168b
  ethosuximide, 171
  felbamate, 169–170t
  gabapentin, 169–170t
  oral side effects, 278b
  phenobarbital, 166t, 169–170t
  phenytoin, 170–171, 171b
  valproate, 167
  vitamin deficiency and, 170
antidepressants, 278b
ANTIFUNGAL AGENTS, 90–92
  for angular cheilitis, 274–275,
      274b
  clotrimazole, 91, 91t
  Diflucan, 91t, 92
  fluconazole, 91t
  imidazole, 90–92
  ketoconazole, 91–92, 91t
  Mycelex, 91
  Mycostatin, 90, 91t
  Nilstat, 90, 91t
  Nizoral, 91, 91t
  nystatin, 90
antihistamines, 24, 278b
antihyperlipidemic agents, 149–152,
    149b
antihypertensive agents, 139–149,
    139–140b
  aspirin interaction and, 49
  oral effects, 278b, 279t
ANTIINFECTIVE AGENTS, 68–89, 278b
  aminoglycosides, 82
  amoxicillin, 71t
  ampicillins, 73t
  antituberculosis agents, 84–85, 84t
    ethambutol, 85
    isoniazid, 84–85
    pyrazinamide, 85
    rifampin, 85
  Atridox, 77t
  azithromycin, 76t
  Biaxin, 76t, 77
  Ceclor, 75b
  cefaclor, 75b
  Ceftin, 75b
  cefuroxime, 75b
  cephalexin, 75b
  cephalosporins, 71t, 75–76, 75b
  Cipro, 83, 83b
  ciprofloxacin, 83, 83b
  clarithromycin, 76t, 77
  clindamycin, 71t, 79–80
  doxycycline, 71t, 77t
  erythromycin, 76, 76t
  Floxin, 83b
  fluoroquinolones, 83–84, 83b
  Keflex, 75b
  Kefurox, 75b
  Laniazid, 84, 84t
  Levaquin, 83b
  levofloxacin, 83b
  macrolides, 69b, 76–77, 76t
    erythromycin, 76, 76t
  metronidazole, 71t, 80–81
  Minocin, 77t
  minocycline, 77t
  Myambutol, 84t, 85

ANTIINFECTIVE AGENTS (Continued)
  Nafcillin, 73t
  nitrofurantoin, 83
  norfloxacin, 83b
  Noroxin, 83b
  ofloxacin, 83b
  Omnipen, 73t
  oxacillin, 73t
  penicillins, 71t, 72–75, 73t
  Periostat, 77t
  piperacillin, 73t, 75
  Priftin, 84t
  quinolones (fluoroquinolones), 83–84,
      83b
  Raniclor, 75b
  Rifadin, 84t, 85
  Rimactane, 84t, 85
  sulfamethoxazole-trimethoprim,
      83
  sulfonamides, 69b, 71t, 82–83
  Sumycin, 77t
  Suprax, 75b
  tetracyclines, 69b, 77–79, 77t
  ticarcillin, 73t, 75
  topical antibiotics, 85–86
    bacitracin, 85
    mupirocin, 85–86
    neomycin, 85
    polymyxin, 85
  vancomycin, 69b
  Vibramycin, 77t
  Zinacef, 75b
  Zithromax, 76t, 77
ANTINEOPLASTIC DRUGS
  aclarubicin, 228b
  Actinomycin-D, 228b
  Actonel, 228b
  adrenocorticosteroids, 228b
  Adriamycin, 228b
  alendronate, 228b
  Alferon N, 228b
  Alkeran, 228b
  alkylating agents, 228b
  altretamine, 228b
  Amethopterin, 228b
  aminobisphosphonates, 228b
  anastrozole, 228b, 229–230t
  androgen, 228b
  antiandrogen, 228b
  antibiotics, 228b
  antiestrogen, 228b
  antimetabolites, 228b
  Aqupla, 228b
  Aredia, 228b
  Arimidex, 228b
  Aromasin, 228b
  aromatase inhibitors, 228b
  asparaginase, 228b, 229t
  azacytidine, 228b
  azathioprine, 231
  bendamustine, 228b
  bicalutamide, 228b
  bisphosphonates, 227–229
  Blenoxane, 228b
  bleomycin, 228b
  Boniva, 228b
  busulfan, 228b
  carboplatin, 228b
  carmustine, 228b
  Casodex, 228b
  Cerubidine, 228b
  chlorambucil, 228b
  cisplatin, 227, 228b, 229t
  cladribine, 228b
  Cosmegen, 228b

ANTINEOPLASTIC DRUGS (Continued)
cyclophosphamide, 228b, 229–230t
cyclosporin, 231
cytosine arabinoside, 228b
dactinomycin, 228b, 229t
daunorubicin, 228b
diethylstilbestrol, 228b
doxorubicin, 228b, 229–230t
Elspar, 228b
Emcyt, 228b
Ergamisol, 228b
Estinyl, 228b
estramustine, 228b
estrogen, 228b
ethinyl estradiol, 228b
etoposide, 228b
Eulexin, 228b
Evista, 228b
exemestane, 228b, 229–230t
Fareston, 228b
Faslodex, 228b
Femara, 228b
floxuridine, 228b
Fludara, 228b
fludarabine, 228b
5-fluorouracil, 228b, 229t
fluoxymesterone, 228b
flutamide, 228b
folic acid analog, 228b
Fosamax, 228b
fulvestrant, 228b
Gleevec, 228b
goserelin, 228b
Halotestin, 228b
Herceptin, 228b
Hexalen, 228b
hormones, 228b
Hydrea, 228b
hydroxyurea, 228b
ibandronate, 228b
Ifex, 228b
ifosfamide, 228b
imatinib mesylate, 228b
immune modulators, 228b
Imuran, 231
interferons, 228b
Intron A, 228b
Keytruda, 228b
letrozole, 228b, 229–230t
Leukeran, 228b
leuprolide, 228b
Leustatin, 228b
levamisole, 228b
lomustine, 228b
Lupron, 228b
Matulane, 228b
mechlorethamine, 228b, 229t
medroxyprogesterone, 228b
Megace, 228b
megestrol, 228b
melphalan, 228b
mercaptopurine, 228b
methotrexate, 228b, 229t
Mithracin, 228b
mithramycin, 228b
mitomycin-C, 228b
Mustargen, 228b
Mutamycin, 228b
Myleran, 228b
nedaplatin, 228b
Nilandron, 228b
nilutamide, 228b
Nipent, 228b
nitrogen mustards, 228b
nitrosoureas, 229t

ANTINEOPLASTIC DRUGS (Continued)
nivolumab, 228b
Nolvadex, 228b
Oncovin, 228b
Opdivo, 228b
oxaliplatin, 228b
paclitaxel, 228b, 229–230t
pamidronate, 228b
Paraplatin, 228b
pembrolizumab, 228b
pentostatin, 228b
pipobroman, 228b
pirarubicin, 228b
plant alkaloids, 227, 228b
Platinol, 228b
plicamycin, 228b
podophyllotoxin derivatives, 228b
prednisone, 228b
procarbazine, 228b, 229t
progestin, 228b
purine analog, 228b
Purinethol, 228b
pyrimidine analog, 228b
raloxifene, 228b
Rheumatrex, 231
risedronate, 228b
Rituxan, 228b
rituximab, 228b
Roferon-A, 228b
Sandimmune, 231
streptozocin, 228b
tamoxifen, 228b, 229t
Taxol, 228b
teniposide, 228b
Teslac, 228b
testolactone, 228b
thioguanine, 228b
thiotepa, 228b
toremifene, 228b
trastuzumab, 228b, 229–230t
Uracil mustard, 228b
uramustine, 228b
Velban, 228b
VePesid, 228b
Vercyte, 228b
Vidaza, 228b
vinblastine, 228b, 229t
vincristine, 228b, 229t
Vumon, 228b
Zanosar, 228b
Zoladex, 228b
zoledronate, 228b
zoledronic acid, 227–229
Zometa, 228b
antipsychotic agents, 175–179, 176t, 278b, 279t
antituberculosis agents, 84–85, 84t
ANTIVIRAL AGENTS, 92–97
Abreva, 92t, 273, 273t
acyclovir, 92–94, 92t
Denavir, 94
docosanol, 94
famciclovir, 94
ganciclovir, 94
for HIV, 93t
abacavir, 93t
Agenerase, 93t
amprenavir, 93t
Aptivus, 93t
atazanavir, 93t
cobicistat, 93t
Crixivan, 93t
darunavir, 93t
delavirdine, 93t
didanosine, 93t
dolutegravir, 93t

ANTIVIRAL AGENTS (Continued)
Edurant, 93t
efavirenz, 93t
elvitegravir, 93t
emtricitabine, 93t
Emtriva, 93t
enfuvirtide, 93t
Epivir, 93t
etravirine, 93t
Fortovase, 93t
fosamprenavir, 93t
Fuzeon, 93t
Hivid, 93t
indinavir, 93t
Intelence, 93t
Invirase, 93t, 95
Isentress, 93t
lamivudine, 93t
Lexiva, 93t
maraviroc, 93t
nelfinavir, 93t
nevirapine, 93t, 94
nonnucleoside reverse transcriptase
  inhibitors, 93t, 94
Norvir, 93t
nucleoside/nucleotide reverse transcriptase
  inhibitors, 93t, 94
Prezista, 93t
protease inhibitors, 93t, 95
raltegravir, 93t
Rescriptor, 93t
Retrovir, 93t, 94
Reyataz, 93t
rilpivirine, 93t
ritonavir, 93t
saquinavir, 93t, 95
Selzentry, 93t
stavudine, 93t
Sustiva, 93t
tenofovir, 93t
tipranavir, 93t
Tivicay, 93t
Tybost, 93t
Videx, 93t
Viracept, 93t
Viramune, 93t, 94
Viread, 93t
Vitekta, 93t
zalcitabine, 93t
Zerit, 93t
Ziagen, 93t
zidovudine, 93t, 94
penciclovir, 92t, 94
Rebetol, 96t
ribavirin, 96t
valacyclovir, 273
Anusol, 185t
Aplenzin, 179–180t
apomorphine, 278b
Apresoline, 140b, 149
Aprinox, 140b
Aptiom, 169–170t
aripiprazole, 176t, 178t
Aristocort, 185t
Arnuity Ellipta, 194–195t
aromatase inhibitors, 221–222t, 223
Artane, 38
articaine, 100t, 102–103t, 105, 108b, 109t
asenapine, 176t, 178t
Asmanex HFA, 194–195t
Asmanex Twisthaler, 194–195t
aspirin1, 2, 3. See also acetylsalicylic acid
  adverse effect of, 24–25
  adverse reactions, 47–49
  pharmacokinetics of, 47

Atacand, 140b
atenolol, 42, 42t, 135t, 140b, 142t
Ativan, 120t, 171
atorvastatin, 151t
Atridox, 22, 77t
atropine
  adverse reactions, 36
  as anticholinergic, 38t
  CNS effects, 37
  uses of, 242
AUTACOIDS AND ANTIHISTAMINES
  acrivastine, 200t
  Alavert, 200t
  Allegra, 200f, 200t
  antihistamines, 199
  Astelin, 201t
  azelastine, 201t
  Benadryl, 200f, 200t
  brompheniramine, 200f, 200t
  cetirizine, 200t
  Chlor-Trimeton, 200f, 200t
  chlorpheniramine, 200f, 200t
  Clarinex, 200t
  Claritin, 200f, 200t
  clemastine, 200t
  desloratadine, 200t
  Dimetane, 200f, 200t
  diphenhydramine, 200f, 200t
  fexofenadine, 200f, 200t
  histamine, 199
  leukotrienes, 201–202
  levocetirizine, 200t
  loratadine, 200f, 200t, 201
  montelukast, 200t
  Semprex, 200t
  Singulair, 200t
  Tavist, 200t
  Xyzal, 200t
  Zyrtec, 200t
AUTONOMIC DRUGS
  acebutolol, 42t
  Adderall, 40t
  Adrenalin, 40t
  adrenergic receptor agonists, 40t
  α-adrenergic receptor antagonists, 42t
  albuterol, 40t
  Aldomet, 40t
  amphetamine, 40t
  anticholinergic agents, 37–38, 38t
  Antilirium, 35t
  Aricept, 35t
  Artane, 38
  atenolol, 42, 42t
  atropine, 36, 38t
  Atrovent, 38t
  autonomic nervous system, 31–33
  Bentyl, 38t
  benztropine, 38
  bethanechol, 35t
  Cardura, 42
  Catapres, 40t
  cholinergic agents, 36
  clonidine, 40t
  Cogentin, 38
  curare, 43
  Dantrium, 43
  dantrolene, 43
  Desoxyn, 40t
  Dexedrine, 40t, 41
  dextroamphetamine, 40t
  Dibenzyline, 42, 42t
  dicyclomine, 38t
  diethylpropion, 41
  dipivefrin, 42
  dobutamine, 40t

AUTONOMIC DRUGS (Continued)
  donepezil, 35t
  dopamine, 42
  doxazosin, 42
  edrophonium, 35t, 36
  ephedrine, 40t, 41–42
  epinephrine, 40, 40t
  EpiPen, 40t
  ergot, 42t
  galantamine, 35t
  glycopyrrolate, 37
  Hytrin, 42
  Inderal, 42, 42t
  insecticides, 36
  ipratropium, 37, 38t
  isoproterenol, 39, 40t
  Isopto Carpine, 35t
  Isuprel, 40t
  labetalol, 42t, 43
  levonordefrin, 41
  Levophed, 40t
  malathion, 35t, 37
  Maldemar, 38t
  Mestinon, 35t
  metaproterenol, 40t
  methamphetamine, 40t
  methyldopa, 40t
  methylphenidate, 40t, 41
  Minipress, 42, 42t
  Neo-Synephrine, 40t, 41
  neostigmine, 35t
  nicotine, 39
  norepinephrine, 40t
  Normodyne, 42t, 43
  OcuClear, 40t
  organophosphates, 36
  oxymetazoline, 40t
  pancuronium, 43
  parasympathetic autonomic nervous
    system, 31
  parathion, 35t, 36
  phenoxybenzamine, 42, 42t
  phentolamine, 42, 42t
  phenylephrine, 40t, 41
  physostigmine, 35t, 36
  pilocarpine, 35t, 36
  pralidoxime, 36
  prazosin, 42, 42t
  Primatene, 40t
  Priscoline, 42
  Pro-Banthine, 37, 38t
  propantheline, 37, 38t
  Propine, 42
  propranolol, 42, 42t
  Prostigmin, 35t
  Protopam, 36
  pseudoephedrine, 40t, 41–42
  pyridostigmine, 35t
  Razadyne, 35t
  Regitine, 42, 42t
  Ritalin, 40t, 41
  rivastigmine, 35t
  Robinul, 37
  Salagen, 35t, 36
  sarin, 35t, 37
  scopolamine, 37, 38t
  Sectral, 42t
  succinylcholine, 43
  Sudafed, 40t, 41–42
  sympathetic autonomic nervous
    system, 31–32
  tabun, 35t
  Tenormin, 42, 42t
  Tensilon, 35t
  Tenuate, 41

AUTONOMIC DRUGS (Continued)
  terazosin, 42
  tetrahydrozoline, 40t
  tolazoline, 42
  Trandate, 42t, 43
  Transderm-Scop, 38t
  trihexyphenidyl, 38
  Tyzine, 40t
  Urecholine, 35t
  vecuronium, 43
  Visine, 40t
  yohimbine, 42t
Avandia, 211–212t, 213
Avapro, 140b
Aventyl, 179–180t
azilsartan, 140b
azithromycin, 76t, 77, 247–248t
AZT, 94

B
bacitracin, 85
baclofen, 127–128
Bactrim, 83
Bactroban, 85, 274–275
Banzel, 169–170t
barbiturates, 124–125, 124t, 126b
bath salts, 254t
BCise, 211–212t
Belsomra, 120t, 127
Benadryl, 162
benazepril, 140b
bendroflumethiazide, 140b
Benicar, 140b
Benzocaine, 100t, 110, 110t
Benzodent, 110
benzodiazepines, 114–115, 114t, 120–121, 120t,
  160, 171–172, 247–248t, 250, 254t
benzothiazepines, 138t
betamethasone, 275–276
betamethasone valerate, 185t, 188, 188t
betaxolol, 140b
biguanides, 210, 211–212t
bile acid sequestrants, 211–212t, 213
bisoprolol, 135t, 140b
bleomycin, 278b
α-blocking agents, 43
β-blocking agents, 43, 126b, 142t, 280b
Breo Ellipta, 194–195t
bretylium, 135t, 278b
Brevicon, 220t
Brevital, 124t
brexpiprazole, 176t, 178t
Brilinta, 155
brivaracetam, 169–170t
Briviact, 169–170t
bumetanide, 140b
Bumex, 140b
bupivacaine, 100t, 102–103t, 104–105, 108b, 109t,
  247–248t
buprenorphine, 59t
bupropion, 179–180t, 181–182, 262
BuSpar, 126
buspirone, 126
butabarbital, 124t
Butisol, 124t
butorphanol, 59t, 65
Bydureon, 211–212t
Byetta, 211–212t, 213
Bystolic, 140b

C
caffeine, 261, 261t
Calan, 137t, 140b
calcitonin, 217
calcium, 78, 98–99

calcium channel blockers, 136–138t, 138, 140b, 142t, 144t, 278b, 280b
canagliflozin, 211–212t, 213
candesartan, 140b, 142t
cannabinoids, 163
Capoten, 140b
captopril, 140b, 280b
carbamazepine, 168–170, 168b, 245–246t
Carbocaine, 100t, 103t, 104
carboxymethylcellulose paste, 276
CARDIOVASCULAR DRUGS
    aldosterone antagonists, 133
    antianginal drugs in, 136–139
        β-adrenergic blocking agents, 138
        calcium channel blocking agents, 138
        nitroglycerin-like compounds, 136–138
        ranolazine, 138
    antiarrhythmic agents, 135–136, 135t
    anticoagulants, 152–153
        alteplase, 155
        clopidogrel, 155
        dipyridamole, 155–156
        heparin, 153
        pentoxifylline, 156
        prasugrel, 155
        streptokinase, 155
        ticagrelor, 155
        ticlopidine, 155
        warfarin, 153–154
    antihyperlipidemic agents, 149–152, 149b
        cholestyramine, 152
        gemfibrozil, 152
        3-hydroxy-3-methylglutaryl coenzyme A reductase, 150–151, 150b
        niacin, 152
    antihypertensive agents
        β-adrenergic blocking agents, 147–148
        angiotensin-converting enzyme inhibitors, 145–146
        angiotensin receptor blockers, 146
        clonidine, 149
        hydralazine, 149
        loop diuretics, 144–145
        methyldopa, 149
        potassium salts, 145
        potassium-sparing diuretics, 145
        renin inhibitors, 146–147
        reserpine, 149
        thiazide diuretics, 142–144
    diuretics, 132
    hemostatic agents, 156
    vasodilators, 133
Cardizem, 140b
Cardura, 42, 140b
cariprazine, 176t, 178t
carisoprodol, 127t, 278b
carvedilol, 140b
Cataflam, 51t
Catapres, 40t, 140b, 149
Catapres-TTS, 22
Celebrex, 54
Celecoxib, 54
Celexa, 179, 179–180t
cephalexin, 75b
cephalosporins, 75–76, 75b, 247–248t, 249
Cerebyx, 169–170t
Cesamet, 163
Cetacaine, 110t
Cetacort, 185t
cetylpyridinium chloride, 287
cevimeline hydrochloride, 277
chemical warfare agents, 37
chlorambucil, 278b
chlordiazepoxide, 120t, 250
chlorhexidine, 276, 278b, 288

chlorhexidine-containing chip, 22
chlorhexidine gluconate, 271, 288, 288f
chlorothiazide, 140b
chlorpromazine, 126b, 176t
chlorpropamide, 210t, 245–246t, 280b
chlorthalidone, 140b
chlorzoxazone, 127, 127t
cholestyramine, 151t, 152
cimetidine, 101, 159
Cinqair, 194–195t, 198
Cipro, 83
ciprofloxacin, 83
cisapride, 278b
cisplatin, 278b
citalopram, 179, 179–180t
Citanest, 100t, 103t, 104
clarithromycin, 76t, 77, 247–248t
clindamycin, 79–80, 247–248t, 249, 278b
clobazam, 171
clobetasol propionate, 185t
Climara, 22
Clomid, 222, 222t
clomiphene, 222, 222t
clonazepam, 120t, 171
clonidine, 140b, 149, 278b
    in transdermal patch, 22
clopidogrel, 155
clorazepate, 120t
clotrimazole, 91, 247–248t, 249
    for angular cheilitis, 274
    for candidiasis, 91b
clozapine, 176t, 178t
Clozaril, 176t
cocaine, 98b, 100t, 254t
codeine, 59–60t
Cogentin, 38
colchicine, 53t, 56
colesevelam, 151t, 211–212t, 213
Colestid, 151t, 152
colestipol, 151t, 152
Compazine, 162, 239
ConZip, 64t
Coreg, 140b
Corgard, 140b
Cortaid, 185t
corticosteroids, 278b
    for aphthous stomatitis, 275–276
    topical administration of, 22
Coumadin, 153
Cozaar, 140b
Crestor, 151t
curare, 43
cyclobenzaprine, 127, 127t, 278b
cyclooxygenase (COX) II-specific agents, 54
cyclosporine, 278b
Cyklokapron, 156
Cymbalta, 179–180t, 180
Cytomel, 217b
Cytotec, 161

D
Dalmane, 120t
danazol, 222t, 223
Danocrine, 222t, 223
Dantrium, 43, 128
dantrolene, 43, 128
dapagliflozin, 211–212t
daunorubicin, 278b
Demadex, 140b
Demerol, 60t, 63, 64t, 258
Denavir, 94, 273, 273t
Depakote, 167–168b
Dermacort, 185t
desflurane, 117
desipramine, 179–180t

Desogen, 220t
desogestrel, 220t
Desoxyn, 260
desvenlafaxine, 179–180t, 180
Desyrel, 179–180t
dexamethasone, 188t
Dexedrine, 40t, 41, 260
dextroamphetamine, 40t, 41, 260
dextromethorphan, 60
dezocine, 59t
DiaBeta, 210t
Diabinese, 210t
diazepam, 114–115, 114t, 120, 120t, 127t, 171, 245–248t
    antiseizure effects of, 121
    for conscious sedation, 124
    in dental procedures, 124
    metabolism of, 16
    as muscle relaxants, 127, 127t
    as premedication, 124
Dibenzyline, 42, 42t
diclofenac, 51t, 154t
dicyclomine, 163
diethylpropion, 41, 260
Diflucan, 92
diflunisal, 46b, 50
digitalis glycosides, 134–135
digoxin, 134, 135b, 136
dihydrocodeine, 60t
dihydropyridines, 138t, 140b
Dilacor, 140b
Dilantin, 279
Dilaudid, 60t, 63–64, 64t, 258
diltiazem, 135t, 138t, 140b, 142t, 278b
Diovan, 140b
dipeptidyl-peptidase-4 inhibitors, 211–212t, 213
Diphen Cough, 273
Diphenhist, 273
diphenhydramine, 162, 200t, 276
diphenoxylate, 60, 163
diphenylalkylamines, 138t
Diprivan, 114, 114t
dipyridamole, 155–156
disopyramide, 135t
disulfiram, 80, 126b
diuretics, 53t, 132, 142t, 280b
Diuril, 140b
divalproex, 167
docosanol, 94, 273, 273t
dofetilide, 135t
Dolobid, 50, 51t
Dolophine, 60t, 64–65, 258
domiphen bromide, 287
dopamine, 42, 42f
Doral, 120t
doxazosin, 42, 140b
doxorubicin, 278b
doxycycline, 126b, 247–248t, 278b
    administration of, 22
    gel, 22
    metabolism of, 16
dronabinol, 163
drospirenone, 220t
DRUG ABUSE
    alcohol, 254–257
    amphetamines, 260–261
    angel dust, 263
    bath salts, 254t
    benzodiazepines, 254t
    Bupropion, 262
    caffeine, 261, 261t
    CHANTIX, 262
    cocaine, 254t
    Demerol, 258
    Desoxyn, 260

DRUG ABUSE *(Continued)*
  Dexedrine, 260
  dextroamphetamine, 260
  diethylpropion, 260
  Dilaudid, 258
  Dolophine, 258
  ethanol, 254*t*
  ethyl alcohol, 254–257
  Habitrol, 262, 262*t*
  heroin, 254*t*, 258
  hydromorphone, 258
  inhalants, 254*t*
  lysergic acid diethylamide, 254*t*, 263
  marijuana, 254*t*, 263
  meperidine, 258
  methadone, 258
  methamphetamine, 254*t*, 260
  1-methyl-4-phenyl-1,2,3,6-tetrahydropyridine, 259
  methylphenidate, 260
  morphine, 258
  naloxone, 258
  Narcan, 258
  NicoDerm, 262, 262*t*
  Nicorette, 262, 262*t*
  nicotine, 261
  Nicotrol, 262, 262*t*
  nitrous oxide, 254*t*, 257–258
  opioid analgesics, 258–259
  oxycodone, 258
  OxyContin, 258
  Percodan, 258
  phencyclidine, 263
  psychedelics (hallucinogens), 262–263
  Ritalin, 260
  sedative-hypnotics, 259–260
  Spice, 254*t*
  Tenuate, 260
  tobacco, 261–262
  Varenicline, 262
  Wellbutrin, 262
  Zyban, 262
dulaglutide, 211–212*t*
Dulera, 194–195*t*
duloxetine, 179–180*t*, 180
Duragesic, 22
Dyclone, 110*t*
dyclonine, 105, 110*t*
dynorphins, 58
Dyrenium, 140*b*

E
Edarbi, 140*b*
Edecrin, 140*b*
Edrophonium, 36
Effexor, 179–180*t*, 180
Effient, 155
Elavil, 179–180*t*
Eligard, 222
EMERGENCY DRUGS
  albuterol, 240*t*, 241
  alprazolam, 240*t*
  antiarrhythmics, 242
  aromatic ammonia spirits, 240*t*, 241
  atropine, 240*t*, 242
  Benadryl, 241
  benzodiazepines, 241–242
  β-blockers, 239, 240*t*, 242
  bretylium, 240*t*, 242
  Compazine, 239
  Dantrium, 239
  dantrolene, 239
  dextrose, 240*t*, 242
  diazepam, 240*t*, 241
  diphenhydramine, 239–241, 240*t*

EMERGENCY DRUGS *(Continued)*
  epinephrine, 239–241, 240*t*, 241*f*
  flumazenil, 240*t*, 242
  glucagon, 240*t*, 242
  glucose, 240*t*, 241, 241*f*
  hydrocortisone, 239, 240*t*, 241–242
  insulin, 235–236
  lidocaine, 237, 240*t*, 242
  midazolam, 241
  morphine, 241
  naloxone, 239, 240*t*, 242
  Narcan, 239, 242
  nitroglycerin, 237, 240*t*, 241, 241*f*
  oxygen, 239–241, 240*t*
  procainamide, 240*t*, 242
  prochlorperazine, 239
  propylthiouracil, 239
  Romazicon, 242
  succinylcholine, 236, 239
  Valium, 241
  Ventolin, 240*t*
  verapamil, 240*t*, 242
  Versed, 241
empagliflozin, 211–212*t*
Empirin, 60*t*, 64*t*
enalapril, 140*b*, 280*b*
encainide, 135*t*
Endocet, 64*t*
Endodan, 64*t*
endorphins, 58
Enduron, 140*b*
enflurane, 114*t*, 115, 117
enkephalins, 58
ephedrine, 40*t*, 41–42
epinephrine, 107*t*, 178–179, 179*b*
  pharmacologic effects of, 40, 40*t*
  uses for, 41
eplerenone, 140*b*
eprosartan, 140*b*
ertugliflozin, 211–212*t*
erythromycin, 70, 76, 76*t*, 247–248*t*, 249
escitalopram, 179, 179–180*t*
Esidrix, 140*b*
Eskalith, 182
eslicarbazepine (Aptiom), 169–170*t*
esmolol, 135*t*
estazolam, 120*t*
esterified estrogens, 218*t*
Estinyl, 218*t*
Estraderm, 22, 218*t*, 219
estradiol transdermal system, 218*t*
estrogens, 218*t*, 219–220, 220*t*
Estropipate, 218*t*
eszopiclone, 120*t*, 126
ethacrynic acid, 140*b*
ethambutol, 84*t*, 85, 280*b*
ethinyl estradiol, 218*t*, 220*t*
ethionamide, 278*b*
ethosuximide, 171, 278*b*
ethyl alcohol, 254–257, 254*t*
ethylaminobenzoate, 100*t*
ethynodiol, 220*t*
etomidate, 114, 114*t*
etonogestrel, 220*t*
Eugenol, 269
eugenol, 269
Euthroid, 217*b*
evolocumab, 151*t*
Evoxac, 277
exenatide, 211–212*t*, 213
ezetimibe, 151–152, 151*t*

F
famciclovir, 94, 273, 273*t*
Fanapt, 176*t*

Fareston, 222*t*
Farxiga, 211–212*t*
felbamate, 169–170*t*
Felbatol, 169–170*t*
felodipine, 140*b*
female sex hormones, 218–221
Femhrt, 218*t*
fenofibrate, 151*t*
fenofibric acid, 151*t*
fenoprofen, 51*t*, 52, 54, 154*t*
fentanyl, 59*t*, 62*b*, 65
  in transdermal patch, 22
Fetzima, 179–180*t*, 180
Fioricet, 64*t*, 128
Fiorinal, 64*t*, 128
flecainide, 135*t*
Flexeril, 127, 127*t*
Flovent Diskus, 194–195*t*
Floxin, 83*b*
fluconazole, 92
flumazenil, 122, 242
flunitrazepam, 259–260
fluocinolone acetonide, 185*t*
fluocinonide, 275–276
fluoride, 278*b*, 284–287, 284–285*b*, 284*t*, 285*f*, 289
fluoroquinolones, 83–84, 83*b*
5-fluorouracil, 228*b*, 229*t*, 278*b*
fluoxetine, 179, 179–180*t*
fluphenazine, 176*t*
flurazepam, 120*t*
flurbiprofen, 51*t*
Flutex, 185*t*
fluticasone propionate, 194–195*t*, 196–197
fluvastatin, 151*t*
folic acid, 83
Forane, 114*t*, 117
Fortamet, 211–212*t*
Fosamax, 228*b*
fosinopril, 140*b*
fosphenytoin (Cerebyx), 169–170*t*
furosemide, 140*b*, 144–145, 280*b*
Fycompa, 169–170*t*

G
gabapentin, 169–170*t*
Gabitril, 169–170*t*
ganciclovir, 94, 273
Garamycin, 82
GASTROINTESTINAL AGENTS
  aluminum hydroxide, 159*t*
  antacids, 161
  anticholinergics, 162
  antidiarrheals, 162
  antiemetics, 162
  antihistamines, 162
  Asacol, 161*t*
  Atarax, 162
  Axid, 159*t*
  azathioprine, 161*t*
  Azulfidine, 161*t*
  Benadryl, 162
  bisacodyl, 162, 162*t*
  Bonine, 161*t*, 162
  calcium carbonate, 159*t*
  cannabinoids, 163
  Carafate, 161
  carboxymethylcellulose, 162*t*
  casanthranol, 162*t*
  cascara sagrada, 162*t*
  castor oil, 162*t*
  Cesamet, 161*t*, 163
  cimetidine, 159, 159*t*
  Citrucel, 162*t*
  clarithromycin, 160*t*
  Colace, 162*t*

GASTROINTESTINAL AGENTS (*Continued*)

Compazine, 161*t*, 162
cyclosporine, 161*t*
Cytotec, 159*t*, 161
dicyclomine, 163
dimenhydrinate, 161*t*, 162
Dipentum, 161*t*
diphenhydramine, 162
diphenoxylate, 161*t*
docusate, 162*t*
Dramamine, 161*t*, 162
dronabinol, 161*t*, 163
Dulcolax, 162*t*
esomeprazole, 159*t*
famotidine, 159, 159*t*
FiberCon, 162*t*
Flagyl, 161*t*
Gas-X, 159*t*, 161
glycerin, 162*t*
histamine$_2$-blocking agents, 159–160
hydroxyzine, 162
hyoscyamine, 163
Imodium, 161*t*, 162
infliximab, 163
itraconazole, 160
Kaopectate, 161*t*, 162
ketoconazole, 160
lactulose, 162*t*
lansoprazole, 159*t*
laxatives, 161–162, 162*t*
Lomotil, 161*t*, 162–163
loperamide, 161*t*, 162–163
magnesium hydroxide, 159*t*, 162*t*
marijuana, 163
Marinol, 161*t*, 163
meclizine, 161*t*, 162
mercaptopurine, 161*t*
mesalamine, 161*t*
Metamucil, 162*t*
methylcellulose, 162*t*
metoclopramide, 159*t*, 161, 163
metronidazole, 161*t*
milk of magnesia, 162*t*
misoprostol, 159*t*, 161
Mylicon, 159*t*, 161
nabilone, 161*t*, 163
nizatidine, 159, 159*t*
nonsteroidal antiinflammatory drugs, 159
olsalazine, 161*t*
omeprazole, 159*t*
pantoprazole, 159*t*
Pentasa, 161*t*, 162
Pepcid, 159*t*
pepto-Bismol, 160, 160*t*
Phenergan, 162
phenolphthalein, 162*t*
phenothiazines, 162
polycarbophil, 162*t*
prednisone, 161*t*
Prevacid, 159*t*
Prilosec, 159*t*
prochlorperazine, 161*t*
promethazine, 162
proton pump inhibitors, 160
psyllium seed, 162*t*
rabeprazole, 159*t*
ranitidine, 159, 159*t*
Reglan, 159*t*, 161, 163
Remicade, 163
Rowasa, 161*t*
scopolamine, 162
senna, 162*t*
simethicone, 159*t*, 161
sodium bicarbonate, 159*t*, 161
sucralfate, 161

GASTROINTESTINAL AGENTS (*Continued*)

sulfasalazine, 161
Tagamet, 159, 159*t*
Tigan, 161*t*, 162–163
Transderm-Scop, 162
trimethobenzamide, 161*t*, 162–163
Zantac, 159*t*
gemfibrozil, 151*t*, 152
Genahist, 273
gentamicin, 82
Geodon, 176*t*
glimepiride, 210*t*
glipizide, 210*t*
glucagon, 214, 240*t*, 242
glucagon-like peptide-1 receptor agonists,
    211–212*t*, 213
Glucophage, 210, 211–212*t*
Glucophage XR, 211–212*t*
α-glucosidase inhibitors, 211–212*t*, 213
Glucotrol, 210*t*
Glucotrol-XL, 210*t*
glucuronic acid, 16
Glumetza, 211–212*t*
glyburide, 210*t*
glycopyrrolate, 37
Glynase PresTab, 210*t*
Glyset, 211–212*t*
gold salts, 278*b*
griseofulvin, 126*b*, 278*b*
guanethidine, 149, 278*b*
guanfacine, 140*b*

H

Habitrol, 262, 262*t*
Halcion, 120*t*
Haldol, 176*t*
haloperidol, 176*t*
halothane, 115*t*, 117
hemostatic agents, 156
heparin, 153
HERBAL PRODUCTS AND DIETARY
    SUPPLEMENTS, 265–270
    angelica, 267*t*
    bilberry, 268*t*
    black cohosh, 268*t*
    bromelain, 268*t*
    chamomile, 268*t*
    chaparral, 267*t*
    clove, 267*t*
    cloves, 268*t*
    coenzyme Q$_{10}$, 267–268*t*
    coleus forskolin, 268*t*
    comfrey, 267*t*
    Cordyceps, 268*t*
    cranberry, 268*t*
    Dong quai, 268*t*
    echinacea, 267*t*
    Echinacea purpurea, 268*t*
    ephedra, 266, 267–268*t*
    evening primrose, 268*t*
    feverfew, 267–268*t*
    garlic, 267–268*t*
    ginger, 268*t*
    ginkgo, 267–268*t*
    ginseng, 268*t*
    goldenseal, 268*t*
    gotu kola, 268*t*
    guar gum, 268*t*
    guggul, 268*t*
    hawthorn, 268*t*
    horse chestnut, 268*t*
    kava, 267–268*t*
    licorice, 268*t*
    Ma-huang, 267*t*
    melatonin, 268*t*

**HERBAL PRODUCTS AND DIETARY
    SUPPLEMENTS** (*Continued*)

    milk thistle, 267*t*
    nettle root, 268*t*
    niacin, 267*t*
    passion flower, 268*t*
    pomegranate, 267*t*
    red clover, 267*t*
    St. John's wort, 266–267, 268*t*
    turmeric, 268*t*
    valerian root, 268*t*
    wormwood, 267*t*
    yohimbe, 267–268*t*
heroin, 254*t*, 258
hexamethonium, 33*t*
histamine, 199
Hurricaine, 110, 110*t*
hydantoins, 278*b*
hydralazine, 133, 140*b*, 149, 278*b*
hydrochlorothiazide, 140*b*, 142, 142*t*
hydrocodone, 60*t*, 63, 64*t*
hydrocortisone, 184, 185*t*, 188, 188*t*
hydrofluorocarbons, 22
hydromorphone, 60*t*, 63–64, 258
3-hydroxy-3-methylglutaryl coenzyme A
    reductase, 150–151, 150*b*
hydroxychloroquine, 280*b*
Hygroton, 140*b*
Hytone, 185*t*
Hytrin, 42, 140*b*

I

ibuprofen, 4, 4*f*, 51*t*, 53–54, 154*t*
iloperidone, 176*t*, 178*t*
imidazole, 90–92
imipramine, 179–180*t*
immunosuppressives, 276
Imuran, 163, 276
indapamide, 140*b*
Inderal, 42, 42*t*, 140*b*
indomethacin, 94, 148, 154*t*
inhalants, 254*t*
insecticides, 36
Inspra, 140*b*
insulins, 208, 208*t*, 209*b*
    inactivation of, 19
interferons, 96*t*, 97
Invega, 176*t*
Invirase, 93*t*, 95
Invokana, 211–212*t*, 213
iodides, 278*b*
ipratropium, 37, 38*t*, 197*t*, 198
irbesartan, 140*b*, 142*t*
iron, 78
Isocaine, 103*t*, 104
isocarboxazid, 179–180*t*
isoflurane, 114*t*, 115, 117
isoniazid, 84–85, 84*t*, 278*b*
isoprenaline, 278*b*
isoproterenol, 39, 40*t*, 278*b*
Isoptin, 137*t*, 140*b*
Isopto Carpine, 35*t*
isosorbide dinitrate, 137*t*
isosorbide mononitrate, 137*t*
isotretinoin, 245, 245–246*t*
isradipine, 140*b*

J

Januvia, 211–212*t*, 213
Jardiance, 211–212*t*

K

Kabikinase, 155
kaolin, 162, 273
Kaopectate, 162, 273

Kelnor, 220*t*
Kenalog, 185*t*, 188
Keppra, 169–170*t*
Kerlone, 140*b*
Ketalar, 114, 114*t*
ketamine, 114, 114*t*, 278*b*
ketoconazole, 91–92, 91*t*, 160, 247–248*t*, 249–250, 280*b*
ketorolac, 51*t*, 54
Klonopin, 120*t*, 171

L
labetalol, 42*t*, 43, 140*b*, 148, 280*b*
lacosamide (Vimpat), 169–170*t*
Lamictal, 169–170*t*
lamotrigine, 169–170*t*
Laniazid, 84–85, 84*t*
Lasix, 140*b*
Latuda, 176*t*
laxatives, 278*b*
Lescol, 151*t*
leuprolide, 222, 222*t*
Levatol, 140*b*
levetiracetam, 169–170*t*
levodopa, 38
levofloxacin, 83*b*
levomilnacipran, 179–180*t*, 180
levonordefrin, 41, 104, 107*t*
Levonorgestrel, 220*t*
Levora, 220*t*
Lexapro, 179, 179–180*t*
Librium, 120*t*
Lidex, 185*t*, 279
lidocaine, 100*t*, 102–103*t*, 108*b*, 109–110*t*, 135*t*, 247–248*t*
linagliptin, 211–212*t*
Lioresal, 127–128
Lipitor, 151*t*
Liptruzet, 151*t*
liraglutide, 211–212*t*
lisinopril, 140*b*, 142*t*
Lispro insulin, 208
lithium, 53*t*, 182, 182*b*, 278*b*
Lithobid, 182
Livalo, 151*t*
lixisenatide, 211–212*t*
Lo/Ovral, 220*t*
Lomotil, 60, 79, 162
Loniten, 140*b*
loop diuretics, 144–145
loperamide, 161*t*, 162
Lopid, 151*t*
Lopressor, 140*b*
lorazepam, 120*t*, 123–124, 171, 247–248*t*
Lorcet, 60*t*
Lortab, 60*t*, 64*t*
losartan, 140*b*
Lotensin, 140*b*
lovastatin, 151, 151*t*
loxapine, 176*t*
Loxitane, 176*t*
Lozol, 140*b*
Luminal, 124*t*
Lunesta, 120*t*, 126
Lupron, 222, 222*t*
lurasidone, 176*t*, 178*t*
Lyrica, 169–170*t*
lysergic acid diethylamide, 254*t*, 263

M
Maalox, 273
macrolides, 76–77, 76*t*
magnesium, 50
male sex hormones, 221–222
Marcaine, 98, 100*t*, 103*t*, 105
marijuana, 254*t*, 263

Marinol, 161*t*, 163
Marplan, 179–180*t*
Mavik, 140*b*
meclofenamate, 51*t*, 154*t*
Meclomen, 51*t*
medroxyprogesterone, 218*t*
mefenamic acid, 51*t*
meglitinides, 210–213, 211–212*t*
melatonin receptor agonist, 120*t*, 126–127
Mellaril, 176*t*
meloxicam, 51*t*
Menest, 218*t*
meperidine, 63, 63*t*, 258
    efficacy of, 60
meperidine, potency of, 11
mepivacaine, 100*t*, 102–103*t*, 108*b*, 109*t*, 247–248*t*
mepolizumab, 194–195*t*, 198
6-mercaptopurine, 278*b*
mercurials, 278*b*
Meritene, 271
mestranol, 220*t*
metformin, 210, 211–212*t*
methadone, 60*t*, 63*t*, 64–65, 258
methamphetamine, 254*t*, 260
methimazole, 278*b*
methocarbamol, 127, 127*t*, 278*b*
methohexital, 124*t*
methotrexate, 49, 53*t*, 229*t*, 278*b*
methoxyflurane, 114–115*t*, 115
methyclothiazide, 140*b*
1-methyl-4-phenyl-1,2,3,6-tetrahydropyridine, 259
methyldopa, 40*t*, 140*b*, 149, 278*b*, 280*b*
methylphenidate, 260
methylprednisolone, 188*t*
metoclopramide, 161, 163, 278*b*
metolazone, 140*b*
metoprolol, 135*t*, 140*b*, 142*t*
metronidazole, 80–81, 245–248*t*, 278*b*
    for oral lesions, 271
    in pregnancy, 72
Mevacor, 151, 151*t*
mexiletine, 135*t*
Micardis, 140*b*
miconazole, 247–248*t*
Micronase, 210*t*
Micronor, 218*t*
Midamor, 140*b*
midazolam, 114, 114*t*, 120–122, 120*t*, 171, 241, 247–248*t*
miglitol, 211–212*t*
Minastrin 24 Fe, 220*t*
Minipress, 42, 140*b*
minocycline, 78, 247–248*t*, 278*b*
minoxidil, 140*b*
mirtazapine, 179–180*t*, 182
misoprostol, 159*t*, 161
Mobic, 51*t*
Modicon, 220*t*
moexipril, 140*b*
Monopril, 140*b*
montelukast (Singulair), 197
morphine, 59*t*, 63, 241, 258
    efficacy of, 60
    potency of, 11
Motrin, 51*t*, 53
mupirocin, 85–86
Myambutol, 84*t*, 85
Mycelex, 91, 91*t*
Mycostatin, 90, 91*t*
Mykrox, 140*b*
Mylanta, 273

N
nabumetone, 51*t*
nadolol, 140*b*

Nafcillin, 73*t*
nalbuphine, 59*t*
Nalfon, 51*t*
nalmefene, 59*t*, 66
naloxone, 59*t*, 65, 258
naltrexone, 59*t*, 66
Naprosyn, 51*t*, 54
naproxen, 51*t*, 54, 154*t*
Narcan, 258
Nardil, 179–180*t*
nateglinide, 210–213, 211–212*t*
Navane, 176*t*
nebivolol, 140*b*
Necon, 220*t*
nefazodone, 179–180*t*, 182
Nembutal, 124*t*
Neo-Cobefrin, 107*t*
Neo-Fradin, 82
Neo-Synephrine, 198–199
neomycin, 82, 85
Neosporin, 85
neostigmine
    cholinergic effects, 35*t*
    oral side effects of, 278*b*
    uses for, 36
Nesina, 211–212*t*
Neurontin, 169–170*t*
nevirapine, 93*t*, 94
niacin, 152
Niaspan, 151*t*
nicardipine, 140*b*
Nicobid, 22
NicoDerm, 22, 262, 262*t*
Nicorette, 262, 262*t*
nicotine, 22, 39, 261
nicotinic acid, 152
Nicotrol, 262, 262*t*
nifedipine, 137–138*t*, 140*b*, 142*t*, 278*b*, 280*b*
Nilstat, 90, 91*t*
niridazole, 278*b*
nisoldipine, 140*b*
nitrazepam, 278*b*
Nitro-Dur, 22
Nitrodisc, 22
nitrofurantoin, 83, 278*b*
nitrogen mustard, 278*b*
nitroglycerin, 136–138
    dosage forms, 137*t*
    in transdermal patch, 22
nitrous oxide, 115–117, 115*t*, 247–248*t*, 250, 254*t*, 257–258
Nizoral, 91, 91*t*
Nolvadex, 222–223, 222*t*
nonbenzodiazepine, benzodiazepine receptor agonists, 126
nonbenzodiazepine-nonbarbiturate sedative-hypnotics, 126
nondihydropyridines, 140*b*
NONOPIOID (NONNARCOTIC) ANALGESICS
    acetaminophen, 46*b*
    acetylsalicylic acid, 45–50
    Advil, 51*t*
    Aleve, 51*t*
    allopurinol, 56
    Anaprox, 51*t*
    Ansaid, 51*t*
    aspirin, 45–46, 46*b*, 48*t*, 49*b*, 50*t*, 53*t*
    Cataflam, 51*t*
    choline salicylate, 46*b*
    colchicine, 56
    cyclooxygenase II-specific agents, 54
    diclofenac, 51*t*
    diflunisal, 46*b*, 51*t*
    Dolobid, 51*t*
    etodolac, 46*b*, 51*t*

NONOPIOID (NONNARCOTIC) ANALGESICS
(Continued)
fenoprofen, 51t
flurbiprofen, 51t
ibuprofen, 46b, 51t
ketoprofen, 46b, 51t
ketorolac, 51t
magnesium salicylate, 46b
meclofenamate, 51t
Meclomen, 51t
mefenamic acid, 51t
meloxicam, 51t
Mobic, 51t
Motrin, 51t
nabumetone, 51t
Nalfon, 51t
Naprosyn, 51t
naproxen, 46b, 51t
naproxen sodium, 51t
nonsteroidal antiinflammatory drugs, 50–54,
    51–53t, 53b, 246, 247–248t
  cyclo-oxygenase II-specific
    agents, 54
  fenoprofen, 54
  ibuprofen, 53–54
  ketorolac, 54
  other, 54
Orudis, 51t
Ponstel, 51t
probenecid, 48t
Relafen, 51t
salicylates, 51t
salsalate, 46b
Toradol, 51t
nonsteroidal antiinflammatory drugs (NSAIDs),
    50–54. See also NONOPIOID
    (NONNARCOTIC) ANALGESICS
  adverse reactions of, 51–52
  classification of, 50, 51t
  contraindications and cautions in, 52,
    53b, 53t
  drug interactions of, 52, 52t
  mechanism of action of, 50
  oral effects, 52
  pharmacokinetics of, 50–51
  pharmacologic effects of, 51
  precautions in, 52
  in pregnancy, 246, 247–248t
  therapeutic uses of, 52–53
Nordette, 220t
norepinephrine
  as neurotransmitter, 34f
  pharmacologic effects of, 40
norethindrone, 218t, 220t
Norflex, 127, 127t
norgestimate, 220t
norgestrel, 220t
Norinyl, 220t
Normodyne, 42t, 43, 148
Norpramin, 179–180t
nortriptyline, 179–180t
Norvasc, 140b
Novocain, 100t, 105
Nucala, 194–195t, 198
Nucynta, 64t, 66
NuvaRing, 220t
nystatin, 90

O
Ocella, 220t
Octocaine, 103, 103t
ofloxacin, 83b
Ogen, 218t
Ogestrel, 220t
olanzapine, 176t, 178t
olmesartan, 140b

omeprazole, 159t
Onfi, 171
Onglyza, 211–212t
Opana, 64t
OPIOID (NARCOTIC) ANALGESICS, 58–67,
    258–259
  agonist-antagonist opioids, 65
  antagonists, 65–66
  Buprenex, 65
  butorphanol, 59t, 65
  Demerol, 60t, 63, 64t
  dextromethorphan, 60
  dezocine, 59t
  Dilaudid, 60t, 63–64, 64t
  diphenoxylate, 60
  Dolophine, 60t, 64–65
  dynorphins, 58
  Empirin, 60t, 64t
  endorphins, 58
  enkephalins, 58
  fentanyl, 59t, 62b, 65
  Fiorinal, 64t
  hydrocodone, 63, 64t
  hydromorphone, 60t, 63–64
  Lomotil, 60
  meperidine (see meperidine)
  methadone (see methadone)
  mixed opioids, 65
  morphine (see morphine)
  nalbuphine, 59t
  nalmefene, 59t
  naloxone, 59t, 65
  naltrexone, 59t, 66
  oxycodone, 60t, 63, 64t
  partial agonists, 65
  pentazocine, 59–60t
  Percocet, 64t
  Percodan, 60t, 64t
  propoxyphene, 63t
  Roxicet, 60t, 64t
  Roxiprin, 60t, 64t
  Subutex, 65
  Synalgos, 60t
  Talwin, 60t
  Tylenol, 60t, 64t
  Tylox, 60t, 64t
  Vicodin, 60t, 64t
opioids, 114, 114t, 247–248t, 249, 278b
Orabase, 276
Orabase-B, 110
Orajel, 110t
oral antidiabetic agents, 209–213, 209b, 209f,
    211–212t
oral contraceptives, 72, 76t, 220, 221t
  oral side effects, 278b
Oraqix, 109–110
orexin receptor antagonist, 127
organophosphates, 36
orphenadrine, 127, 127t, 278b
Ortho-Cept, 220t
Ortho-Cyclen, 220t
Ortho-Novum, 220t
Ortho Tri-Cyclen, 220t
Orudis, 51t
Ovcon-35, 220t
Ovcon-50, 220t
oxalates, 289
oxazepam, 120t
oxcarbazepine, 169–170t
Oxecta, 64t
Oxycocet, 64t
oxycodone, 60t, 63, 64t, 258
OxyContin, 64t, 258
oxygen, 239–241, 240t
oxyphenbutazone, 278b
Ozempic, 211–212t

P
paliperidone, 176t, 178t
Pamelor, 179–180t
PANCREATIC HORMONES, 204
Pancuronium, 43
Paraflex, 127
Parafon Forte DSC, 127t
Parathion, 36
Parnate, 179–180t
paroxetine, 179, 179–180t
partial agonists, 65
Paxil, 179, 179–180t
penbutolol, 140b
penciclovir, 92t, 94, 247–248t, 273, 273b, 273t
Penecort, 185t
penicillamine, 278b, 280b
penicillin V, 247–248t
penicillin VK, 75
penicillins, 72–75, 72f, 73t, 268t, 278b
  allergic reactions to, 70
pentaerythritol tetranitrate, 137t
pentazocine, 59–60t
pentobarbital, 124t
Pentothal, 124t
pentoxifylline, 156
perampanel (Fycompa), 169–170t
Percocet, 60t, 64t
Percodan, 60t, 64t, 258
Peridex, 276
perindopril, 140b
PerioChip, 22
perphenazine, 176t
Persantine, 155–156
Pertofrane, 179–180t
phencyclidine, 263
phenelzine, 179–180t
phenobarbital, 124t, 166t, 169–170t,
    278b
  metabolism of, 168
phenothiazines, 107t, 162, 280b
phenoxybenzamine, 42, 42t
phentolamine, 42, 42t
phenylbutazone, 278b
phenylephrine, 40t, 41
phenytoin, 126b, 135t, 170–171, 171b, 245–246t,
    278b, 280b
physostigmine, 35t, 36
pilocarpine
  acetylcholine response to, 277
  oral side effects of, 278b
  for xerostomia, 36
pindolol, 140b
pioglitazone, 211–212t, 213
piroxicam, 154t
pitavastatin, 151t
PITUITARY HORMONES, 215–217
  anterior pituitary, 215–217
  posterior pituitary, 217
Plavix, 155
Polocaine, 104
polymyxin, 85
Ponstel, 51t
Pontocaine, 100t, 105, 110t
potassium salts, 145
potassium-sparing diuretics, 145
practolol, 280b
pralidoxime, 36
pramlintide, 211–212t, 213
Prandin, 210–213, 211–212t
prasugrel, 155
Pravachol, 151t
pravastatin, 151t
prazosin, 42, 42t, 140b
Precose, 211–212t, 213
prednisolone, 188t
prednisone, 280

Prefest, 218t
pregabalin (Lyrica), 169–170t
PREGNANCY AND BREASTFEEDING
    acetaminophen, 247–248t, 249
    acyclovir, 247–248t
    alcohol, 251
    alprazolam, 247–248t
    amoxicillin, 247–248t, 249
    amphetamines, 245–246t
    ampicillin, 247–248t, 249
    androgens, 245–246t
    angiotensin-converting enzyme inhibitors,
        245–246t
    anticoagulants, 245
    antidepressants, 245–246t
    antiepileptic agents, 245
    antineoplastic agents, 245, 245–246t
    aspirin, 246, 247–248t
    augmentin, 247–248t
    azithromycin, 247–248t
    barbiturates, 245–246t
    benzodiazepines, 247–248t, 250
    bupivacaine, 247–248t
    carbamazepine, 245–246t
    cephalosporins, 247–248t, 249
    chlorpropamide, 245–246t
    clarithromycin, 247–248t
    clindamycin, 247–248t, 249
    clomipramine, 245–246t
    clotrimazole, 247–248t, 249
    cocaine, 245–246t
    diazepam, 245–248t
    diethylstilbestrol, 245–246t
    doxycycline, 247–248t
    epinephrine, 246, 247–248t
    erythromycin, 247–248t, 249
    estazolam, 247–248t
    ethanol, 245–246t
    etretinate, 245–246t
    halazepam, 247–248t
    heroin, 245–246t
    ibuprofen, 246
    iodide, 245–246t
    isotretinoin, 245–246t
    ketoconazole, 247–248t, 249–250
    lidocaine, 247–248t
    lithium, 245–246t
    lorazepam, 247–248t
    mepivacaine, 247–248t
    methadone, 245–246t
    methylthiouracil, 245–246t
    metronidazole, 247–248t
    miconazole, 247–248t
    midazolam, 247–248t
    minocycline, 247–248t
    nitrous oxide, 247–248t, 250
    nonsteroidal antiinflammatory drugs
        (NSAIDs), 246, 247–248t
    nystatin, 247–248t, 249
    opioids, 247–248t, 249
    penciclovir, 247–248t
    penicillamine, 245–246t
    penicillin V, 247–248t
    phencyclidine, 245–246t
    phenytoin, 245–246t
    propylthiouracil, 245–246t
    quazepam, 247–248t
    streptomycin, 245–246t
    tamoxifen, 245–246t
    temazepam, 247–248t
    tetracycline, 245–246t
    thalidomide, 245–246t
    triazolam, 247–248t
    valproic acid, 245–246t
    vitamin A analogs, 245
    warfarin, 245–246t

Premphase, 218t
Prempro, 218t
Prevalite, 151t
prilocaine, 100t, 102–103t, 108b, 109–110, 109t
Primaquine, 27
Prinivil, 140b
Priscoline, 42
Pristiq, 179–180t, 180
Pro-Banthine, 37, 38t
ProAir HFA, 194–195t
probenecid, 48t, 49
procainamide, 135t, 240t, 242, 278b, 280b
procaine, 100t, 105
procaine penicillin G, 105
Procardia, 137t
prochlorperazine, 161t, 178, 239
progestins, 218t, 220, 220t
Prolixin, 176t
propafenone, 135t
propantheline, 37, 38t
Propine, 42
propofol, 114, 114t
propoxycaine, 100t
propoxyphene, 63t, 126b
propranolol, 135t, 137t, 140b, 280b
propylthiouracil, 217b, 278b
ProSom, 120t
Prostaglandins, 47
Protopam, 36
Provera, 218t
Prozac, 179, 179–180t
Pseudoephedrine, 40t, 41–42, 198–199
PSYCHEDELICS (HALLUCINOGENS),
    262–263
    angel dust, 263
    2,5-dimethoxy-4-methylamphetamine, 262
    dimethyltryptamine, 262
    lysergic acid diethylamide, 263
    marijuana, 263
    mescaline, 262
    peyote, 262
    phencyclidine, 263
    psilocybin, 262
PSYCHOTHERAPEUTIC AGENTS
    Abilify, 176t
    amitriptyline, 179–180t
    antipsychotic agents, 175–179
    Aplenzin, 179–180t
    aripiprazole, 176t, 178t
    asenapine, 176t
    Aventyl, 179–180t
    brexpiprazole, 176t
    bupropion, 179–180t, 181–182
    cariprazine, 176t
    Celexa, 179, 179–180t
    chlorpromazine, 176t
    citalopram, 179, 179–180t
    clozapine, 176t, 178t
    Clozaril, 176t
    Cymbalta, 179–180t, 180
    desipramine, 179–180t
    desvenlafaxine, 179–180t
    Desyrel, 179–180t
    duloxetine, 179–180t, 180
    Effexor, 179–180t, 180
    Effexor XR, 179–180t
    Elavil, 179–180t
    epinephrine, 178–179, 179b
    escitalopram, 179, 179–180t
    Eskalith, 182
    Fanapt, 176t
    Fetzima, 179–180t
    fluoxetine, 179, 179–180t
    fluphenazine, 176t
    Geodon, 176t
    Haldol, 176t

PSYCHOTHERAPEUTIC AGENTS (Continued)
    haloperidol, 176t
    iloperidone, 176t
    imipramine, 179–180t
    Invega, 176t
    isocarboxazid, 179–180t
    Latuda, 176t
    levomilnacipran, 179–180t
    Lexapro, 179, 179–180t
    lithium, 182, 182b
    Lithobid, 182
    loxapine, 176t
    Loxitane, 176t
    lurasidone, 176t
    Marplan, 179–180t
    Mellaril, 176t
    mirtazapine, 179–180t, 182
    monoamine oxidase inhibitors, 179–180t, 181
    Nardil, 179–180t
    Navane, 176t
    nefazodone, 179–180t, 182
    Norpramin, 179–180t
    nortriptyline, 179–180t
    olanzapine, 176t, 178t
    paliperidone, 176t
    Pamelor, 179–180t
    Parnate, 179–180t
    paroxetine, 179, 179–180t
    Paxil, 179, 179–180t
    perphenazine, 176t
    Pertofrane, 179–180t
    phenelzine, 179–180t
    Pristiq, 179–180t, 180
    prochlorperazine, 178
    Prolixin, 176t
    Prozac, 179, 179–180t
    quetiapine, 176t, 178t
    Remeron, 179–180t
    Rexulti, 176t
    Risperdal, 176t
    Risperdal M-TAB, 176t
    risperidone, 176t, 178t
    Saphris, 176t
    selective serotonin reuptake inhibitors, 179–180
    Seroquel, 176t
    Seroquel XR, 176t
    sertraline, 179, 179–180t
    Serzone, 179–180t, 182
    thioridazine, 176t
    thiothixene, 176t
    Thorazine, 176t
    Tofranil, 179–180t
    tranylcypromine, 179–180t
    trazodone, 179–180t, 182
    tricyclic antidepressants, 179–180t, 180–181
    Trilafon, 176t
    Trintellix, 179–180t
    venlafaxine, 179–180t, 180
    Viibryd, 179–180t
    vilazodone, 179–180t
    vortioxetine, 179–180t
    Vraylar, 176t
    Wellbutrin, 179–180t, 181–182
    ziprasidone, 176t, 178t
    Zoloft, 179–180t
    Zyprexa, 176t
    Zyprexa Zydis, 176t
Psychotropics, 280b
Pulmicort Flexhaler, 194–195t
pyrazinamide, 84t, 85
pyridoxine (vitamin B$_6$), 84t, 85
pyrimethamine, 280b

Q
quazepam, 120t, 247–248t
Questran, 151t, 152

quetiapine, 176t, 178t
quinapril, 140b
quinidine, 126b, 135t, 278b, 280b
quinolones, 83–84

R
ramelteon, 120t, 126
ramipril, 140b
ranolazine, 138
Ravocaine, 100t
Rebetol, 96t
Regitine, 42, 42t
Reglan, 163
Relafen, 51t
Remeron, 179–180t
renin inhibitor, direct, 140b, 146–147
repaglinide, 210–213, 211–212t
reserpine, 140b, 149
reslizumab, 194–195t, 198
RESPIRATORY DRUGS
    Accolate, 194–195t, 197
    acetylcysteine, 199
    aclidinium, 197t
    β2-adrenergic agonist
        long acting, 194–195t
        short acting, 194–195t
    Advair Diskus, 194–195t, 197t
    Advair HFA, 194–195t, 197t
    Aerospan HFA, 194–195t
    AirDuo RespiClick, 194–195t, 197t
    albuterol, 194–195t, 196, 197t
    Allerest, 198–199
    Alupent, 194–195t
    Alvesco, 194–195t
    aminophylline, 198
    antitussives, 199
    Arcapta Neohaler, 197t
    arformoterol, 197t
    Arnuity Ellipta, 194–195t
    Asmanex HFA, 194–195t
    Asmanex Twisthaler, 194–195t
    Atrovent, 197t, 198
    β2-adrenergic agonist
        long acting, 196
        short acting, 196
    beclomethasone, 194–195t, 196–197
    Breo Ellipta, 194–195t, 197t
    Brovana, 197t
    budesonide, 194–195t, 197t
    chlorofluorocarbons as, 196
    ciclesonide, 194–195t
    Cinqair, 194–195t
    Combivent, 197t, 198
    Combivent Respimat, 197t
    corticosteroids, 196–197
    cromolyn, 194–195t, 198
    Daliresp, 197t
    Deltasone, 194–195t
    dextromethorphan, 199
    Dulera, 194–195t
    DuoNeb, 197t
    expectorants, 199
    Flovent Diskus, 194–195t
    Flovent HFA, 194–195t, 196–197
    flunisolide, 194–195t
    fluticasone furoate, 194–195t, 196–197, 197t
    fluticasone propionate, 194–195t, 197t
    Foradil Aerolizer, 194–195t, 197t
    formoterol, 194–195t, 197t
    glycopyrrolate, 197t
    guaifenesin, 199
    hydrofluoroalkane, 196
    indacaterol, 197t
    Intal, 194–195t, 198
    ipratropium, 197t, 198
    leukotriene modifiers, 197–198

RESPIRATORY DRUGS (Continued)
    levalbuterol, 194–195t
    mepolizumab, 194–195t
    metaproterenol, 194–195t
    methylxanthines, 194–195t
    Meticorten, 194–195t
    mometasone furoate, 194–195t
    montelukast, 194–195t, 197
    mucolytics, 199
    Mucomyst, 199
    nasal decongestants, 198–199
    NasalCrom, 194–195t, 198
    nedocromil, 194–195t, 198
    Neo-Synephrine, 198–199
    olodaterol, 197t
    omalizumab, 194–195t, 198
    Perforomist, 197t
    phenylephrine, 198–199
    prednisone, 194–195t
    ProAir HFA, 194–195t
    ProAir RespiClick, 194–195t
    Proventil HFA, 194–195t
    pseudoephedrine, 198–199
    Pulmicort Flexhaler, 194–195t
    reslizumab, 194–195t
    Robitussin, 199
    roflumilast, 197t
    salmeterol, 194–195t, 197t
    Seebri Neohaler, 197t
    Serevent Diskus, 194–195t, 197t
    Sinex, 198–199
    Singulair, 194–195t, 197
    Slo-Bid, 194–195t, 198
    Spiriva, 197t
    Spiriva HandiHaler, 197t
    Striverdi Respimat, 197t
    Sucrets, 198–199
    Sudafed, 198–199
    Symbicort, 194–195t, 197t
    sympathomimetic agents, 196
    Theo-Dur, 194–195t, 198
    theophylline, 194–195t, 198
    Tilade, 194–195t, 198
    tiotropium, 197t
    tiotropium bromide, 197t, 198
    Tudorza, 197t
    Ventolin HFA, 194–195t
    vilanterol, 197t
    Xolair, 194–195t, 198
    Xopenex HFA, 194–195t
    zafirlukast, 194–195t, 197
    zileuton, 194–195t, 197
    Zyflo, 194–195t, 197
    Zyflo CR, 194–195t
Restoril, 120t
Retrovir, 93t
Revex, 66
ReVia, 66, 255
Rexulti, 176t
riboflavin (vitamin B2), 275
Rifadin, 84t, 85
rifampin, 69b, 84t, 85
Rimactane, 84t, 85
Rimimcatane, 84t, 85
Rimactane, 84t, 85
Risperdal, 176t
risperidone, 176t, 178t
Ritalin, 41, 260
Robaxin, 127, 127t
Robinul, 37
Romazicon, 122
rosiglitazone, 211–212t, 213
rosuvastatin, 151t
Roxicet, 60t, 64t
Roxiprin, 60t, 64t
Rozerem, 120t, 126
rufinamide (Banzel), 169–170t
Rybix, 64t

S
Sabril, 169–170t
Salagen, 35t, 36
salicylates1, 2. See also acetylsalicylic acid
Sandimmune, 69b, 231, 276
Saphris, 176t
saquinavir, 95
sarin, 35t, 37
saxagliptin, 211–212t
Saxenda, 211–212t
scopolamine, 37
    as anticholinergic, 38t
    CNS effects, 38
    in transdermal patch, 22, 162
Seasonale, 220, 220t
secobarbital, 124t
Seconal, 124t
Sectral, 140b
SEDATIVE-HYPNOTICS, 259–260, 278b
    barbiturates, 259
    benzodiazepines, 259
    chloral hydrate, 259–260
    chlordiazepoxide, 259
    diazepam, 259
    flunitrazepam, 259–260
    meprobamate, 259
    Miltown, 259
    Rohypnol, 259–260
    Valium, 259
selective serotonin reuptake inhibitors, 179–180
semaglutide, 211–212t
Septocaine, 100t, 103t, 105
Septra, 83
Serax, 120t
Serophene, 222, 222t
Seroquel, 176t
serotonin, 126
sertraline, 179, 179–180t
Serzone, 179–180t, 182
sevoflurane, 117
Siladryl, 273
simethicone, 159t, 161
simvastatin, 151t
Sinex, 198–199
sitagliptin, 211–212t, 213
Slo-Niacin, 151t
sodium glucose transporter-2 inhibitors, 211–212t, 213
sodium valproate, 278b
Soma, 127t
Sonata, 120t, 126
sotalol, 135t
Spice, 254t
spironolactone, 140b, 145, 280b
St. John's wort, 266–267
stannous fluoride, 278b
Starlix, 210–213, 211–212t
statins, 150–151, 151t
stavudine, 93t
Steglatro, 211–212t
steroids, 126b
Streptase, 155
streptokinase, 155
streptomycin, 84t, 245–246t, 280b
succinylcholine, 43
Sucrets, 198–199
Sudafed, 40t, 41–42, 198–199
Sufenta, 114, 114t
sufentanil, 114, 114t
Sular, 140b
sulfamethoxazole-trimethoprim, 83
sulfasalazine, 161t, 280b
sulfonamides, 69b, 71t, 82–83, 278b
sulfonylureas, 209–210, 210f, 210t
    aspirin interaction and, 49
    oral effects, 78–79

sulfuric acid, 16
sulindac, 154t
Sustacal, 271
Sustagen, 271
suvorexant, 120t, 127
Symlin, 211–212t, 213
Synalar, 185t
Synalgos, 60t
Synthroid, 217b

T
Talwin, 60t
Talwin-NX, 65
tamoxifen, 222–223, 222t
Tanzeum, 211–212t
Tapazole, 217b
Tekturna, 140b
telmisartan, 140b
temazepam, 120t
Temovate, 185t
Tenex, 140b
Tenormin, 138, 140b
Tenuate, 41, 260
terazosin, 140b, 148
testosterone, 221
tetracaine, 100t, 105, 110t
tetracycline, 69b, 71t, 77–79, 77t
    for candidiasis, 78
    in gingival crevicular fluid, 18, 77
    oral side effects of, 278b
    in pregnancy, 245–248t, 249
Teveten, 140b
thalidomide, 245–246t, 276
theophylline, 198
thiazides, 142t, 280b
thiazolidinediones, 211–212t, 213, 213b
thiopental
    in blood-brain barrier, 15
    redistribution of, 16
thiopental sodium, 124t
thioridazine, 176t
thiothixene, 176t
thiouracil, 278b
THYROID HORMONES, 217–218
Thyrolar, 217b
tiagabine (Gabitril), 169–170t
ticagrelor, 155
Ticlid, 155, 278b
ticlopidine, 155, 278b
timolol, 135t, 140b
tizanidine, 128
tobramycin, 82
Tobrex, 82
Tofranil, 179–180t

tolazoline, 42
tolbutamide, 107t, 280b
Topamax, 169–170t
topiramate, 169–170t
Toradol, 51t, 54
toremifene, 222t
torsemide, 140b
Tradjenta, 211–212t
Trandate, 148
trandolapril, 140b
tranexamic acid, 156
Transderm-Nitro, 22
Transderm-Scop, 22, 38t
Tranxene, 120t
tranylcypromine, 179–180t
trazodone, 179–180t, 182
Trental, 156
Tri-Norinyl, 220t
triamcinolone acetonide, 185t, 188, 188t, 280
triamterene, 140b, 145
triazolam, 120t
triclosan, 269
tricyclic antidepressants, 126b, 179–180t, 180–181
trihexyphenidyl, 38
Trilafon, 176t
Trileptal, 169–170t
Trilipix, 151t
trimethoprim, 69b, 83
Trintellix, 179–180t
Triphasil, 220t
triprolidine, 280b
Trulicity, 211–212t
Tylenol, 25, 54, 60t, 64t
Tylox, 60t, 64t

U
Ultram, 64t
Univasc, 140b

V
valacyclovir, 273
Valisone, 185t
Valium, 114, 114t, 120t, 171, 241
    metabolism of, 16
    as muscle relaxant, 127, 127t
valproate, 167
valproic acid, 168b, 278b
valsartan, 140b
Vancocin, 81
varenicline, 262
vasoconstrictors, 105–107
vasodilators, 133, 149
Vasotec, 140b
vecuronium, 43

venlafaxine, 180
verapamil, 135t, 138t, 140b, 142t, 278b
Versed, 114–115, 114t, 120t, 171, 241
Vicodin, 60t, 64t
Vicoprofen, 64t
Victoza, 211–212t
vigabatrin, 169–170t
Viibryd, 179–180t
vilazodone, 179–180t, 182
Vimpat, 169–170t
Viramune, 94
vitamin A, 245
vitamin D, 170
vitamin E, 267t
vitamin K, 72
Vivitrol, 66
vortioxetine, 179–180t, 182
Vraylar, 176t
Vytorin, 151t

W
warfarin, 48t, 49, 53t, 76t, 126b, 153–154, 154b,
    154t, 245–246t, 278b
Welchol, 151t, 211–212t, 213
Wellbutrin, 179–180t, 181–182, 262

X
xylitol, 269, 287–288, 288b
Xylocaine, 98, 100t, 103t, 109, 110t

Z
zafirlukast (Accolate), 197
zaleplon, 120t, 126
Zanaflex, 128
Zarontin, 171
Zaroxolyn, 140b
Zebeta, 140b
Zestril, 140b
Zetia, 151–152, 151t
zidovudine, 93t, 94
zileuton (Zyflo), 197
zinc, 78
ziprasidone, 176t, 178t
Zocor, 151t
Zohydro, 64t
Zoloft, 179, 179–180t
zolpidem, 120t, 126
Zonegran, 169–170t
zonisamide, 169–170t
Zovia, 220t
Zovirax, 92, 92t, 273
Zyban, 262
Zyloprim, 56
Zyprexa, 176t

Note: Page numbers followed by *f* indicate figures, *t* indicate tables and *b* indicate boxes.

A

Abbreviations, in prescription writing, 8*t*, 9
Absorption, of drug, 14–15
Abstinence syndrome, 252
Abuse, of nitrous oxide, 116–117
Acetaminophen, 54–55
  adverse reactions of, 54–55
    hepatic effects, 54–55, 55*t*
    nephrotoxicity, 55
    skin reactions, 55
  doses and preparations of, 55, 56*t*
  drug interactions of, 55
  pharmacokinetics of, 54
  pharmacologic effects of, 54, 54*b*
  in pregnancy, 249, 249*b*
  toxicity of, 55
  uses of, 55, 55*b*
Acetylcholine
  formula for, 35*f*
  as neurotransmitter, 33
  receptor sites, 35*b*
Acetylcholinesterase, 35
Acetylsalicylic acid, 45–50
  adverse reactions of, 47–49, 48*t*
    bleeding, 48
    gastrointestinal, 47–48, 47*b*
    hepatic and renal, 48
    hypersensitivity (allergy), 48–49, 48*b*
    pregnancy and nursing considerations, 48
    Reye syndrome, 48
  chemistry of, 45–46, 46*f*
  common agents, 50
  diflunisal, 50
  doses and preparations of, 49–50, 50*t*
  drug interactions of, 49
  mechanism of action of, 46, 47*f*
  pharmacokinetics of, 47
  pharmacologic effects of, 47
    analgesic effects, 47, 47*f*
    antiinflammatory effect, 47
    antiplatelet effect, 47, 48*f*
    antipyretic effect, 47
    uricosuric effect, 47
  toxicity of, 49, 49*b*
  uses of, 49
Acid urine, 17
Acids, weak, ionization and, 15
Acquired immunodeficiency syndrome, 94–96
Actinic lip changes, 277
Active transport, 14
Acute adrenocortical insufficiency, 239
Acute myocardial infarction, 237
Acute necrotizing ulcerative gingivitis (ANUG), 271, 271*b*, 272*f*
Acute poisoning, in barbiturates, 125
Acyclovir, 92–94, 92*b*
Addiction
  to drugs, 252
  to opioid analgesics, 61–62, 62*b*
Addison disease, 184
Adhesives, for tooth hypersensitivity, 289
Adrenal cortex, 184
Adrenal crisis, corticosteroid effects on, 187, 189, 189*b*
Adrenal medulla, 32
Adrenergic (sympathomimetic) agents, 40–42, 40*t*
α-Adrenergic blocking agents, 42

α₁-Adrenergic blocking agents, 148, 148*b*
β-Adrenergic blocking agents, 42, 147–148, 148*b*
  dental drug interactions of, 148
  for heart failure, 133, 138
  oral, 43
Adrenocortical insufficiency, acute, 239
Adrenocorticosteroids, 184–191
  academic skills assessment for, 191
  adverse reactions of, 185–187, 189
  classification of, 184, 184*b*
  clinical case study for, 191
  corticosteroid products and, 188, 188*t*
  definitions of, 184–185
  dental hygiene considerations for, 191
  dental implications of, 189–190, 189*b*
  mechanism of action of, 185, 185*b*
  mechanism of release of, 184, 184*b*, 185*f*
  metabolic changes of, 186, 187*f*
  pharmacologic effects of, 185, 186*f*
  routes of administration of, 185, 185*t*
  steroid supplementation of, 190, 190*b*, 190*f*
  topical use of, 190
  uses of, 187–188, 187*b*
    dental, 188
    medical, 187–188
Adrenocorticotropic hormone (ACTH), 184
Adverse reactions, 24–29
  of acetaminophen, 54–55
  of acetylsalicylic acid, 47–49, 48*t*
  of acyclovir, 93
  of α₁-adrenergic blocking agents, 148
  of aminoglycosides, 82
  of angiotensin-converting enzyme inhibitors, 145, 146*b*
  of angiotensin receptor blockers, 146
  of antidepressant agents, 181*f*
  of antiepileptic agents, 167
  of antihistamine, 201
  of antihypertensive agents, 149
  of antiinfective agents
    allergic reactions as, 70
    cost, 72, 72*f*
    dose forms in, 72
    drug reactions as, 70–72
    gastrointestinal complaints, 72
    pregnancy considerations in, 72
    superinfection (suprainfection), 70
  of antipsychotic agents, 176–177, 177*f*
    anticholinergic, 177–178, 177*b*
    antiemetic, 176
    antipsychotic, 175–176
    cardiovascular, 177
    extrapyramidal, 176–177
    metabolic, 177
    orthostatic hypotension as, 177–178
    sedation as, 176, 178
    seizures as, 177
    tachycardia as, 177
  of barbiturates, 125
  of benzodiazepines, 121–122
  of calcium channel blocking agents, 147
  of carbamazepine, 168–170
  of cephalosporins, 75–76
  from cholinergic agents, 35–36, 35*b*
  of cimetidine, 159–160
  of clindamycin, 79
  clinical manifestations of, 25–27
    drug interactions and, 25–26, 26*t*
    on fetal development, 25
    hypersensitivity as, 26–27, 27*t*

Adverse reactions (*Continued*)
  idiosyncrasy in, 27
  interference with natural defense mechanism, 27
  local effect, 25
  on nontarget tissues, 25
  on target tissues, 25
  of clonidine, 149
  of corticosteroids, 185–187, 189
  definitions and classifications of, 24–25, 25*f*
  dental hygiene considerations and, 28
  of erythromycin, 76
  of 3-hydroxy-3-methylglutaryl coenzyme A reductase inhibitors, 151
  of intranasal antihistamine, 201–202
  of isoniazid, 85
  of lamotrigine, 168
  of leukotriene modifiers, 197–198
  of levetiracetam, 168
  of local anesthetics, 101–103, 104*f*
  of metronidazole, 80
  of nitrous oxide, 116, 116*b*, 257–258
  of NSAIDs, 51–52
  of opioid analgesics, 60–63, 60*t*
  of oxcarbazepine, 168
  of penicillin, 73–74
  of phenytoin, 170–171
  of quinolones, 83–84
  recognizing, 28
  of rifampin, 85
  of second-generation antipsychotics, 178*t*
  of selective serotonin reuptake inhibitors, 179–180
  of sulfonamides, 82–83, 82*b*
  of tetracyclines, 77–78
  of thiazide diuretics, 143–144, 143*b*, 144*t*
  toxicologic evaluation of drugs for, 27–28, 27–28*b*, 27*f*
  of tricyclic antidepressants, 181
  of valproate, 167
  of vancomycin, 82
Age and weight, and drug effects, 19
Agonists, in drug action, 13, 14*f*
Agonist-antagonist opioids, 65
β₂-Agonists
  long-acting, 194–195*t*, 196
  short-acting, 194–195*t*, 196, 196*b*
Agranulocytosis, 231
  with antipsychotic agents, 177
Airplane glue, 253
Airway obstruction, acute, 236
Akathisia, 176*b*, 177
Akinesia, 176*b*, 177
Albuterol
  in emergency kit, 241
  for respiratory treatment, 196, 196*b*
Alcohol, 252*b*, 255*f*
  acetaminophen toxicity and, 55, 55*t*
  alcohol use disorder, 254–255, 255*b*
  cimetidine interaction with, 160
  dental management of alcoholic patient, 257*t*
  dental treatment and, 256–257
  ethyl, 254–257, 254*b*
  intoxication, acute, 254
  long-term effects of, 254
  pharmacokinetics, 254
  in pregnancy, 251, 251*b*
  treatment, 255–256, 255*b*
  withdrawal, 254, 254*b*, 255*f*
Alcoholic liver disease, signs of advanced, 257*b*
Alcoholics Anonymous, 255

Alcoholism, benzodiazepines in, 124
Aldosterone antagonists, for heart failure, 133
Alkaline urine, 17
Allergic reactions
  as adverse reaction, 24
  of antiinfective agents, 70
  to opioid analgesics, 62, 62b, 62f
  of sulfonamides, 83
Allergic rhinitis, 199–202, 199f
  drugs for treatment of, 192–203, 200t
    academic skills assessment in, 202
    clinical case study for, 203
    dental hygiene considerations for, 202
  selected nasal sprays for, 201t
Allergy
  from cephalosporins, 75–76
  from clindamycin, 79
  corticosteroids for, 188
  from tetracyclines, 78
Allopurinol, for gout, 56
Alopecia, from carbamazepine, 170, 170b
Aluminum salts, in antacids, 161
Alveolar osteitis, 275, 275b
Amblyopia, phenytoin and, 170, 170b
American Academy of Pediatric Dentistry, 284
American Academy of Pediatrics, 284
American College of Cardiology (ACC), 132
American Dental Association (ADA)
  cartridge color codes, for local anesthetics, 103b
  on fluoride products, 284
  prophylactic antibiotics, 70
American Heart Association (AHA), prophylactic antibiotics, 70, 86
Amides, 103–105
γ-Aminobutyric acid (GABA), benzodiazepines and, 121, 121f
Aminoglycosides, 82
  adverse reactions of, 82
  pharmacokinetics of, 82
  spectrum of, 82
  uses of, 82
Amoxicillin, in pregnancy, 249
Amphetamines, 260–261
  management of acute overdose and withdrawal, 261
  pattern of abuse, 260–261, 260f
Anabolic agents, 221, 221–222t
Analgesia, 59, 59b, 60f
  barbiturates and, 125
Analgesic-sedative combinations, 128, 128b
Analgesics
  nonopioid (nonnarcotic) (see Nonopioid (nonnarcotic) analgesics)
  opioid (nonnarcotic) (see Opioid analgesics)
  in pregnancy, 246–249
Anaphylactic shock, 26, 236, 236b
Anaphylaxis, 26
Androgenic anabolic steroids, 222b
Androgens, 221–222, 221–222t
Anencephaly, 250f
Anesthesia
  general (see General anesthetics)
  local (see Local anesthetics)
  topical, 23
Angel dust, 263
Angina pectoris, 136, 136b, 137f, 137t, 237
  prevention of, 139
  treatment of acute attack, 139
Angiotensin-converting enzyme inhibitors, 133, 139, 145–146, 145–146b
Angiotensin receptor blockers, 133, 139, 146
Angular cheilitis/cheilosis, 274–275, 274b, 274f
Antacids, 161

Antagonists, in drug action, 13, 14f
Anterograde amnesia, from benzodiazepines, 121–122
Anti-immunoglobulin E antibodies, in respiratory diseases, 198
Antiandrogens, 221–222t
Antianginal drugs, 136–139
  β-adrenergic blocking agents, 138
  for angina pectoris, 136, 136b, 137f, 137t
  angiotensin-converting enzyme inhibitors, 139
  angiotensin receptor blockers, 139
  calcium channel blocking agents, 138, 138b, 138t
  dental implications of, 139
    myocardial infarction, 139
    prevention of anginal attack, 139
    treatment of acute anginal attack, 139
  nitroglycerin-like compounds, 136–138, 138b
    adverse reactions of, 136
    drug interactions and contraindications to, 136–138
    mechanism of, 136, 136b
    storage of, 138
  ranolazine, 138
Antianxiety agents, 119b, 120f
  academic skills assessment, 129
  baclofen in, 127–128
  barbiturates in, 124–125, 124t
    adverse reactions of, 125
    chemistry of, 125
    contraindications for, 125
    drug interactions with, 125, 126b
    long-term use of, 125
    mechanism of action of, 125
    pharmacokinetics of, 125
    pharmacologic effects of, 125
    uses of, 125
  benzodiazepines in, 120–121, 120t
    abuse and tolerance of, 122, 122b
    adverse reactions of, 121–122
    chemistry of, 120
    dental patient taking, management of, 124, 124b
    drug interactions with, 123
    mechanism of action of, 121–124, 121f
    medical uses of, 123–124
    pharmacokinetics of, 120–121
    pharmacologic effects of, 121
  centrally acting muscle relaxants in, 127, 127t
  clinical case study on, 129
  dantrolene in, 128
  definitions of, 119–120
  dental hygiene considerations for, 129
  general comments about, 128
    analgesic-sedative combinations, 128, 128b
    precautions, 128
    special considerations, 128, 128b
  increased anxiety levels and, 119, 120f
  melatonin in, 127
  melatonin receptor agonist in, 126–127
  nonbenzodiazepine, benzodiazepine receptor agonists in, 126
  nonbenzodiazepine-nonbarbiturate sedative-hypnotics in, 126
  orexin receptor antagonist in, 127
  tizanidine in, 128
Antiarrhythmic agents, 135–136, 135b
  for arrhythmias, 135
  automaticity of, 135, 135b
  classification of, 135t
  digoxin, 136
  in emergency kit, 242
  management of dental patients taking, 136t
  mechanism of action of, 135t

Antibiotic interactions, tetracyclines and, 79
Anticholinergic effects
  of antipsychotic agents, 177–178, 177b
  of respiratory drugs, 201–202, 201b
  of tricyclic antidepressants, 181
Anticholinergics, 37–38, 37f
  adverse reactions of, 37
  contraindications to, 38
  dental hygiene considerations for, 43
  drug interactions with, 38
  intranasal, 202
  pharmacologic effects of, 37
  uses of, 38, 38t
  for vomiting, 162
Anticoagulants, 152–153
  alteplase, 155
  antibiotics and, 72
  clopidogrel, 155, 155b
  dipyridamole, 155–156
  direct thrombin inhibitor in, 155
  factor Xa inhibitors, 154–155
  for hemostasis, 153
  heparin, 153
  pentoxifylline, 156
  prasugrel, 155
  streptokinase, 155
  ticagrelor, 155
  ticlopidine, 155
  warfarin, 153–154, 153f, 154b, 154t
Anticonvulsant effect, of barbiturates, 125
Antidepressant agents, 179–182, 179–180t, 180–181f
  adverse reactions of, 181f
  bupropion, 181–182
  dental implications of, 182, 182b
  monoamine oxidase inhibitors, 181, 181b
  nefazodone, mirtazapine, vilazodone, and vortioxetine, 182
  selective serotonin reuptake inhibitor, 179–180, 180f
  serotonin-norepinephrine reuptake inhibitors, 180
  suicide and, 182
  trazodone, 182
  tricyclic antidepressants, 180–181
Antidiabetic agents, oral, 209–213, 209b, 209f, 211–212t
Antidiarrheals, 162
Antidiuretic hormone (ADH), opioid effects, 61
Antiemetic effects, antipsychotic agents and, 176
Antiemetics
  anticholinergics, 162
  antihistamines, 162
  cannabinoids, 163
  chemoreceptor trigger zone, 162f
  metoclopramide, 163
  trimethobenzamide, 162–163
Antiepileptics, 169t. See also Epilepsy
  adverse reactions of, 167
    central nervous system depression, 167
    for epilepsy, dental management of, 166, 166b, 166t
    gastrointestinal distress, 167
  for bipolar disorder, 182–183
  carbamazepine, 168–170, 168b
  drug interactions of, 167, 167b
  ethosuximide, 171
  lamotrigine, 168
  levetiracetam, 168
  nonseizure uses of, 172
    for neurologic pain, 172
    psychiatric use, 172, 172b
  oxcarbazepine, 168
  phenytoin, 170–171
  valproate, 167, 167b

Antiestrogens, 221–222t
Antifungal agents, 90–92, 90b
  cimetidine interaction with, 160
  imidazoles, 90–92
    clotrimazole, 91, 91b
    ketoconazole, 91–92, 92b
  mechanism of action of, 91f
  nystatin, 90
  for oral candidiasis, 91t
Antihistamines, 199
  academic skills assessment of, 202
  adverse reactions to, 201
  anticholinergic effects of, 201
  clinical case study on, 203
  dental hygiene considerations for, 202
  pharmacologic effects of, 200, 200f
  toxicity of, 201
  for vomiting, 162
Antihyperlipidemic agents, 149–152, 149b, 150f, 151t
  cholesterol absorption inhibitors, 151–152
  cholestyramine, 152
  fibric acid derivatives, 152
  fish oils, 152
  3-hydroxy-3-methylglutaryl coenzyme A reductase inhibitors, 150–151, 150b
  niacin, 152
Antihypertensive agents, 139–149, 139–140b, 141–142t, 143b, 143f, 144t
  management of dental patient taking, 149, 149b
Antiinfective agents, 68–89
  academic skills assessment, 88
  adverse reactions with, 70–72
  ampicillins, 74–75
  antibiotic prophylaxis, 86–88, 87t
  antituberculosis agents, 84–85, 84t
  cephalosporins, 75–76, 75b
  clindamycin, 79–80
  clinical case study, 88
  definitions, 69, 69b
  dental hygiene considerations for, 88
  dental infection, 68, 69b
    "evolution," 68–69
    stages of, 81
  failure of, 81
  indications for, 70, 71t
  for infection, 69
  macrolides, 76–77
    azithromycin, 77
    clarithromycin, 77
    erythromycin, 76
  metronidazole, 80–81
  in pregnancy, 249–250
  resistance to, 69–70
  tetracyclines, 77–79
  topical antibiotics, 85–86
Antimicrobial agents, for nondental use, 81–84
  aminoglycosides, 82
  nitrofurantoin, 83
  penicillins (see Penicillins)
  quinolones (fluoroquinolones), 83–84, 83b
  sulfamethoxazole-trimethoprim, 83
  sulfonamides, 82–83
  vancomycin, 81–82, 81b
Antimuscarinic drugs, 37, 198, 198b
Antineoplastic drugs, 225–232
  academic skills assessment, 232
  adverse drug effects, 227–231, 229t
    bone marrow suppression, 227
    dermatologic effects, 230
    gastrointestinal effects, 230
    germ cells, 230
    hepatotoxicity, 230
    immunosuppression, 230
    nephrotoxicity, 230, 230b

Antineoplastic drugs (Continued)
    neurologic effects, 230
    oral effects, 230–231, 230–231b, 230t, 231f
    osteonecrosis, 227–230
  classification of, 226t, 227, 227f, 228b
  clinical case study, 232
  combinations of, 231
  dental hygiene considerations for, 232
  dental implications of, 231, 231b
  mechanism of action of, 225–226, 226b, 226f
  use of, 225, 225b
Antioxidant, in local anesthetics, 103
Antipsychotic agents
  dental implications of, 178–179, 178b
  drug interactions of, 177–178
  effects of, 175–176, 178
  first-generation, 175–177
  mechanism of action of, 175, 177f
  pharmacologic effects of, 175–177
  for psychiatric disorders, 175–179, 176t
  second-generation, 177, 182
    for bipolar disorder, 183
  uses of, 178
Antisialagogue action, 162
Antithyroglobulin antibody, 217
Antithyroid agents, 217b, 218
Antituberculosis agents, 84–85, 84t
  ethambutol, 85
  isoniazid, 84–85
  pyrazinamide, 85
  rifampin, 85
Antitussives, 199
Antiviral agents, 92–97, 93f
  academic skills assessment and, 97
  for acquired immunodeficiency syndrome, 94–96
    fusion/entry inhibitors, 95
    highly active antiretroviral therapy, 95–96, 96b
    integrase inhibitors, 95
    nonnucleoside reverse transcriptase inhibitors, 94
    nucleoside/nucleotide reverse transcriptase inhibitors, 94, 94t, 95f
    pharmacokinetic enhancers, 95
    postexposure prophylaxis, 96
    protease inhibitors, 95
  for chronic hepatitis, 96–97, 96t
    interferons, 97
    nucleoside/nucleotide analogs, 96–97
    protease inhibitors, 97
  clinical case study and, 97
  dental hygiene considerations and, 97
  for herpes simplex, 92–94, 92t
    acyclovir, 92–94, 92b
    docosanol 10 %, 94
    famciclovir, 94
    penciclovir, 94
Anxiety control, benzodiazepines for, 123
Anxiety disorders, 174–175
APF 1.23%, 286
Aphthous stomatitis, corticosteroids for, 188
Appointment scheduling, 3
Aromatase inhibitors, 221–222t, 223
Aromatic ammonia spirits, in emergency kit, 241, 242f
Arrhythmias, 238–239
Arthritis, drugs for, 56–57
Articaine, 105
Aspirin
  adverse effects of, 24–25
  in pregnancy, 246, 246b
  regular, 50
Asthma, 192, 192b, 193f, 236
  aspirin effects, 48–49
  dental patient with, management of, 199b

Asthma (Continued)
  treatment of, 193t
  US Food and Drug Administration-approved, 194–195t
Atherosclerosis, 149–150
Atropine, in emergency kit, 242
Attitude of patient, and drug effects, 19
Aura, 165
Autonomic drugs, 30–44, 31b
Autonomic nervous system, 31–33
  adrenergic blocking agents, 42–43, 42t
  anatomy of, 31, 32f
  dental hygiene considerations for, 43
  effects on effector organs, 33t
  functional organization of, 32, 32b, 32f
  neurotransmitters in, 32–33, 32b, 33t
  parasympathetic (see Parasympathetic autonomic nervous system)
  sympathetic (see Sympathetic autonomic nervous system)

B
Bacitracin, 85
Baclofen, 127–128
Bactericidal, definitions of, 69
Bacteriostatic, definition of, 69
Balanced anesthesia, 112
Barbiturates, 124–125, 124t
  adverse reactions of, 125
  anesthetic doses of, 125
  chemistry of, 125
  contraindications for, 125
  drug interactions with, 125, 126b
  long-term use of, 125
  mechanism of action of, 125
  pharmacokinetics of, 125
  pharmacologic effects of, 125
  uses of, 125
Barrett esophagus, 158
Bases, weak, ionization and, 15
Bath salts, 261
Behavior
  adrenocorticosteroid effects on, 189
  benzodiazepine effects on, 121
Benadryl, in emergency kit, 241
Benzocaine, as topical anesthetic, 110
Benzodiazepine receptor agonists, 126
Benzodiazepines, 114–115, 120–121, 120t, 171–172
  abuse and tolerance of, 122, 122b
    overdose, treatment of, 122, 122b
  adverse reactions of, 121–122
  antiseizure effects of, 121
  chemistry of, 120
  cimetidine interaction with, 160
  dental patient taking, management of, 124, 124b
  drug interactions with, 123
  in emergency kit, 241–242
  mechanism of action of, 121–124, 121b, 121f
  medical uses of, 123–124, 123b
  pharmacokinetics of, 120–121
  pharmacologic effects of, 121
  in pregnancy, 250, 250f
Biguanides, 210
Bile acid sequestrants, 213
Bile salts, 161
Biliary excretion, of drugs, 18
Biliary tract constriction, opioid effects, 61
Biologic response modifiers, 57
Biologically equivalent drugs, 5
Biotransformation. See Metabolism
Bipolar disorders
  antiepileptics for, 172b
  antipsychotic agents for, 178
  drugs for treatment of, 182–183

Birth defects. *See also* Pregnancy and breastfeeding
  aspirin effects, 48
Bisphosphonate-related osteonecrosis of the jaw (BRONJ), 229, 229f
Black box warning, 6–7
Bladder, sympathomimetic agent effects on, 40
Bleeding
  aspirin effects, 48
  valproate and, 167, 167b
β-Blockers, in emergency kit, 242
Blood-brain barrier, drug distribution and, 15
Blood clotting
  drugs increasing, 156
  NSAID effects on, 51
Blood coagulation, drugs affecting, 152–155
Blood pressure
  changes in, corticosteroid effects on, 189
  classification of, 141t
  sympathomimetic effect on, 40
Bone
  fetal, tetracycline effects on, 249
  tetracycline effects on, 78
Bone marrow suppression, by antineoplastic drugs, 227
Botanical medicine, 265
Brain, cholinergic agent effects on, 35
Breastfeeding. *See* Pregnancy and breastfeeding
Brivaracetam (Briviact), 169–170t
Bromocriptine, 217
Bronchial asthma, cholinergic agents and, 36
Bronchodilation, adrenergic agents for, 41
Bulk laxatives, 161
Bupivacaine, 104–105, 104b
Buprenorphine, 65
Bupropion, 179–180t, 181–182, 262
Burkitt lymphoma, 225
Burning mouth or tongue syndrome, 276
Buspirone, 126

C
Caffeine, with aspirin, 50
Calcitonin, 217
Calcium channel blocking agents, 138, 138b, 138t, 147, 147b
  adverse reactions of, 147
  drug interactions of, 147
  mechanism of action of, 138, 147
  oral manifestations of, 147
  pharmacologic effects of, 147
Calcium salts, in antacids, 161
Cancer cell response, to chemotherapy, 226f
Candida albicans, 273–274
Candidiasis (Moniliasis), 273–274, 273b, 274f
Cannabinoids, for vomiting, 163
Carbamazepine, 168–170, 168b
  adverse reactions of, 168–170
  drug interactions of, 170, 170b
  pharmacologic effects of, 168
Carbohydrates, membrane, 14
Cardiac arrest, 237–238
  adrenergic agents for, 41
  bupivacaine and, 105
Cardiopulmonary resuscitation (CPR), 234
  building blocks of, 237f
Cardiovascular disease, drugs for, 131, 131b
Cardiovascular drugs
  academic skills assessment in, 156
  β-adrenergic blockers in, 133, 147–148, 148b
  aldosterone antagonists in, 133
  angiotensin-converting enzyme inhibitors in, 133, 139, 145–146, 145–146b, 146f
  angiotensin receptor blockers in, 133, 139, 146
  angiotensin II receptor neprilysin inhibitor in, 134

Cardiovascular drugs (*Continued*)
  antianginal drugs, 136–139
    β-adrenergic blocking agents, 138
    angina pectoris, 136, 136b, 137f, 137t
    calcium channel blocking agents, 138, 138b, 138t
    nitroglycerin-like compounds, 136–138, 136b, 137t, 138b
    ranolazine, 138
  antiarrhythmic agents in, 135–136, 135b, 136t
  anticoagulants, 152–153
    alteplase, 155
    clopidogrel, 155, 155b
    dipyridamole, 155–156
    direct thrombin inhibitor in, 155
    factor Xa inhibitors, 154–155
    for hemostasis, 153
    heparin, 153
    pentoxifylline, 156
    prasugrel, 155
    streptokinase, 155
    ticagrelor, 155
    ticlopidine, 155
    warfarin, 153–154, 153f, 154b, 154t
  antihyperlipidemic agents in, 149–152, 149b, 150f, 151f
    cholesterol absorption inhibitors, 151–152
    cholestyramine, 152
    fibric acid derivatives, 152
    fish oils, 152
    3-hydroxy-3-methylglutaryl coenzyme A reductase inhibitors, 150–151, 150b
    niacin, 152
  antihypertensive agents in, 139–149, 139–140b, 141–142t, 143b, 143f, 144t
  clinical case study in, 156–157
  dental hygiene considerations for, 156
  dental implications of, 131–132, 139
    contraindications to, 131–132, 132b
    periodontal disease, 132
    vasoconstrictor limit, 132, 132b
  diuretics in, 132, 142–146, 144f
  hemostatic agents in, 156
  I_F channel inhibitor in, 134
  vasodilators in, 133
Cardiovascular system
  anticholinergic agent effects on, 37–38
  antipsychotic agent effects on, 177
  benzodiazepine effects on, 122
  cholinergic agent effects on, 35
  complications, of diabetes mellitus, 207
  local anesthetic effects in, 102
  NSAID effects on, 51
  opioid effects on, 61
  tricyclic antidepressant effects on, 181
Caries, 68, 282–288, 282b
  prevention of, 282–288
    nonpharmacologic therapies in, 283, 283b, 283f
    pharmacologic therapies, 283–288
      chlorhexidine, 288, 288f
      fluoride, 284–287, 284–285b, 284t, 285–287f, 286–287t, 287b
      xylitol, 287–288, 288b
  risk categories for, 283b
Cataracts, corticosteroid effects on, 186
Catecholamine, 39
Cations, tetracyclines and, 78
Celiac disease, 163
Cell cycle, 225–226, 226b, 226–227f
Cell division, antineoplastic drugs and, 226
Central α-adrenergic agonists, 149
Central nervous system
  adrenergic agents for, 41
  anticholinergic agent effects on, 37, 37f

Central nervous system (*Continued*)
  antihypertensive agents in, 149
  benzodiazepines in, 121
  calcium channel blocking agents in, 147
  carbamazepine effect on, 168
  corticosteroid effects on, 186
  depressants, 254–259
    antipsychotic agents and, 177
    ethyl alcohol, 254–257, 254b
    nitrous oxide, 257–258
    opioid analgesics, 258–259
    opioid street drug, 259
    sedative-hypnotics, 259–260
  depression
    from antiepileptic agents, 167
    antihistamine and, 201
    barbiturates in, 125
  disorders of, drugs for treatment of, 174–183
  local anesthetic effects on, 102
  metronidazole on, 80
  NSAID effects on, 51
  opioid effects on, 61
  phenytoin effects on, 170, 170b
  quinolones on, 83
  selective serotonin reuptake inhibitor effect on, 179
  stimulants, 260–262
    amphetamines, 260–261
    caffeine, 261, 261t
    cocaine, 260
    lysergic acid diethylamide, 263
    marijuana, 263
    phencyclidine, 263
    psychedelics (hallucinogens), 262–263
    tobacco, 261–262
  sympathomimetic effect on, 40
  tolerance of, 122
  tricyclic antidepressant effects on, 181
Centrally acting muscle relaxants, 127, 127t
Cephalosporins
  adverse reaction, 75–76
  local reaction from, 75
  mechanism of action of, 75
  oral, 75, 75b
  pharmacokinetics of, 75
  in pregnancy, 249
  spectrum of, 75
  uses of, 76
Cerebrovascular accident, 238–239
Chain of survival, 235f
Chemical name, of drug, 4, 4f
Chemically equivalent drugs, 5
Chemoreceptor trigger zone (CTZ), opioid effects, 61
Chemotherapy. *See also* Antineoplastic drugs
  sensitivity of neoplastic diseases to, 226b
Chewing gum, xylitol, 287–288
Chewing tobacco, 261
Children, aspirin toxicity, 49
Chlorhexidine, 288, 288b, 288f
Chloride channel activator, 162
Chlorofluorocarbons (CFCs), in metered-dose inhalers, 196
Cholesterol
  elevated, dental implications of, 152, 152b
  intestinal absorption of, inhibitors of, 151–152
Cholestyramine, 152
Cholinergic (parasympathomimetic) agents, 35–37, 35t
  adverse reactions from, 35–36, 35b
  contraindications to, 36
  dental hygiene considerations for, 43
  pharmacologic effects of, 35
  uses of, 36–37

Cholinesterase inhibitors, 37
Choriocarcinoma, antineoplastic drugs for, 225
Chronic dental pain, opioid use, 67
Chronic obstructive pulmonary disease (COPD), 192–195, 192b
  drugs for, approved by US Food and Drug Administration, 197t
  from nitrous oxide, 116
  treatment of, 195t
Cigar smoking, 261. See also Tobacco
Cimetidine, for gastrointestinal disease, 159–160
Cirrhosis, clinical manifestations of, 256f
Cleft palate and lip, 249f, 250
Clindamycin, 79–80
  adverse reactions with, 79
  pharmacokinetics of, 79
  in pregnancy, 249
  spectrum of, 79
  uses of, 80
Clomiphene, 222, 222t
Clonidine, 149
Clotrimazole, 91, 91b
  in pregnancy, 249
Coagulation factors, 256
Cocaine, in central nervous system, 260
Codeine, 63, 64t
Colchicine, for gout, 56
Coma, diabetic, 236
Communication, 175
Compazine, 176
Competitive antagonist, 13, 14f
Compliance, 175
Computer resources, of information, 4
Congenital heart disease, prophylactic antibiotics and, 70
Conscious sedation, benzodiazepines and, 123–124
Consciousness, lost or altered, 235–236
Constipation
  from antihypertensive agents, 149
  opioid effects, 61
Contraceptive drugs, 220t
Controlled Substance Act of 1970, 6
Convulsion, emergency drugs and, 239
Coronary artery disease, 149–150
Corticosteroids, 184, 196–197, 196b
  for asthma, 196–197
  candidiasis of oral cavity and, 197
  for chronic obstructive pulmonary disease, 197
  for oral conditions, 279–280
  for recurrent aphthous stomatitis, 275–276
Corticotropin-releasing hormone (CRH), 184
Cost, of antiinfective agents, 72, 72f
Cough, suppression, by opioid analgesics, 60
Cretinism, 217
Cricothyrotomy, 236
Crohn disease, 163, 163f
Cromolyn, 198, 198b
Cross-tolerance, 19
Crystal meth, 260, 260f
Cushing syndrome, 184
Cyclobenzaprine, 127
Cycloplegia
  from anticholinergic agents, 37
  from cholinergic agents, 35
Cytochrome P-450
  enzymes, cimetidine effects on, 160
  induction and inhibition of, 16–17, 17f, 17t
Cytolytic reactions, 26

D
Danazol, 222t, 223
Dantrolene, 128
Databases, about herbal supplements, 269b

Date rape, 259–260
Decongestants
  intranasal, 202
  oral, 202
Decongestion, nasal, sympathomimetic agents for, 41
Defibrillation, 237–238
Delayed hypersensitivity reactions, 27
Delirium tremens, 254, 254b
Delusions, 174
Dental floss, 283, 283b
Dental hygiene considerations
  for adrenocorticosteroids, 191
  adverse reactions and, 28
  for antianxiety agents, 129
  for anticholinergics, 43
  for anticonvulsants, 172
  for antihistamines, 202
  for antiinfective agents, 88
  for antineoplastic drugs, 232
  for cardiovascular drugs, 156
  for diabetes mellitus, 214
  for drug abuse, 264
  for emergency drugs, 243
  for endocrine disorders, 223
  for epilepsy, 172
  for gastrointestinal drugs, 164
  for general anesthetics, 117
  for local anesthetics, 111
  for natural/ herbal products and dietary supplements, 265–270
  for nonopioid (nonnarcotic) analgesics, 57
  for opioid analgesics, 67
  for oral conditions, 281
  for oral disorders, hygiene-related, 290
  for pregnancy and breastfeeding, 251
  for psychotherapeutic agents, 183
  for seizures, 172
Dental hygienist
  adverse reactions and, 28
  ANS drugs and, 31
  drug names and, 4–5
  impaired, 264
  patient adherence to medication therapy and, 9–10
  in prescription writing, 7–10
  role of, 2–3, 2b
  sources of information of, 3–4, 3–4b
Dental infections, stages of, 81
Dentifrices, 284, 286, 286f, 286t
Dentinal hyperalgesia, 288–289
Dentistry
  antibiotic prophylaxis for, 86–88
    cardiac conditions, 86, 87b
    dental procedures, 86, 86b
    for infective endocarditis, 86–87, 86b
    noncardiac medical conditions, 88
    prosthetic joint prophylaxis, 87–88
  antiinfective agents, use of, 81
  cardiovascular disease (see Cardiovascular drugs)
  corticosteroids and, 188
  metronidazole for, 81
  office emergency (see Emergency drugs)
  patient management in, peptic ulcer disease and GERD, 159, 159b
  tetracyclines for, 79
Dependence, 253
Depolarizing agents, 43
Depression, 174
  antipsychotic agents for, 178
Dermatologic effects
  of antineoplastic drugs, 230
  of carbamazepine, 170
  of phenytoin, 170

Desflurane, 117, 117b
Dextrose, in emergency kit, 242
Diabetes mellitus, 204–208, 204b, 206f
  academic skills assessment, 214
  clinical case study on, 214
  dental evaluation of, 207–208, 208t
  dental implications of, 205–207
  drugs for treatment of, 204–214
    biguanides, 210
    bile acid sequestrants, 213
    cautions and contraindications of, 207
    dipeptidyl-peptidase-4 inhibitors, 213
    glucagon-like peptide-1 receptor agonists, 213
    α-glucosidase inhibitors, 213
    insulins, 208, 208t, 209b
    meglitinides, 210–213
    oral antidiabetic agents, 209–213, 209b, 209f, 211–212t
    pramlintide, 213
    sodium glucose transporter-2 inhibitors, 213
    sulfonylureas, 209–210, 210f, 210t
    thiazolidinediones, 213, 213b
  goals of therapy for, 208
  oral complications of, 206, 207t
  periodontal disease and, 205–206
  systemic complications of, 207
  types of, 204–205, 205t
  xerostomia and, 205
Diabetic coma, 236
Diazepam, 120–121, 123
Dietary Supplement Health and Education Act, 265–266, 265b
Digitalis glycosides, 134–135, 134b
  adverse reactions in, 134
  dental drug interactions of, 134
  management of dental patient taking, 134–135, 135b
  pharmacologic effects of, 134
  uses of, 134
Dipeptidyl-peptidase-4 inhibitors, 213
Diphenhydramine (DPH)
  in emergency kit, 239–241
  for herpes infections, 272–273
  for recurrent aphthous stomatitis, 276
Direct-acting sympathomimetic agents, 35, 36f
Disease-modifying antirheumatic drugs, 56–57
Disintegration, in oral absorption of drugs, 15
Dispersion, in oral absorption of drugs, 15
Disruption, in oral absorption of drugs, 15
Dissociation of drug (pKa), local anesthetics and, 107–108
Dissolution, in oral absorption of drugs, 15
Distribution, of drugs, 15–16
Disulfiram, for alcoholism, 255
Disulfiram-like reaction, of cephalosporins, 75
Diuretic agents, 142–146, 144f
  for heart failure, 132
  loop, 144–145
  potassium salts, 145, 145b
  potassium-sparing, 145
  thiazide, 142–144
    adverse reactions of, 143–144, 143b, 144t
    mechanism of action of, 143, 144t
Docosanol 10 %, 94
Dopamine, 42, 42f
Dosage forms, 23
Dose effect curve log, 11, 12f
Dose forms, of antiinfective agents, 72
Dose-response curve, 27–28, 27f
Doses
  of acetaminophen, 55, 56t
  of acetylsalicylic acid, 49–50, 50t

Doxycycline, tetracyclines and, 79
Drug abuse
  academic skills assessment in, 264
  addiction and habituation, 253, 253b
  by category, 254t
  central nervous system depressants, 254–259
    ethyl alcohol, 254–257, 254b
    nitrous oxide, 257–258
    opioid analgesics, 258–259
    opioid street drug, 259
    sedative-hypnotics, 259–260
  central nervous system stimulants, 260–262
    amphetamines, 260–261
    caffeine, 261, 261t
    cocaine, 260
    lysergic acid diethylamide, 263
    marijuana, 263
    phencyclidine, 263
    psychedelics (hallucinogens), 262–263
    tobacco, 261–262
  clinical case study in, 264
  definition of, 252
  dental hygiene considerations in, 264
  identifying, 263–264, 263b
  impaired dental hygienist, 264
  physical dependence, 253
  psychological dependence, 253
  tolerance, 253, 253b
Drug Abuse Control Amendments of 1965, 6
Drug action
  characterization of, 11–12
    efficacy in, 11, 11b, 12f
    log dose effect curve in, 11, 12f
    potency in, 11, 11b, 12f
    therapeutic index, 12, 12b
  dosage forms and, 23
  factors altering, 18–19
  and handling, 11–23
  mechanism of, 12–13
  pharmacokinetics and, 14–18
    absorption, 14–15
    clinical, 18
    distribution, 15–16
    metabolism (biotransformation) in, 16–18, 16b, 16f
    passage across body membranes in, 14
    redistribution in, 16
  routes of administration and, 19–23, 19b, 20t
    inhalation, 22, 22b, 22f
    intradermal, 20–22, 22f
    intramuscular, 20, 22f
    intraperitoneal, 22
    intrathecal, 22
    intravenous, 20
    oral, 19–20, 19b
    rectal, 20
    subcutaneous, 20
    topical, 22–23
Drug allergy, 24
Drug Amendments of 1962, 6
Drug Enforcement Administration (DEA), 5
Drug interactions
  of acetaminophen, 55
  of acetylsalicylic acid, 49
  with adrenergic agonists, 43
  with α_1-adrenergic blocking agents, 148
  with β-adrenergic blocking agents, 148
  adverse reactions and, 25–26
  with angiotensin-converting enzyme inhibitors, 146
  with angiotensin receptor blockers, 146
  with anticholinergic agents, 38
  of antiepileptics, 167b
  of antiinfective agents, 70–72
  of antipsychotic agents, 177–178

Drug interactions (Continued)
  with barbiturates, 125, 126b
  of benzodiazepines, 123
  with calcium channel blocking agents, 147
  of carbamazepine, 170
  drug effects and, 19
  with erythromycin, 76, 76t
  of herbal products, 266–267
  of ketoconazole, 92
  of lamotrigine, 168
  of levetiracetam, 168
  of metronidazole, 80, 80b
  of nitroglycerin-like compounds, 136–138
  between nonsteroidal antiinflammatory drugs and warfarin, 154t
  of NSAIDs, 52, 52t
  of opioid analgesics, 63, 63t
  of oxcarbazepine, 168
  of tetracyclines, 78–79
  of tricyclic antidepressants, 181
  of valproate, 167
  between warfarin and antiinfectives, 154t
Drug Price Competition and Patent Term Restoration Act, 5
Drugs. *See also specific drugs in* Drug Index
  adverse reaction from (*see* Adverse reactions)
  biologically equivalent, 5
  chemically equivalent, 5
  clinical evaluation of, 5–6
  definition of, 2
  development of new, 5f
  in emergency kit for dental office, 239–242, 240f, 240t
  federal regulations and regulatory agencies for, 5
  labeled and off-label uses, 7
  legislation, 6–7
  medication administration of, 3
  names of, 4–5, 4b, 4f
  recall of, 7
  scheduled, 6, 6t
  substitution of, 5, 5b
  therapeutically equivalent, 5
  toxicologic evaluation of, 27–28, 27–28b
Duration, of drug action, 19
Durham-Humphrey Law of 1952, 6
Dyclonine, 105
Dysgeusia, from antihypertensive agents, 149
Dysmorphology, 251
Dyspnea, in heart failure, 132
Dystocia, 249–250

E
Efferent nerve, typical, 32f
Efficacy, of drug, 11, 11b, 12f
Electroconvulsive therapy, 175
Electrolyte, corticosteroid effects on, 187
Emergencies, corticosteroids for, 188
Emergency drugs, 233–243
  academic skills assessment in, 243
  categories of emergencies in, 235–239
    adrenocortical insufficiency, acute, 239
    cardiovascular system, 236–239
      acute myocardial infarction as, 237
      angina pectoris as, 237
      arrhythmias, 238–239
      cardiac arrest as, 237–238
      cerebrovascular accident, 238–239
    consciousness
      diabetic coma, 236
      hypoglycemia, 235–236
      lost or altered, 235–236
      seizures, 236, 236b
      syncope, 235, 235b
    drug-related, 239
    extrapyramidal reactions as, 239

Emergency drugs (Continued)
    hyperthermia, malignant, 239
    respiratory emergencies, 236
      acute airway obstruction, 236
      anaphylactic shock, 236, 236b
      asthma, 236
      hyperventilation, 236
    thyroid storm as, 239
  clinical case study for, 243
  dental hygiene considerations for, 243
  devices for, 242b
  emergency kit for dental office, 239–243
    drugs in, 239–242, 240f, 240t
    equipment for, 242–243
  general measures for, 234–235
    preparation for treatment, 234–235, 234b
    steps indicated in, 234, 234–235b
Emergency situations, dental hygienist in, 3
Emesis, opioid effects, 61
Emollients, 162
Emotional instability, nitrous oxide and, 116
Emphysema, adrenergic agents for, 41
Emptying time, stomach, 161
Enabling, 253
Endocarditis, infective, prophylactic antibiotics and, 70
Endocrine disorders, drugs for treatment of, 215–224
  academic skills assessment, 223
  clinical case study on, 223–224
  dental hygiene considerations, 223
Endocrine glands, 204, 215, 216f
Enflurane, 117
Enteral administration, 19
Enteric-coated aspirin, 50
Enterohepatic circulation, drug distribution and, 16
Environmental factors
  birth defects and, 244
  carcinogens, 225, 225b
  drug effects and, 19
Epilepsy, 165–166, 165b
  benzodiazepines for, 123–124
  classification of, 165
  dental treatment of patient with, 172
  drug therapy of patients with, 166–172, 166b, 166t
    adverse reactions of, 167
    carbamazepine, 168–170, 168b
    dental hygiene considerations in, 172
    drug interactions of, 167, 167b
    ethosuximide, 171
    lamotrigine, 168
    levetiracetam, 168
    oxcarbazepine, 168
    phenytoin, 170–171
    valproate, 167
  generalized seizures, 165–166
    absence, 165, 165b
    status epilepticus, 166, 166b
    tonic-clonic, 165–166, 165b
  partial (focal seizures), 166, 166t
Epinephrine
  antipsychotic agents and, 178–179, 179b
  in cardiovascular patients, 132
  drug interactions with, 107, 107t
  in emergency kit, 239–241, 241f
  local anesthetics and, 104, 106f, 107b
  as neurotransmitter, 39
  in pregnancy, 246
  toxic reactions to, 239
Epinephrine reversal, 42
Equipment, for dental emergencies, 242–243
Erectile dysfunction, 237
Erythromycin, in pregnancy, 249

Eslicarbazepine (Aptiom), 169–170t
Esters, 105
Estrogens, 219–220
Eszopiclone, 126
Ethambutol, 85
Ethosuximide, 171
Ethyl alcohol, 245. *See also* Alcohol
Etomidate, 114
Euphoria, by opioid analgesics, 59
Excretion, of drugs, 17–18
Exfoliative dermatitis, 230
Exocrine glands, anticholinergic agent effects on, 37
Exophthalmos, 218
Expectorants, for respiratory infections, 199
Extended-release hydrocodone, 63, 64t
Extrapyramidal effects, 176–177
Extrapyramidal reactions, 239
Extrarenal routes, drug excretion by, 17–18
Eye
    anticholinergic agent effects on, 37
    cholinergic agent effects on, 35
    sympathomimetic agent effects on, 40

F
Facilitated diffusion, 14
Famciclovir, 94
Febuxostat, for gout, 56
Federal Food and Drug Administration (FDA), acetaminophen and, 55
Federal Patent Law, 4
Federal Trade Commission (FTC), 5, 269
Federal Trademark Law, 4
Feedback, negative, 215
Felbamate (Felbatol), 169–170t
Fentanyl, 65
Fetal alcohol syndrome (FAS), 251, 251f
Fetal development, adverse reactions on, 25
Fetal hydantoin syndrome, 171, 171f
Fibric acid derivatives, 152
First-generation antipsychotic agents
    adverse reactions, 176–177, 177f
    antiemetic effects, 176
    antipsychotic effect of, 175–176
    extrapyramidal effects, 176–177
    orthostatic hypotension, 177
    pharmacologic effects of, 175–177
    sedation as, 176, 178
    seizures, 177
First-order kinetics, 18, 18f
First-pass effect, 16
Fish oils, 152
Floppy infant syndrome, 122
Fluconazole, 92
Fluid balance, corticosteroid effects on, 187
Flumazenil
    benzodiazepines and, 122
    in emergency kit, 242
Fluoride, 284–287
    mechanism of action of, 284
    preparations of, 284–287
        dentifrices, 286, 286f, 286–287t
        patient-applied, 286–287
        professionally applied, 284–286, 284t, 285b, 285f
        rinses, 287b, 287f, 287t
    for tooth hypersensitivity, 289
    toxicity of, 284, 284b, 284t
Follicle-stimulating hormone (FSH), 215
Food, Drug and Cosmetic Act of 1938, 6
Food and Drug Act of 1906, 6
Food and Drug Administration (FDA), 5
    opioid classification, 61
Foreign body, aspiration of, 236
Fosphenytoin (Cerebyx), 169–170t

Fungal infections. *See* Antifungal agents
Fusion/entry inhibitors, for HIV, 95

G
Gabapentin (Neurontin), 169–170t
Gallstones, opioid effects, 61
Gastroesophageal reflux disease (GERD), 158, 158b
Gastrointestinal diseases, 158–159
    anticholinergic agents for, 38
    drugs for, 158–164
Gastrointestinal distress, 167
Gastrointestinal drugs, 158–159, 159f
    academic skills assessment in, 164
    antacids, 161, 161t
    anticholinergics, 162
    antidiarrheals, 162
    antiemetics, 162
    antihistamines, 162
    cannabinoids, 163
    for chronic inflammatory bowel disease, 163, 163b
    clinical case study in, 164
    dental hygiene considerations in, 164
    dental implications of, 159, 159b
    for gastroesophageal reflux disease, 158
    histamine$_2$-blocking agents, 159–160, 159t
    5-HT$_3$ receptor antagonists, 163
    laxatives, 161–162, 162t
    metoclopramide, 161
    miscellaneous, 161
    misoprostol, 161
    mixed antiinfective therapy for ulcer treatment, 160, 160t
    phenothiazines, 162
    proton pump inhibitors, 159t, 160
    simethicone, 161
    sucralfate, 161
    trimethobenzamide, 162–163
    for ulcers, 159
Gastrointestinal effects
    of acetylsalicylic acid, 47–48, 47b
    of adrenocorticosteroids, 189
    of antiinfective agents, 72
    of antineoplastic drugs, 230
    of calcium channel blocking agents, 147
    of carbamazepine, 168
    of cephalosporins, 75
    of cholinergic agents, 35
    of clindamycin, 79, 79b
    of erythromycin, 76
    of metronidazole, 80, 80b
    of NSAIDs, 51
    of opioid analgesics, 60
    of phenytoin, 170
    of quinolones, 83
    of selective serotonin reuptake inhibitor, 180
    of tetracyclines, 78
Gastroparesis, diabetic, 161
Gels, fluoride, 286
Gemfibrozil, 152
General anesthetics, 112–118, 112b
    academic skills assessment and, 117
    adverse reactions of, 113, 113b, 114t
    balanced, 117
    classification of, 113, 114t
    clinical case study and, 118
    dental hygiene considerations and, 117
    halogenated hydrocarbons, 117
    history of, 112
    induction anesthesia, 113–115
        benzodiazepines, 114–115
        etomidate, 114
        inhalation anesthetics, 115, 115b
        intravenous anesthetics, 113

General anesthetics (*Continued*)
        ketamine, 114, 114b
        opioids, 114
        physical factors, 115, 115t
        propofol, 114, 114b
        ultrashort-acting barbiturates, 113–114
    mechanism of action of, 112–113
        levels of, 113f
        stages and planes of, 112–113, 112b, 113t
    nitrous oxide, 115–117, 115b, 115t
        abuse of, 116–117
        adverse reactions of, 116, 116b
        contraindications for, dental issues and, 116–117
        emotional instability, 116
        pharmacokinetics of, 116
        pharmacologic effects of, 116
        pregnancy considerations for, 116, 116b
Generic name, of drug, 4f
Genetic variation, and drug effects, 19
Geographic tongue, 276
GERD. *See* Gastroesophageal reflux disease
Germ cells, antineoplastic drugs and, 230
German Federal Health Agency, 265
German measles, in pregnancy, 244
Gestation, 246
Gingival crevicular fluid, drug excretion in, 18
Gingival enlargement, 279, 281f
    from antihypertensive agents, 149
    phenytoin and, 171, 171b
Gingivectomy, 171
Gingivitis, 288
Glaucoma
    adrenocorticosteroid effects on, 189
    anticholinergic and, 38
Glomerular filtration, of drugs, 17
Glucagon, 204, 214
    in emergency kit, 242
Glucagon-like peptide-1 (GLP-1) receptor agonists, 213
Glucocorticoids, 184b, 185, 186f, 187b
Glucose, in emergency kit, 241, 241f
α-Glucosidase inhibitors, 213
Glucuronic acid, 16
Glucuronidation, 16
Goiter, 217b
Gonadotropin-releasing hormone (GnRH), 215, 221–222t
Gonadotropins, 215
Good Manufacturing Practice (GMP), 268–269, 269b
Gout, drugs for, 56
    allopurinol, 56
    colchicine, 56
    febuxostat, 56
    NSAIDs for, 51
    probenecid, 56
Graves disease, 217
Growth hormone, 215
Guanethidine, 149

H
H$_1$-receptor blocking effects, 201, 201b
Habituation, 253
Half-life (t$_{1/2}$), of drug, 18
Hallucinogens. *See* Psychedelics
Halogenated hydrocarbons, 117
Halothane, 117
Hapten, 26
Harrison Narcotic Act, 5
Hashimoto disease, 217
Healing, diabetes mellitus and, 207
Health care worker. *See also* Dental hygienist; Dentistry
    mental disorders and, 174

Health history, 2
  adverse reactions and, 24
Heart
  anatomy of, 132, 132f
  sympathomimetic agent effects on, 40
Heart failure, 132–133, 132b
  β-adrenergic blockers for, 133
  aldosterone antagonists for, 133
  angiotensin-converting enzyme inhibitors for, 133
  angiotensin receptor blockers for, 133
  diuretics for, 132
  treatment of, 132–133, 133f
  vasodilators for, 133
Heart valve prosthesis, prophylactic antibiotics, 70
Heartburn, 158, 161
Heimlich maneuver, 236, 237f
Helicobacter pylori, related to ulcer, 159
Hematologic effects
  of carbamazepine, 168
  of tetracyclines, 78
Hemorrhoids, 20
Hemostasis
  adrenergic agents for, 41
  cephalosporins and, 75
Hemostatic agents, 156
Hepatitis, chronic, 96–97, 96t
Hepatitis B, opioid abuse, 259
Hepatotoxicity. *See also* Liver
  from antineoplastic drugs, 230
  of tetracyclines, 78
  of valproate, 167
Herbal medicine. *See* Natural/herbal products and
  dietary supplements
Heroin, 258
Herpes infections, 271–273, 271b, 272f
  antiviral agents for, dosing of, 273t
  symptoms, treatment of, 273, 273b
  treatment for, 272–273
    acyclovir, 273, 273b
    docosanol, 273
    famciclovir and valacyclovir, 273, 273b
    penciclovir, 273, 273b
Herpes simplex virus, 92–94, 92t
Highly active antiretroviral therapy (HAART),
  95–96
Histamine, 199
Histamine release, opioid effects, 61
Histamine₂-blocking agents, for gastrointestinal
  diseases, 159–160, 159t
Hormonal contraceptives, 220–221, 220t
Hormone replacement therapy, 217
Hospitalizations, adverse reactions and, 24
5-HT₃ receptor antagonists, for gastrointestinal
  diseases, 163
"Huffing," 253, 253b
Human chorionic gonadotropin (hCG), 215–217
Human immunodeficiency virus (HIV), 93–94t, 94
  sulfonamide and, 83
Human menopausal gonadotropin (hMG), 215–217
Hydralazine, 149
Hydrocodone, 63, 64t
Hydrocortisone, in emergency kit, 241–242
Hydromorphone, 63–64, 64t
3-Hydroxy-3-methylglutaryl coenzyme A
  reductase inhibitors, 150–151, 150b
Hyperprolactinemia, 217
Hypersensitivity. *See also* Allergic reactions
  to aspirin, 48
  to NSAIDs, 52
  quinolone and, 83
  tooth, 288–289
Hypersensitivity reactions, 27t, 278
Hypertension, 139, 139b
  α₁-adrenergic blocking agents in, 148, 148b
  β-adrenergic blocking agents in, 147–148, 148b

Hypertension (Continued)
  angiotensin-converting enzyme inhibitors in,
    145–146, 145–146b, 146f
  angiotensin receptor blockers in, 146
  calcium channel blocking agents in, 147, 147b
  central α-adrenergic agonists in, 149
    clonidine as, 149
    direct vasodilators as, 149
    methyldopa as, 149
  direct renin inhibitors in, 146–147
  diuretic agents for, 142–146, 144f
  patient evaluation in, 141
  peripheral adrenergic neuron antagonist in, 149
  treatment of, 141–142, 141f, 142t, 143b, 143f
Hyperthermia, malignant, 239
Hyperthyroidism, 217–218, 217b
  cholinergic agents and, 36
Hyperventilation, 236
Hypnotic doses, of barbiturates, 125
Hypoglycemia, 235–236
  treatment of, 214
Hypophysis, 215
Hypopituitarism, 215
Hypothalamus, 184, 215
Hypothyroidism, 217, 217b

I
Ibuprofen, 4, 4f
Idiosyncratic reaction, 27
Imidazoles, 90–92
Immune system, hypersensitivity of, 26
Immunoglobulin E (IgE), in allergic reaction, 26
Immunosuppression, by antineoplastic drugs, 230
Immunosuppressives, 56
  for recurrent aphthous stomatitis, 276, 276b
Indirect-acting sympathomimetic agents, 35, 36f
Induction, of cytochrome P-450, 16–17, 17f, 17t
Induction anesthesia, 113–115
  benzodiazepines, 114–115
  etomidate, 114
  inhalation anesthetics, 115, 115b
  intravenous anesthetics, 113
  ketamine, 114, 114b
  opioids, 114
  physical factors, 115, 115t
  propofol, 114, 114b
  ultrashort-acting barbiturates, 113–114
Infections
  corticosteroid effects on, 186, 189
  diabetes mellitus and, 207
Inflammation, corticosteroids for, 188
Inflammatory bowel disease (IBD), 163
Information, sources of, 3–4, 3–4b
Inhalation anesthetics, 115, 115b
Inhalation route, of drug administration, 22, 22b,
  22f
Inhibition, of cytochrome P-450, 16–17, 17f, 17t
Injection site, absorption of drug from, 15
Insomnia
  benzodiazepines for, 123, 123b
  nonpharmacologic management of, 123b
  phenytoin and, 170, 170b
  zolpidem for, 126
Insulin, 204, 208, 208t, 209b. *See also* Diabetes
  mellitus
Insulin shock, 208
Integrase inhibitors, 95
Interference, with natural defense mechanisms, 24
  as adverse reaction, 27
Interferons, 97
Interleukin-5 antibody antagonists, 198
International Classification of Epileptic Seizures,
  165, 166t
International normalized ratio (INR), 72, 256
  formula for, 153f

Intoxication, acute, 254
Intradermal route, of drug administration, 20–22,
  22f
Intramuscular route, of drug administration, 20, 22f
Intranasal corticosteroids, 201
Intraperitoneal route, of drug administration, 22
Intrathecal route, of drug administration, 22
Intrauterine device (IUD), 220
Intravenous anesthetics, 113
Intravenous route, of drug administration, 20
Investigational new drug application (INDA), 5
Iodine, 217, 217b
Ionization, of drugs, 15
Irreversible cholinesterase inhibitors, 37
Islets of Langerhans, 204
Isoenzymes, 16–17, 17t
Isoflurane, 117
Isoniazid, 84–85

J
Jaundice, cholestatic, 76
Journals
  about herbal supplements, 269b
  as source of information, 4

K
Kefauver-Harris Bill, 6
Ketamine, 114, 114b
Ketoconazole, 91–92, 92b
  in pregnancy, 249–250
Kidney
  acetaminophen effects on, 55
  aminoglycoside effects on, 82
  drug excretion and, 22
  NSAID effects on, 51–52
Kinetics
  first-order, 18, 18f
  zero-order, 18, 18f
Kinetics, drug, 18

L
Lacosamide (Vimpat), 169–170t
Lactation, benzodiazepines in, 122
Lamotrigine, 168, 169–170t
Laryngospasm, 236
Laxatives, 161–162, 162t
Legislation of drugs, 6–7
Lethal dose, 27–28
Leukopenia, 227
Leukotriene modifiers, 197–198, 201–202, 201b
Leuprolide, 222, 222t
Levetiracetam, 168, 169–170t
Lichen planus, 276, 276f
Lidocaine, 103–104, 103b
  and prilocaine (injection-free local anesthesia),
    109–110
  as topical anesthetic, 109
  vasodilating effect of, 107–108
Lipids, membrane, 14
Lipoproteins, high-density, 150
β-Lipotropin, 215
Lithium
  for bipolar disorder, 182
  management of dental patient taking., 182b
Liver
  acetaminophen effects on, 54–55, 55t
  in drug distribution, 16
  tetracyclines and, 78
Liver function test (LFT), azithromycin and, 77
Local anesthetics, 98–111, 98b
  academic skills assessment in, 111
  adverse reactions of, 101–103, 104f
    allergy, 102–103, 102b
    local effects, 102
    malignant hyperthermia, 102, 102b

Local anesthetics *(Continued)*
    pregnancy and nursing considerations, 102
    toxicity of, 102
  amides, 103–105
    articaine, 105
    bupivacaine, 104–105, 104*b*
    lidocaine, 103–104, 103*b*
    mepivacaine, 104, 104*b*
    prilocaine, 104, 104*b*
  cardiovascular effects of, 102
  central nervous system effects of, 102
  by chemical structure, 100*t*
  chemistry of, 98
  choice of, 107–108, 107*b*, 108–109*f*
  clinical case study in, 111
  composition of solutions, 103, 103*b*
  contraindications to, 109*t*
  in dental cartridges, 103*b*, 103*t*
  dental hygiene considerations, 111
  doses of, and vasoconstrictor, 110, 110*b*
  duration of action of, 107–108, 108*b*
  dyclonine, 105
  esters, 105
    procaine, 105
    tetracaine, 105
  history of, 98, 98*b*, 99*f*
  ideal, 98, 99*b*
  maximum safe doses of, 102*t*, 107*t*
  mechanism of action of, 98–99
    ionization factors, 99, 99*b*, 100–101*f*,
      100*t*
    on nerve fibers, 98–99, 98*b*, 100*b*, 100*f*
  nerve function loss and, 101*b*
  pain and, 99*f*
  patients receiving, instructions for, 103*b*
  pharmacokinetics of, 99–101
    absorption, 99–101, 99*b*
    distribution, 101
    excretion, 101
    metabolism, 101, 101*b*
  pharmacologic effects of, 101
    antiarrhythmic, 101
    peripheral nerve conduction (blocker), 101
  physical properties of, 109*t*
  in pregnancy, 246
  reaction to, 239
  topical anesthetics, 108–110, 110*t*
    benzocaine, 110
    lidocaine, 109
    precautions in, 110, 110*b*
  vasoconstrictors in, 105–107, 105*b*, 106*f*,
    107*b*
    drug interactions with, 107, 107*b*, 107*t*
Local reaction, from cephalosporins, 75
Local tissue irritation, 25
Log dose effect curve, 11, 12*f*
Loop diuretics, 144–145
Lorazepam, 123–124
Lubricants, 161–162
Luteinizing hormone, 215
Lysergic acid diethylamide, 262–263

M
Macroangiopathy, diabetes mellitus and, 207
Macrolides, 76–77, 76*t*
  azithromycin and clarithromycin, 77
  erythromycin, 76
    adverse reactions of, 76
    drug interactions of, 76
    mechanism and spectrum of, 76
    pharmacokinetics of, 76
    uses of, 76
Magnesium salts, in antacids, 161
Malignant hyperthermia, 239
  local anesthetics and, 102, 102*b*

Manic-depressive disorder, 174
Marijuana, 163, 263
  medical, 263
  synthetic, 263
Mask, oxygen, 242
Mast cell stabilizers, 202
Measurement
  household measures, 7
  metric system for, 7, 7*b*
Mechanism of action. *See also* Drug action
  of acetylsalicylic acid, 46, 47*f*
  of α_1-adrenergic blocking agents, 148
  of adrenocorticosteroids, 185, 185*b*
  of angiotensin-converting enzyme inhibitors,
    145
  of antineoplastic drugs, 225–226, 226*b*, 226*f*
  of barbiturates, 125
  of benzodiazepines, 121–124, 121*b*, 121*f*
  of calcium channel blocking agents, 147
  of cephalosporins, 75
  of erythromycin, 76
  of local anesthetics, 98–99
    ionization factors, 99, 99*b*, 100–101*f*, 100*t*
    on nerve fibers, 98–99, 98*b*, 100*b*, 100*f*
  of nitroglycerin-like compounds, 136, 136*b*
  of NSAIDs, 50
  of opioid analgesics, 58, 58*b*, 59*f*, 59*t*
  of penicillins, 73
  of sulfonamides, 82–83, 82*b*, 82*f*
  of thiazide diuretics, 143, 144*t*
Median effective dose, 27–28
Medication history, 2, 3*b*
Medication therapy, dental hygienist and patient
  adherence, 9–10
Medroxyprogesterone, 220
Meglitinides, 210–213
Melanoma, 225
Melatonin, 127
Melatonin receptor agonist, 126–127
Membranes, passage of drugs across, 14
Menopause, 219
Menotropins, 221–222*t*
Menstruation
  menstrual cycle, 219*f*
  NSAID effects on, 51
Mental illness, classification of, 175*f*
Meperidine, 63, 63–64*t*
Mepivacaine, 104, 104*b*
Mescaline, 253
Metabolism
  of drug, 16–18, 16*b*, 16*f*
    cytochrome P-450 induction and inhibition
      in, 16–17, 17*f*, 17*t*
    excretion in, 17–18
    first-pass effect in, 16
    mechanisms of, 16*f*
    sympathomimetic agent effects on, 39–40
Metabolite, 16
Metered-dose inhalers, 195–196, 195*b*, 196*f*
Methadone, 63*t*, 64–65
Methemoglobinemia
  articaine and, 105
  prilocaine and, 104
1-methyl-4-phenyl-1,2,3,6-tetrahydropyridine
  (MPTP), 259
Methyldopa, 149
Methylxanthines, for respiratory treatment, 198
Metoclopramide
  for gastrointestinal diseases, 161
  for vomiting, 163
Metronidazole, 80–81
  adverse reactions of, 80
  drug interactions of, 80, 80*b*
  pharmacokinetics of, 80
  in pregnancy, 249

Metronidazole *(Continued)*
  spectrum of, 80
  uses of, 81
Microangiopathy, diabetes mellitus and, 207
Microcephaly, 251
Micronor, 220
Microphthalmia, 251
Midazolam, 121–122
Milk, drug excretion by, 18
Mineralocorticoids, 184*b*, 185, 187*b*
Miosis, 32
  opioid effects, 61
Mirtazapine, 179–180*t*, 182
Misoprostol, for ulcer treatment, 161
Misuse of drug, 253
Monoamine oxidase inhibitors (MAOIs), 181,
  181*b*
  epinephrine and, 107
  opioid interactions with, 63
Montelukast (Singulair), 197
Mood stabilizers, 172
Morning glory seeds, 253
Morphine, 63
  in emergency kit, 241
Motion sickness, anticholinergic agents for, 38
Mouth rinses, 287, 287*b*, 287*f*, 287*t*
Mu receptor antagonists, 162
Mucolytics, for respiratory infections, 199
Multiple myeloma, antineoplastic drugs for, 225
Mupirocin, 85–86
Muscle relaxation, in benzodiazepines, 121
Muscle spasms, control of, benzodiazepines in,
  124
Myasthenia gravis, cholinergic agents and, 36
Mycelex, 91, 91*b*
Mydriasis, 32
  from anticholinergic agents, 37
Myeloneuropathy, from nitrous oxide, 258, 258*b*
Myocardial infarction
  acute, 237
  contraindications, to dental implications, 131
  dental implications of, 139
Myxedema, 217

N
Nalmefene, 66, 66*b*
Naloxone, 65, 65*b*
  in emergency kit, 242
Naltrexone, 66, 66*b*
  for alcoholism, 255
Narcolepsy, 41
Narcotic drugs. *See* Opioid analgesics
Nasal decongestants, 198–199
National Asthma Education and Prevention
  Program Expert Panel Report 3, 192
National Cancer Institute, tobacco abuse, 262
National Health and Nutrition Examinations
  Survey (NHANES), 139
Natural/herbal products and dietary supplements,
  265–270, 265*b*, 266–267*f*
  academic skills assessment on, 270
  adverse effects of, 266, 267*t*
  clinical case study on, 270
  dental hygiene considerations and, 270
  dental hygiene implications of, 267–268*t*
  drug interactions of, 266–267
  Good Manufacturing Practice, 268–269, 269*b*
  limited regulation of, 265–266
    Dietary Supplement Health and Education
      Act, 265–266, 265*b*
    package labeling, 266
  in oral health care, 269
    acemannan, 269
    essential oil mouth rinse, 269
    oil of cloves (eugenol), 269

Natural/herbal products and dietary supplements (Continued)
    triclosan, 269
    xylitol, 269, 270f
  recommendations for discontinuing, 268t
  safety of, 266, 266b
  standardization of, 267–268
Nausea, opioid effects, 61
Necrosis, as adverse reaction, 25
Nefazodone, 179–180t, 182
Neomycin, 85
Neostigmine, cholinergic agents and, 36
Nephrotoxicity
  of aminoglycoside, 82
  of antineoplastic drugs, 230, 230b
  of cephalosporin, 75
  of tetracyclines, 78
Nerve action potential, 98–99, 100f
Neurologic effects, of antineoplastic drugs, 230
Neurologic pain, antiepileptics for, 172
Neuromuscular blocking drugs, 43
Neuromuscular junction, 33, 33–34f
Neuropathy, diabetes mellitus and, 207
Neurotransmitters, 32–33, 32b, 33t
Niacin, 152
Nicotine-containing products, 262t
Nicotinic agonists and antagonists, 39
Nilstat, 90, 91t
Nitrofurantoin, 83
Nitroglycerin. See also Antianginal drugs
  in emergency kit, 241, 241f
Nitrolingual spray, 241f
Nitrous oxide, 112, 115–117, 115b, 115t, 257–258, 258f
  abuse of, 116–117
  adverse reactions to, 116, 116b, 257–258
  contraindications for, dental issues and, 116–117
  emotional instability, 116
  patterns of abuse, 257
  pharmacokinetics of, 116
  pharmacologic effects of, 116
  pregnancy considerations for, 116, 116b
Nitrous oxide-oxygen mixture, in pregnancy, 250
Nizoral, 91–92, 92b
Nonbenzodiazepine, benzodiazepine receptor agonists, 126
Nonbenzodiazepine-nonbarbiturate sedative-hypnotics, 126
Noncompetitive antagonist, 13, 14f
Nondepolarizing (competitive) blockers, 43
Nonnucleoside reverse transcriptase inhibitors, 94
Nonopioid (nonnarcotic) analgesics, 45–57
  academic skills assessment, 57
  acetaminophen (see Acetaminophen)
  acetylsalicylic acid (see Acetylsalicylic acid)
  classification of, 45, 46b
  clinical case study on, 57
  dental hygiene considerations for, 57
  gout drugs, 56
    allopurinol, 56
    colchicine, 56
    febuxostat, 56
    probenecid, 56
  nonsteroidal antiinflammatory drugs (see Nonsteroidal antiinflammatory drugs)
  pain and, 45, 46f
  salicylates, 45–50, 46b
Nonpituitary chorionic gonadotropin, 221–222t
Nonprescription medication, 3
Nonsteroidal antiinflammatory drugs (NSAIDs), 50–54
  adverse reactions of, 51–52
    blood clotting, 51
    cardiovascular effects, 51
    central nervous system effects, 51

Nonsteroidal antiinflammatory drugs (NSAIDs) (Continued)
    gastrointestinal effects, 51
    hypersensitivity reactions, 52
    oral effects, 52
    pregnancy and nursing considerations, 52, 52b
    renal effects, 51–52
  classification of, 50, 51t
  contraindications and cautions in, 52, 53b, 53t
  cyclooxygenase II-specific agents, 54
  drug interactions of, 52, 52t
  fenoprofen, 54
  ibuprofen, 53–54
  ketorolac, 54
  mechanism of action of, 50
  naproxen sodium, 54, 54b
  pharmacokinetics of, 50–51
  pharmacologic effects of, 51
  precautions in, 52
  in pregnancy, 246, 246b
  therapeutic uses of, 52–53
    dental, 52–53, 53f
    medical, 52
Nontarget tissues, adverse reactions on, 25
NSAIDs. See Nonsteroidal antiinflammatory drugs
Nucleoside analogs, 96–97
Nucleoside/nucleotide reverse transcriptase inhibitors, 94, 94t, 95f
Nucleotide analogs, 96–97
Nursing
  aspirin effects, 48
  local anesthetics and, 102
  metronidazole and, 80
  NSAID effects, 52, 52b
  opioid effects, 61
  quinolone and, 84
Nutritional supplements. See Natural/herbal products and dietary supplements
Nystatin, 90, 91t
  in pregnancy, 249

O
Obsessive-compulsive disorder, 174–175
Oils, essential, 288
Oligodactyly, 249–250, 250f
Omnibus Budget Reconciliation Act (OBRA), 5
Online resources, of information, 4
Ophthalmic effects, of corticosteroids, 186
Ophthalmologic examination, anticholinergic agents for, 38
Opioid analgesics, 58–67, 258–259
  abuse-deterrent opioids, 65, 65t
  academic skills assessment for, 67
  acute overdose and withdrawal from, management of, 258, 258b
  addiction to, 61–62, 62b
  adverse reactions of, 60–63, 60t
  agonists, 63–65, 64t
    codeine, 63
    extended-release hydrocodone, 63
    fentanyl family, 65
    hydrocodone, 63
    hydromorphone, 63–64
    meperidine, 63, 63t
    methadone, 63t, 64–65
    morphine, 63
    oxycodone, 63, 64t
    oxymorphone, 63
    propoxyphene, 63t
  allergic reactions to, 62, 62b, 62f
  antagonists, 65–66
    nalmefene, 66, 66b
    naloxone, 65, 65b
    naltrexone, 66, 66b

Opioid analgesics (Continued)
  classification of, 58, 59t
  clinical case studies on, 67
  dental hygiene considerations in, 67
  dental implications of, 259
    chronic pain, 259
    increased incidence, 259
    pain control, 259
    prescriptions for opioids, 259, 259b
  dental use of, 66, 66b
  drug interactions of, 63, 63t
  efficacy of, 60t
  history of, 58
  mechanism of action of, 58, 58b, 59f, 59t
  mixed opioids, 65
  partial agonists, 65
  pattern of abuse, 258
  pharmacokinetics of, 58–59, 58b, 60t
  pharmacologic effects of, 59–60
  tapentadol, 66
  tramadol, 66, 66b
Opioids, 114
  overdose in, 239
  in pregnancy, 249, 249f
Oral absorption, of drugs, 15
Oral conditions, 271–281
  agents used in treatment of, 279–281
    corticosteroids in, 279–280
    palliative treatment, 280–281
  burning mouth or tongue syndrome, 276
  dental hygiene considerations for, 281
  drug-induced side effects, 277–279, 278b
    gingival enlargement, 279, 281f
    hypersensitivity-type reactions, 278
    oral lesions resembling autoimmune-type reactions, 279, 280b
    osteonecrosis of the jaw, 279
    sialorrhea, 277
    stains, 279, 280f
    xerostomia, 277, 279f
  geographic tongue, 276
  immune reactions, 275–276
    lichen planus, 276, 276f
    recurrent aphthous stomatitis, 275–276, 275b, 275f
  infectious lesions, 271–275
    acute necrotizing ulcerative gingivitis (ANUG), 271, 271b, 272f
    alveolar osteitis, 275, 275b
    angular cheilitis/cheilosis, 274–275, 274b, 274f
    candidiasis (Moniliasis), 273–274, 273b, 274f
    herpes infections, 271–273, 271b, 272f
  inflammation, 277
    actinic lip changes, 277
    pericoronitis, 277
    postirradiation caries, 277
    root sensitivity, 277
    stomatitis, 277
Oral contraceptives, 220, 221b
  antibiotics and, 72
  dental drug interactions with, 221t
Oral decongestants, adverse effects of, 202
Oral disorders, hygiene-related, 282–291
  academic skills assessment in, 291
  clinical case study in, 291
  dental caries, 282–288, 282b
    prevention of, 282–288, 283b, 283f
    risk categories for, 283b
  dental hygiene considerations in, 290
  gingivitis, 288
    prevention, 288
  tooth hypersensitivity, 288–289

Oral effects
    of antineoplastic drugs, 230–231, 230–231b,
        230t, 231f
    of carbamazepine, 170
    of estrogen, 220
    of metronidazole, 80, 80b
    of NSAIDs, 52
    of selective serotonin reuptake inhibitor, 180
Oral glucose gels, 241f
Oral lesions
    corticosteroids for, 188
    resembling autoimmune-type reactions, 279,
        280b
        erythema multiforme-like, 279
        lichenoid-like eruptions, 279, 280b
        lupus-like reactions, 279
Oral mucositis, 230, 231f
Oral route, of drug administration, 19–20, 19b
Oral surgery, adrenocorticosteroids for, 188,
        188b
Orexin receptor antagonist, 127
Orphan drugs, 7
Orthopnea, in heart failure, 132
Orthostatic hypotension
    from antihypertensive agents, 149
    with antipsychotic agents, 177–178
Osmotic laxatives, 162
Osteonecrosis
    by antineoplastic drugs, 227–230
    of the jaw, 279
Osteoporosis, corticosteroid effects on, 186, 189
Ototoxicity, of aminoglycosides, 82
Ovaries, 218–219
Over-the-counter (OTC) drugs. See also
        Nonprescription medication
    nasal decongestants as, 198–199
Overactive bladder
    adrenergic agents for, 41
    anticholinergic agents for, 38
Overdose
    of amphetamines, 261
    of benzodiazepines, 122, 122b
    of heroin, 258
    of opioids, 61, 258, 258b
    of sedative-hypnotics, 260
Oxalates, for tooth hypersensitivity, 289
Oxcarbazepine, 168, 169–170t
Oxycodone, 63, 64t
Oxygen, in emergency kit, 239–241
Oxygen tank, 242
Oxytocin, 217

P
Package inserts (PIs), 6
Package labeling, 266
Pain
    local anesthetics and, 99f
    nonopioid (nonnarcotic) analgesics and, 45,
        46f
Palliative treatment, 273, 280–281
Palpebral fissures, 251
Pancreas, 205f
Pancreatic hormones, 204
Panic disorder, benzodiazepines for, 123
Paralysis, from cholinergic agents, 36
Paranoia, 174
Parasympathetic autonomic nervous system
        (PANS), 31, 34f, 35–39, 35b
    anticholinergic (parasympatholytic) agents in,
        37–38, 37f
        adverse reactions of, 37
        contraindications to, 38
        drug interactions with, 38
        pharmacologic effects of, 37
        uses of, 38, 38t

Parasympathetic autonomic nervous system
        (PANS) (Continued)
    cholinergic (parasympathomimetic) agents in,
        35–37, 35t
        adverse reactions from, 35–36, 35b
        contraindications to, 36
        pharmacologic effects of, 35
        uses of, 36–37
    nicotinic agonists and antagonists in, 39
Parasympatholytic agents, 37–38, 37f
Parasympathomimetic agents, 35–37, 35t
Parenteral administration, 19
Paresthesia, 105
Parkinson disease, 259
    anticholinergic agents for, 38
Parkinsonism, 177
Passive transfer, 14, 14f
Patent ductus arteriosus, side effects, 48
Pathologic state, drug effects and, 19
Patient adherence, drug effects and, 19
Penciclovir, 94
Penicillins, 72–75, 72f, 73t
    adverse reactions of, 73–74
        allergy and hypersensitivity in, 74
        toxicity of, 73–74
    mechanism of action of, 73, 73t
    pharmacokinetics of, 72–73, 72b
    resistance to, 73
    specific, 74–75
        ampicillins, 74–75
        extended-spectrum, 75
        penicillin G, 74
        penicillin V, 74
        penicillinase-resistant, 74
    spectrum of, 73
    uses of, 74
Pentazocine, 65
Peptic ulcer
    cholinergic agents and, 36
    corticosteroid effects on, 186
Perampanel (Fycompa), 169–170t
Perception, 45
Pericoronitis, 277
Periodontal disease, 68
    cardiovascular disease and, 132
    corticosteroid effects on, 189
    diabetes mellitus and, 205–206
Peripheral adrenergic neuron antagonist,
        149
Personality disorders, 174–175
Peyote, 253
Pharmacodynamics, 3t
Pharmacokinetics, 3t. See also Drug action
    of acetaminophen, 54
    of acetylsalicylic acid, 47
    of acyclovir, 92
    of aminoglycosides, 82
    of barbiturates, 125
    of benzodiazepines, 120–121
    of cephalosporins, 75
    of clindamycin, 79
    of erythromycin, 76
    of ethyl alcohol, 254, 255f
    of isoniazid, 85
    of local anesthetics, 99–101
        absorption, 99–101, 99b
        distribution, 101
        excretion, 101
        metabolism, 101, 101b
    of metronidazole, 80
    of nitrous oxide, 116
    of NSAIDs, 50–51
    of opioid analgesics, 58–59, 58b, 60t
    of penicillins, 72–73, 72b
    of quinolones, 83

Pharmacokinetics (Continued)
    of rifampin, 85
    of tetracyclines, 77
Pharmacologic effects
    of acetaminophen, 54, 54b
    of acetylsalicylic acid, 47
    of adrenocorticosteroids, 185, 186f
    of antihistamines, 200, 200f
    of antipsychotic agents, 175–177, 176t
    of barbiturates, 125
    of benzodiazepines, 121
    of calcium channel blocking agents, 147
    of carbamazepine, 168
    of centrally acting muscle relaxants, 127
    of local anesthetics, 101
    of nitrous oxide, 116
    of NSAIDs, 51
    of opioid analgesics, 59–60
Pharmacology
    definition of, 2
    disciplines related to, 3t
    history of, 2, 2b
Pharmacotherapy, 3t
Pharmacy, 3t
Phencyclidine, 263
Phenobarbital, 169–170t
Phenothiazines
    epinephrine and, 107
    for vomiting, 162
Phenytoin, 170–171
    adverse reactions of, 24, 170–171
    dental management of patients taking, 171b
Phobia, 174–175
Phocomelia, 244
Photosensitivity, tetracyclines and, 78
Physical dependence, 253
Physiologic antagonist, 13
Phytomedicine, 265
Pigmentation, minocycline on, 78
Pituitary gland, 184, 215
Pituitary hormones, 215–217, 216f
    anterior pituitary, 215–217, 215b
    posterior pituitary, 217, 217b
Placebo effect, 19
Placenta, drug distribution and, 15
Plaque buildup, 282
Plasma, drug distribution by, 15
Plummer disease, 217
Polymyxin, 85
Postirradiation caries, 277
Postural hypotension, 61
Potassium salts, 145, 145b
Potassium-sparing diuretics, 145
Potency, of drug, 11, 11b, 12f
Pramlintide, 213
Preclinical testing, of drugs, 5
Pregabalin (Lyrica), 169–170t
Pregnancy and breastfeeding, 244–251
    academic skills assessment for, 251
    adverse effects on fetus, 245–246t
    antibiotic effects on, 72
    aspirin effects on, 48, 246, 246b
    benzodiazepines and, 122
    clinical case study on, 251
    dental drugs during, 246–251, 247–248t
        acetaminophen, 249, 249b
        analgesics, 246–249
        antianxiety agents, 250–251
            alcohol, 251, 251b
            benzodiazepines, 250, 250f
            nitrous oxide-oxygen mixture, 250
        antiinfective agents, 249–250
            amoxicillin, 249
            cephalosporins, 249
            clindamycin, 249

Pregnancy and breastfeeding (Continued)
clotrimazole, 249
erythromycin, 249
ketoconazole, 249–250
metronidazole, 249
nystatin, 249
tetracyclines, 249
dental hygiene considerations for, 251
epinephrine, 246
general principles of, 244, 244b
history of, 244
local anesthetics and, 102, 246
management of, 244, 245b
metronidazole effects on, 80
nitrous oxide and, 116, 116b
NSAID effects, 52, 52b, 246, 246b
opioid effects on, 61, 249, 249f
quinolone effects on, 84
teratogenicity, 244–245, 245b
trimesters, 244
US Food and Drug Administration pregnancy
categories, 245–246, 245b, 246f
Premedication, with benzodiazepines, 124
Prescription
abbreviations used in, 8t, 9
electronic and fax, 9, 9f
format of, 7–8, 8f
body, 7–8
closing, 8
heading, 7
label regulations, 8–9, 9f
writing of, 7–10
Prilocaine, 104, 104b
Printed resources, of information, 3
Probenecid, for gout, 56
Procaine, 105
Prodrug, 16
Progesterone, 218–219
Progestins, 220
Prophylactic indications
for antibiotics, used in dentistry, 70
for infective endocarditis, 86–87, 86b
for prosthetic joint, 87–88
Propofol, 114, 114b
Propoxyphene, 63t
Proprotein convertase subtilisin/kexin type 9
inhibitors, 152
Propylparaben, in local anesthetics, 103
Prostatic hypertrophy, anticholinergic agents and, 38
Protease inhibitors
for chronic hepatitis, 97
for HIV, 95
Proteins, membrane, 14
Prothrombin time, acetaminophen effects, 54–55
Proton pump inhibitors, 159t, 160
Psychedelics (hallucinogens), 262–263
lysergic acid diethylamide, 263
marijuana, 263
phencyclidine, 263
Psychiatric disorders, 174–175, 174–175b
Psychologic factors, drug effects and, 19
Psychological dependence, 253
Psychoses, symptoms of, 175b
Psychotherapeutic agents
academic skills assessment for, 183
antidepressant agents as, 179–182, 179–180t,
180–181f
adverse reactions of, 181f
bupropion, 181–182
dental implications of, 182, 182b
monoamine oxidase inhibitors, 181, 181b
nefazodone, mirtazapine, vilazodone, and
vortioxetine, 182
selective serotonin reuptake inhibitor, 179–180,
180f

Psychotherapeutic agents (Continued)
serotonin-norepinephrine reuptake
inhibitors, 180
suicide and, 182
trazodone, 182
tricyclic antidepressants, 180–181
antipsychotic agents as
dental implications of, 178–179, 178b
drug interactions of, 177–178
first-generation, 175–177
mechanism of action of, 175, 177f
pharmacologic effects of, 175–177
for psychiatric disorders, 175–179, 176t
second-generation, 177, 182–183
uses of, 178
for bipolar disorders, 182–183
antiepileptic drugs, 182–183
lithium, 182
second-generation antipsychotics, 183
clinical case study for, 183
dental hygiene considerations for, 183
Pulmonary edema, in heart failure, 132
Pulp procedures, adrenocorticosteroids for, 188
Pyrazinamide, 85

Q
Quinolones (fluoroquinolones), 83–84, 83b

R
Ramelteon, 126
Ranolazine, 138
Rapid eye movement (REM) sleep, reduction of,
benzodiazepines in, 121
Reaction, 45
α-Receptors, 39
β-Receptors, 39, 39f
Receptors, in drug action, 13, 13f
Rectal route, of drug administration, 20
Recurrent aphthous stomatitis (RAS), 275–276,
275b, 275f
corticosteroids for, 275–276
diphenhydramine for, 276
immunosuppressives for, 276, 276b
Redistribution, of drug, 16
Relapse, 253
Renal route, drug excretion by, 17
Renal toxicity, of metronidazole, 80
Renin inhibitors, direct, 146–147
Reserpine, 149
Resins, for tooth hypersensitivity, 289
Resistance
to antibiotics, 69–70
of penicillins, 73
Respiratory depression, opioid effects, 60–61, 60b
Respiratory diseases, 192–195, 193f
academic skills assessment for, 202
clinical case study on, 203
drugs for treatment of, 192–203, 193f
anti-immunoglobulin E antibodies as, 198
antimuscarinic drugs, 198, 198b
corticosteroids as, 196–197, 196b
cromolyn, 198, 198b
dental hygiene considerations for, 202
dental implications of, 199
interleukin-5 antibody antagonists, 198
leukotriene modifiers, 197–198
metered-dose inhalers, 195–196, 195b, 196f
methylxanthines, 198
sympathomimetic agents as, 196
long-acting β₂-agonists, 194–195t, 196
short-acting β₂-agonists, 194–195t, 196, 196b
for upper respiratory infections, 198–199
antitussives, 199
expectorants and mucolytics, 199
nasal decongestants, 198–199

Respiratory emergencies, 236
Respiratory obstruction, from nitrous oxide,
116
Respiratory system
benzodiazepine effects on, 122
sympathomimetic agent effects on, 40
Resuscitation bag, 242
Retinopathy, diabetes mellitus and, 207
ReVia, 255
Reye syndrome
acetaminophen and, 55
acetylsalicylic acid effects on, 48
aspirin effects on, 48
Rifampin, 85
Romazicon, in emergency kit, 242
Root sensitivity, 277
Route of administration
of adrenocorticosteroids, 185
drug effects and, 19
Rufinamide (Banzel), 169–170t

S
Salicylates, 45–50, 46b. See also Nonopioid
(nonnarcotic) analgesics
Salicylism, 49
Saliva, drug excretion in, 18
Salivary glands, sympathomimetic agent effects
on, 40
Salmeterol, for respiratory treatment, 196
Salt, iodized, 217
Schizophrenia, 174, 174b
Sedation
anticholinergic drugs and, 43
by opioid analgesics, 59
Sedative doses, of barbiturates, 125
Sedative-hypnotics, 259–260
management of acute overdose and withdrawal,
260
pattern of abuse, 259–260, 259b
Sedatives, with aspirin, 50
Seizures, 236, 236b. See also Epilepsy
drugs for, 165–173
academic skills assessment in, 172
benzodiazepines for, 123–124
clinical case study, 173
dental hygiene considerations in, 172
with first-generation antipsychotics, 177
Selective estrogen receptor modulators (SERMs),
223
Selective serotonin reuptake inhibitors (SSRIs),
179–180, 179–180t, 180f
adverse reactions of, 179–180
Self-made emergency kits, 240f
Serotonin-norepinephrine reuptake inhibitors
(SNRIs), 179–180t, 180
Sevoflurane, 117
Sex, drug effects and, 19
Sex hormones
agents affecting, 222–223
female, 218–221
dose forms and doses, 218t
estrogens, 219–220
hormonal contraceptives, 220–221, 220t
progestins, 220
male, 221–222
agonists, and antagonists, 221–222t
androgens, 221–222
Sexually transmitted disease, 259
Shock, adrenergic agents for, 41
Shock therapy, 175
Sialorrhea, 277
Side effect, 24, 25f. See also Adverse reactions
Simethicone, 161
Simplified Adult Basic Life Support (BLS)
algorithm, 238f

Smoking. *See also* Tobacco
 benzodiazepines and, 123
 chronic obstructive pulmonary disease and, 192–193
 gastrointestinal disease and, 163
Smooth muscle, anticholinergic agent effects on, 37
Sodium bicarbonate, 161
Sodium chloride, in local anesthetics, 103
Sodium fluoride (NaF) varnish, 285
Sodium glucose transporter-2 inhibitors, 213
Sodium hydroxide, in local anesthetics, 103
Spectrum
 of acyclovir, 93
 of aminoglycosides, 82
 of cephalosporins, 75
 of clindamycin, 79
 of erythromycin, 76
 of metronidazole, 80
 of penicillins, 73
 of quinolones, 83
 of sulfonamides, 82
 of tetracyclines, 77
 of vancomycin, 81–82
Sphygmomanometer, 242
Spina bifida, 250f
Staining of teeth, 279, 280f
Stannous fluoride (SnF), 286
Starling's law, 132
Statins. *See* 3-Hydroxy-3-methylglutaryl coenzyme A reductase inhibitors
Status asthmaticus, 192
Steroids, 184
 supplementation of, 190, 190b, 190f
Stevens-Johnson syndrome, 230
Stimulants, 162
Stomatitis, 277
Stool softeners, 162
Stroke, 238–239
Subcutaneous route, of drug administration, 20
Subgingival strips and gels, 22
Sublingual and buccal routes, of drug administration, 23, 23b
Substance use disorders, 252–264. *See also* Drug abuse
Sucralfate, for ulcer treatment, 161
Suicide, 175
 antidepressant agents and, 182
Sulfamethoxazole-trimethoprim, 83
Sulfite, 103b
Sulfonamides, 82–83
Sulfonylureas, 209–210, 210f, 210t
Superinfection
 from antiinfective agents, 70
 from cephalosporins, 75
 from clindamycin, 79
 from tetracyclines, 78
Suvorexant, 127
Sweat, drug excretion by, 18
Sympathetic autonomic nervous system (SANS), 31–32, 34f, 39–43, 39f
 adrenergic blocking agents in, 42–43
 adrenergic (sympathomimetic) agents in, 40–42, 40t
  adverse reactions from, 41
  contraindications to, 41
  pharmacologic effects of, 40
  uses of, 41
 neuromuscular blocking drugs in, 43
 receptors of, 39
Sympathomimetic agents, 40–42, 40t, 196
 long-acting β$_2$-agonists, 194–195t, 196
 short-acting β$_2$-agonists, 194–195t, 196, 196b
Sympathomimetic amines, 182
Synaptic cleft, 31
Syncope, 235, 235b
Syndactyl, 249–250, 250f

T
Tachycardia
 adrenergic agonists and, 43
 anticholinergic agents and, 38
 cholinergic agents and, 36
Tamoxifen, 222–223, 222t
Tapentadol, 66
Tardive dyskinesia, 176b, 177, 179
Target tissues, adverse reactions on, 25
Teeth, tetracyclines and, 78, 78f
Temporomandibular disease (TMD), 67
Temporomandibular joint
 arthritis of, adrenocorticosteroids for, 188
 pain in, antipsychotic agents and, 179
Teratogenic effect, 25
Teratogenicity
 of antiepileptics, 167
 of dental drugs, 244–245, 245b, 245–246t
 of NSAIDs, 52
 of phenytoin, 171, 171f
 of valproate, 167
Tetracaine, 105
Tetracyclines, 77–79, 77t
 adverse reaction of, 77–78
  allergy, 78
  gastrointestinal effects, 78
  hematologic effects, 78
  hepatotoxicity, 78
  nephrotoxicity, 78
  photosensitivity, 78
  superinfection, 78
  on teeth and bones, 78
 drug interactions, 78–79
 pharmacokinetics of, 77
 in pregnancy, 249
 spectrum of, 77
 teeth staining and, 279
 uses of, 79
Tetrahydrocannabinol, 263
Tetraiodothyronine (T$_4$), 217
Thalidomide, 244
The Complete German Commission E Monographs: Therapeutic Guide to Herbal Medicines, 265
Therapeutic effect, of drug, 13
Therapeutic index, 12, 12b
 of benzodiazepines, 122, 122b
 of drug, 27–28f, 28
Therapeutically equivalent drugs, 5
Thiazide diuretics, 142–144
 adverse reactions of, 143–144, 143b, 144t
 mechanism of action of, 143, 144t
Thiazolidinediones, 213, 213b
Thrombophlebitis, in benzodiazepines, 122
Thyroid hormones, 217–218
 antithyroid agents, 217b, 218
 hyperthyroidism, 217–218, 217b
 hypothyroidism, 217, 217b
 iodine, 217, 217b
Thyroid-stimulating hormone (TSH), 215
Thyroid storm, 239
Thyroidectomy, 218
Thyrotoxicosis, 218
Thyrotropin, 215
Tiagabine (Gabitril), 169–170t
Tic douloureux, 168
Time of administration, drug effects and, 19
Tizanidine, 128
Tobacco, 252b, 261–262
 dental hygienist's role in cessation of, 262
 management and withdrawal in, 262
 nicotine, 261
 pattern of abuse, 261, 261b
 smokeless, 261–262

Tolerance
 drug effects and, 19
 to drugs, 253, 253b
  to benzodiazepines, 122, 122b
Tooth hypersensitivity, 288–289
 pathophysiology of, 289, 289b, 289f
 treatment of, 289, 289–290f, 289t
Toothbrushes, 283, 283b
Toothpastes, 286t
 without sodium lauryl sulfate, 275t
Topical anesthetics, local, 108–110, 110t
Topical corticosteroids, 188, 188b
Topical NaF, 285
Topical route, of drug administration, 22–23
Topiramate (Topamax), 169–170t
Toremifene, 222t
Toxic reaction, 24, 25f
Toxicity
 of acetaminophen, 55
 of acetylsalicylic acid, 49, 49b
 of fluoride, 284, 284b, 284t
Toxicology, 3t
Tracheotomy, 236
Trade name, of drugs, 4f, 5
Tramadol, 66, 66b
Transdermal patch, 22–23, 22f
Transferases, 16
Trazodone, 182
Tremors, adrenergic agonists and, 43
Trendelenburg position, 235, 235f
Triclosan, 288
Tricyclic antidepressants, 180–181
 adverse reactions of, 181
 dental implications of, 182
 drug interactions of, 181
Trigeminal neuralgia, carbamazepine for, 168b
Triiodothyronine (T$_3$), 217
Trimethobenzamide, for vomiting, 162–163
Tuberculosis. *See* Antituberculosis agents
Tubular diffusion, passive, of drugs, 17
Tubular secretion, active, of drugs, 17
Tumor necrosis factor (TNF), 163
Tumor necrosis factor (TNF)-α inhibitors, 57
Type 1 diabetes, 204, 205t
Type 2 diabetes, 205, 205t, 206b

U
Ulcerative colitis, 163, 163f
Ulcers, 159
 peptic, cholinergic agents and, 36
Ultrashort-acting barbiturates, 113–114
United States Adopted Name Council, 4
United States Pharmacopeia Convention, 269
Urinary retention, opioid effects, 61
Urinary tract, obstruction of
 anticholinergic agents and, 38
 cholinergic agents and, 36
US Food and Drug Administration, pregnancy categories, 245–246, 245b, 246f

V
Valproate, 167
Valproic acid, dental management of patients taking, 168b
Vancomycin, 81–82, 81b
 adverse reactions of, 82
 spectrum of, 81–82
Varenicline, 262
Vasoconstriction, sympathomimetic agents for, 41
Vasoconstrictors, in local anesthetics, 105–107, 105b, 106f, 107b
 doses of, 110, 110b
 drug interactions with, 107, 107b, 107t

Vasodilators
  direct, 149
  for heart failure, 133
Vasopressin, 217
Vessels, sympathomimetic agents on, 40
Vigabatrin (Sabril), 169–170t
Vilazodone, 179–180t, 182
Viral infections. *See* Antiviral agents
Visual system, benzodiazepine effects
      on, 122
Vitamin deficiency, phenytoin and, 170
Vitamin K, in alcoholism, 256
Vomiting, opioid effects, 61
Vortioxetine, 179–180t, 182

W
Warfarin, 153–154
  management of dental patient taking, 154b
Water fluoridation, 284

Websites, about herbal supplements, 269b
Wellbutrin, 181–182
Wernicke-Korsakoff syndrome, 254
Withdrawal
  from alcohol, 254, 254b, 255f
  of amphetamines, 261
  of antiepileptics, 167
  of drug, 253
  from opioids, 61, 258, 258b
  of sedative-hypnotics, 260
  of tobacco, 262, 262t
Wound healing
  delayed, corticosteroid effects on, 189
  impaired, corticosteroid effects on, 186

X
Xerostomia, 177b, 182, 277, 279f
  as adverse reaction, 24
  agents producing, 279t

Xerostomia *(Continued)*
  anticholinergic drugs and, 43
  from antihypertensive agents, 149
  diabetes mellitus and, 205
Xylitol, 287–288, 288b

Z
Zafirlukast (Accolate), 197
Zaleplon, 126
Zanaflex, 128
Zarontin, 171
Zero-order kinetics, 18, 18f
Zileuton (Zyflo), 197
Zinc, 78
Zolpidem, 126
Zonisamide (Zonegran),
      169–170t
Zovirax, 92, 92b
Zyloprim, 230